Reviewers

REVIEWERS OF THE UK EDITION

Ian Beech, Rgn, RMN, BA, MA, PGCE
Head of Mental Health Division
Faculty of Health, Sport and Science
University of Glamorgan

David Bell, RMN, BSc, MA, PGCert
Senior Mental Health Lecturer
School of Health,
University of Wolverhampton

Heather Brundrett, BSc, MA
Senior Lecturer
Department of Applied Mental Health
University of Derby

Julie Dixon, Dip N (Mental Health), MA
Lecturer
School of Nursing
University of Nottingham

Willie McDonald, RMN, Bsc, MSc, PgCLTHE
Lecturer in Mental Health Nursing
School of Nursing
Midwifery and Community Health
Glasgow Caledonian University

Jim Turner, HND, RMN, BA, MA, Dip CAT, PG Dip Ed, RNT
Principal Lecturer in Nursing (Mental Health)
Faculty of Health and Wellbeing
Sheffield Hallam University

Neil Withnell, BSc, MSc
Lecturer in Mental Health Nursing
School of Nursing
University of Salford.

REVIEWERS OF THE US EDITION

Barbara Amendola, APN-C
Professor of Nursing
Ocean County College
Toms River, New Jersey

Judy A. Bourrand, RN, MSN
Assistant Professor (Course Coordinator, Psychiatric-Mental
    Health Nursing)
Samford University, Ida V. Moffett School of Nursing
Birmingham, Alabama

Janice Caie-Lawrence
Instructor
Henry Ford Community College
Dearborn, Michigan

Janet Niemi Chubb, MS, RN (DHSc candidate)
Assistant Professor of Nursing
North Georgia College and State University
Dahlonega, Georgia

Judith A. Collins, BSN, MA, ARNP, BC
Lecturer; Clinical Instructor
University of Iowa, College of Nursing
Iowa City, Iowa

Cindy Cunningham, MSN, APRN, BC
Nursing Instructor
Delaware Technical & Community College
Georgetown, Delaware

Jan Dalsheimer, MS, RN
Associate Clinical Professor
Texas Woman's University
Dallas, Texas

Karen S. Dearing
Assistant Professor
Brigham Young University
Provo, Utah

Leona F. Dempsey, RN, APNP, PhD
Assistant Professor
University of Wisconsin, Oshkosh and Medication
Prescriber, Oshkosh Counseling and Wellness Center
University of Wisconsin Oshkosh
Oshkosh, Wisconsin

Jewel Diller, RN, MSEd, MSN, FNP
Associate Professor
Ivy Tech Community College of Indiana
Fort Wayne, Indiana

Denise Doliveira, RN MSN
Assistant Professor
Community College of Allegheny County,
    Boyce Campus
Monroeville, Pennsylvania

Janet Duffey, RN, MS, APRN, BC
Assistant Professor of Nursing
Napa Valley College
Napa, California

Allison Edmonds, MS, ARNP
Faculty Clinical Instructor
University of South Florida
College of Nursing
Tampa, Florida

Mental Health Nursing

Sheila L. Videbeck, PhD, RN

Des Moines Community College
Ankeny, Iowa

Adapted for the UK
by

**Kevin Acott, MA, RMN, BSc (Hons),
PGCE (PCET), Dip.PTSC, Dip.EH.P**

Tutor and Branch Leader (Mental Health),
University of Surrey

Illustrations by Cathy J Miller

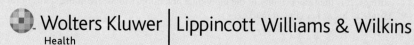 Wolters Kluwer | Lippincott Williams & Wilkins
Health

Philadelphia • Baltimore • New York • London
Buenos Aires • Hong Kong • Sydney • Tokyo

First UK edition
Publisher: Cathy Peck
Academic Marketing Executive: Alison Major
Production Director: Chris Curtis
Senior Production Manager: Richard Owen
Project Manager: Cosmas Georgallis
Copy Editor: Linda Antoniw
Proofreader: Cosmas Georgallis
Indexer: Thomson Digital
Typesetter: Thomson Digital
Printed and bound by timesprinters

US edition
Acquisitions Editor: Pete Darcy
Development Editor: Katherine Burland
Production Editor: Mary Kinsella
Director of Nursing Production: Helen Ewan
Senior Managing Editor / Production: Erika Kors
Art Director, Design: Joan Wendt
Art Director, Illustration: Brett MacNaughton
Manufacturing Coordinator: Karin Duffield
Indexer: Angie Weil
Typesetter: Circle Graphics

First UK Edition

British Library Cataloging-in-Publication Data. A catalogue record for this book is available from the British Library.

ISBN-10: 1-901831-02-7

ISBN-13: 978-1-901831-02-3

Videbeck, Sheila L.
   Psychiatric-mental health nursing / Sheila L. Videbeck; illustrations by Cathy J. Miller. — 4th ed.
      p.; cm.
   Includes bibliographical references and index.
      ISBN-13: 978-0-7817-6425-4
   1. Psychiatric nursing. I. Title.
      [DNLM: 1. Psychiatric Nursing. 2. Mental Disorders—nursing. WY 160 V652p 2008]
      RC440.V536 2008
      616.89'0231—dc22

Care has been taken to confirm the accuracy of the information presented and to describe generally accepted practices. However, the authors, editors and publisher are not responsible for errors or omissions or for any consequences from application of the information in this book and make no warranty, expressed or implied, with respect to the currency, completeness or accuracy of the contents of the publication. Application of this information in a particular situation remains the professional responsibility of the practitioner; the clinical treatments described and recommended may not be considered absolute and universal recommendations.

The authors, editors and publisher have exerted every effort to ensure that drug selection and dosage set forth in this text are in accordance with the current recommendations and practice at the time of publication. However, in view of ongoing research, changes in regulations and the constant flow of information relating to drug therapy and drug reactions, the reader is urged to check the package insert for each drug for any change in indications and dosage and for added warnings and precautions. This is particularly important when the recommended agent is a new or infrequently employed drug.

Some drugs and medical devices presented in this publication have clearance for limited use in restricted research settings. It is the responsibility of the individual practitioner to ascertain the status of each drug or device planned for use in his or her clinical practice.

Preface

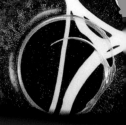

This first UK adaptation of *Mental Health Nursing* maintains the strong student focus of the US editions, presenting sound nursing theory, therapeutic modalities and clinical applications across the care and treatment continuum. The chapters are concise, carefully structured and the writing style kept direct – without being over-simplistic – in order to facilitate learning for students with a range of prior knowledge and experience.

The text draws on an adapted nursing process framework and emphasizes the necessity for collaborative, respectful and compassionate engagement that underpins comprehensive holistic assessment, negotiated care planning, effective therapeutic interventions and rigorous evaluation of care and treatment. A multidisciplinary approach, drawing on neurobiological theory, psychology and pharmacology is taken throughout. Interventions focus on contexts of client care, including group and one-to-one communication, client, carer and community education, and the need to work with formal and informal resources, as well as their practical application across a variety of clinical settings.

This UK edition is supported with a newly enhanced ancillary package – including chapter-specific group discussion topics – designed to assist teachers, trainers and mentors with programme delivery and student evaluation, and to assist students to build on their strengths, develop self-awareness and work towards a comprehensive knowledge and practice synthesis.

ORGANIZATION OF THE TEXT

Unit 1: Current Theories and Practice provides a strong foundation for students. It addresses the history and current contexts of – and key issues in – mental health nursing. It thoroughly explores neurobiological theories, psychopharmacology and psychosocial concepts as a basis for understanding mental health problems and their care and treatment. Recent changes in service configuration and roles are discussed.

Unit 2: Building the Nurse–Client Relationship presents the basic elements essential for the practice of effective and compassionate mental health nursing. Chapters on therapeutic relationships and therapeutic communication prepare students to begin working with people both in specialist mental health settings and in other areas of health care. The chapter on responses to stress, health and illness provides a framework for understanding the individual client within his or her cultural and sub-cultural context. An entire chapter is devoted to assessment approaches, emphasizing the importance in mental health nursing of assessment that is flexible, collaborative, thorough and therapeutic.

Unit 3: Key Social, Cultural and Psychological Issues covers topics that are not exclusive to mental health settings, including legal and ethical issues; anger, aggression and hostility; abuse and violence; and grief and loss. Nurses in all practice settings find themselves confronted with issues related to these topics. Additionally, many legal and ethical concerns are interwoven with explorations of violence and loss.

Unit 4: Nursing Practice for Specific Mental Health Problems covers the major 'disorders' confronted by nurses. Each chapter provides current information on possible aetiologies, onset and clinical course, care and treatment, and the role of the nurse in a multidisciplinary approach to validating client experience and working towards satisfactory solutions.

PEDAGOGICAL FEATURES

Mental Health Nursing incorporates several pedagogical features designed to facilitate student learning:

- Learning Objectives focus the students' reading and study.

- Key Terms identify new terms used in the chapter. Each term is identified in bold and defined in the text.

- Application of the Nursing Process sections use the assessment framework presented in Chapter 8, so students can compare and contrast various disorders more easily.

- Critical Thinking Questions stimulate students' thinking about current dilemmas and issues in mental health.

- Key Points summarize chapter content to reinforce important concepts.

- Chapter Study Guides provide workbook-style questions for students to test their knowledge and understanding of each chapter

SPECIAL FEATURES

- Clinical Vignettes are provided for each major disorder discussed in the text to 'paint a picture' for better understanding.

- Drug Alerts highlight essential points about psychotropic drugs.

- Cultural Considerations sections appear in each chapter, as part of an attempt to raise awareness of issues of diversity and difference.

- Therapeutic Dialogues give specific examples of nurse–client interaction to promote therapeutic communication skills.

- Internet Resources to further enhance study are located at the end of each chapter.

- Client/Family Education boxes provide information that help strengthen students' roles as educators.

- Symptoms and Interventions are highlighted for chapters in Units 3 and 4.

- Sample Nursing Care Plans are provided for chapters in Units 3 and 4.

- Self-awareness features appear at the end of each chapter and encourage students to reflect on themselves, their thoughts and feelings and their attitudes as a way to foster both personal and professional development.

- Group Discussion Topics are provided

Acknowledgements

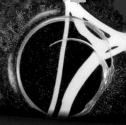

ACKNOWLEDGEMENTS (SV)

I am grateful to all the students in my classes who have taught me what I need to know to be a better teacher. Their continued input helps make this text practical, interesting and focused on student learning.

I also want to thank the dedicated people at Lippincott Williams & Wilkins who provide all the assistance and resources I need to make this text a success. To Renee Gagliardi, Katherine Burland, Season Evans, Candice Davis, Mary Kinsella and Margaret Zuccarini, I extend my appreciation for a job well done.

And as always, my friends continue to be a major part of my life – their support, encouragement, criticism and loyalty help me in everything I do. My relationships with them help make this text possible.

ACKNOWLEDGEMENTS (KA)

Thanks firstly to Sheila for her hugely impressive text, a labour of love that provided such a solid, richly thoughtful and humane foundation for me to work on – I had by far the easier job simply tweaking, shifting and fiddling about with her words (and then throwing in a few bits of my own!). Mental health nursing in the rest of the world owes so much to the US, and Sheila is one in a long and distinguished line of American pragmatists and thinkers who have immeasurably improved the lives of educators, students, nurses and clients globally.

Thanks to Sue Hodge for doing what I certainly could never have done and producing a concise, clear, accurate and thoughtful chapter on mental health law and ethics; thanks also to Mike Ramsay for his invaluable comments on that chapter and to other reviewers who have pointed out some of my many errors, omissions and peculiar way with the English language.

I'd like also to thank my clients, my students, my colleagues, my family and my friends: you've each helped me understand better the complex, contradictory, bewildering, uplifting, frustrating and life-enhancing nature of mental health care and mental health nursing: I hope some of that understanding is transmitted here in my adaptation of Sheila's exceptional work.

Contents

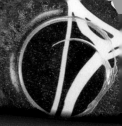

1

Current Theories and Practice

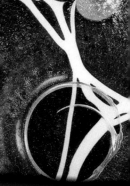

Chapter

1

Foundations of Mental Health Nursing

Key Terms

- **asylum**
- **Care Programme Approach**
- **compassion**
- **curiosity**
- ***International Classification of Diseases*, 2nd edition (*ICD-10*)**
- **mental disorder**
- **mental health**
- **psychotropic drugs**
- **recovery**
- **risk**
- **self-awareness**
- **standards of care**

Learning Objectives

After reading this chapter, you should be able to:

1. Describe characteristics of 'mental health' and 'mental illness'.

2. Identify important historical landmarks in mental health care.

3. Discuss current trends in the treatment of people with mental health problems.

4. Discuss the Department of Health's *From values to action: The Chief Nursing Officer's review of mental health nursing* (2006).

5. Describe common concerns within mental health nursing.

6. Discuss the purpose, use and limitations of the World Health Organization's *International Classification of Diseases*, 2nd edition (*ICD-10*) and the American Psychiatric Association's *Diagnostic and Statistical Manual of Mental Disorders*, 4th edition, Text Revision (*DSM-IV-TR*).

7. Begin to recognize the importance of self-awareness and to work to build on your compassion, your empathy and your curiosity.

As you begin – or deepen – your study of mental health nursing, you're likely to feel a range of emotions: you may – at different times – be excited, uncertain, apprehensive or anxious, lost. The field of mental health often seems – regardless of how much experience we have – confusing, contradictory, unfamiliar and mysterious, a political and linguistic battleground, with images from the media and the arts often confusing our perceptions. It's frequently hard to pin down what the experience is really like – for professionals and for clients, what nurses and other clinicians actually do in this area and how the system has developed in the way it has. This chapter starts to address these concerns – and others – by providing an overview of the history of mental health care, offering a sketch of advances in care and treatment and current issues in mental health, and attempting to define the role of the mental health nurse.

MENTAL HEALTH AND MENTAL ILLNESS

Mental Health

The World Health Organization (1948) defines 'health' as a state of complete physical, mental and social wellness, not merely the absence of disease or infirmity. This definition emphasizes health as a positive state of well-being. People in a state of emotional, physical and social well-being fulfil life responsibilities (on the whole), function effectively in daily life (on the whole) and are satisfied with their interpersonal relationships and themselves (on the whole).

No single, universally-accepted definition of '**mental health**' exists. Generally, a person's behaviour can provide clues to his or her mental health. Because each person (and each professional discipline) can have a different view or interpretation of behaviour (depending on their own history,

values and beliefs), the determination of what exactly mental health is may be difficult. In most cases, though, mental health can be agreed as a state of emotional, psychological and social 'wellness', evidenced by satisfying interpersonal relationships, effective social behaviour and coping, positive self-concepts and emotional stability.

Mental health has many components, and an array of interlinking factors influences it. A person's mental health is never set in stone: it is always in a dynamic, ever-changing, state of flux. Elements influencing someone's mental health positively can be categorized as individual, interpersonal and social/cultural:

- *Individual,* or personal, factors include a person's genetic make-up, qualities of autonomy and independence, self-esteem, the capacity and willingness to grow, develop and take risks, vitality, crisis-management skills, the ability to find meaning and purpose in life, the capacity to tolerate distress, a sense of belonging and reality orientation.
- *Interpersonal,* or relationship, factors include effective communication skills, the willingness and ability to help others, intimacy, and a balance of separateness and connectedness.
- *Social/cultural,* or environmental, factors include power and control issues, economic and political issues, a sense of community, access to adequate resources, the intolerance of violence, support for diversity, and a positive, yet realistic, view of – and from – one's world.

Mental Illness/Mental Disorder

For the purposes of this book, we will usually use the term 'mental health problem' when referring to any kind of behavioural, emotional or cognitive difficulty and '**mental disorder**' to describe a diagnosable difficulty or impairment. It is important to remember that 'mental illness' is a widely accepted concept and a much-used phrase still in modern mental health care. Both the terms 'mental illness' and 'mental disorder' are widely used in practice, and it's important to remember that in the UK they are *also* applied in a legal context: in England and Wales, for example, according to the Mental Health Act, 2007, 'mental disorder' now means any disorder or disability of the mind: a far less restrictive (or far more all-encompassing) definition than found in the previous (1983) Act and one that has changed from a rigidly defined meaning that previously included 'mental illness'. In Scotland, 'mental disorder' means 'any mental illness, personality disorder, or learning disability, however caused or manifested.'

'Psychiatry' and 'psychiatric' are terms we will use when referring specifically to the branch of medicine that aims to research and treat mental disorders/mental illness: it is one of the key major contributing factors to the understanding for nurses of mental health, mental health difficulties and their care and treatment problems.

Factors contributing to mental health problems (whether defined as mental illnesses or mental disorders or neither) can – as with 'mental health' – be viewed through the lenses of individual, interpersonal and social/cultural categories. Individual factors include genetic make-up, intolerable or unrealistic worries or fears, inability to distinguish reality from fantasy, intolerance of life's uncertainties, a sense of disharmony in life, and a loss of meaning or purpose. Interpersonal factors include ineffective communication, excessive dependency on or withdrawal from relationships, inadequate sense of belonging, inadequate social support and loss of emotional control. Social/cultural factors include lack of resources, violence, homelessness, poverty, an unwarranted negative view of the world, and discrimination such as stigma, racism, classism, ageism and sexism.

It may be apparent already that 'mental health' and 'mental illness' are difficult to define precisely: they have long been very controversial and contested concepts. People who can carry out their roles in society and whose behaviour is appropriate and adaptive can be viewed as healthy. Conversely, those who fail to fulfil roles and carry out responsibilities, or whose behaviour is deemed inappropriate, may be viewed as 'ill'. The culture of any society strongly influences its values and beliefs, and this in turn affects how that society defines health and illness. What one society (or group in society) may view as acceptable and appropriate, another society (or group) may see as maladaptive and inappropriate. As mentioned, the term 'mental illness' is still widely used in the UK, but, as a concept, it has many critics and there are many problems associated with the term (see Box 1.1).

When – and how – do difficulties or problems become defined as 'mental disorder' or 'mental illness'?

We need to be careful about the potentially objectifying and reductionist aspects of categorization. Nevertheless, categorizations and classifications can help in building evidence, ensuring appropriate treatment and care and in understanding the interplay between psychological, biological and social factors in someone's life; they are to be found everywhere and students need to begin to understand their use, as well as the challenges that that use brings to the provision of person-centred, genuinely holistic care.

DSM-IV-TR (American Psychiatric Association, 2000) defines a **mental disorder** as 'a clinically significant behavioural or psychological syndrome or pattern that occurs in an individual and is associated with present distress (e.g., a painful symptom) or disability (i.e., impairment in one or more important areas of functioning) or with a significantly increased risk of suffering death, pain, disability or an important loss of freedom' (p. xxxi). It may appear clear to the student from this definition just how complex definition can be: what *is* 'clinically significant'? Who defines it? What is the meaning of – and relationship between – the 'behavioural' and the 'psychological'?

INTERNATIONAL CLASSIFICATION OF DISEASES

The *International Classification of Diseases*, 2nd edition (*ICD-10*) is produced by the World Health Organization (1994). It tends to be used more in the UK than *DSM-IV-TR*. It classifies mental disorders into the following 'blocks':

F00–F09 Organic, including symptomatic, mental disorders
F10–F19 Mental and behavioural disorders due to psychoactive substance use
F20–F29 Schizophrenia, schizotypal and delusional disorders
F30–F39 Mood [affective] disorders
F40–F48 Neurotic, stress-related and somatoform disorders
F50–F59 Behavioural syndromes associated with physiological disturbances and physical factors
F60–F69 Disorders of adult personality and behaviour
F70–F79 Mental retardation
F80–F89 Disorders of psychological development
F90–F98 Behavioural and emotional disorders with onset usually occurring in childhood and adolescence
F99 Unspecified mental disorder

Each block is further subdivided twice, e.g.

F42 Obsessive-Compulsive Disorder
F42.0 Predominantly obsessional thoughts or ruminations
F42.1 Predominantly compulsive acts (obsessional rituals)
F42.2 Mixed obsessional thoughts and acts
F42.3 Other obsessive-compulsive disorders
F42.3 Obsessive-compulsive disorder (unspecified).

Box 1.1 THE TERM 'MENTAL ILLNESS'

When someone experiences severe and/or enduring mental health problems, they are sometimes described as 'mentally ill', but there are difficulties with this term. They include:

- The lack of a universally agreed cut-off point between normal behaviour and behaviour associated with mental illness.
- The label 'mental illness' is highly stigmatizing.
- The term 'mental illness' can misleadingly imply that all mental health problems are solely caused by medical or biological factors.
- For many people, the existing systems of categorizing illnesses do not relate closely enough to their experiences.

From *http://www.mentalhealth.org.uk/information/mental-health-overview/mental-illness*. Copyright © Mental Health Foundation.

DIAGNOSTIC AND STATISTICAL MANUAL OF MENTAL DISORDERS

The *Diagnostic and Statistical Manual of Mental Disorders*, 4th edition, Text Revision (*DSM-IV-TR*) is a taxonomy published by the American Psychiatric Association. The *DSM-IV-TR* has three stated purposes:

- To provide a standardized nomenclature and language for all mental health professionals
- To present defining characteristics or symptoms that differentiate specific diagnoses
- To assist in identifying the underlying causes of disorders.

A 'multi-axial' classification system that involves assessment on several axes, or domains of information, it allows the practitioner to identify all the factors that relate to a person's condition:

- Axis I is for identifying all major psychiatric disorders except 'mental retardation' and 'personality disorders'. Examples include depression, schizophrenia, anxiety and substance-related disorders.
- Axis II is for reporting mental retardation and personality disorders as well as prominent maladaptive personality features and defence mechanisms.
- Axis III is for reporting current medical conditions that are potentially relevant to understanding or managing the person's mental disorder as well as medical conditions that might contribute to understanding the person.
- Axis IV is for reporting psychosocial and environmental problems that may affect the diagnosis, treatment and prognosis of mental disorders. Included are problems with the primary support group, the social environment, education, occupation, housing, economics, access to health care and the legal system.
- Axis V presents a Global Assessment of Functioning, which rates the person's overall psychological functioning on a scale of 0–100. This represents the clinician's assessment of the person's current level of functioning; the clinician may also give a score for prior functioning (e.g. highest Global Assessment of Functioning in past year or 6 months ago).

It is worth pointing out that, in the UK, classification of 'personality disorders' in particular (see Chapter 16) often uses *DSM-IV* rather than *ICD-10*.

WESTERN HISTORICAL PERSPECTIVES ON THE TREATMENT OF MENTAL HEALTH PROBLEMS

Throughout history, people across a wide variety of cultures believed (and many still believe) that any sickness indicated the displeasure of the gods or spirits and was, in fact, punishment for sins and wrongdoing. Those with what would now be seen in Western cultures as mental disorders were frequently viewed as being either divine or demonic,

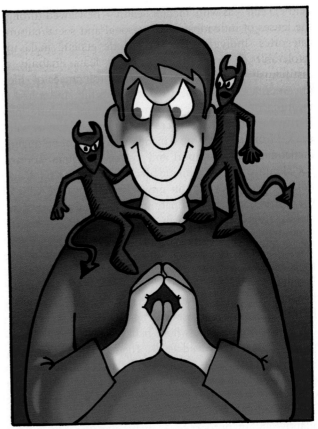

Possessed by demons?

depending on their behaviour. Individuals seen as divine were worshipped and adored; those seen as demonic were ostracized, punished and sometimes burned at the stake. There are interesting parallels here to the way in which contemporary societies relate- both 'positively' and 'negatively' to people with apparent mental disorders . . .

Aristotle (382–322 BC) attempted to relate mental disorders to physical disorders and developed a theory that the amounts of blood, water, and yellow and black bile in the body controlled the emotions. These four substances, or humours, corresponded with happiness, calmness, anger and sadness. Imbalances of the four humours were believed to cause mental disorders, so treatment was aimed at restoring balance through blood-letting, starving and purging. Such 'treatments' persisted well into the 19th century (Baly, 1982).

In early Christian times (AD 1–1000), primitive beliefs and superstitions were strong. All diseases were again blamed on demons, and the mentally ill were viewed as possessed. Priests performed exorcisms to rid evil spirits. When that failed, they used more severe and brutal measures, such as incarceration in dungeons, flogging and starving.

During the Renaissance (1300–1600), people with mental health problems were distinguished from criminals, particularly in England. Those considered harmless were allowed to wander the countryside or live in rural communities, but the more 'dangerous lunatics' were thrown in prison, chained and starved (Rosenblatt, 1984). In 1547, the Hospital of St. Mary of Bethlehem ('Bedlam') was officially declared a hospital for the insane, the first of its kind. By 1775, visitors at the institution were charged a fee for the privilege of viewing and ridiculing the inmates, who were seen as animals, less than human (McMillan, 1997). During this same period in the colonies (in particular what were to become the United States), the mentally disordered were considered evil or possessed and were punished. Witch-hunts were conducted, and offenders were burned at the stake.

Period of Enlightenment and Creation of Mental Institutions

In the 1790s, a period of relative enlightenment concerning people with mental health problems began. Phillippe Pinel in France and William Tuke in England formulated the concept of **asylum** as a safe refuge or haven offering protection at institutions where people had been whipped, beaten and starved just because they had mental health problems (Gollaher, 1995). With this movement began the 'moral treatment' of people seen as 'mad'. In the US, Dorothea Dix (1802–1887) began a crusade to reform the treatment of 'mental illness' after a visit to Tuke's institution in England. Dix believed that society had obligations to those who had mental health problems and promoted adequate shelter, nutritious food and warm clothing, influencing nursing and mental health care generally in the US, in Europe and in the UK (Gollaher, 1995).

The period of 'enlightenment' was, however, short-lived. Within 100 years of the establishment of the first asylum, many hospitals had become places of fear and alienation. Attendants were frequently guilty of abusing the residents, the rural locations of hospitals were viewed as isolating patients from their families and homes, and the phrase *insane asylum* took on a negative connotation: places that cared for the 'mad' entered modern consciousness as sites of Gothic horror and suffering.

Sigmund Freud and Treatment of Mental Disorders

A period of scientific study and treatment of mental disorders began with Sigmund Freud (1856–1939) and his contemporaries, such as Emil Kraepelin (1856–1926) and Eugene Bleuler (1857–1939). With these men, the study of psychiatry and the diagnosis and treatment of mental health problems started in earnest. Freud challenged society to view human beings objectively. He studied the mind, its disorders and their treatment as no one had before, and many other theorists built on Freud's pioneering work (see Chapter 2), which, despite periods of being 'unfashionable', remains hugely influential. Kraepelin, meanwhile, began classifying mental disorders according to their 'symptoms' and Bleuler – crucially – coined the term *schizophrenia*, both influencing the still-hegemonic 'medical' approach to mental health.

Development of Psychopharmacology

A great leap in the treatment of mental disorders began in about 1950 with the development of **psychotropic drugs.** Chlorpromazine (Largactil), an antipsychotic drug, and lithium, an antimanic agent, were the first drugs to be developed. Over the following 10 years, monoamine oxidase inhibitor antidepressants; haloperidol (Haldol), an antipsychotic; tricyclic antidepressants; and anti-anxiety agents, specifically benzodiazepines, were introduced. For the first time, drugs actually reduced agitation, psychotic thinking and depression in many people. Perhaps equally importantly, attitudes to the 'mad' had begun to change amongst professionals, politicians and lay-people – more positive, tolerant and enlightened views became more common. In the UK, the 1959 Mental Health Act sought to make hospital admissions for mental health problems as similar as possible to those for physical problems, to reduce significantly the number of compulsory admissions and to ensure that local councils took responsibility for those who didn't need admission. Hospital stays were shortened and many people – previously confined for years in institutions – were able to go home.

There was a flip-side, however, to this apparent progress: the side-effects of the new medications were often – in the shorter term – unpleasant (a battery of effects such as weight gain, sedation, distressing extrapyramidal side-effects) and frequently – in the longer term – could lead to crippling conditions such tardive dyskinesia. In some cases, the effects of taking psychotropic medication were fatal. Although the increasingly assertive voices of people with mental health problems have helped lead to drug companies, prescribers and non-medical professionals becoming more careful about, and sensitive to, the impact of medication, unpleasant and dangerous side-effects can still occur; the nurse's role as educator about, monitor of and advocate for and against psychotropic medication remains crucial.

Movement Toward Community Mental Health

The movement toward treating those with mental health problems in less restrictive environments gained further momentum in the UK in 1961 with Enoch Powell's famous 'water tower' speech, which announced the proposed closure of the large psychiatric institutions and the development of 'care in the community'. This process took the best part of the next four decades to achieve as community services – often poorly resourced – began to develop to replace the old system. In the 1970s and 1980s, Community Mental Health Teams (CMHTs) were established and new, smaller Acute Units built (often on General Hospital sites). Pressure groups (such as MIND) developed more political power, having some influence on the 1983 Mental Health Act which further enshrined certain rights in law and, in particular, aimed to prevent the abuse of medical power.

Despite these changes, mental health care remained poorly resourced – and something of a 'Cinderella' service – but, in part as a result of a number of high-profile murders by people with mental health problems (for example, the case of Jonathan Zito's murder by Christopher Clunis in 1992 and the subsequent Ritchie Report (Ritchie, 1994)), it began to receive greater and greater attention from successive governments and from the population as a whole. Over the past decade, mental health services have rarely been out of the public eye.

MENTAL HEALTH IN THE 21ST CENTURY

Developments in the UK have been patchy, inconsistent and confusing: influences such as devolved parliaments in Scotland and Wales, changing political configurations in Northern Ireland and wide historical regional differences have meant that services have changed (and continue to change) at different paces and with different emphases. By the end of the 1990s, though, it was generally agreed that 'community care' (and the patchy community services that had developed) had had negative as well as positive effects. A number of high-profile murders by people with diagnosed mental health problems led to increasing media, public and government disquiet with services, much of it justified. There were – justified – criticisms that CMHTs – particularly nurses – had been focusing more on those with short-term problems than those – often much more challenging people – with more complex, 'chronic' problems. Often, those responsible for the shift to a community-based mental health system had not accurately anticipated the extent of the needs of people with severe and persistent mental health problems. Many people did not have all the skills – emotional, cognitive, interactional – necessary to live fully independently in the community: learning these skills is often time-consuming and labour-intensive, requiring sustained, prolonged staff input. In addition, the nature of some mental health problems made learning these skills more difficult. For example, a client who is experiencing hallucinations or paranoid ideas can have difficulty listening to or comprehending instructions. Other clients may experience drastic shifts in mood, being unable to get out of bed one day and unable to concentrate or pay attention a few days later. Psychotic disorders – as we will see later – can lead to 'cognitive deficits' which can hamper the development of new ways of living.

Although the move towards the community reduced the number of hospital beds, in many areas the number of *admissions* to those beds often increased, and although people with severe and persistent mental health problems now had shorter hospital stays, they were now often admitted to hospitals more frequently. The continuous flow of clients being admitted and discharged often threatened to overwhelm acute psychiatric units. In addition, more and more people had a dual problem of both severe mental health problems and substance abuse: use of alcohol and

drugs exacerbated symptoms of mental ill-health, again making return to hospital more likely.

Meanwhile, CMHTs were accused – with some justification – of focusing on a group of people dismissively termed 'the worried well': people whose problems were painful and distressing but who were not seen as experiencing severe mental health problems. GPs – under huge pressure themselves – frequently referred this client-group into the services. People with a huge range of social and mental health needs were seen as 'falling through the net' – ignored until they came to the attention of emergency services.

The **Care Programme Approach** (CPA), initially introduced in England in 1991 and in Wales, Scotland and Northern Ireland in the following few years, did begin (after a painfully faltering start) to ensure that an appointed Care Coordinator (more often than not, a nurse) took responsibility for overseeing care for people, whether within or outside hospital. The CPA aims to prevent people 'falling through the net' and to ensure that everyone who comes into contact with services has their needs assessed, a plan of care drawn up by the multidisciplinary team and regular reviews of that care undertaken.

The CPA was never a panacea to all the systemic problems in mental health care – indeed, its overemphasis on documentation often proved counter-productive. Over the past decade, therefore, attempts have been made to 'reconfigure' services so that they better meet the needs of the whole population. New approaches to delivering services, evolving from the 'North Birmingham' model and the National Service Frameworks (Department of Health, 1999, 2006; Appleby, 2007) have led to the development of new teams – such as 'Assertive Outreach Teams', 'Crisis Resolution and Home Treatment' teams, 'Early Intervention in Psychosis' teams and 'Primary Care Mental Health' teams – and a breakdown of the division between acute inpatient services (neglected and frequently seen as the 'worst', least-resourced and most embattled part of the system) and community services.

Crucially, an increasing emphasis on 'evidence-based practice' and a shift towards the employment of both cognitive-behavioural and **'recovery'**-focused strategies and principles within mental health care have moved the therapeutic focus of services and shifted power relationships between professionals and between professionals and 'service users'. At the same time as this increase in focus on collaborative partnerships in care, on evidence and research and on genuine user involvement (and somewhat paradoxically) – there has come an increasing interest in (some would say an obsession with) the assessment and management of **risk**, exemplified – in England and Wales – by the governmental pressure for, the wrangles over and the final legislative compromises contained within the Mental Health Act (2007).

Despite all these changes, mental health problems remain a significant social, economic and personal issue (see Box 1.2). MIND – the National Association for Mental Health – suggests that 'one in four of us will experience a mental health

Box 1.2 MENTAL HEALTH STATISTICS

- Stress-related illness is costing the NHS between £300 and £400 million every year.
- According to the Sainsbury Centre for Mental Health, the total cost of mental health problems is around £77 billion per year.
- Around 6.8 million people of working age in the UK are disabled. This is around 20% of the working age population.
- More than 2.5 million individuals receive incapacity benefit and/or severe disability allowance.
- Close to 1 million people are claiming incapacity benefit due to mental ill-health.
- People who are disabled because of mental health problems have lower employment rates than all other disabled groups.
- Only around 20% of people with mental health problems are in employment.

From MIND *http://www.mind.org.uk/Information/Factsheets/Statistics/Statistics+6.htm.* © 2007 Mind (National Association for Mental Health).

problem at some point in our lives' and that 'each year more than 250,000 people are admitted to psychiatric hospitals and over 4,000 people take their own lives' (MIND, 2008).

In England and Wales, the tortuous, bitter, decade-long debates before the eventual 2007 Royal Assent and 2008 general implementation of the Mental Health Act (2007) illustrate some of the many tensions still inherent in mental health systems: in particular, the issues of public safety versus individuals' rights, and the social control role versus the therapeutic role of mental health professionals. Readers will have to confront their own thoughts and feelings about these complex issues and develop ways to respond effectively and compassionately.

Mental Health Care and Diversity

The UK Census (Office of National Statistics, 2001) found that 86% of the population considered themselves 'White British' but concluded that this figure would almost certainly decrease as the numbers of people viewing themselves as non-White British, Black African, Asian or Caribbean in origin, for example, increases. In the 10 years from 1991 to 2001 Great Britain's ethnic minority population increased from 3.1 million to 4.6 million. As a *proportion* of the population, the ethnic minority population also increased – from 5.6 per cent to 8.1 per cent. The Black African population – the group with the largest increase – *doubled* between 1991 and 2001

Many people from ethnic minority populations experience major economic, social and educational deprivation as well as the fear and reality of racist attack. Women, in particular, in some communities are far less likely to be economically and socially active and more likely to be vulnerable to mental health problems. Nurses must be fully prepared to care for this growing culturally diverse population, care which includes becoming far more aware of cultural differences and the complex social and economic factors that influence mental health and the treatment of mental health problems (see Chapter 7 for a discussion of cultural differences).

Diversity is not limited to culture; the structure of families has changed as well. With divorce rates remaining at between 140,000 and 160,000 a year, single parents head many families, and many 'blended' families are created when divorced persons remarry. According to the Office of National Statistics, nearly a quarter of children (24%) in Britain were living in 'lone-parent' families in 2006, more than three times the proportion in 1972. Twenty-nine per cent of households consist of a single person (Office of National Statistics, 2007) and increasing numbers of people live together without being married. Gay men and lesbians form partnerships more confidently and openly than ever before, and sometimes adopt children. The face of the family in the UK is fascinating, complex and ever-changing and provides a constant challenge to nurses to provide sensitive, competent care.

Mental Health and Homelessness

Homelessness is a major problem in the UK today. Between 1991 and 2006 the percentage of homeless people who were vulnerable due to mental health problems tripled. Those who are homeless and have mental health problems can be found in parks, airports and bus terminals, on the streets, in police stations and prisons. Some use shelters, halfway houses, or 'B & B's; others rent cheap hotel rooms when they can afford it. Homelessness worsens problems for many people with mental health problems, who end up on the streets, contributing to a vicious cycle.

Many of the problems of the homeless, as well as those who pass through the revolving door of mental health care, stem from an historical lack of adequate community resources. Inpatient psychiatric treatment still accounts for most of the spending for mental health in the UK, and community mental health has never been given the secure financial base it needs to be effective. In addition, mental health services provided in the community must be individualized, available and culturally relevant to be effective.

Despite the flaws in the system, community-focused services have hugely positive aspects that make them preferable for most people with mental health problems. People can remain in their own communities, maintain contact with family and friends, and enjoy personal freedom that is not possible in an institution, where people often lose motivation and hope

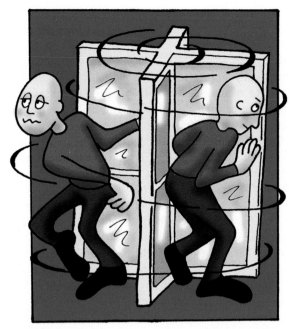

Revolving door

as well as functional daily living skills, such as shopping and cooking. Treatment in the community is a trend that will – hopefully – continue; that community, though, is changing and bringing with it new challenges.

THE FUTURE

In early 2006, *The future of mental health: A vision for 2015* set out a 'radical but realistic agenda for the next 10 years' (Sainsbury Centre for Mental Health, 2006). It emphasized the need for enhanced integration of mental health services – and those with mental health problems – into everyday community life, real autonomy and choice for clients, accessible and flexible care and treatment options, the elimination of fear, intolerance and exclusion. In some parts of the service, we're well on the way there. It will be – in part – down to mental health nurses to decide whether the objectives in this, the vision, are comprehensively achieved.

Factors such as devolution and ever-evolving political, economic, social and ideological contexts across the UK and the wider world will ensure that the future for mental health services remains fluid and contestable and that it will undoubtedly – while retaining some essential shared elements – continue to involve different configurations, ideologies and practices from region to region and country to country.

Policy drivers such as Scotland's *Better health better care: Action plan* (Scottish Government, 2007) and England's *High quality care for all* report (Professor the Lord Darzi of Denham KBE, 2008) made it clear that wide variations in health care – including mental health care – needed to be tackled rigorously; good practice – already existing in places – needed to be spread to reduce variations. Genuine, effective patient and public involvement, the extension

of 'choice' and increased accountability were, the report said, necessary in all sectors of health care. Demographic changes, the development of new information technologies and changing expectations will all impact on this process: it will be fascinating to see how mental health services will develop and evolve in response.

MENTAL HEALTH NURSING PRACTICE

In the 19th century, Florence Nightingale, famously, helped set nurses and the practice of nursing on its way to professionalism and its key contemporary role in modern health care; though of course the act of nursing – caring for people effectively in a way that is respectful, compassionate and collaborative – has been with us since human beings first evolved.

Nursing of people with mental health problems has long had a close, complex, overlapping, sometimes tense, relationship to both its physical health-care counterpart and to the medical profession. Up until the late 19th century, 'attendants' in asylums had little or no training or education; they were chosen for their strength – both 'moral' and physical. They were mostly men, mostly working-class, and their efforts to be considered professionals – or nurses – in any way were firmly resisted by the resolutely middle-class (and female) nursing establishment. Gradually – and painfully slowly – and with more emphasis on practical and academic education (usually led by doctors), the need for some kind of registration, and with shifts in social attitudes, attendants' training and development needs began to be recognized. From 1885, when the Medico-Psychological Association published the very first textbook for attendants – *The handbook for the instruction of attendants on the insane* – until 1951, when the General Nursing Council finally 'won', control of attendant training was fought over by psychiatrists and general nurses.

The very first UK university degree in psychiatric nursing (as it was commonly termed up until the late 1990s) was established at the University of Manchester in 1969, but it wasn't until the controversial 'Project 2000' in the 1990s that general and psychiatric nurse training fully 'merged' with a 'Common Foundation Programme' as part of a course based in higher education. The move into academia – controversial from the start – has helped facilitate a wider and deeper research base and some much needed professional 'self-esteem', although critics continue to argue that the essence of nursing – a pragmatic, common-sense and compassionate desire to understand and help – has been lost.

Throughout its history, psychiatric (later, 'mental health') nursing has been influenced by a number of innovative, energetic and courageous individuals. Two American nursing theorists shaped psychiatric nursing practice significantly: Hildegard Peplau and June Mellow. Peplau published *Interpersonal relations in nursing* in 1952 and *Interpersonal techniques: The crux of psychiatric nursing* in 1962. She described the therapeutic nurse–client relationship and identified its key phases and

Box 1.3   RECOMMENDATIONS OF THE CHIEF NURSING OFFICER'S REVIEW OF MENTAL HEALTH NURSING

- Positive, user-centred values form the bedrock of good practice.
- Carers and families need to have their contribution recognized and valued and their information and support needs appropriately met by mental health nurses (MHNs).
- Mental health nursing needs to develop its practice in many areas.
- Mental health nursing needs to move away from a traditional model of care towards a biopsychosocial and values-based approach.

- Good pre-registration education is key to ensuring that MHNs are equipped with appropriate fundamental skills and attitudes.
- Clinical supervision is essential underpinning for good practice.
- Professional leadership and support structures are required to promote good and confident nursing practice.

Department of Health. (2006). *From values to action: The Chief Nursing Officer's review of mental health nursing*, p. 13. Available: *http://www.dh.gov.uk/en/ Publicationsandstatistics/Publications/PublicationsPolicyAndGuidance/DH_4133839*. © 2006 Crown Copyright.

tasks, and wrote extensively about anxiety (see Chapter 13). The interpersonal dimension that was crucial to her beliefs forms the foundations of good practice today. Mellow's 1968 work, *Nursing therapy,* described her approach of focusing on clients' psychosocial needs and strengths. She contended that the nurse as therapist is particularly suited to working with those with severe mental illness in the context of daily activities, focusing on the here and now to meet each person's psychosocial needs (Mellow, 1986). Both Peplau and Mellow substantially contributed to the practice of psychiatric nursing and influenced later US and UK nursing theorists, such as Dorothy Orem, Phil Barker and Kevin Gournay

Many social, political and legislative changes have impacted on mental health nursing, some of which will be explored in more detail later. The political and attitudinal changes to society and to health care wrought in part by Margaret Thatcher in the 1980s and her New Labour successors in the 1990s and 2000s have influenced nursing and nurses hugely and, for the first time, mental health care has seemed to take centre stage in policy-making. Perhaps the key driving document was the *National service framework for mental health*, first published in 1999, a 10-year strategy aimed at clarifying national standards for the provision of mental health services and a configuration of services that would help attain those standards. A five-year review (Appleby, 2004) highlighted the progress that had been made and some of the problems that remained and attempted to take into account both recent and potential changes in need and in service configuration.

In 2006, the *Chief Nursing Officer's review of mental health nursing* (Department of Health, 2006) pointed the way forward for the profession in an attempt to answer the question *'How can mental health nursing best contribute to the care of service users in the future?'* Its findings and recommendations can be found in Box 1.3.

The *CNO's review* emphasized – alongside a focus on the need to develop the notoriously poor physical health-care skills of mental health nurses (MHNs) – the need for the values and principles of recovery-optimism, collaboration, active participation in care and a focus on strengths rather than deficits – to be embedded in mental health nursing, and, similarly, the review of mental health nursing in Scotland in 2006 (Scottish Executive/ NHS Scotland, 2006) has attempted to focus nursing on 'rights, relationships and recovery'. It is to be hoped that the principles outlined in these two initiatives – historically underpinning all good nursing practice – will become the norm.

The Nursing and Midwifery Council published, in 2007, *Standards of proficiency for nursing* (available at http://www. nmc-uk.org/aFrameDisplay.aspx?DocumentID=328) which defined the principles of practice for nurses in the UK. To become registered as a mental health nurse, people must achieve these standards.

The Millan principles underpinned the development of the new Mental Health (Care and Treatment) (Scotland) Act 2003 and are outlined in Box 1.4. This is an excellent set of principles which students – in whatever setting – could usefully adopt to inform their practice.

CONCERNS

People beginning a clinical experience in the mental health field often have a variety of fears and worries; these are normal – and often lurk even in the mind of the most experienced nurse.

Some common concerns (and 'helpful hints'):

- *What if I say the wrong thing?* No one magic phrase can solve a client's problems; likewise, no single statement can significantly worsen them. Listening carefully, feeling – and

Box 1.4   THE TEN MILLAN PRINCIPLES

1. Non-discrimination – people with mental health and substance misuse problems should, wherever possible, retain the same rights and entitlements as those with other health needs.
2. Equality – all interventions will be exercised without any direct or indirect discrimination on the grounds of physical disability, age, gender, sexual orientation, language, religion, or national, ethnic or social origin.
3. Respect for diversity – service users should receive care, treatment and support in a manner that accords respect for their individual qualities, abilities and diverse backgrounds, and properly takes into account their age, gender, sexual orientation, ethnic group, and social, cultural and religious background.
4. Reciprocity – where society imposes an obligation on an individual to comply with a programme of treatment of care, it should impose a parallel obligation on the health and social care authorities to provide safe and appropriate services, including ongoing care following discharge from compulsion.
5. Informal care – wherever possible, care, treatment and support should be provided to people with substance misuse problems without the use of compulsory powers.
6. Participation – service users should be fully involved, so far as they are able to be, in all aspects of their assessment, care, treatment and support. Their past and present wishes should be taken into account. They should be provided with all the information and support necessary to enable them to participate fully. Information should be provided in a way that makes it most likely to be understood.
7. Respect for carers – those who provide care to service users on an informal basis should receive respect for their role and experience, receive appropriate information and advice, and have their views and needs taken into account.
8. Least restrictive alternative – service users should be provided with any necessary care, treatment and support, both in the least invasive manner and in the least restrictive manner and environment compatible with the delivery of safe and effective care, taking account, where appropriate, of the safety of others.
9. Benefit – any intervention should be likely to produce for the service user a benefit that cannot reasonably be achieved other than by the intervention.
10. Child welfare – the welfare of a child affected by substance misuse or mental health problems should be paramount in any interventions imposed on the child under mental health legislation.

Adapted from *Essential Care: A Report on the Approach Required to Maximise Opportunity for Recovery from Problem Substance Use in Scotland.* http://openscotland.gov.uk/Publications/2008/03/20144059/8

showing – genuine interest, and caring about the client are extremely important. A nurse who possesses these elements but says something that sounds out of place could simply restate it by saying, 'That didn't come out right. What I meant was . . .': honesty and genuineness are at the very heart of nursing care.

- *What should I be doing?* In many mental health settings, clearly defined tasks and responsibilities may appear minimal. The idea of 'just talking to people' may make us feel as though we're not really doing anything. Each of us must deal with our own anxiety about approaching a stranger to talk about very sensitive and personal issues. Development of the therapeutic nurse–client relationship and trust takes time, skill and patience.
- *What if no one seems to want to talk in any depth to me?* Both inexperienced and experienced practitioners sometimes fear that clients will reject them or refuse to have anything to do with them. Some clients may not want to talk or are reclusive; we shouldn't see that necessarily as a personal insult or failure. Generally, many people in emotional distress welcome the opportunity to have someone listen to them and show a genuine interest in their situation. Being available and willing to listen is often all it takes to begin a significant interaction with someone. At the same time, it's vital to respect clients' right to refuse to talk to us. The use of tools, assessment forms and other documentation can offer a bridge between two people: but they can also act as a barrier.
- *Am I prying when I ask personal questions?* Listen: and follow the client's lead. We can all sometimes feel awkward discussing personal or distressing issues and it's important to remember that questions involving personal matters should rarely be the first thing we say to a client. More comfort with discussing these issues (on both sides) usually arises after some trust and rapport have been established, built on a foundation of **compassion** and genuine **curiosity**. When emotional or personal issues are addressed in the context of a collaborative nurse–client

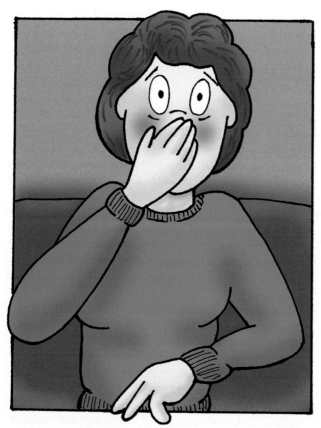

'What if I say the wrong thing?'

easier to manage. It's vital to protect the client's privacy and dignity when he or she cannot do so.

- *Is it dangerous? Am I likely to get hurt working with people with mental health problems?* Media coverage – and cultural myths – about those with 'mental illness' are widespread and pernicious, leaving the impression (conscious or unconscious) for all of us that clients with mental health problems are potentially violent. Actually, statistically, clients hurt themselves far more often than they harm others. Collaborative risk and safety assessments – and agreed, transparent, risk-management plans – are essential, however, and when physical aggression does occur, we should all feel competent to handle aggressive clients in a safe manner. Learners should not become involved in the physical restraint of an aggressive client, because it's likely that he or she has not had the training and experience required. When talking to or approaching clients who are potentially aggressive, it may be helpful to sit in an open area rather than in a closed room, provide plenty of space for the client, or request that someone else be present.

- *What if I come across someone I know being cared for on a unit or in the community?* In any clinical setting, it is possible that we might see someone we know. People often have additional fears because of the stigma that is still associated with seeking mental health treatment. It is essential in mental health that the client's identity and treatment be kept confidential. If we recognize someone we know, we should notify a senior member of staff, who can decide how to handle the situation. It is usually best for someone to talk with the client and reassure him or her about confidentiality. The client should be reassured that the professional will not read the client's record and will not be assigned to work directly with the client; if necessary, the member of staff should be moved to another clinical area.

- *What if I realize I have similar problems or issues to a client?* We all discover that some of the problems, family dynamics, or life events of particular clients are similar to our own or those of people close to us. It can be a shock for us to discover – and difficult to admit – that there are far more similarities between 'us' and 'them' than there are differences. There is no easy answer for this concern. Many of us have stressful lives or abusive childhood experiences; some cope – at least superficially – fairly successfully, whereas others appear devastated emotionally. There is no clear dividing line between the 'healthy' nurse and the 'ill' client . . . we need to be able to identify when our own experiences, beliefs and feelings are being used to help the client and when they are potentially harmful: clinical supervision is essential to help this process of identification. We're all human beings: the essence of nursing is to use our common humanity, our experience and our skills to help others and to learn from each other. Chapter 7 discusses these factors in more detail.

relationship, asking sincere – and seemingly necessary – questions is not prying but is an attempt to use therapeutic communication skills to help validate the person's experiences and to begin to work towards solutions.

- *How will I handle behaviour that seems to me to be bizarre or inappropriate?* The behaviour and statements of some clients may be shocking or distressing. It's important to monitor one's facial expressions and emotional responses so that clients don't feel rejected or ridiculed, though, at the same time, honest, human-to-human feedback may be essential to help someone begin to change. Senior clinical and educational staff *should* always be available to assist us in – or after – such situations: we should never feel as if we have to handle situations alone.

- *What happens if a client asks me for a date or displays sexually aggressive or inappropriate behaviour?* Some clients have difficulty recognizing or maintaining interpersonal boundaries. When a client seeks contact of any type outside the nurse–client relationship, it is important for the nurse (with the assistance of other staff) to clarify the boundaries of the professional relationship (see Chapter 5). Likewise, setting limits and maintaining boundaries are needed when a client's behaviour is sexually inappropriate. Most of us feel uncomfortable dealing with such behaviour, but with practice and the assistance of others it becomes

SELF-AWARENESS ISSUES

The development of **self-awareness** is an ongoing process by which someone attempts to gain recognition of his or her own feelings, beliefs and attitudes, and to ensure his or her ability to remain curious, to be compassionate and to be effective. Self-awareness is particularly important in mental health nursing. Everyone, professionals, clients and learners, has values, ideas and beliefs that are unique and different from those of others. At times, a nurse's values and beliefs will conflict with those of the client or with the client's behaviour. The nurse must learn to accept these differences among people and view each client as a worthwhile person regardless of that client's opinions and lifestyle. The nurse does not need to condone the client's views and behaviour; he or she merely needs to accept them as different from his or her own and not let them interfere with care.

As an example, a nurse who believes that abortion is wrong may be assigned to care for a client who has recently had an abortion. If the nurse is going to help the client, he or she must be able to separate his or her own beliefs about abortion from those of the client: the nurse must make sure that personal feelings and beliefs do not interfere with or hinder the client's care.

The nurse can accomplish enhanced self-awareness through formal or informal reflection, spending time consciously focusing on how one feels and what one values or believes. Although we all have values and beliefs, we may not have really spent time discovering how we feel or what we believe about certain issues, such as suicide or a client's refusal to take needed medications. The nurse needs to discover himself or herself and what he or she believes before trying to help others with different views.

Points to Consider When Working on Self-Awareness

- Keep a diary or journal that focuses on experiences and related thoughts and feelings. Work on identifying thoughts and feelings and the circumstances from which they arose. Review the diary or journal periodically to look for patterns or changes.
- Talk to someone you trust about your experiences, thoughts and feelings. This might be a family member, friend, co-worker or tutor. Discuss how he or she might feel in a similar situation, or ask how he or she deals with uncomfortable situations or feelings.
- Engage in formal clinical supervision. Even experienced clinicians need a supervisor with whom they can discuss personal feelings and challenging client situations, to gain insight and new approaches.
- Seek alternative points of view. Put yourself in the client's situation and think about his or her feelings, thoughts and actions.

- Don't necessarily be critical of yourself (or others) for having certain values or beliefs. Accept them as a part of yourself, or work to change those values and beliefs you wish to be different.

KEY POINTS

- Mental health and mental disorder/mental illness are difficult to define and are heavily influenced by one's culture and society.
- The World Health Organization defines health as a state of complete physical, mental and social wellness, not merely the absence of disease or infirmity.
- Historically, mental disorder was often viewed as demonic possession, sin or weakness, and people were punished accordingly.
- Today, mental disorder is most commonly seen as a multifaceted problem with 'symptoms' causing dissatisfaction with one's characteristics, abilities and accomplishments; ineffective or unsatisfying interpersonal relationships; dissatisfaction with one's place in the world; ineffective coping with life events; and lack of personal growth.
- Factors contributing to mental health include a person's genetic make-up, qualities of autonomy and independence, self-esteem, the capacity and willingness to grow, develop and take risks, vitality, crisis-management skills, the ability to find meaning and purpose in life, the capacity to tolerate distress, a sense of belonging and reality orientation; effective communication skills, the willingness and ability to help others, intimacy, and a balance of separateness and connectedness; and power and control issues, economic and political issues, a sense of community, access to adequate resources, the intolerance of violence, support for diversity, and a positive, yet realistic, view of – and from – one's world.
- Factors contributing to mental health problems are genetic make-up and childhood experiences; anxiety, worries and fears; ineffective communication; excessive dependence or withdrawal from relationships; loss of emotional control; lack of resources; and violence, homelessness, poverty and discrimination.
- The *ICD-10* and *DSM-IV* are taxonomies used to provide a standard nomenclature of mental disorders, define characteristics of disorders, and assist in identifying underlying causes of disorders.
- A significant advance in treating people with mental health problems was the development of psychotropic drugs in the early 1950s.
- The shift from institutional care to care in the community began in the 1960s, allowing many people to leave institutions for the first time in years.
- There have been many changes in attitude and policy in the past two decades, in particular renewed emphasis on evidence-based care, on recovery and optimism, on risk and

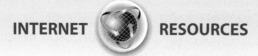

INTERNET RESOURCES

RESOURCE	INTERNET ADDRESS
Centre for Evidence-Based Mental Health	http://www.cebmh.com/
Center for the Study of the History of Nursing	http://www.nursing.upenn.edu/history
Mental Health Alliance	http://www.mentalhealthalliance.org.uk/
Mental Health History Timeline	http://www.mdx.ac.uk/www/study/mhhtim.htm
Mental Health Nurse	http://www.mentalhealthnurse.co.uk/
MIND	http://www.mind.org.uk/
National Institute for Mental Health in England	http://nimhe.csip.org.uk/index.html
National Library for Health	http://www.library.nhs.uk/mentalhealth/
RETHINK	http://www.rethink.org/
Royal College of Psychiatrists	http://www.rcpsych.ac.uk
Sainsbury Centre for Mental Health	http://www.scmh.org.uk/
Tidal Model	http://www.tidal-model.com/
World Health Organization	http://www.who.int

safety, and in policy drivers such as the Care Programme Approach and the National Service Frameworks.

• Mental health nursing was recognized as such in the late 1800s, although it only fairly recently became a distinct profession.

• Mental health nursing practice has been profoundly influenced by Hildegard Peplau and June Mellow (and in the UK by Phil Barker), who wrote about the nurse–client relationship, anxiety, nurse therapy and interpersonal nursing theory.

• The *Chief Nursing Officer's review of mental health nursing* has published **standards of care** that should guide mental health nursing clinical practice.

• Common concerns of mental health nurses include fear of saying the wrong thing, not knowing what to do, being rejected by clients, being threatened physically, recognizing someone they know as a client, and sharing similar problems or backgrounds with clients.

• Awareness of one's feelings, beliefs, attitudes, values and thoughts, called self-awareness, is absolutely essential to the practice of mental health nursing.

• The goal of self-awareness is to know oneself so that one's values, attitudes and beliefs do not negatively affect clients, and so we can maintain and develop our curiosity, our compassion and our effectiveness.

REFERENCES

American Psychiatric Association. (2000). *Diagnostic and Statistical Manual of Mental Disorders* (4th edn, text revision). Washington, DC: American Psychiatric Association.

Appleby, L. (2004). *The national service framework for mental health: Five years on.* London: Department of Health.

Appleby, L. (2007). *Mental health ten years on: Progress on mental health care reform.* London: Department of Health. Available: http://www.dh.gov.uk/en/Publicationsandstatistics/Publications/PublicationsPolicyAndGuidance/DH_07424

Baly, M. (1982). A leading light. *Nursing Mirror, 155*(19), 49–51.

Department of Health. (1999). *National service framework for mental health: Modern standards and service models.* Available: http://www.dh.gov.uk/en/Publicationsandstatistics/Publications/PublicationsPolicyAndGuidance/DH_4009598

Department of Health. (2006). *From values to action: The Chief Nursing Officer's review of mental health nursing.* Available: http://www.dh.gov.uk/en/Publicationsandstatistics/Publications/PublicationsPolicyAndGuidance/DH_4133839

Gollaher, D. (1995). *Voice for the mad: The life of Dorothea Dix.* New York: Free Press.

McMillan, I. (1997). Insight into bedlam: One hospital's history. *Journal of Psychosocial Nursing, 3*(6), 28–34.

Mellow, J. (1986). A personal perspective of nursing therapy. *Hospital and Community Psychiatry, 37*(2), 182–183.

Mental Health Act (as amended). (2007). London: OPSI. Available: http://www.dh.gov.uk/en/Healthcare/NationalServiceFrameworks/Mentalhealth/DH_089882

MIND. (2008). *MIND factsheet: The social contexts of mental distress.* Available: http://www.mind.org.uk/Information/Factsheets/Statistics/Statistics+6.htm

Nursing and Midwifery Council. (2007). Standards of proficiency for nursing. Available: http://www.nmc-uk.org/aFrameDisplay.aspx?DocumentID=328

Office of National Statistics. (2001). *UK census.* Available: http://www.statistics.gov.uk/census/default.asp

Office of National Statistics. (2007). *Focus on families.* Basingstoke: Palgrave Macmillan.

Professor the Lord Darzi of Denham KBE. (2008). *High quality care for all: NHS Next Stage Review final report.* London: Department of Health. Available: http://www.dh.gov.uk/en/publicationsandstatistics/publications/publicationspolicyandguidance/DH_085825

Ritchie, J. (1994). *The inquiry into the care and treatment of Christopher Clunis.* London: Department of Health.

Rosenblatt, A. (1984). Concepts of the asylum in the care of the mentally ill. *Hospital and Community Psychiatry, 35,* 244–250.

Sainsbury Centre for Mental Health. (2006). *The future of mental health: A vision for 2015.* Available: http://www.scmh.org.uk/pdfs/mental+health+futures+policy+paper.pdf

Scottish Executive/NHS Scotland. (2006). *Rights, relationships and recovery: The Report of the National Review of Mental Health Nursing in Scotland.* Available: http://www.scotland.gov.uk/Publications/2006/04/18164814/0

Scottish Executive. (2003). *The Mental Health (Care and Treatment) (Scotland) Act 2003*. Available: http://www.nes.scot.nhs.uk/mhagp/index.htm

Scottish Government. (2007). *Better health better care: Action plan*. Available: http://www.scotland.gov.uk/Publications/2007/12/11103453/0

World Health Organization. (1948). Preamble to the constitution of the World Health Organization. Available at: http://www.who.int/suggestions/faq/en/

World Health Organization. (1994). *International Classification of Diseases* (2nd edn) (*ICD-10*). Available: http://www.who.int/classifications/icd/en/

ADDITIONAL READING

Barker, P. & Buchanan-Barker, P. (2005). *The Tidal Model: A guide for mental health professionals*. Brunner-Routledge

Nolan, P. (1993). *A history of mental health nursing*. Cheltenham: Nelson-Thornes.

Chapter Study Guide

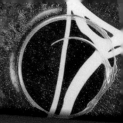

MULTIPLE-CHOICE QUESTIONS

Select the best answer for each of the following questions.

1. Approximately how many of us will experience a mental health problem at some time in our lives?
   a. 1 in 5
   b. 1 in 4
   c. 1 in 3
   d. 1 in 2

2. Hospitals established by Dorothea Dix were designed to provide which of the following?
   a. Asylum
   b. Confinement
   c. Therapeutic milieu
   d. Public safety

3. Hildegard Peplau is best known for her writing about which of the following?
   a. Community-based care
   b. Humane treatment
   c. Psychopharmacology
   d. Therapeutic nurse–client relationship

4. According to MIND, how many people with mental health problems are in employment?
   a. 10%
   b. 20%
   c. 30%
   d. 40%

FILL-IN-THE-BLANK QUESTIONS

Indicate what type of information is recorded for each axis of the DSM-IV.

_____ Axis I

_____ Axis II

_____ Axis III

_____ Axis IV

_____ Axis V

GROUP DISCUSSION TOPICS

1. Discuss why the definition of mental health and mental illness is controversial.

2. Examine recent trends in mental health care in the UK.

3. Explore three different concerns nursing students might have as they begin mental health nursing clinical experiences.

Psychosocial Theories and Therapeutic Approaches

Key Terms

- alternative medicine
- behaviour modification
- behaviourism
- client-centred therapy
- closed group
- cognitive and cognitive-behavioural therapies
- complementary medicine
- counselling
- countertransference
- crisis
- crisis intervention
- dialectical behaviour therapy
- dream analysis
- education group
- ego
- ego defence mechanisms
- family therapy
- free association
- group therapy
- hierarchy of needs
- humanism
- id
- individual psychotherapy
- integrative medicine
- milieu therapy
- mindfulness
- negative reinforcement

Learning Objectives

After reading this chapter, you should be able to:

1. Explain the basic beliefs and approaches of the following psychosocial theories: psychoanalytic, developmental, interpersonal, humanistic, behavioural and crisis intervention.

2. Describe the following psychosocial treatment modalities: individual psychotherapy, group psychotherapy, family therapy, behaviour modification, systematic desensitization, token economy, self-help groups, support groups, educational groups, cognitive-behavioural therapies, solution-focused therapies, milieu therapy and psychiatric rehabilitation and recovery.

3. Identify the psychosocial theory on which each treatment strategy is based.

4. Identify how several of the theoretical perspectives have influenced current nursing practice.

- open group
- operant conditioning
- parataxic mode
- participant observer
- positive reinforcement
- prototaxic mode
- psychiatric rehabilitation
- psychoanalysis
- psychosocial interventions
- psychotherapy
- psychotherapy group
- recovery
- self-actualization
- self-help group
- solution-focused
- subconscious
- superego
- support group
- syntaxic mode
- systematic desensitization
- therapeutic community or milieu
- therapeutic nurse–patient relationship
- Tidal Model
- transference

Today's mental health nursing has an eclectic approach, one that incorporates concepts and strategies from a variety of sources. This chapter presents an overview of major psychosocial theories, highlights the ideas and concepts in current practice and explains the various psychosocial treatment modalities. Psychosocial theories have generated many models currently used in individual and group therapy and various treatment settings. The 'medical model' of treatment is based on the neurobiological theories discussed in Chapter 3, though contemporary psychiatric practice usually incorporates psychosocial ideas and practices, just as many psychosocial approaches will embrace the careful, collaborative use of medication.

PSYCHOSOCIAL THEORIES AND PRACTICE

Many theories attempt to explain human behaviour, health and mental health problems. Each theory suggests how 'normal' development occurs, based on the theorist's beliefs, assumptions and view of the world. These theories suggest strategies that the clinician can use to work with clients. Many theories discussed in this chapter were not based on empirical or research evidence; rather, they evolved from individual experiences and might more appropriately be called conceptual models or frameworks. Which theory is most widespread in a particular area at a particular time is dependent on a variety of factors: economic, social and political. Theories are intimately connected to power, particularly the power of certain occupational groups or disciplines to have their view of the world accepted. The student is encouraged to maintain a curious scepticism towards these theories and to consider carefully the evidence for them.

This chapter discusses the following types of psychosocial theories:

A. Psychoanalytic
B. Developmental
C. Interpersonal
D. Behavioural
E. Humanistic
F. Cognitive-behavioural.

A. Psychoanalytic Theories

SIGMUND FREUD: THE FATHER OF PSYCHOANALYSIS

Sigmund Freud (1856–1939; Figure 2.1) developed psychoanalytic theory in the late 19th and early 20th centuries in Vienna, where he spent most of his life. Several other noted psychoanalysts and theorists have contributed to this body of knowledge, but Freud is its undisputed founder. Many clinicians and theorists did not agree with much of Freud's psychoanalytic theory and later developed their own theories and styles of treatment.

Psychoanalytic theory supports the notion that all human behaviour is caused and can be explained (it is, in essence, a

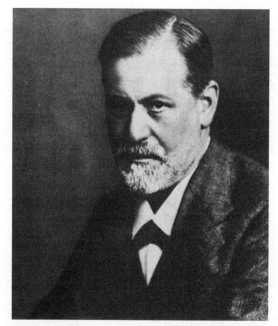

Figure 2.1. Sigmund Freud: the father of psychoanalysis.

'deterministic' theory). Freud believed that *repressed* (driven from conscious awareness) sexual impulses and desires motivate much human behaviour. He developed his initial ideas and explanations of human behaviour from his experiences with a few clients, all of them women who displayed unusual behaviours such as disturbances of sight and speech, inability to eat, and paralysis of limbs. These symptoms had no physiological basis, so Freud considered them to be the 'hysterical' or neurotic behaviour of women. After several years of working with these women, Freud concluded that many of their problems resulted from childhood trauma or failure to complete tasks of psychosexual development. These women repressed their unmet needs and sexual feelings as well as traumatic events. The 'hysterical' or neurotic behaviours resulted from these unresolved conflicts.

Personality Components: Id, Ego and Superego. Freud conceptualized personality structure as having three components: id, ego, and superego (Freud, 1923/1962). The **id** is the part of one's nature that reflects basic or innate desires, such as pleasure-seeking behaviour aggression and sexual impulses. The id seeks instant gratification, causes impulsive, unthinking behaviour and has no regard for rules or social convention. The **superego** is the part of a person's nature that reflects moral and ethical concepts, values and parental and social expectations; therefore, it is in direct opposition to the id. The third component, the **ego,** is the balancing or mediating force between the id and the superego. The ego represents mature and adaptive behaviour that allows a person to function successfully in the world. Freud believed that anxiety resulted from the ego's attempts to balance the impulsive instincts of the id with the stringent rules of the superego. The accompanying drawing demonstrates the relationship of these personality structures.

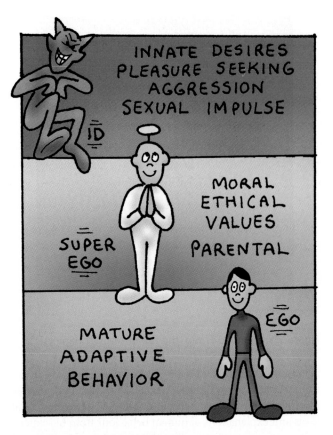

Freud's components of personality

Behaviour Motivated by Subconscious Thoughts and Feelings. Freud believed that the human personality functions at three levels of awareness: conscious, preconscious and unconscious (Freud, 1923/1962). *Conscious* refers to the perceptions, thoughts and emotions that exist in the person's awareness, such as being aware of happy feelings or thinking about a loved one. *Preconscious* thoughts and emotions are not currently in the person's awareness, but he or she can recall them with some effort – for example, an adult remembering what he or she did, thought or felt as a child. The *unconscious* is the realm of thoughts and feelings that motivate a person even though he or she is totally unaware of them. This realm includes most defence mechanisms (see discussion to follow) and some instinctual drives or motivations. According to Freud's theories, the person represses into the unconscious the memory of traumatic events that are too painful to remember.

Freud believed that much of what we do and say is motivated by our **subconscious** thoughts or feelings (those in the preconscious or unconscious level of awareness). A 'Freudian slip' is a term we commonly use to describe slips of the tongue – for example, saying 'You look portly today' to an overweight friend instead of 'You look pretty today'. Freud believed that these slips are not accidents or coincidences but rather are indications of subconscious feelings or thoughts that accidentally emerge in casual day-to-day conversation.

Freud's Dream Analysis. Freud believed that a person's dreams reflect his or her subconscious and have significant meaning, although sometimes the meaning is hidden or symbolic (Loden, 2002). **Dream analysis**, a primary method used in **psychoanalysis**, involves discussing a client's dreams to discover their true meaning and significance. For example, a client might report having recurrent frightening dreams about snakes chasing her. Freud's interpretation might be that the woman fears intimacy with men; he would view the snake as a phallic symbol, representing the penis.

Another method used to gain access to subconscious thoughts and feelings is **free association**, in which the therapist tries to uncover the client's true thoughts and feelings by saying a word and asking the client to respond quickly with the first thing that comes to mind. Freud believed that such quick responses would be likely to uncover subconscious or repressed thoughts or feelings

Ego Defence Mechanisms. Freud believed the self, or ego, uses **ego defence mechanisms**, which are methods of attempting to protect the self and cope with basic drives or emotionally painful thoughts, feelings or events. Defence mechanisms are explained in Table 2.1. For example, a person who has been diagnosed with cancer and told he has 6 months to live but refuses to talk about his illness is using the defence mechanism of denial, or refusal to accept the reality of the situation. If a person dying of cancer exhibits continuously cheerful behaviour, he could be using the defence mechanism of reaction formation to protect his emotions. Most defence mechanisms operate at the unconscious level of awareness, so people are not aware of what they are doing and often need help to see the reality.

Five Stages of Psychosexual Development. Freud based his theory of childhood development on the belief that sexual energy, termed *libido,* was the driving force of human behaviour. He proposed that children progress through five stages of psychosexual development: oral (birth to 18 months), anal (18 to 36 months), phallic/oedipal (3 to 5 years), latency (5 to 11 or 13 years) and genital (11 to 13 years). Table 2.2 describes these stages and the accompanying developmental tasks. Psychopathology results when a person has difficulty making the transition from one stage to the next, or when a person remains stalled at a particular stage or regresses to an earlier stage. Freud's open discussion of sexual impulses, particularly in children, was considered shocking for his time (Freud, 1923/1962).

Transference and Countertransference. Freud developed the concepts of transference and countertransference. **Transference** occurs when the client displaces on to the therapist attitudes and feelings that the client originally experienced in other relationships (Freud, 1923/1962). Transference patterns are automatic and unconscious in the therapeutic relationship. For example, an adolescent female client working with a nurse who is about the same age as the teen's parents might react to the nurse like she reacts to her parents. She might experience intense feelings of rebellion or make sarcastic remarks; these reactions are actually based on her experiences with her parents, not the nurse.

Table 2.1 EGO DEFENCE MECHANISMS (AFTER FREUD)

Compensation	Overachievement in one area to offset real or perceived deficiencies in another area • Napoleon complex: diminutive man becoming emperor • Nurse with low self-esteem works double shifts so her ward manager will like her
Conversion	Expression of an emotional conflict through the development of a physical symptom, usually sensorimotor in nature • Teenager forbidden to see X-rated movies is tempted to do so by friends and develops blindness, and he is unconcerned about the loss of sight
Denial	Failure to acknowledge an unbearable condition; failure to admit the reality of a situation or how one enables the problem to continue • Diabetic person eating a lot of chocolate • Spending money freely when broke • Waiting 3 days to seek help for severe abdominal pain
Displacement	Ventilation of intense feelings toward people less threatening than the one who aroused those feelings • Person who is angry at his boss yells at his wife • Child who is harassed by a bully at school mistreats a younger sibling
Dissociation	Dealing with emotional conflict by a temporary alteration in consciousness or identity • Amnesia that prevents recall of yesterday's car accident • Adult remembers nothing of childhood sexual abuse
Fixation	Immobilization of a portion of the personality resulting from unsuccessful completion of tasks in a developmental stage • Never learning to delay gratification • Lack of a clear sense of identity as an adult
Identification	Modelling actions and opinions of influential others while searching for identity, or aspiring to reach a personal, social or occupational goal • Nursing student becoming a CPN because this is the speciality of a mentor she admires
Intellectualization	Separation of the emotions of a painful event or situation from the facts involved; acknowledging the facts but not the emotions • Person shows no emotional expression when discussing a serious car accident
Introjection	Accepting another person's attitudes, beliefs and values as one's own • Person who dislikes guns becomes an avid hunter, just like a best friend
Projection	Unconscious blaming of unacceptable inclinations or thoughts on an external object • Man who has thought about same-gender sexual relationship, but never had one, assaults a man who is gay • Person with many prejudices loudly identifies others as bigots
Rationalization	Excusing own behaviour to avoid guilt, responsibility, conflict, anxiety or loss of self-respect • Student blames failure on teacher being mean • Man says he beats his wife because she doesn't listen to him
Reaction formation	Acting the opposite of what one thinks or feels • Woman who never wanted to have children becomes a super-mum • Person who despises the boss tells everyone what a great boss he or she is
Regression	Moving back to a previous developmental stage to feel safe or have needs met • Five-year-old asks for a bottle when new baby brother is being fed • Man pouts like a 4-year-old if he is not the centre of his girlfriend's attention
Repression	Excluding emotionally painful or anxiety-provoking thoughts and feelings from conscious awareness • Woman has no memory of the mugging she suffered yesterday • Woman has no memory before age 7, when she was removed from abusive parents
Resistance	Overt or covert antagonism toward remembering or processing anxiety-producing information • Nurse is too busy with tasks to spend time talking to a dying patient • Person attends court-ordered treatment for alcoholism but refuses to participate
Sublimation	Substituting a socially acceptable activity for an impulse that is unacceptable • Person who has quit smoking sucks on boiled sweets when the urge to smoke arises • Person goes for a 15-minute walk when tempted to eat junk food
Substitution	Replacing the desired gratification with one that is more readily available • Woman who would like to have her own children opens a day care centre
Suppression	Conscious exclusion of unacceptable thoughts and feelings from conscious awareness • Student decides not to think about a parent's illness to study for a test • Woman tells a friend she cannot think about her son's death right now
Undoing	Exhibiting acceptable behaviour to make up for or negate unacceptable behaviour • Person who cheats on a spouse brings the spouse a bouquet of roses • Man who is ruthless in business donates large amounts of money to charity

Table 2.2	FREUD'S DEVELOPMENTAL STAGES	

Phase	Age	Focus
Oral	Birth to 18 months	Major site of tension and gratification is the mouth, lips and tongue; includes biting and sucking activities Id present at birth Ego develops gradually from rudimentary structure present at birth
Anal	18–36 months	Anus and surrounding area are major source of interest. Acquisition of voluntary sphincter control (toilet training)
Phallic/oedipal	3–5 years	Genital focus of interest, stimulation and excitement Penis is organ of interest for both sexes Masturbation is common Penis envy (wish to possess penis) seen in girls; oedipal complex (wish to marry opposite-sex parent and be rid of same-sex parent) seen in boys and girls
Latency	5–11 or 13 years	Resolution of oedipal complex Sexual drive channelled into socially appropriate activities such as school work and sports Formation of the superego Final stage of psychosexual development
Genital	11–13 years	Begins with puberty and the biological capacity for orgasm; involves the capacity for true intimacy

Adapted from Freud, S. (1962). The ego and the id (*The standard edition of the complete psychological works of Sigmund Freud;* J. Strachey, Trans.). New York: W. W. Norton & Company.

Countertransference occurs when the therapist displaces on to the client attitudes or feelings from his or her past. For example, a female nurse who has teenage children and who is experiencing extreme frustration with an adolescent client may respond by adopting a parental or chastising tone. The nurse is countertransferring her own attitudes and feelings toward her children on to the client. Nurses can deal with countertransference by examining their own feelings and responses, using self-awareness and talking with colleagues.

CURRENT PSYCHOANALYTIC PRACTICE

Psychoanalysis focuses on discovering the causes of the client's unconscious and repressed thoughts, feelings and conflicts believed to cause anxiety, and on helping the client to gain insight into and resolve these conflicts and anxieties. The analytic therapist uses the techniques of free association, dream analysis and interpretation of behaviour.

'Pure' psychoanalysis is still practised today but on a very limited basis. Analysis is lengthy, with weekly or more frequent sessions for several years. It is costly and not covered by conventional health insurance programmes; thus, it has become known as 'therapy for the wealthy'. However, many practitioners, including many nurses, use psychodynamic psychotherapy, based to a greater or lesser extent on Freud's ideas; and many other therapeutic approaches, and many cultural ideas and practices – including the media, business and arts, have been profoundly influenced by Freud.

B. Developmental Theories

ERIK ERIKSON AND PSYCHOSOCIAL STAGES OF DEVELOPMENT

Erik Erikson (1902–1994) was a German-born psychoanalyst who extended Freud's work on personality development across the life span while focusing on social and psychological development in the life stages. In 1950, Erikson published *Childhood and society,* in which he described eight psychosocial stages of development. In each stage, the person must complete a life task that is essential to his or her well-being and mental health. These tasks allow the person to achieve life's virtues: hope, purpose, fidelity, love, caring and wisdom. The stages, life tasks and virtues are described in Table 2.3.

Erikson's eight psychosocial stages of development are still used in a variety of disciplines. In his view, psychosocial growth occurs in sequential phases, and each stage is dependent on completion of the previous stage and life task. For example, in the infant stage (birth to 18 months), trust versus mistrust, the infant must learn to develop basic trust (the positive outcome), such as that he or she will be fed and taken care of. The formation of trust is essential: mistrust, the negative outcome of this stage, will impair the person's development throughout his or her life.

JEAN PIAGET AND COGNITIVE STAGES OF DEVELOPMENT

Jean Piaget (1896–1980) explored how intelligence and cognitive functioning develop in children. He believed that human intelligence progresses through a series of stages

Table 2.3	ERIKSON'S STAGES OF PSYCHOSOCIAL DEVELOPMENT	
Stage	**Virtue**	**Task**
Trust vs. mistrust (infant)	Hope	Viewing the world as safe and reliable; relationships as nurturing, stable and dependable
Autonomy vs. shame and doubt (toddler)	Will	Achieving a sense of control and free will
Initiative vs. guilt (preschool)	Purpose	Beginning development of a conscience; learning to manage conflict and anxiety
Industry vs. inferiority (school age)	Competence	Emerging confidence in own abilities; taking pleasure in accomplishments
Identity vs. role confusion (adolescence)	Fidelity	Formulating a sense of self and belonging
Intimacy vs. isolation (young adult)	Love	Forming adult, loving relationships and meaningful attachments to others
Generativity vs. stagnation (middle adult)	Care	Being creative and productive; establishing the next generation
Ego integrity vs. despair (maturity)	Wisdom	Accepting responsibility for one's self and life

based on age, with the child at each successive stage demonstrating a higher level of functioning than at previous stages. In his schema, Piaget strongly believed that biological changes and maturation were responsible for cognitive development.

Piaget's four stages of cognitive development are as follows:

1. Sensorimotor – birth to 2 years. The child develops a sense of self as separate from the environment and the concept of object permanence; that is, tangible objects do not cease to exist just because they are out of sight. He or she begins to form mental images.
2. Preoperational – 2 to 6 years. The child develops the ability to express self with language, understands the meaning of symbolic gestures, and begins to classify objects.
3. Concrete operations – 6 to 12 years. The child begins to apply logic to thinking, understands spatiality and reversibility, and is increasingly social and able to apply rules; however, thinking is still concrete.
4. Formal operations – 2 to 15 years and beyond. The child learns to think and reason in abstract terms, further develops logical thinking and reasoning, and achieves cognitive maturity.

Piaget's theory suggests that individuals reach cognitive maturity by middle to late adolescence. Some critics of Piaget believe that cognitive development is less rigid and more individualized than his theory suggests. Piaget's theory is useful when working with children. The nurse may better understand what the child means if the nurse is aware of his or her level of cognitive development. Also, teaching, for children, is often structured with their cognitive development in mind.

C. Interpersonal Theories

HARRY STACK SULLIVAN: INTERPERSONAL RELATIONSHIPS AND MILIEU THERAPY

Harry Stack Sullivan (1892–1949) was an American psychiatrist who extended the theory of personality development to include the significance of interpersonal relationships. Sullivan believed that one's personality involves more than individual characteristics, particularly how one interacts with others. He thought that inadequate or non-satisfying relationships produce anxiety, which he saw as the basis for all emotional problems (Sullivan, 1953). The importance and significance of interpersonal relationships in one's life is probably Sullivan's greatest contribution to the field of mental health.

Five Life Stages. Sullivan established five life stages of development – infancy, childhood, juvenile, pre-adolescence and adolescence, each focusing on various interpersonal relationships (Table 2.4). Sullivan also described three developmental cognitive modes of experience and believed that mental disorders are related to the persistence of one of the early modes. The **prototaxic mode**, characteristic of infancy and childhood, involves brief, unconnected experiences that have no relationship to one another. Adults with schizophrenia exhibit persistent prototaxic experiences. The **parataxic mode** begins in early childhood as the child begins to connect experiences in sequence. The child may not make logical sense of the experiences and may see them as coincidence or chance events. The child seeks to relieve anxiety by repeating familiar experiences, although he or she may not understand what he or she is doing. Sullivan explained paranoid ideas and slips of the tongue as a person operating in the parataxic mode. In the **syntaxic mode**, which begins to appear in school-aged children and

Table 2.4	SULLIVAN'S LIFE STAGES	

Stage	Ages	Focus
Infancy	Birth to onset of language	Primary need for bodily contact and tenderness Prototaxic mode dominates (no relation between experiences) Primary zones are oral and anal If needs are met, infant has sense of well-being; unmet needs lead to dread and anxiety
Childhood	Language to 5 years	Parents viewed as source of praise and acceptance Shift to parataxic mode (experiences are connected in sequence to each other) Primary zone is anal Gratification leads to positive self-esteem Moderate anxiety leads to uncertainty and insecurity; severe anxiety results in self-defeating patterns of behaviour
Juvenile	5–8 years	Shift to the syntaxic mode begins (thinking about self and others based on analysis of experiences in a variety of situations) Opportunities for approval and acceptance of others Learn to negotiate own needs Severe anxiety may result in a need to control or in restrictive, prejudicial attitudes
Preadolescence	8–12 years	Move to genuine intimacy with friend of the same sex Move away from family as source of satisfaction in relationships Major shift to syntaxic mode Capacity for attachment, love and collaboration emerges or fails to develop
Adolescence	Puberty to adulthood	Lust is added to interpersonal equation Need for special sharing relationship shifts to the opposite sex New opportunities for social experimentation lead to the consolidation of self-esteem or self-ridicule If the self-system is intact, areas of concern expand to include values, ideals, career decisions and social concerns

Adapted from Sullivan, H. S. (1953). *The interpersonal theory of psychiatry.* New York: W. W. Norton & Company.

becomes more predominant in pre-adolescence, the person begins to perceive him or herself and the world within the context of the environment and can analyse experiences in a variety of settings. Maturity may be defined as predominance of the syntaxic mode (Sullivan, 1953).

Therapeutic Community or Milieu. Sullivan envisioned the goal of treatment as the establishment of satisfying interpersonal relationships. The therapist provides a corrective interpersonal relationship for the client. Sullivan coined the term **participant observer** for the therapist's role, meaning that the therapist both participates in and observes the progress of the relationship.

Sullivan is also credited with developing the first **therapeutic community or milieu** with young men with schizophrenia in 1929 (although the term *therapeutic community* was not used extensively until Maxwell Jones published *The therapeutic community* in 1953). In the concept of therapeutic community or milieu, the interaction among clients is seen as beneficial in itself, and treatment emphasizes the role of this client-to-client interaction. Until this time, it was believed that the interaction between the client and the psychiatrist was the one essential component to the

client's treatment. Sullivan, and later Jones, observed that interactions among clients in a safe, therapeutic setting provided great benefits to clients. The concept of **milieu therapy**, originally developed by Sullivan, involved clients' interactions with one another, including practising interpersonal relationship skills, giving one another feedback about behaviour and working co-operatively as a group to solve day-to-day problems.

Milieu therapy was one of the primary modes of treatment in the acute hospital setting. In today's health-care environment, however, inpatient hospital stays are often too short for clients to develop meaningful relationships with one another. The concept of milieu therapy receives little attention as such, although management of the milieu, or environment, is still a primary role for the nurse in terms of providing safety and protection for all clients and promoting social interaction. Following the generally acknowledged failure of much inpatient care in the UK, practice approaches such as the Star Wards Project (2006; 2008) have begun to re-emphasize this vital part of the nursing role and the value of environments that are themselves therapeutic.

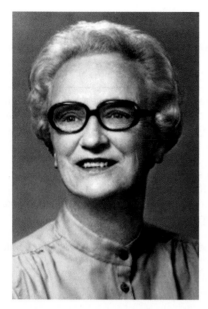

Figure 2.2. Hildegard Peplau, who developed the phases of the nurse–client therapeutic relationship, which has made great contributions to the foundation of nursing practice today.

HILDEGARD PEPLAU: THERAPEUTIC NURSE–PATIENT RELATIONSHIP

Hildegard Peplau (1909–1999; Figure 2.2) was a nursing theorist and clinician who built on Sullivan's interpersonal theories and also saw the role of the nurse as a participant observer. Peplau developed the concept of the **therapeutic nurse–patient relationship**, which includes four phases: orientation, identification, exploitation and resolution (Table 2.5).

During these phases, the client accomplishes certain tasks and makes relationship changes that help the healing process (Peplau, 1952).

1. The *orientation phase* is directed by the nurse and involves engaging the client in treatment, providing explanations and information and answering questions.
2. The *identification phase* begins when the client works interdependently with the nurse, expresses feelings and begins to feel stronger.
3. In the *exploitation phase,* the client makes full use of the services offered.
4. In the *resolution phase,* the client no longer needs professional services and gives up dependent behaviour. The relationship ends.

Peplau's concept of the nurse–client relationship, with tasks and behaviours characteristic of each stage, has been modified but remains in use today (in particular in its influence on the Tidal Model) (see Chapter 5).

Roles of the Nurse in the Therapeutic Relationship. Peplau also wrote about the roles of the nurse in the therapeutic relationship and how these roles help meet the client's needs. The primary roles she identified are as follows:

- *Stranger*: offering the client the same acceptance and courtesy that the nurse would to any stranger
- *Resource person*: providing specific answers to questions within a larger context
- *Teacher*: helping the client to learn formally or informally
- *Leader*: offering direction to the client or group
- *Surrogate*: serving as a substitute for another, such as a parent or sibling
- *Counsellor*: promoting experiences leading to health for the client, such as expression of feelings.

Table 2.5   PEPLAU'S STAGES AND TASKS OF RELATIONSHIPS

Stage	Tasks
Orientation	Clarification of patient's problems and needs
	Patient asks questions
	Explanation of hospital routines and expectations
	Patient harnesses energy toward meeting problems
	Patient's full participation is elicited
Identification	Patient responds to persons he or she perceives as helpful
	Patient feels stronger
	Expression of feelings
	Interdependent work with the nurse
	Clarification of roles of both patient and nurse
Exploitation	Patient makes full use of available services
	Goals such as going home and returning to work emerge
	Patient's behaviours fluctuate between dependence and independence
Resolution	Patient gives up dependent behaviour
	Services are no longer needed by patient
	Patient assumes power to meet own needs, set new goals and so forth

Adapted from Peplau, H. (1952). *Interpersonal relations in nursing.* New York: G. P. Putnam's Sons.

Table 2.6 ANXIETY LEVELS

Mild	Moderate	Severe	Panic
Sharpened senses	Selectively attentive	Perceptual field reduced to one detail or scattered details	Perceptual field reduced to focus on self
Increased motivation	Perceptual field limited to the immediate task	Cannot complete tasks	Cannot process environmental stimuli
Alert	Can be redirected	Cannot solve problems or learn effectively	Distorted perceptions
Enlarged perceptual field	Cannot connect thoughts or events independently	Behaviour geared toward anxiety relief and is usually ineffective	Loss of rational thought
Can solve problems	Muscle tension	Feels awe, dread, horror	Personality disorganization
Learning is effective	Diaphoresis	Doesn't respond to redirection	Doesn't recognize danger
Restless	Pounding pulse	Severe headache	Possibly suicidal
Gastrointestinal 'butterflies'	Headache	Nausea, vomiting, diarrhoea	Delusions or hallucination possible
Sleepless, irritable	Dry mouth	Trembling	Can't communicate verbally
Hypersensitive to noise	Higher voice pitch	Rigid stance	Either cannot sit (may bolt and run) or is totally mute and immobile
	Increased rate of speech	Vertigo	
	Gastrointestinal upset	Pale	
	Frequent urination	Tachycardia	
	Increased automatisms (nervous mannerisms)	Chest pain	
		Crying	
		Ritualistic (purposeless, repetitive) behaviour	

Adapted from Peplau, H. (1952). *Interpersonal relations in nursing.* New York: G. P. Putnam's Sons.

Peplau also believed that the nurse could take on many other roles, including consultant, tutor, safety agent, mediator, administrator, observer and researcher. These were not defined in detail but were 'left to the intelligence and imagination of the readers' (Peplau, 1952, p. 70).

Four Levels of Anxiety. Peplau defined anxiety as the initial response to a psychological threat. She described four levels of anxiety: mild, moderate, severe and panic (Table 2.6). These serve as the foundation for working with clients with anxiety in a variety of contexts (see Chapter 13).

1. *Mild anxiety* is a positive state of heightened awareness and sharpened senses, allowing the person to learn new behaviours and solve problems. The person can take in all available stimuli (perceptual field).
2. *Moderate anxiety* involves a decreased perceptual field (focus on immediate task only); the person can learn new behaviour or solve problems only with assistance. Another person can redirect the person to the task.
3. *Severe anxiety* involves feelings of dread or terror. The person cannot be redirected to a task; he or she focuses only on scattered details and has physiological symptoms of tachycardia, diaphoresis and chest pain. A person with severe anxiety may go to an emergency department, believing he or she is having a heart attack.
4. *Panic anxiety* can involve loss of rational thought, delusions, hallucinations and complete physical immobility and muteness. The person may bolt and run aimlessly, often exposing himself or herself to injury.

THE TIDAL MODEL

In the UK, Ireland, Australia, New Zealand and Japan especially, Peplau's ideas have been further developed and refined by Phil Barker and Poppy Buchanan-Barker in the 'Tidal Model'– a highly successful and influential approach to mental health nursing that has drawn even more heavily than Peplau on humanistic- and solution-focused ideas (Barker & Buchanan-Barker, 2005). The **Tidal Model** developed from nursing research that addressed what people perceived as their 'need for psychiatric nursing'. Its values are outlined in Box 2.1.

SYSTEMIC AND FAMILY THEORIES

Systemic therapies focus on the individual as part of a system. **Family therapy**, one form of systemic therapy, is a type of **group therapy** in which the client and his or her family members (or significant others) participate. Different cultures and different groups of individuals, of course, have very different notions of what 'family' means. The Association For Family Therapy takes 'family' to mean 'any group of people who define themselves as such, who care about and care for each other'. Developed from the work of Bateson, Minuchin, the Milan School and De Shazer, goals include understanding how family dynamics contribute to the client's psychopathology, mobilizing the family's inherent strengths and functional resources, restructuring maladaptive family behavioural styles and strengthening family problem-solving behaviours (Sadock & Sadock, 2004). Family therapy can be used both to assess and to

Box 2.1 THE TIDAL MODEL 'TEN COMMITMENTS'

The nurse needs to:

1. Value The Voice
2. Respect The Language
3. Develop Genuine Curiosity
4. Become The Apprentice
5. Reveal Personal Wisdom
6. Be Transparent
7. Use The Available Toolkit
8. Craft The Step Beyond
9. Give The Gift Of Time
10. Know That Change Is Constant

Reproduced with permission from *http://www.tidal-model.com/Ten%20 Commitments.htm*

treat various psychiatric disorders. Although one family member usually has been identified initially as the one who has problems and needs help, it often becomes evident through the therapeutic process that other family members also have emotional problems and difficulties and, indeed, that the problem often lies within the system – *between* people – rather than *within* individuals.

ERIC BERNE: TRANSACTIONAL ANALYSIS

Eric Berne (who, like many other founders of 'post-Freudian' therapies was psychoanalytically trained) developed Transactional Analysis in the late 1950s, and some of its key principles remain highly relevant – and much valued in nursing – today. He shifted the focus of psychoanalysis from individual dynamics to the dynamics between people, brought into psychotherapy the practice of using contracts and posited the existence of three 'ego states' – the 'Parent', the 'Adult' and the 'Child' – which affected and shaped people's 'transactions'. It is an often-used criticism of nurses that they adopt a 'parent–child' approach to their clients way beyond when this might be beneficial (for example, in the early hours of an admission) and that we should strive, always, to develop 'adult–adult' relationships with our clients and our colleagues.

D. Behavioural Theories

Behaviourism grew out of a reaction to introspective models that focused on the contents and operations of the mind. Behaviourism is a school of psychology that focuses on observable behaviours and what one can do externally to bring about behaviour changes. It does not attempt to explain how the mind works.

Behaviourists believe that behaviour can be changed through a system of rewards and punishments. For adults, receiving a regular payslip at the end of the month is a constant positive reinforcer that motivates people to continue to go to work every day and to try to do a good job. It helps motivate positive behaviour in the workplace. If someone stops receiving a payslip, he or she is most likely to stop working.

If a motorist consistently speeds (negative behaviour) and does not get caught, he or she is likely to continue to speed. If the driver receives a speeding ticket (a negative reinforcer), he or she is likely to slow down. However, if the motorist does not get caught for speeding for the next 4 weeks (negative reinforcer is removed), he or she is likely to resume speeding.

IVAN PAVLOV: CLASSICAL CONDITIONING

Laboratory experiments with dogs provided the basis for the development of Ivan Pavlov's theory of classical conditioning: behaviour can be changed through conditioning with external or environmental conditions or stimuli. His experiment with dogs involved his observation that dogs naturally began to salivate (response) when they saw or smelled food (stimulus). Pavlov (1849–1936) set out to change this salivating response or behaviour through conditioning. He would ring a bell (new stimulus), then produce the food, and the dogs would salivate (the desired response). Pavlov repeated this ringing of the bell along with the presentation of food many times. Eventually he could ring the bell and the dogs would salivate without seeing or smelling food. The dogs had been 'conditioned', or had learned a new response – to salivate when they heard the bell. Their behaviour had been modified through classical conditioning, or a conditioned response.

B. F. SKINNER: OPERANT CONDITIONING

One of the most influential behaviourists was B. F. Skinner (1904–1990), an American psychologist. He developed the theory of **operant conditioning**, which says people learn their behaviour from their history or past experiences, particularly those experiences that were repeatedly reinforced. Although some criticize his theories for not considering the role that thoughts, feelings or needs play in motivating behaviour, his work has provided several important principles still used today. Skinner did not deny the existence of feelings and needs in motivation; however, he viewed behaviour as only that which could be observed, studied and learned or unlearned. He maintained that if the behaviour could be changed, then so, too, could the accompanying thoughts or feelings. Changing the behaviour was what was important.

The following principles of operant conditioning described by Skinner (1974) form the basis for behaviour techniques in use today:

1. All behaviour is learned.
2. Consequences result from behaviour – broadly speaking, reward and punishment.

3. Behaviour that is rewarded with reinforcers tends to recur.
4. Positive reinforcers that follow a behaviour increase the likelihood that the behaviour will recur.
5. Negative reinforcers that are removed after a behaviour increase the likelihood that the behaviour will recur.
6. Continuous reinforcement (a reward every time the behaviour occurs) is the fastest way to increase that behaviour, but the behaviour will not last long after the reward ceases.
7. Random intermittent reinforcement (an occasional reward for the desired behaviour) is slower to produce an increase in behaviour, but the behaviour continues after the reward ceases.

These behavioural principles of rewarding or reinforcing behaviours are used to help people change their behaviours, in a therapy known as behaviour modification. **Behaviour modification** is a method of attempting to strengthen a desired behaviour or response by reinforcement, either positive or negative. For example, if the desired behaviour is assertiveness, whenever the client uses assertiveness skills in a communication group, the group leader provides **positive reinforcement** by giving the client attention and positive feedback. **Negative reinforcement** involves removing a stimulus immediately after a behaviour occurs so that the behaviour is more likely to occur again. For example, if a client becomes anxious when waiting to talk in a group, he or she may volunteer to speak first to avoid the anxiety.

In a residential setting, operant principles would, in the past, often come into play in a 'token economy', a way to involve residents in performing activities of daily living. A chart of desired behaviours, such as getting up on time, taking a shower and getting dressed, was kept for each resident. Each day the chart was marked when the desired behaviour occurs. At the end of the day or the week, the resident got a reward or token for each time each of the desired behaviours occurred. The resident could redeem the tokens for items such as snacks, TV time or time away from the ward. This somewhat crude – and potentially demeaning – approach seems (thankfully) to be becoming less and less popular as the principles of the far more sophisticated and empowering humanistic and cognitive-behavioural therapies and of person-centred approaches to mental heath care have taken more of a hold in the UK.

Conditioned responses, such as fears or phobias, are sometimes, though, still treated with behavioural techniques. **Systematic desensitization** can be used to help clients overcome irrational fears and anxiety associated with phobias. The client is asked to make a list of situations involving the phobic object, from the least to the most anxiety provoking. The client learns and practises relaxation techniques to decrease and manage anxiety. The client then is exposed to the least anxiety-provoking situation and uses the relaxation techniques to manage the resulting anxiety. The client is gradually exposed to more and more anxiety-provoking situations until he or she can manage the most anxiety-provoking situation.

Behavioural techniques can be used for a variety of different problems. In the treatment of anorexia nervosa, the goal is weight gain. A behavioural contract between the client and therapist or physician is initiated when treatment begins. Initially, the client has little unsupervised time and is restricted to the hospital unit. The contract may specify that if the client gains a certain amount of weight, such as 0.2 kg/day, in return he or she will get increased unsupervised time, or time off the unit, as long as the weight gain progresses. When working with children with attention deficit hyperactivity disorder, goals include task completion for homework, hygiene tasks, turn-taking when talking and so forth. The child is given a 'star' or sticker when tasks are completed. Upon reaching a specified number of stars, the child receives a reward. These techniques can be powerful and effective; they can also, though, end up being (or being seen as) punitive and abusive and reinforcing someone's problems.

E. Humanistic ('Person-centred' or 'Client-centred') Theories

Humanistic ideas represent a significant shift away from the psychoanalytic view of the individual as a neurotic, impulse-driven person with repressed psychic problems and away from the focus on and examination of the client's past experiences. **Humanism**, in psychological terms, focuses instead on a person's positive qualities, his or her capacity to change (human potential), and the promotion of self-esteem. Humanists do consider the person's past experiences, but they direct more attention toward the present and future. Behaviour is seen as both 'internal' and 'external', i.e. what can't be observed may be as important, on the whole, as what can.

ABRAHAM MASLOW: HIERARCHY OF NEEDS

Abraham Maslow (1921–1970) was an American psychologist who studied the needs or motivations of the individual. He differed from previous theorists in that he focused on the total person, not just on one facet of the person, and emphasized health instead of simply illness and problems. Maslow (1954) formulated the **hierarchy of needs**, in which he used a pyramid to arrange and illustrate the basic drives or needs that motivate people. The most basic needs – the physiological needs of food, water, sleep, shelter, sexual expression and freedom from pain – must be met first. The second level involves safety and security needs, which include protection, security and freedom from harm or threatened deprivation. The third level is love and belonging needs, which include enduring intimacy, friendship and acceptance. The fourth level involves esteem needs, which include the need for self-respect and esteem from others. The highest level is self-actualization, the need for beauty, truth and justice.

Maslow hypothesized that the basic needs at the bottom of the pyramid would dominate the person's behaviour until those needs were met, at which time the next level of needs

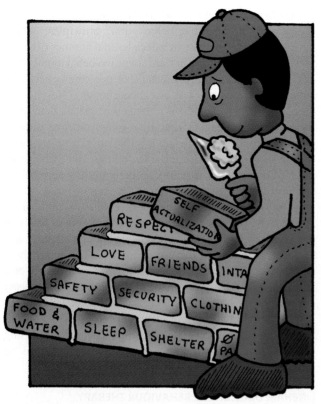

Maslow's hierarchy of needs

would become dominant. For example, if needs for food and shelter are not met, they become the overriding concern in life: the hungry person risks danger and social ostracism to find food.

Maslow used the term **self-actualization** to describe a person who has achieved all the needs of the hierarchy and has developed his or her fullest potential in life. Few people ever become fully self-actualized.

Maslow's theory explains individual differences in terms of a person's motivation, which is not necessarily stable throughout life. Traumatic life circumstances or compromised health can cause a person to regress to a lower level of motivation. For example, if a 35-year-old woman who is functioning at the 'love and belonging' level discovers she has cancer, she may regress to the 'safety' level to undergo treatment for the cancer and preserve her own health. This theory helps nurses understand how clients' motivations and behaviours change during life crises (see Chapter 7).

CARL ROGERS: CLIENT-CENTRED THERAPY

Carl Rogers (1902–1987) was a humanistic American psychologist who focused on the therapeutic relationship and developed a new method of client-centred therapy. He remains a crucial figure in mental health nursing and his ideas are an integral part of both education and practice in the field. Rogers was one of the first to use the term *client* rather than *patient*. **Client-centred therapy** focuses on the role of the client, rather than the therapist, as the key to the

healing process. Rogers believed that each person experiences the world differently and knows his or her own experience best (Rogers, 1961). According to Rogers, clients do 'the work of healing', and within a supportive and nurturing client–therapist relationship, clients can cure themselves. Clients are in the best position to know their own experiences and make sense of them, to regain their self-esteem, and to progress toward self-actualization.

The therapist takes a person-centred approach, a supportive role, rather than a directive or expert role, because Rogers viewed the client as the expert on his or her life. The therapist must promote the client's self-esteem as much as possible through three central concepts:

- *Unconditional positive regard* – a non-judgemental caring for the client that is not dependent on the client's behaviour
- *Genuineness* – realness or congruence between what the therapist feels and what he or she says to the client
- *Empathetic understanding* – in which the therapist senses the feelings and personal meaning from the client and communicates this understanding to the client

Unconditional positive regard promotes the client's self-esteem and decreases his or her need for defensive behaviour. As the client's self-acceptance grows, the natural self-actualization process can continue.

Rogers also believed that the basic nature of humans is to become self-actualized, or to move toward self-improvement and constructive change. We are all born with a positive self-regard and a natural inclination to become self-actualized. If relationships with others are supportive and nurturing, the person retains feelings of self-worth and progresses toward self-actualization, which is healthy. If the person encounters repeated conflicts with others or is in non-supportive relationships, he or she loses self-esteem, becomes defensive and is no longer inclined toward self-actualization; this is not healthy.

VIKTOR FRANKL: LOGOTHERAPY

Viktor Frankl based his beliefs on his observations of people in Nazi concentration camps during the Second World War. His curiosity about why some survived and others did not led him to conclude that survivors were able to find meaning in their lives even under miserable conditions. Hence, the search for meaning (*logos*) is the central theme in logotherapy. Counsellors and therapists who work with clients in spirituality and grief counselling often use the concepts that Frankl developed.

FRITZ PERLS: GESTALT THERAPY

Gestalt therapy, founded by Frederick 'Fritz' Perls, emphasizes identifying the person's feelings and thoughts in the here and now. Perls believed that self-awareness leads to self-acceptance and responsibility for one's own thoughts and feelings. Therapists often use gestalt therapy techniques to increase clients' self-awareness by having them write and read letters, keep journals and perform other activities – such as talking to empty chairs – designed to help put the past to rest and focus on the present.

DE SHAZER AND O'HANLON: SOLUTION-FOCUSED THERAPY

'Solution-focused' ideas have become increasingly influential in the UK over the past two decades as the Brief Therapy Practice in London (and others) have disseminated and adapted the work of De Shazer (De Shazer *et al.*, 2007) and O'Hanlon (1996) in the US to the NHS, Social Services and Probation Departments. It is a pragmatic approach that draws on both humanistic principles and systems theory and emphasizes the 'socially constructed' nature of problems – and their solutions. It attempts to validate current distress but forsakes what it sees as an 'archaeological' approach to problems – a desire to directly link the past and present and assume the existence of 'pathology' buried deep – and instead seeks to elicit strengths, competencies and exceptions to the problem areas in someone's life, building on those elements and moving towards a clearly defined set of behavioural, cognitive, affective and social goals.

F. Cognitive Therapies

More and more therapists and mental health professionals use **cognitive therapies**, which focus on immediate thought processing: how a person perceives or interprets his or her experience determines how he or she feels and behaves. For example, if a person interprets a situation as dangerous, he or she experiences anxiety and tries to escape. Basic emotions of sadness, elation, anxiety and anger are reactions to perceptions of loss, gain, danger and wrongdoing by others (Beck & Rush, 1995).

ALBERT ELLIS: RATIONAL-EMOTIVE BEHAVIOUR THERAPY

Albert Ellis, from the 1950s on, the founder of rational emotive therapy (later called rational-emotive behaviour therapy), identified 11 'irrational beliefs' that people use to make themselves unhappy. An example of an irrational belief is 'If I love someone, he or she must love me back just as much'. Ellis claimed that continuing to believe this patently untrue statement will make the person utterly unhappy, but he or she will blame it on the person who does not return his or her love. Ellis also believed that people have 'automatic thoughts' that cause them unhappiness in certain situations, and he used the ABC technique to help people identify these automatic thoughts: *A* is the activating stimulus or event, *C* is the excessive inappropriate response, and *B* is the blank in the person's mind that he or she must fill in by identifying the automatic thought. In the UK, Dr Windy Dryden has done a great deal to help popularize and develop Ellis's ideas (Dryden, 2001).

AARON BECK: COGNITIVE THERAPY AND 'CBT'

Aaron Beck was the second great pioneer of cognitive therapy, initially focused on people with depression, and

he has been at the forefront of the rapid and widespread acceptance of 'cognitive-behavioural' principles, which have emerged in the past two decades in a number of therapies now grouped together as 'cognitive-behavioural therapy' (CBT). Beck conceptualized that the 'core beliefs' that emerge in childhood ('I'm not good enough', 'No-one will ever love me', 'The world is a dangerous place') determine the 'automatic thoughts' that arise when someone is faced with a potentially challenging situation. These thoughts then give rise to uncomfortable feelings and behaviours that – ultimately – can reinforce the unhealthy core beliefs and lead to mental health problems.

Cognitive-behavioural therapists employ a number of approaches, but collaboration and transparency, teaching the client cognitive principles, using thought diaries and activity schedules and the use of homework all typify these approaches. They tend to be focused, time-limited and structured. Recent government guidance (and investment) is proof of the present general acceptance of CBT in the UK as helpful in all sorts of mental health problems – from depression and anxiety to psychosis. There is increasing pressure (and some training and support) for nurses to develop skills in CBT.

LINEHAN: DIALECTICAL BEHAVIOUR THERAPY

Dialectical behaviour therapy (DBT) emerged first in the UK in the 1990s, following the successful work of Marsha Linehan (1993) in the US with people diagnosed with borderline personality disorder (BPD). It has become increasingly popular as a way of helping this very challenging group of people and its principles – a combination of CBT, psychodynamic ideas and the concept of 'mindfulness' from Zen Buddhism – are accepted increasingly in mental health care.

MINDFULNESS-BASED COGNITIVE THERAPY

Increasingly, **mindfulness** – the development of here-and-now non-judgemental observation of, and full awareness of, thoughts, feelings and behaviour, married with meditative techniques – is used in combination with cognitive therapies in order to deal with distress, help people regulate their emotions and interact in a more satisfying way. The work of Jon Kabat-Zinn (2001) has been particularly influential.

STRESS-VULNERABILITY MODEL

The stress-vulnerability model of working with people with psychosis adopts a flexible, broadly cognitive-behavioural approach to reducing the likelihood of 'breakdown' in those with a physical and psychological vulnerability. It adopts a person-centred, psycho-educational approach to helping people minimize the presence and impact of environmental, physical and emotional stresses. People learn how to recognize signs of impending stress and ways to tackle it before it overwhelms their defences.

Crisis Intervention

A **crisis** is a turning point in an individual's life that produces an overwhelming emotional response. Individuals experience a crisis when they confront some life circumstance or stressor that they cannot effectively manage through use of their customary coping skills. Caplan (1964) identified the stages of crisis: (1) the person is exposed to a stressor, experiences anxiety and tries to cope in a customary fashion; (2) anxiety increases when customary coping skills are ineffective; (3) the person makes all possible efforts to deal with the stressor, including attempts at new methods of coping; and (4) when coping attempts fail, the person experiences disequilibrium and significant distress.

Crises occur in response to a variety of life situations and events and fall into three categories:

- *Maturational crises,* sometimes called *developmental crises,* are predictable events in the normal course of life, such as leaving home for the first time, getting married, having a baby and beginning a career.
- *Situational crises* are unanticipated or sudden events that threaten the individual's integrity, such as the death of a loved one, loss of a job and physical or emotional illness in the individual or family member.
- *Adventitious crises,* sometimes called social crises, include natural disasters like floods, earthquakes or hurricanes; war; terrorist attacks; riots; and violent crimes such as rape or murder.

Note that not all events that result in crisis are 'negative' in nature. Events like marriage, retirement and childbirth are often desirable for the individual but may still present overwhelming challenges. Equally, apparently traumatic events such as bereavement, redundancy or a psychotic episode may prove to be a trigger for personal growth and development. Aguilera (1998) identified three factors that influence whether or not an individual experiences a crisis: the individual's perception of the event, the availability of emotional supports and the availability of adequate coping mechanisms. When the person in crisis seeks assistance, these three factors represent a guide for effective intervention. The person can be assisted to view the event or issue from a different perspective, for example, as an opportunity for growth or change rather than as a threat. Assisting the person to use existing supports or helping the individual find new sources of support can decrease the feelings of being alone or overwhelmed. Finally, assisting the person to learn new methods of coping will help to resolve the current crisis and give him or her new coping skills to use in the future.

Crisis is described as self-limiting; that is, the crisis does not last indefinitely but usually exists for 4–6 weeks. At the end of that time, the crisis is resolved in one of three ways. In the first two, the person either returns to his or her pre-crisis level of functioning or begins to function at a higher level; both are positive outcomes for the individual. The third resolution is that the person's functioning stabilizes at a level lower than pre-crisis functioning, which is a negative outcome for the individual. Positive outcomes are more likely when the problem (crisis response and precipitating event or issue) is clearly and thoroughly defined. Likewise, early intervention is associated with better outcomes.

Persons experiencing a crisis are usually distressed and likely to seek help for their distress. They are ready to learn and even eager to try new coping skills as a way to relieve their distress. This is an ideal time for intervention that is likely to be successful. **Crisis intervention** includes a variety of techniques based on the assessment of the individual. *Directive interventions* are designed to assess the person's health status and promote problem-solving, such as offering the person new information, knowledge or meaning; raising the person's self-awareness by providing feedback about behaviour; and directing the person's behaviour by offering suggestions or courses of action. *Supportive interventions* aim at dealing with the person's needs for empathetic understanding, such as encouraging the person to identify and discuss feelings, serving as a sounding board for the person and affirming the person's self-worth. Techniques and strategies that include a balance of these different types of intervention are the most effective.

CULTURAL CONSIDERATIONS

The major psychosocial theorists were white and born in Europe or the US, as were many of the people whom they treated. What they considered normal or typical may not apply equally well to people with different racial, ethnic or cultural backgrounds. For example, Erikson's developmental stages focus on autonomy and independence for toddlers, but this focus may not be appropriate for people from other cultures in which early individual independence is not a developmental milestone. Therefore, it is important that the nurse avoids reaching faulty conclusions when working with clients and families from other cultures. Chapter 7 discusses cultural factors in depth.

TREATMENT MODALITIES

Benefits of Community Mental Health Treatment

Recent changes in culture, political ideologies and public attitudes have affected mental health treatment, as they have all areas of medicine, nursing and related health disciplines (see Chapter 4). Inpatient treatment is – or, perhaps more accurately, *should be* – the last, rather than the first, mode of treatment for mental health problems. Current 'best practice' reflects the belief that it is more beneficial and certainly more cost-effective for clients to remain in the community and receive care and treatment there whenever possible. The client can often continue to work and can stay connected to family, friends and other support systems while participating in care. Care focused in the community also takes into account that a person's personality or behaviour patterns, such as coping skills, styles of communication and level of self-esteem, gradually develop over the course of a lifetime and cannot be changed in a relatively short inpatient course of treatment. Hospital admission may still be indicated when the person is severely depressed and suicidal, severely psychotic, experiencing alcohol or drug withdrawal, or exhibiting behaviours that require close supervision in a safe, supportive environment.

Recent developments in the UK have led to the establishment of Crisis Recovery and Home Treatment teams, who span the gap between inpatient and outpatient teams and are able to offer intensive, short-term support, previously only possible in hospital, in someone's home. This section briefly describes the 'talking therapy' modalities currently used in both 'inpatient' and 'community' settings.

The terms '**psychotherapy**' and '**counselling**' are increasingly used interchangeably. The general consensus, though, is that 'psychotherapy' tends to be longer term and aimed far more on fundamental change in the way someone lives and thinks and feels, whereas counselling is considered to be more focused on the resolution of particular problems. For the purpose of this book, we will usually use the more commonly used term 'therapy' to encompass both the 'psychotherapy' and 'counselling' offered within mental health services.

Therapies offered in the NHS should – according to policy and general agreement – be increasingly based on 'evidence', although evidence for the effectiveness of particular therapies with particular mental health problems is often scarce and fiercely debated. Nurses frequently use *adaptations* of these therapies, drawing on a variety of theories and evidence to apply CBT, DBT and solution-focused principles to the 'real-world' environments they have to work in (which are rarely quiet, private, uninterrupted or time-secured in the way that those of psychotherapists or counsellors are). Nursing adaptations of therapies have a far less robust evidence-base than 'pure' therapies: CBT has an excellent evidence-base when used by therapists in contained, regular settings; when used in its inevitably adapted forms in busy inpatient units or in people's own homes, it has little concrete evidence to back it up. This said, the work of Scott Miller and Barry Duncan may be helpful here, and point to issues relevant both to therapists and to nurses. The work of Miller and others at the Institute for Therapeutic Change, based on – among other things – meta-analyses of psychotherapies, suggests that there are 'common factors' that determine the outcome of therapy, factors that are independent of the particular form of therapy being offered. They suggest that '. . . change principally results from factors common to all approaches and from the client's pre-existing abilities and participation—the client is the hero of the therapeutic drama'. These common factors are 'extra-therapeutic' or client factors (that is, what the client does or doesn't do), the therapeutic alliance/relationship, the therapist's allegiance to a model and the model or technique itself (Duncan *et al.*, 2007). 'The probability for success,' says Miller, 'is greater when the treatment offered fits with or is complementary to the *client's* theory' (Miller, 2008).

Individual Psychotherapeutic Work

Individual psychotherapeutic work is a method of bringing about change in a person by exploring his or her feelings, attitudes, thinking and behaviour. It involves a one-to-one relationship between the therapist and the client and may be based on any of the theoretical perspectives outlined earlier in this chapter, although most frequently on psychodynamic, CBT or DBT principles. Outside the NHS, people generally seek this kind of therapy based on their desire to understand themselves and their behaviour, to make personal changes, to improve interpersonal relationships or to get relief from emotional pain or unhappiness. Within the NHS, people with mental health problems may be referred for psychotherapy to address their particular issues, usually to a psychologist, a psychotherapist or a nurse therapist. The relationship between the client and the therapist proceeds through stages similar to those of the nurse–client relationship: introduction, working and termination.

The therapist–client relationship is seen as key to the success of this type of therapy, although there are different emphases depending on the type of therapy offered. The client and the therapist must be compatible for therapy to be effective. Therapists vary in their formal credentials, experience and model of practice. Selecting a therapist is extremely important in terms of successful outcomes for the client, though this is rarely an option within the NHS. The client needs, ideally, to be able to select a therapist whose theoretical beliefs and style of therapy are congruent with the client's needs and expectations of therapy. The client may also have to try different therapists to find a 'good match'.

A therapist's (or nurse's) theoretical beliefs, professional experience and personal history strongly influence his or her style of therapy (discussed earlier in this chapter). A therapist grounded in interpersonal theory may emphasize relationships, whereas an existential therapist may focus more on the client's self-responsibility. Equally, someone who themselves has benefited from CBT, say, in the past may favour that approach for their clients.

The nurse or other professional who is familiar with the client may be in a position to recommend a therapist or a choice of therapists from inside or outside the NHS. He or she also may help the client understand what different therapists have to offer.

The client should select a therapist carefully (where this is possible) and should ask about the therapist's treatment approach and area of specialization. At present, there are no laws as such that regulate the practice and licensing of therapists, and a few therapists have little or no formal education, credentials or experience but still practise entirely within legal limits. A client can ensure some protection by ensuring a therapist is a member of one of a number of organizations, in particular the British Association for Counselling and Psychotherapy (BACP), the British Association for Cognitive and Behavioural Therapies (BACBP), the British Psychological Society (BPS) or the United Kingdom Council for Psychotherapy (UKCP). Calling the local community mental health services, the person's GP or NHS Direct is another way for a client to check a therapist's credentials and ethical practices.

THE NURSE AND PSYCHOTHERAPEUTIC WORK

It is important to note that the majority of psychotherapeutic work undertaken by nurses is 'embedded' or 'informal', integrated into a broader relationship rather than narrow 'psychotherapy' *per se*. This does not make it any less valuable – indeed, the psychotherapeutic work undertaken by nurses in inpatient units, specialist teams and CMHTs (among others) is highly valued by clients and often exceptionally effective in validating past and current experiences and empowering people to change and find solutions to their problems. CBT is increasingly being used as a guide to this kind of work, though recovery principles are also underpinning it. Key elements of a less formal psychotherapeutic approach are:

- **Engagement**: establishing rapport; negotiating boundaries (time, place, person); acknowledging and validating current feelings and concerns; ensuring openness, transparency and agreement on concrete objectives within a focused conversation; asking about people's dreams, hopes and desires; agreeing achievable goals for the conversation.
- **Exchanging information**: offering and receiving information about someone's life, about their fears, about their strengths, competencies, achievements, about the exceptions – when the problem doesn't happen, when it happens less, when it bothers the person less; eliciting clients' thoughts and beliefs about themselves, about other people and about the world; maintaining a pragmatic optimism.
- **Action planning**: agreeing clear steps forward – steps which, if completed, will leave the person with a sense of mastery; trying something out that's neither too hard nor too easy.
- **Evaluation**: checking out both the outcome of the action plan and the usefulness of the psychotherapeutic process so far – what's been helpful, what's been less helpful?

These four phases are rarely completely discrete; nevertheless, they will usually be present in most effective therapeutic conversations in any setting.

Groups

A group is a number of people who gather in a face-to-face setting to accomplish tasks that require co-operation, collaboration or working together. Each person in a group is in a position to influence, and to be influenced by, other group members. Group *content* refers to what is said in the context of the group, including educational material, feelings and emotions, or discussions of the project to be completed. Group *process* refers to the behaviour of the group and its individual members, including seating arrangements, tone of voice, who speaks to whom, who is quiet and so forth. Content and process occur continuously throughout the life of the group.

STAGES OF GROUP DEVELOPMENT

A group may be established to serve a particular purpose in a specified period, such as a work group to complete an assigned project or a therapy group that meets with the same members to explore ways to deal with depression. These groups develop in observable stages. In the pre-group stages, members are selected, the purpose or work of the group is identified and group structure is addressed. Group structure includes where and how often the group will meet, identification of a group leader and the rules of the group; for example, whether individuals can join the group after it begins, how to handle absences and expectations for group members.

The beginning stage of group development, or the initial stage, commences as soon as the group begins to meet. Members introduce themselves, a leader can be selected (if not done previously), the group purpose is discussed and rules and expectations for group participation are reviewed. Group members begin to 'check out' one another and the leader as they determine their levels of comfort in the group setting.

The working stage of group development begins as members begin to focus their attention on the purpose or task the group is trying to accomplish. This may happen relatively quickly in a work group with a specific assigned project, but may take two or three sessions in a therapy group because members must develop some level of trust before sharing personal feelings or difficult situations. During this phase, several group characteristics may be seen. Group cohesiveness is the degree to which members work together co-operatively to accomplish the purpose. Cohesiveness is a desirable group characteristic and is associated with positive group outcomes. Cohesiveness is evidenced when members value one another's contributions to the group; members think of themselves as 'we' and share responsibility for the work of the group. When a group is cohesive, members feel free to express all opinions, positive and negative, with little fear of rejection or retribution. If a group is 'overly cohesive', in that uniformity and agreement become the group's implicit goals, there may be a negative effect on the group outcome. In a therapy group, members do not give one another needed feedback if the group is overly cohesive. In a work group, critical thinking and creative problem-solving are unlikely, which may make the work of the group less meaningful.

Some groups exhibit competition, or rivalry, among group members. This may positively affect the outcome of the group if the competition leads to compromise, improved group performance and growth for individual members. Many times, however, competition can be destructive for the group; when conflicts are not resolved, members become hostile, or the group's energy is diverted from accomplishing its purpose to bickering and power struggles.

The final stage, or termination, of the group occurs before the group disbands. The work of the group is reviewed, with the focus on group accomplishments, growth of group members, or both, depending on the purpose of the group.

Observing the stages of group development in groups that are ongoing is difficult, with members joining and leaving the group at various times. Rather, the group involvement of new members as they join the group evolves as they feel accepted by the group, take a more active role and join in the work of the group. An example of this type of group would be Alcoholics Anonymous, a self-help group with stated purposes. Members may attend Alcoholics Anonymous meetings as often or infrequently as they choose; group cohesiveness or competition can still be observed in ongoing groups.

GROUP LEADERSHIP

Groups often have an identified or formal leader – someone designated to lead the group. In therapy groups and education groups, a formal leader is usually identified based on his or her education, qualifications and experience. Some work groups have formal leaders appointed in advance, whereas other work groups select a leader at the initial meeting. Support groups and self-help groups usually do not have identified formal leaders; all members are seen as equals. An informal leader may emerge from a 'leaderless' group or from a group that has an identified formal leader. Informal leaders are generally members recognized by others as having the knowledge, experience or characteristics that members admire and value.

Effective group leaders focus on group process as well as on group content. Tasks of the group leader include giving feedback and suggestions; encouraging participation from all members (eliciting responses from quiet members, placing limits on members who may monopolize the group's time); clarifying thoughts, feelings and ideas; summarizing progress and accomplishments; and facilitating progress through the stages of group development.

GROUP ROLES

Roles are the parts that members play within the group. Not all members are aware of their 'role behaviour', and changes in members' behaviour may be a topic that the group will need to address. Some roles facilitate the work of the group, whereas other roles can negatively affect the process or outcome of the group. Growth-producing roles include the information-seeker, opinion-seeker, information-giver, energizer, coordinator, harmonizer, encourager and elaborator. Growth-inhibiting roles include the monopolizer, aggressor, dominator, critic, recognition-seeker and passive follower.

GROUP THERAPY

In **group therapy**, clients participate in sessions with a group of people. The members share a common purpose and are expected to contribute to the group to benefit others and receive benefit from others in return. Group rules are established that all members must observe. These rules vary according to the type of group. Being a member of a group allows the client to learn new ways of looking at a problem or ways of coping with or solving problems, and also helps him or her to learn important interpersonal skills. For example, by interacting with other members, clients often receive feedback on how others perceive and react to them and their behaviour. This is extremely important information for many clients with mental disorders, who often have difficulty with interpersonal skills.

The therapeutic results of group therapy (Yalom, 1995) include the following:

- Gaining new information, or learning
- Gaining inspiration or hope
- Interacting with others
- Feeling acceptance and belonging

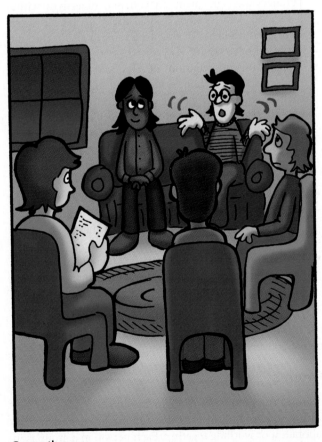

Group therapy

- Becoming aware that one is not alone and that others share the same problems
- Gaining insight into one's problems and behaviours and how they affect others
- Giving of oneself for the benefit of others (altruism).

Therapy groups vary with different purposes, degrees of formality and structures. Our discussion includes psychotherapy groups, family therapy, family education, education groups, support groups and self-help groups.

Psychotherapy Groups. The goal of a **psychotherapy group** is for members to learn about their behaviour and to make positive changes in their behaviour by interacting and communicating with others as a member of a group. Groups may be organized around a specific diagnosis, such as depression, or a particular issue, such as improving interpersonal skills or managing anxiety. Group techniques and processes are used to help group members learn about their behaviour with other people and how it relates to core personality traits. Members also learn they have responsibilities to others and can help other members achieve their goals.

Psychotherapy groups are often formal in structure, with one or two therapists as the group leaders. One task of the group leader or the entire group is to establish the rules for the group. These rules deal with confidentiality, punctuality, attendance and social contact between members outside of group time.

There are two types of groups: open groups and closed groups. **Open groups** are ongoing and run indefinitely, allowing members to join or leave the group as they need to. **Closed groups** are structured to keep the same members in the group for a specified number of sessions. If the group is closed, the members decide how to handle members who wish to leave the group and the possible addition of new group members (Yalom, 1995).

Educational ('Psycho-educational') Groups. The goal of an education group is to provide information to members on a specific issue – for instance, **individual psychotherapy** (sometimes offered within the NHS) is a method of bringing about change in a person by exploring his or her feelings, attitudes, thinking and behaviour. It involves a one-to-one relationship between the therapist and the client and may be based on any of the theoretical perspectives outlined earlier in this chapter, though most frequently on psychodynamic or CBT principles. Outside the NHS, people generally seek this kind of therapy based on their desire to understand themselves and their behaviour, to make personal changes, to improve interpersonal relationships or to get relief from emotional pain or unhappiness. Within the NHS, people with mental health problems may be referred for therapy to address their particular issues, usually to a psychologist, a psychotherapist or a nurse therapist. The relationship between the client and the therapist proceeds through stages similar to those of the nurse–client relationship: introduction, working and termination.

Self-Help Groups. In a **self-help** group, members share a common experience, but the group is not a formal or structured therapy group. Although professionals organize some self-help groups, many are run by members and do not have a formally identified leader. Various self-help groups are available. Some are locally organized and announce their meetings in local newspapers. Others are nationally organized, such as Alcoholics Anonymous, Parents Without Partners, Gamblers Anonymous and Al-Anon (a group for spouses and partners of alcoholics), and have national headquarters and Internet websites (see Internet Resources).

Most self-help groups have a rule of confidentiality: whoever is seen and whatever is said at the meetings cannot be divulged to others or discussed outside the group. In many 12-step programmes, such as Alcoholics Anonymous and Gamblers Anonymous, people use only their first names so their identities are not divulged (although in some settings, group members do know one another's names).

Complementary and Alternative Therapies

Complementary medicine includes therapies *used with* conventional medicine practices (the medical model). **Alternative medicine** is therapies *used in place* of conventional treatment. **Integrative medicine** combines conventional medical therapy and complementary and alternative medicine (CAM) therapies that have scientific evidence supporting their safety and effectiveness.

There is a wide variety of complementary and alternative therapies:

- *Alternative medical systems* such as homeopathic medicine and naturopathic medicine in Western cultures, and traditional Chinese medicine that includes herbal and nutritional therapy, restorative physical exercises (yoga, *Tai chi*), meditation, acupuncture and remedial massage.
- *Mind–body interventions* include meditation, prayer, mental healing and creative therapies that use art, music or dance.
- *Biologically-based therapies* use substances found in nature such as herbs, food and vitamins. Dietary supplements, herbal products, medicinal teas, aromatherapy and a variety of diets are included.
- *Manipulative and body-based therapies* are based on manipulation and/or movement of one or more parts of the body, such as therapeutic massage and chiropractic or osteopathic manipulation.
- *Energy therapies* include two types of therapy: biofield therapies, intended to affect energy fields that are believed to surround and penetrate the body, such as therapeutic touch, *qi gong* and *Reiki*; and bioelectric-based therapies involving the unconventional use of electromagnetic fields, such as pulsed fields, magnetic fields and AC or DC fields. *Qi gong* is part of Chinese medicine that combines movement, meditation and regulated breathing to enhance the flow of vital energy and promote healing. *Reiki* (Japanese, meaning 'universal life energy') is based on the belief that when spiritual energy is channelled through a *Reiki* practitioner, the patient's spirit and body are healed.

There is as yet little or no evidence that any of these therapies have clear beneficial effects, and clients may be reluctant to tell professionals about the use of CAM. Therefore, it is important that the nurse ask clients specifically about use of herbs, vitamins or other health practices in a non-judgemental way.

Psychiatric Rehabilitation and Recovery

Until very recently, **psychiatric rehabilitation** in the UK involved providing services to people with severe and persistent mental health problems to help them to live in the community. These programmes were often called *community support services* or *community support programmes*. Psychiatric rehabilitation was meant to focus on the client's strengths, not just on his or her illness. The client actively participated in programme planning. The programmes were designed to help the client manage the illness and symptoms, gain access to needed services and live successfully in the community

Psychiatric rehabilitation programmes assist clients with activities of daily living such as transportation, shopping, food preparation, money management and hygiene. Social support and interpersonal relationships are recognized as a primary need for successful community living. Psychiatric rehabilitation programmes provide opportunities for socialization, such as drop-in centres and places where clients can go to be with others in a safe, supportive environment. Vocational referral, training, job coaching and support are available for clients who want to seek and maintain employment. Community support programmes also provide education about the client's illness and treatment, and help the client to obtain health care when needed.

Lecomte *et al.* (2005) emphasized the importance of including the client in identifying rehabilitation goals. There is often a disparity between what health-care professionals view as the client's needs and what the client perceives as valuable. Offering services that meet each client's most important goals can significantly improve their quality of life and promote recovery and well-being.

RECOVERY PRINCIPLES

Over the past few years there has been a shift in emphasis from 'rehabilitation' models (which adopt a fairly limited, medicalized approach to the reintegration of people who have been 'ill') to models that adopt the more positive principles of '**recovery**', principles that have developed in part from the increasingly assertive voice of service users in the UK, who have consistently argued that existing models are restricting, pessimistic and demeaning to people who have mental health problems. The notion of recovery encompasses far more than its lay meaning: it encapsulates a positive, optimistic, inclusive approach to mental ill-health, one that demands collaboration, hope and empowerment and one that strives to find meaning and purpose in the lives

Box 2.2

Recovery is the awakening of hope after despair
Recovery is breaking through denial and achieving understanding and acceptance
Recovery is moving from withdrawal to engagement and active participation in life
Recovery is active coping rather than passive adjustment
Recovery means no longer viewing oneself primarily as a mental patient and reclaiming a positive sense of self
Recovery is a journey from alienation to purpose
Recovery is a complex journey
Recovery is not accomplished alone – it involves support and partnership

Allott, P. & Loganathan, L. (2002). Discovering hope for recovery from a British perspective – A review of a sample of recovery literature, implications for practice and systems change. West Midlands Partnerships for Mental Health, Birmingham www.wmpmh.org.uk. Available: *http://www.critpsynet.freeuk.com/LITERATUREREVIEWFinal.htm*

of all, regardless of whether they have been diagnosed with 'schizophrenia', 'bipolar disorder' or any other medical label (Box 2.2). The nurse's role is to facilitate this process: by being compassionate and by being effective.

THE NURSE AND PSYCHOSOCIAL INTERVENTIONS

Bridging the gap between 'recovery' and more traditional medical approaches to psychosis, the Thorn initiative, which began in 1992, has trained nurses and supported nursing work in interventions with people who are diagnosed with schizophrenia (and, latterly, those with severe depression and bipolar disorders), interventions that place someone's 'illness' in its social context (more in Chapter 14).

SELF-AWARENESS ISSUES

Whether directly employing counselling/psychotherapy, using adapted or embedded counselling or psychotherapeutic techniques, or referring to/supporting other professionals in their psychotherapeutic work, the nurse must examine his or her beliefs about the theories of psychosocial development, develop knowledge about different approaches and their evidence-base, and realize that many treatment approaches are available. Different treatments may work for different clients: no one approach works for everyone. Sometimes the nurse's personal opinions may not

Critical Thinking Questions

1. Can sound parenting and nurturing in a loving environment overcome a genetic or biological predisposition to mental 'illness'?
2. Can children raised in a hostile environment, without parental love, support and consistency, avoid mental health problems as adults? If so, how? What factors could help a person overcome a neglectful or traumatic childhood?

agree with those of the client, but the nurse must make sure that those beliefs do not inadvertently affect the therapeutic process. For example, an overweight client may be working on accepting herself as being overweight rather than trying to lose weight, but the nurse believes the client really just needs to lose weight. The nurse's responsibility is to support the client's needs and goals, not to promote the nurse's own ideas about what the client should do. Hence, the nurse must support the client's decision to work on self-acceptance. For the nurse who believes that being overweight is simply a lack of willpower, it might be difficult to support a client's participation in a self-help weight-loss group, such as Overeaters Anonymous, that emphasizes overeating as a disease and accepting oneself.

Points to Consider When Working on Self-Awareness

Points to consider regarding psychosocial theories and treatment:

- No one theory explains all human behaviour. No one approach will work with all clients.
- Becoming familiar with the variety of psychosocial approaches for working with clients will increase the nurse's effectiveness in promoting the client's health and well-being.
- The client's feelings and perceptions about his or her situation are the most influential factors in determining his or her response to therapeutic interventions, rather than what the nurse believes the client should do.

 KEY POINTS

- Psychosocial theories help to explain human behaviour – both mental health and mental illness. There are several types of psychosocial theories, including psychoanalytic theories, interpersonal theories, humanistic theories, behavioural theories and cognitive theories.
- Freud believed that human behaviour is motivated by repressed sexual impulses and desires and that childhood development is based on sexual energy (libido) as the driving force.
- Erik Erikson's theories focused on both social and psychological development across the life span. He proposed eight stages of psychosocial development; each stage includes a developmental task and a virtue to be achieved (hope, will, purpose, fidelity, love, caring and wisdom). Erikson's theories remain in wide use today.
- Jean Piaget described four stages of cognitive development: sensorimotor, preoperational, concrete operations and formal operations.
- Harry Stack Sullivan's theories focused on development in terms of interpersonal relationships. He viewed the therapist's role (termed *participant observer*) as key to the client's treatment.
- Hildegard Peplau is a nursing theorist whose theories formed much of the foundation of modern nursing practice, including the therapeutic nurse–patient relationship, the role of the nurse in the relationship and the four anxiety levels.
- Abraham Maslow developed a hierarchy of needs, stating that people are motivated by progressive levels of needs; each level must be satisfied before the person can progress to the next level. The levels begin with physiological needs and then proceed to safety and security needs, belonging needs, esteem needs and finally self-actualization needs.
- Carl Rogers developed client-centred therapy in which the therapist plays a supportive role, demonstrating unconditional positive regard, genuineness and empathetic understanding to the client.
- Therapists such as De Shazer and O'Hanlon have built on Rogers's principles and those of systemic and family practitioners to develop solution-focused brief therapies.
- Behaviourism focuses on the client's observable performance and behaviours and external influences that can bring about behaviour changes, rather than on feelings and thoughts.
- Systematic desensitization is an example of conditioning in which a person who has an excessive fear of something, such as frogs or snakes, learns to manage his or her anxiety response through being exposed to the feared object.
- B. F. Skinner was a behaviourist who developed the theory of operant conditioning in which people are motivated to learn or change behaviour with a system of rewards or reinforcement.
- A crisis is a turning point in an individual's life that produces an overwhelming response. Crises may be maturational, situational or adventitious. Effective crisis intervention includes engagement with, and collaborative assessment of, the person in crisis, promotion of problem-solving and the provision of empathetic understanding.
- Ellis and Beck developed cognitive therapies which are based on the premise that how a person thinks about or

INTERNET RESOURCES

RESOURCES	INTERNET ADDRESS
Albert Ellis Institute (Rational Emotive Behaviour Therapy)	http://www.rebt.org
Alcoholics Anonymous	http://www.alcoholics-anonymous.org.uk
Beck Institute for Cognitive Therapy and Research	http://www.beckinstitute.org
Behavioural Tech (DBT)	http://behaviouraltech.org/
Brief Therapy Practice	http://www.brieftherapy.org.uk
British Association for Cognitive and Behavioural Therapies (BACBP)	http://www.babcp.com
British Association for Counselling and Psychotherapy (BACP)	http://www.bacp.co.uk
British Psychological Society (BPS)	http://www.bps.org.uk
Institute for the Study of Therapeutic Change	http://www.talkingcure.com
Institute of Transactional Analysis	http://www.ita.org.uk/
RETHINK	http://www.rethink.org
Scottish Recovery Network	http://www.scottishrecovery.net
Star Wards	http://starwards.org.uk/
United Kingdom Council For Psychotherapy (UKCP)	www.psychotherapy.org.uk

interprets life experiences determines how he or she will feel or behave. It seeks to help the person change how he or she thinks about things to bring about an improvement in mood and behaviour.

- Linehan and Kabat-Zinn have incorporated concepts and practices of mindfulness into cognitive approaches.
- Treatment of mental disorders and emotional problems can include one or more of the following: individual psychotherapeutic approaches, group psychotherapeutic work, family therapy, family/carer education, psychiatric rehabilitation and recovery work, self-help groups, support groups, education groups and other **psychosocial interventions**.
- An understanding of psychosocial theories and treatment modalities can help the nurse select appropriate and effective intervention strategies to use with clients.

REFERENCES

Aguilera, D. C. (1998). *Crisis intervention: Theory and methodology* (7th edn). St. Louis: Mosby.

Allott, P. & Loganathan, L. (2002). Discovering hope for recovery from a British perspective – A review of a sample of recovery literature, implications for practice and systems change. West Midlands Partnerships for Mental Health, Birmingham. Available: http://www.crispynet.freeuk.com/LITERATUREREVIEWFinal.htm

Barker, P. & Buchanan-Barker, P. (2005). *The Tidal Model.* Brunner-Routledge.

Beck, A. T. & Rush, A. J. (1995). Cognitive therapy. In H. I. Kaplan & B. J. Sadock (Eds.), *Comprehensive textbook of psychiatry, Vol. 2* (6th edn, pp. 1847–1856). Philadelphia: J. B. Lippincott.

Bright. (2006). Star Wards: Practical ideas for improving the daily experiences and treatment outcomes of acute mental health in patients. Available: http://starwards.org.uk/?page_id=8

Bright. (2008). Star Wards 2: The Sequel—Loads more practical ideas for improving the daily experiences and treatment outcomes of mental health inpatients. Available: http://starwards.org.uk/?page_id=8

Caplan, G. (1964). *Principles of preventive psychiatry.* New York: Basic Books.

De Shazer, S., Dolan, Y., & Korman, H. (2007). *More than miracles: The state of the art of solution-focused brief therapy.* Philadelphia: Haworth Press.

Dryden, W. (2001). *Reason to change: A rational emotive behaviour therapy workbook.* Hove: Brunner-Routledge.

Duncan, B., Miller, S., & Sparks, J. (2007). Common factors and the uncommon heroism of youth. *Psychotherapy in Australia, 13,* 2.

Erikson, E. H. (1995). *Childhood and Society: New Edition.* London: Vintage Books.

Freud, S. (1962). *The ego and the id (The standard edition of the complete psychological works of Sigmund Freud;* J. Strachey, Trans.). New York: W. W. Norton & Company. (Original work published 1923.)

George, E., Iveson, C., & Ratner, H. (2001). *Problem to solution.* London: BT Press.

Jones, M. (1953). *The therapeutic community.* New York: Basic Books.

Kabat-Zinn, J. (2001). *Full catastrophe living: How to cope with stress, pain and illness using mindfulness meditation.* London: Piatkus.

Lecomte, T., Wallace, C. J., Perreault, M., & Caron, J. (2005). Consumer's goals in psychiatric rehabilitation and their concordance with existing services. *Psychiatric Services, 56*(2), 209–211.

Linehan, M. (1993). *Cognitive behavioural treatment of borderline personality disorder (diagnosis & treatment of mental disorders).* New York: Guilford.

Loden, S. (2002). The fate of the dream in contemporary psychoanalysis. *Journal of the American Psychoanalytic Association, 5*(1), 43–70.

Maslow, A. H. (1954). *Motivation and personality.* New York: Harper & Row.

Miller, S. (2008). 'What Works' in Therapy? Available: www.talkingcure.com/docs/What_Works.doc

O'Hanlon, W. (1996). *A field guide to Possibility Land.* London: BT Press.

Peplau, H. (1952). *Interpersonal relations in nursing.* New York: G. P. Putnam's Sons.

Rogers, C. R. (1961). *On becoming a person: A therapist's view of psychotherapy.* Boston: Houghton Mifflin.

Sadock, B. J. & Sadock, V. A. (2004). *Concise textbook of clinical psychiatry* (3rd edn). Philadelphia: Lippincott Williams & Wilkins.

Skinner, B. F. (1974). *About behaviourism.* New York: Alfred A. Knopf, Inc.

Sullivan, H. S. (1953). *The interpersonal theory of psychiatry.* New York: Norton.

Yalom, I. D. (1995). *The theory and practice of group psychotherapy.* New York: Basic Books.

ADDITIONAL READING

Beck, A. T. (1976). *Cognitive therapy and the emotional disorders.* New York: New American Library, Inc.

Berne, E. (1964). *Games people play.* New York: Grove Press.

Caplan, G. (1964). *Principles of preventive psychiatry.* New York: Basic Books.

Crain, W. C. (1980). *Theories of development: Concepts and application.* Englewood Cliffs, NJ: Prentice Hall, Inc.

Dimeff, L. & Koerner, K. (2007). *Dialectical behaviour therapy in clinical practice: applications across disorders and settings.* New York: Guilford.

Frankl, V. E. (1959). *Man's search for meaning: An introduction to logotherapy.* New York: Beacon Press.

Glasser, W. (1965). *Reality therapy: A new approach to psychiatry.* New York: Harper & Row.

Grant, A., Mills, J., Mulhern, R., & Short, N. (2004) .*Cognitive behavioural therapy in mental health care.* London: Sage.

Hendrick, S. S. (2004). Close relationships research: A resource for couple and family therapists. *Journal of Marital and Family Therapy, 30*(1), 13–27.

Miller, P. H. (1983). *Theories of developmental psychology.* San Francisco: W. H. Freeman & Co.

Millon, T. (Ed.). (1967). *Theories of psychopathology.* Philadelphia: W. B. Saunders.

National Center for Complementary and Alternative Medicine. (2006). *What is complementary and alternative medicine?* Available: http://nccam.nih.gov/health.

Perls, F. S., Hefferline, R. F., & Goodman, P. (1951). *Gestalt therapy: Excitement and growth in the human personality.* New York: Dell Publishing Co., Inc.

Sugarman, L. (1986). *Life-span development: Concepts, theories and interventions.* London: Methuen & Co., Ltd.

Szasz, T. (1961). *The myth of mental illness.* New York: Hoeber-Harper.

Viscott, D. (1996). *Emotional resilience: Simple truths for dealing with the unfinished business of your past.* New York: Harmony Books.

Watkins, P. (2007). *Recovery: A guide for mental health practitioners.* Oxford: Butterworth-Heinemann.

Chapter Study Guide

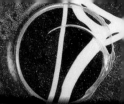

MULTIPLE-CHOICE QUESTIONS

Select the best answer for each of the following questions.

1. Which of the following theorists believed that a corrective interpersonal relationship with the therapist was the primary mode of treatment?
   a. Sigmund Freud
   b. Hildegard Peplau
   c. Harry Stack Sullivan

2. Dream analysis and free association are techniques in which of the following?
   a. Client-centred therapy
   b. Gestalt therapy
   c. Logotherapy
   d. Psychoanalysis

3. Four levels of anxiety were described by
   a. Erik Erikson
   b. Sigmund Freud
   c. Hildegard Peplau
   d. Carl Rogers

4. Correcting how one thinks about the world and oneself is the focus of
   a. Behaviourism
   b. Cognitive therapy
   c. Psychoanalysis

5. The personality structures of id, ego and superego were described by
   a. Sigmund Freud
   b. Hildegard Peplau
   c. Frederick Perls
   d. Harry Stack Sullivan

6. Recovery principles focus on
   a. A client's strengths
   b. Medication compliance
   c. Social skills deficits
   d. Symptom reduction

7. When a nurse develops feelings toward a client that are based on the nurse's past experience, it is called
   a. Countertransference
   b. Role reversal
   c. Transference
   d. Unconditional regard

8. A facilitated group that was designed for the same people to meet weekly for 10 sessions to learn cognitive-behavioural strategies to deal with their depression would be a(n)
   a. Closed psychoeducational group
   b. Psychodynamic psychotherapy group
   c. Open therapy group
   d. Self-help support group

FILL-IN-THE-BLANK QUESTIONS

Write the name of the appropriate theorist beside the statement or theory. Names may be used more than once.

1. The client is the key to his or her own healing. _____

2. Social and psychological factors influence development. _____

3. Behaviour change occurs through conditioning with environmental stimuli. _____

4. People make themselves unhappy by clinging to irrational beliefs. _____

5. Behaviour is learned from past experience that is reinforcing. _____

6. Client-centred therapy _____

7. Gestalt therapy _____

8. Hierarchy of needs _____

9. Logotherapy _____

10. Rational emotive therapy _____

GROUP DISCUSSION TOPICS

Describe each of the following types of groups, and give an example.

1. What might be the benefits of group psychotherapy over individual psychotherapy?

2. What should be seen as valid evidence of a therapeutic approach working?

3. What makes us favour one approach over another?

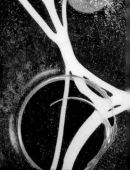

Chapter

3

Neurobiological Theories, the Nurse and Psychopharmacology

Key Terms

- adrenaline
- akathisia
- anticholinergic side-effects
- antidepressant drugs
- antipsychotic drugs
- anxiolytic drugs
- collaborative prescribing
- computed tomography (CT)
- depot injection
- dopamine
- dystonia
- efficacy
- ethical prescribing
- extrapyramidal symptoms (EPS)
- half-life
- kindling process
- limbic system
- magnetic resonance imaging (MRI)
- mood-stabilizing drugs
- neuroleptic malignant syndrome (NMS)
- neurotransmitter
- noradrenaline
- nurse prescribing
- off-label use

Learning Objectives

After reading this chapter, you should be able to:

1. Discuss the structures, processes and functions of the brain.

2. Describe the current neurobiological research and theories that are the basis for current psychopharmacological treatment of mental disorders.

3. Discuss the nurse's role in educating clients and families about current neurobiological theories and medication management.

4. Discuss the categories of drugs used to treat mental health problems and their mechanisms of action, side-effects and special nursing considerations.

5. Identify client responses that indicate treatment effectiveness.

6. Discuss common barriers for clients in maintaining their medication regime.

7. Develop a teaching plan for clients and families for implementation of the prescribed therapeutic regime.

- positron emission tomography (PET)
- potency
- pseudoparkinsonism
- psychoimmunology
- psychopharmacology
- psychotropic drugs
- rebound
- serotonin
- serotonin syndrome
- stimulant drugs
- tardive dyskinesia
- withdrawal

Much remains unknown about what causes mental health problems. Their aetiology remains much-debated, but there seems little doubt that an array of genetic, environmental, interpersonal, intrapersonal and neurobiological features contributes to their development. Science in the past 20 years has made great strides in helping us understand how the brain works and in presenting possible causes to explain why some brains work differently from others. Such advances in neurobiological research are continually expanding the knowledge base in the field of psychiatric medicine and are, inevitably, greatly influencing clinical practice. The mental health nurse must have a core understanding of how the brain functions and of the current theories regarding 'mental illness'. This chapter includes an overview of the major anatomical structures of the nervous system and how they work – the neurotransmission process. It presents the major current neurobiological theories regarding what causes 'mental illness', including genetics and heredity, stress and the immune system and infectious agents.

The use of medications to treat 'mental illness' (**psychopharmacology**) is related to these neurobiological theories. These medications directly affect the central nervous system (CNS) and, subsequently, behaviour, perceptions, thinking and emotions. This chapter discusses five categories of drug, including their mechanisms of action, their side-effects and the roles of the nurse in administration and client teaching. Although pharmacological interventions seem to be an effective treatment for many disorders in many different people, social interventions and approaches, such as cognitive-behavioural therapies, family therapy and other psychotherapies, greatly enhance the success of that pharmacological treatment, as well as offering effective 'stand-alone' help. Chapters 2 and 4 discuss these psychosocial modalities.

Nurses should NEVER administer any medication without an awareness of the contraindications and possible side-effects.

This chapter provides an overview of key drugs but reference to senior practitioners, national and local policies, to the BNF and to medical and pharmacist colleagues must always be made if any doubt about a prescription exists.

THE NERVOUS SYSTEM AND HOW IT WORKS

Central Nervous System

The CNS is composed of the brain, the spinal cord and associated nerves that control voluntary acts. Structurally, the brain is divided into the cerebrum, cerebellum, brain stem and limbic system. Figures 3.1 and 3.2 show the locations of brain structures.

CEREBRUM

The cerebrum is divided into two hemispheres; all lobes and structures are found in both halves except for the pineal body, or gland, which is located between the hemispheres. The pineal body is an endocrine gland that influences the activities of the pituitary gland, islets of Langerhans, parathyroids, adrenals and gonads. The corpus callosum is a pathway connecting the two hemispheres and co-ordinating their functions. The left hemisphere controls the right side of the body and is the centre for logical reasoning and analytical functions such as reading, writing and mathematical tasks. The right hemisphere controls the left side of the body and is the centre for creative thinking, intuition and artistic abilities.

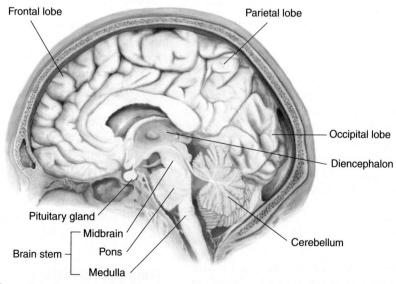

Figure 3.1. Anatomy of the brain.

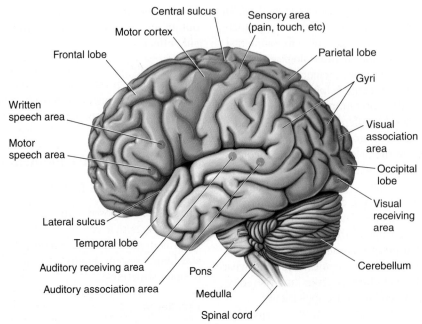

Figure 3.2. The brain and its structures.

The cerebral hemispheres are divided into four lobes: frontal, parietal, temporal and occipital. Some functions of the lobes are distinct; others are integrated. The frontal lobes control the organization of thought, body movement, memories, emotions and moral behaviour. The integration of all this information regulates arousal, focuses attention and enables problem solving and decision making. Abnormalities in the frontal lobes seem to be associated with some schizophrenias, attention deficit hyperactivity disorder (ADHD) and some dementias. The parietal lobes interpret sensations of taste and touch, and assist in spatial orientation. The temporal lobes are centres for the senses of smell and hearing, and for memory and emotional expression. The occipital lobes assist in co-ordinating language generation and visual interpretation, such as depth perception.

CEREBELLUM

The cerebellum is located below the cerebrum and is the centre for co-ordination of movements and postural adjustments. The cerebellum receives and integrates information from all areas of the body, such as the muscles, joints, organs and other components of the CNS. Research has shown that inhibited transmission of dopamine, a neurotransmitter, in this area is associated with the lack of smooth, co-ordinated movements in diseases such as Parkinson's disease and some dementias.

BRAIN STEM

The brain stem includes the midbrain, pons and medulla oblongata and the nuclei for cranial nerves III through XII. The medulla, located at the top of the spinal cord, contains vital centres for respiration and cardiovascular functions.

Above the medulla and in front of the cerebrum, the pons bridges the gap both structurally and functionally, serving as a primary motor pathway. The midbrain connects the pons and cerebellum with the cerebrum. It measures only 0.8 inches (2 cm) in length and includes most of the reticular activating system and the extrapyramidal system. The reticular activating system influences motor activity, sleep, consciousness and awareness. The extrapyramidal system relays information about movement and co-ordination from the brain to the spinal nerves. The locus ceruleus, a small group of noradrenaline-producing neurons in the brain stem, is associated with stress, anxiety and impulsive behaviour.

LIMBIC SYSTEM

The **limbic system** is an area of the brain located above the brain stem that includes the thalamus, hypothalamus, hippocampus and amygdala (although some sources differ regarding the structures that this system includes). The thalamus regulates activity, sensation and emotion. The hypothalamus is involved in temperature regulation, appetite control, endocrine function, sexual drive and impulsive behaviour associated with feelings of anger, rage or excitement. The hippocampus and amygdala are involved in emotional arousal and memory. Disturbances in the limbic system have been implicated in a variety of mental disorders, such as the memory loss that accompanies some dementias and the poorly controlled emotions and impulses seen with psychotic or manic behaviour.

Neurotransmitters

Approximately 100 billion brain cells form groups of neurons, or nerve cells, that are arranged in networks. These

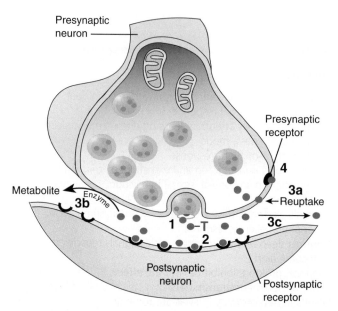

Figure 3.3. Schematic illustration of (1) neurotransmitter (T) release; (2) binding of transmitter to postsynaptic receptor; termination of transmitter action by (3a) reuptake of transmitter into the presynaptic terminal, (3b) enzymatic degradation, or (3c) diffusion away from the synapse; and (4) binding of transmitter to presynaptic receptors for feedback regulation of transmitter release.

neurons communicate information with one another by sending electrochemical messages from neuron to neuron, a process called *neurotransmission*. These electrochemical messages pass from the dendrites (projections from the cell body), through the soma or cell body, down the axon (long extended structures), and across the synapses (gaps between cells) to the dendrites of the next neuron. In the nervous system, the electrochemical messages cross the synapses

between neural cells by way of special chemical messengers called neurotransmitters.

Neurotransmitters are the chemical substances manufactured in the neuron that aid in the transmission of information throughout the body. They either excite or stimulate an action in the cells (excitatory) or inhibit or stop an action (inhibitory). These neurotransmitters fit into specific receptor cells embedded in the membrane of the dendrite, just like a certain key shape fits into a lock. After neurotransmitters are released into the synapse and relay the message to the receptor cells, they are either transported back from the synapse to the axon to be stored for later use (re-uptake) or are metabolized and inactivated by enzymes, primarily monoamine oxidase (MAO) (Figure 3.3).

These neurotransmitters are necessary in just the right proportions to relay messages across the synapses. Studies are beginning to show differences in the amount of some neurotransmitters available in the brains of people with certain mental disorders compared with people who have no signs of mental disorder (Figure 3.4).

Major neurotransmitters have been found to play a role in mental health problems as well as in the actions and side-effects of **psychotropic drugs**. Table 3.1 lists the major neurotransmitters and their actions and effects. Dopamine and serotonin have received the most attention in terms of the study and treatment of psychiatric disorders (Tecott & Smart, 2005). The following is a discussion of the major neurotransmitters associated with mental disorders.

DOPAMINE

Dopamine, a neurotransmitter located primarily in the brain stem, has been found to be involved in the control of complex movements, motivation, cognition and regulation of

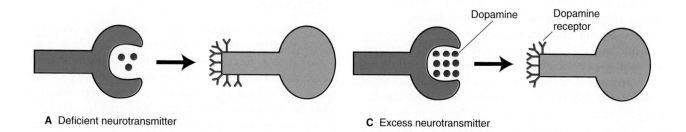

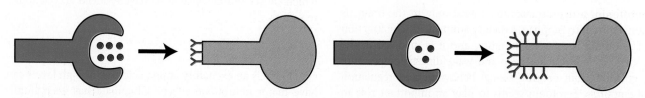

A Deficient neurotransmitter

C Excess neurotransmitter

B Deficient receptor

D Excess receptors

Figure 3.4. Abnormal neurotransmission causing some mental disorders because of excess transmission or excess responsiveness of receptors.

Table 3.1   MAJOR NEUROTRANSMITTERS

Type	Mechanism of Action	Physiological Effects
Dopamine	Excitatory	Controls complex movements, motivation, cognition; regulates emotional response
Noradrenaline (norepinephrine)	Excitatory	Causes changes in attention, learning and memory, sleep and wakefulness, mood
Adrenaline (epinephrine)	Excitatory	Controls fight-or-flight response
Serotonin	Inhibitory	Controls food intake, sleep and wakefulness, temperature regulation, pain control, sexual behaviours, regulation of emotions
Histamine	Neuromodulator	Controls alertness, gastric secretions, cardiac stimulation, peripheral allergic responses
Acetylcholine	Excitatory or inhibitory	Controls sleep and wakefulness cycle; signals muscles to become alert
Neuropeptides	Neuromodulators	Enhance, prolong, inhibit or limit the effects of principal neurotransmitters
Glutamate	Excitatory	Results in neurotoxicity if levels are too high
Gamma-aminobutyric acid (GABA)	Inhibitory	Modulates other neurotransmitters

emotional responses. Dopamine is generally excitatory and is synthesized from tyrosine, a dietary amino acid. Dopamine is implicated in schizophrenias and other psychotic disorders as well as in movement disorders such as Parkinson's disease. Antipsychotic medications work by blocking dopamine receptors and reducing dopamine activity.

NORADRENALINE AND ADRENALINE

Noradrenaline, the most prevalent neurotransmitter in the nervous system, is located primarily in the brain stem and plays a role in changes in attention, learning and memory, sleep and wakefulnes and mood regulation. Noradrenaline and its derivative, **adrenaline**, also are known as norepinephrine and epinephrine, respectively. Excess noradrenaline has been implicated in several anxiety disorders; deficits may contribute to memory loss, social withdrawal and depression. Some antidepressants block the reuptake of noradrenaline, whereas others inhibit MAO from metabolizing it. Adrenaline has limited distribution in the brain but controls the fight-or-flight response in the peripheral nervous system.

SEROTONIN

Serotonin, a neurotransmitter found only in the brain, is derived from tryptophan, a dietary amino acid. The function of serotonin is mostly inhibitory, and it is involved in the control of food intake, sleep and wakefulness, temperature regulation, pain control, sexual behaviour and regulation of emotions. Serotonin seems to play an important role in anxiety and mood disorders and the schizophrenias. It has been found to contribute to the delusions, hallucinations and withdrawn behaviour often seen in people diagnosed

with schizophrenia. Some antidepressants block serotonin reuptake, thus leaving it available longer in the synapse, which results in improved mood.

HISTAMINE

The role of histamine in mental health is under investigation. It is involved in peripheral allergic responses, control of gastric secretions, cardiac stimulation and alertness. Some psychotropic drugs block histamine, resulting in weight gain, sedation and hypotension.

ACETYLCHOLINE

Acetylcholine is a neurotransmitter found in the brain, spinal cord and peripheral nervous system, particularly at the neuromuscular junction of skeletal muscle. It can be excitatory or inhibitory. It is synthesized from dietary choline found in red meat and vegetables and has been found to affect the sleep-wake cycle and to signal muscles to become active. Studies have shown that people with Alzheimer's disease have decreased acetylcholine-secreting neurons, and people with myesthenia gravis (a muscular disorder in which impulses fail to pass the myoneural junction, which causes muscle weakness) have reduced acetylcholine receptors.

GLUTAMATE

Glutamate is an excitatory amino acid that at high levels can have major neurotoxic effects. Glutamate has been implicated in the brain damage caused by stroke, hypoglycaemia, sustained hypoxia or ischaemia, and some degenerative diseases such as Huntington's or Alzheimer's.

Table 3.2	BRAIN IMAGING TECHNOLOGY		
Procedure	**Imaging Method**	**Results**	**Duration**
Computed tomography (CT)	Serial X-rays of brain	Structural image	20–40 min
Magnetic resonance imaging (MRI)	Radio waves from brain detected from magnet	Structural image	45 min
Positron emission tomography (PET)	Radioactive tracer injected into bloodstream and monitored as client performs activities	Functional	2–3 h
Single photon emission computed tomography (SPECT)	Same as PET	Functional	1–2 h

GAMMA-AMINOBUTYRIC ACID

Gamma-aminobutyric acid (γ-aminobutyric acid, or GABA), an amino acid, is the major inhibitory neurotransmitter in the brain and has been found to modulate other neurotransmitter systems rather than to provide a direct stimulus (Plata-Salaman *et al.*, 2005). Drugs that increase GABA function, such as benzodiazepines, are used to treat anxiety and to induce sleep.

BRAIN IMAGING TECHNIQUES

At one time, the brain could be studied only through surgery or autopsy. During the past 25 years, however, several brain imaging techniques have been developed that now allow visualization of the brain's structure and function. These techniques are useful for diagnosing some disorders of the brain and have helped to correlate certain areas of the brain with specific functions. Brain imaging techniques are also useful in research to find the causes of mental disorders. **Computed tomography** (CT or 'CAT' scans), **magnetic resonance imaging (MRI)** and **positron emission tomography (PET)** are all examples of procedures intended to help us understand brain functioning (Table 3.2).

NEUROBIOLOGICAL CAUSES OF 'MENTAL ILLNESS'

Genetics and Heredity

Unlike many physical illnesses that have been found to be hereditary, such as cystic fibrosis, Huntington's disease and Duchenne's muscular dystrophy, the genetic origins of mental disorders do not seem to be straightforward. Current theories and studies indicate that several mental disorders may be linked to a specific gene or combination of genes but that the source is not solely genetic; non-genetic factors also play important roles.

To date, one of the most promising discoveries is the identification in 2007 of variations in the gene *SORL1* that may be a factor in late-onset Alzheimer's disease. Research

is continuing in an attempt to find genetic links to other 'diseases' such as the schizophrenias and mood disorders. This is the focus of ongoing research in the Human Genome Project, funded by the US National Institutes of Health (NIH) and the US Department of Energy. This international research project, started in 1988, is the largest of its kind. It has identified all human DNA and continues with research to discover the human characteristics and diseases each gene is related to (encodes). In addition, the project also addresses the ethical, legal and social implications of human genetics research. This programme (known as ELSI) focuses on privacy and fairness in the use and interpretation of genetic information, clinical integration of new genetic technologies, issues surrounding genetics research and professional and public education (National Institutes of Health, 2007). The researchers publish their results in the journal *Science;* further information can be obtained at www.genome.gov and at http://genome.wellcome.ac.uk

Three types of studies are commonly conducted to investigate the genetic basis of 'mental illness':

1. *Twin studies* are used to compare the rates of certain 'mental illnesses' or traits in monozygotic (identical) twins, who have an identical genetic make-up, and dizygotic (fraternal) twins, who have a different genetic make-up. Fraternal twins have the same genetic similarities and differences as non-twin siblings.
2. *Adoption studies* are used to determine a trait among biological versus adoptive family members.
3. *Family studies* are used to compare whether a trait is more common among first-degree relatives (parents, siblings, children) than among more distant relatives or the general population.

Although some genetic links have been found in certain mental disorders, studies have not shown that these illnesses are solely genetically linked. Investigation continues about the influence of inherited traits versus the influence of the environment – the 'nature versus nurture' debate. The influence of environmental or psychosocial factors is discussed in Chapter 2.

Stress and the Immune System (Psychoimmunology)

Researchers are following many avenues to discover possible causes of 'mental illness'. **Psychoimmunology**, a relatively new field of study, examines the effect of psychosocial stressors on the body's immune system. A compromised immune system could contribute to the development of a variety of illnesses, particularly in populations already genetically at risk. So far, efforts to link a specific stressor with a specific disease have been unsuccessful.

Infection as a Possible Cause

Some researchers are focusing on infection as a cause of 'mental illness'. Most studies involving viral theories have focused on 'schizophrenia', but so far none has provided specific or conclusive evidence. Theories that are being developed and tested include the existence of a virus that has an affinity for tissues of the CNS, the possibility that a virus may actually alter human genes and maternal exposure to a virus during critical foetal development of the nervous system.

Swedo and colleagues (2004) studied the relation of streptococcal bacteria and obsessive-compulsive disorder (OCD) and tics. They found enlarged basal ganglia, indicating a possible autoimmune response to streptococcal infection. When blood plasma (high in streptococcal antibodies) was replaced by transfusion with healthy donor plasma, the incidence of tics decreased by 50%, and other OCD symptoms were reduced by 60%. Studies such as this are promising in discovering a link between infection and some mental disorders.

THE NURSE'S ROLE IN RESEARCH AND EDUCATION

Amid all the reports of research in these areas of neurobiology, genetics and heredity, the implications for clients and their families are still not clear or specific. Often, reports in the media regarding new research and studies are confusing, contradictory or difficult for clients and their families to understand. The nurse must ensure that clients and families are well informed about progress in these areas and must also help them to distinguish between facts and hypotheses. The nurse can explain if or how new research may affect a client's treatment or prognosis. The nurse is, potentially, an excellent resource for exchanging information and answering questions.

PSYCHOPHARMACOLOGY

The Nurse's Role

The mental health nurse's role is vital in ensuring the effective, **collaborative** and **ethical prescribing**, administration and monitoring of pharmacological interventions in mental distress. As with all mental health nursing interventions, the three overlapping phases of rapport-building and *engagement*, the exchange of *information* and an agreed, negotiated plan of *action* are vital in ensuring that this aspect of care and treatment actually enhances people's lives. The nursing role is NOT merely about ensuring 'compliance' or 'concordance': it is about facilitating the informed, safe and person-centred use of psychopharmacology *when necessary and indicated by evidence*, and it is about integrating that use of medications in a wider package of care and treatment that takes its lead from *what the person wants*, not what the services want to provide.

Nurse Prescribing

Independent **nurse prescribing** remains controversial – both within and outside the profession – but has developed rapidly over the past few years. There are now well over 10,000 nurse prescribers practising in the UK, around 1% of whom work in mental health care (Snowden, 2006). Nurses who can prescribe are divided into two groups: 'independent' and 'supplementary' prescribers. At present all independent prescribers are either district nurses (DNs), health visitors (HVs) or practice nurses (PNs) with a DN/HV qualification. From 2007, all first-level nurses and

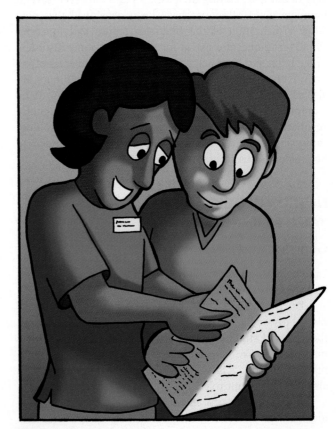

Keeping clients informed

midwives (including MHNs) were able to prepare to train to prescribe from a restricted formulary, although there is no validated training programme for this extended group as yet. Some mental health nurses are supplementary prescribers and are able – after thorough professional training and with ongoing support and supervision – to change the drug, dosage, frequency and timing of a patient's medication as agreed within a clinical management plan (CMP). This medication will have been prescribed initially by a GP or a psychiatrist.

Principles That Guide Pharmacological Treatment

The following are several principles that guide the use of medications to treat psychiatric disorders:

- A medication is selected based on its effect on the client's 'target symptoms', such as delusional thinking, panic attacks or hallucinations. The effectiveness of the medication is evaluated largely by its ability to diminish or eliminate the target symptoms.
- Many psychotropic drugs must be given in adequate dosages for some time before their full effect is realized. For example, tricyclic antidepressants can require 4 to 6 weeks before the client experiences optimal therapeutic benefit.
- The dosage of medication is often adjusted to the lowest effective dosage for the client. Sometimes a client may need higher dosages to stabilize his or her target symptoms, whereas lower dosages can be used to sustain those effects over time.
- As a rule, older adults require lower dosages of medications than do younger clients to experience therapeutic effects. It also may take longer for a drug to achieve its full therapeutic effect in older adults.
- Psychotropic medications are often decreased gradually (tapering) rather than abruptly. This is because of potential problems with **rebound** (temporary return of symptoms), recurrence of the original symptoms or **withdrawal** (new symptoms resulting from discontinuation of the drug).
- Follow-up care is essential to ensure 'concordance' with the medication regime, to make needed adjustments in dosage and to manage side-effects.
- Concordance with the medication regime is often enhanced when that regime is as simple as possible in terms of both the number of medications prescribed and the number of daily doses.

Regulation

The Medicines and Healthcare Products Regulatory Agency (MHRA) is the government agency responsible for ensuring that medicines and medical devices work and are 'acceptably safe'.

There are two ways that drugs can be licensed for use in the UK, either

- through the European Medicines Evaluation Agency (EMEA) (for Europe-wide licences); or
- through the MHRA (for UK-only licences).

According to the MHRA, 'There is widespread confusion between the roles of MHRA and NICE (the National Institute for Health and Clinical Excellence). MHRA is concerned about the relationships between benefits and risks; NICE is concerned, *inter alia*, about the relationships between benefits and costs'. 'As a considerable over-simplification', the MHRA says, 'a product can be sold while NICE says it can be bought [by the NHS]' (http://www.mhra.gov.uk/home/idcplg?IdcService=GET_FILE&dDocName=con2030689&RevisionSelectionMethod=Latest)

The MHRA or EMEA approves each drug for use in a particular population and for specific diseases. At times, a drug will prove effective for a disease that differs from the one involved in original testing and MHRA or EMEA approval. This is called **'off-label' use**. An example is some anticonvulsant drugs (approved to prevent seizures) that are prescribed for their effects in stabilizing the moods of clients with bipolar disorder The General Medical Council has produced Guidelines in Good Practice in Prescribing Medicines (2006) (http://www.gmc-uk.org/guidance/current/library/prescriptions_faqs.asp#5d) which ensure that off-label use is carried out safely and responsibly.

The Post Licensing Division of the MHRA monitors the occurrence and severity of drug side-effects. Spontaneous reports of adverse reactions are received from UK doctors under the voluntary 'Yellow Card' scheme. The physicians, pharmacists and scientists working in the Pharmacovigilance Group of the MHRA Post Licensing Division use data from Yellow Card reports to assess the causal relationship between the drugs and reported reactions, and to identify possible risk factors contributing to the occurrence of reactions, for example, age or underlying disease.

In the US, when a drug is found to have serious or life-threatening side-effects, even if such side-effects are rare, the Food and Drug Administration (FDA) may issue a black box warning. This means that package inserts must have a highlighted box, separate from the text, which contains a warning about the serious or life-threatening side-effect(s). The FDA – controversially – recently required a black box warning be placed on all antidepressant medications because of a fear of an increased suicide risk in children and adolescents.

Antipsychotic Drugs

Antipsychotic drugs, also known as *neuroleptics,* are used to treat the symptoms of psychosis, such as the delusions and hallucinations seen in some people diagnosed with schizophrenia, schizoaffective disorder and the manic phase of bipolar disorder. Off-label uses of antipsychotics include treatment of anxiety and insomnia; aggressive

Table 3.3   ANTIPSYCHOTIC DRUGS

Generic (Trade) Name	Routes	Normal Daily Dosage*	Maximum Dose (mg)
Conventional Antipsychotics			
Phenothiazines			
Chlorpromazine hydrochloride (Largactil)	O, IM	O 75–300, IM 25–50 every 6–8 h	1000
Levomepromazine hydrochloride (Nozinan)	O, IM	O 100–200, IM 25–50 every 6–8 h	1000
Promazine hydrochloride	O	O 400–800 as short-term adjunctive	800
Pericyazine (Neulactil)	O	O 75–300 and O 15–30 daily as short-term adjunctive	300
Pipotiazine (Piportil)	D	D 50–100 every 4 weeks	25 test dose; max. 200
Fluphenazine (Modecate)	D	D 12.5–100 every 2–4 weeks	12.5 test dose; max. 100
Perphenazine (Fentazin)	O	O 12	24
Prochlorperazine	O, IM	O 75–100, IM 12.5–25 tds	100
Trifluoperazine (Stelazine)	O	O 10–15	20+
Butyrophenones			
Benperidol (Anquil)	O	O 0.25–1.25	1.25
Haloperidol (Haldol, Dozic, Serenace)	O/IV/IM/D	O 3–30, IV/IM 2–10 every 4–8 h up to max 18 daily	30
Diphenylbutylpiperidines			
Pimozide (Orap)	O	O 2–20	20
Thioxanthenes			
Flupentixol (Depixol)	O, D	O 3–9, D 50 every 4 weeks to 300 every 2 weeks	Oral 18, D 400 weekly
Zuclopenthixol (Clopixol)	O, D	O 20–50, D 200–500 every 1–4 weeks	O 150, D 600 weekly
Substituted Benzamides			
Sulpiride (Dolmatil, Sulpor)	O	O 400–800	800 in predominantly negative symptoms; 2400 in predominantly positive symptoms
Atypical Antipsychotics			
Clozapine (Clozaril)**	O	200–450**	900**
Risperidone (Risperdal Consta)	O, D	O 4–6, D 25–37.5	O 16, D 50 every 2 weeks
Olanzapine (Zyprexa)	O	O 5–20	20
Quetiapine (Seroquel)	O	O 300–450	750
Amisulpride (Solian)	O	Acute episode: 400–800 Negative symptoms: 50–300	1200
Zotepine (Zoleptil)	O	75–300	300
Sertindole (Serdolect)	O	12–20	24
New-generation Antipsychotic			
Aripiprazole (Abilify)	O	10–15	30

O, Oral; IM, intramuscular injection (usually when required); D, IM depot injection; IV, intravenous injection. tds, three times daily.

*Values are mg/day for oral doses only; IM dosage in mg for working-age adults, doses adjusted in children or the elderly (see *British National Formulary* (BNF)).

** Note special warnings (p. 53).

Table adapted using British National Formulary (BNF) Online. (2008). http://www.bnf.org/bnf/bnf/55/

behaviour; and delusions, hallucinations and other disruptive behaviours that sometimes accompany Alzheimer's disease. Antipsychotic drugs work by blocking receptors of the neurotransmitter dopamine. They have been in clinical use since the 1950s. They are the primary medical treatment for schizophrenia and also are used in psychotic episodes of acute mania, psychotic depression and drug-induced psychosis. Clients with dementia who have psychotic symptoms sometimes respond to low dosages of conventional antipsychotics. Atypical antipsychotics can cause increased mortality rate in elderly clients with dementia-related psychosis. Short-term therapy with antipsychotics may be useful for transient psychotic symptoms such as those seen in some clients with borderline personality disorder.

Table 3.3 lists available dosage forms, usual daily oral dosages and extreme dosage ranges for conventional and atypical antipsychotic drugs. The low end of the extreme range typically is used with older adults or children with psychoses, aggression or extreme behaviour management problems.

MECHANISM OF ACTION

The major action of all antipsychotics in the nervous system is to block receptors for the neurotransmitter dopamine; however, the therapeutic mechanism of action is only partially understood. Dopamine receptors are classified into subcategories (D1, D2, D3, D4 and D5), and D2, D3 and D4 have been associated with mental illness. The typical antipsychotic drugs are potent antagonists (blockers) of D2, D3 and D4. This makes them effective in treating target symptoms but also produces many extrapyramidal side-effects (discussion to follow) because of the blocking of the D2 receptors. Newer, atypical antipsychotic drugs such as clozapine (Clozaril) are relatively weak blockers of D2, which may account for the lower incidence of extrapyramidal side-effects. In addition, atypical antipsychotics inhibit the reuptake of serotonin, as do some of the antidepressants, increasing their effectiveness in treating the depressive aspects of schizophrenia. Other 'atypicals' include amisulpride, aripiprazole, olanzapine, quetiapine, risperidone and zotepine.

Six antipsychotics are currently available for **depot injection,** a time-release form of medication for maintenance therapy and for clients whose 'concordance' with oral medication may be erratic. These are haloperidol (as decanoate) (Haldol), flupentixol decanoate (Depixol), fluphenazine decanoate (Modecate), zuclopenthixol decanoate (Clopixol) and pipotiazine palmitate (Piportil). The newest depot injection is risperidone (Risperdal Consta). Depot antipsychotics are administered by deep intramuscular injection into the gluteal muscle at intervals of 1 to 4 weeks.

Equivalent Doses of Depot Antipsychotics. These equivalences are intended only as an approximate guide; individual dosage instructions should also be checked; patients should be carefully monitored after any change in medication:
Important: these equivalences must not be extrapolated beyond the maximum dose for the drug.

Antipsychotic drug	Dose (mg)	Interval
Flupentixol decanoate	40	2 weeks
Fluphenazine decanoate	25	2 weeks
Haloperidol (as decanoate)	100	4 weeks
Pipotiazine palmitate	50	4 weeks
Zuclopenthixol decanoate	200	2 weeks

From British National Formulary (BNF) Online: http://www.bnf.org/bnf/bnf/current/3263.htm

WARNING ⬢

Elderly patients with dementia-related psychosis treated with atypical antipsychotic drugs are at an increased risk of death. Causes of death are varied, but most of the deaths appear to be either cardiovascular or infectious in nature.

SIDE-EFFECTS

Extrapyramidal Side-effects. **Extrapyramidal symptoms (EPS),** serious neurological symptoms, are the major side-effects of antipsychotic drugs. They include acute dystonia, pseudoparkinsonism and akathisia. Although often collectively referred to as EPS, each of these reactions has distinct features. One client can experience all the reactions in the same course of therapy, which makes distinguishing between them difficult. Blockade of D2 receptors in the midbrain region of the brain stem is responsible for the development of EPS. Conventional antipsychotic drugs cause a greater incidence of EPS than do atypical antipsychotic drugs (Daniel *et al.*, 2006).

Therapies for acute dystonia, pseudoparkinsonism and akathisia are similar and include lowering the dosage of the antipsychotic, changing to a different antipsychotic or administering anticholinergic medication (discussion to follow). Whereas anticholinergic drugs also produce side-effects, atypical antipsychotic medications are often prescribed because the incidence of EPS side-effects associated with them is decreased.

Acute **dystonia** includes acute muscular rigidity and cramping, a stiff or thick tongue with difficulty swallowing and, in severe cases, laryngospasm and respiratory difficulties. Dystonia is most likely to occur in the first week of treatment, in clients younger than 40 years, in males, and in those receiving high-potency drugs such as haloperidol, although it can occur as a result of taking a whole variety of neuroleptic medications, including antidepressants, anxiolytics and lithium. Spasms or stiffness in muscle groups can produce *torticollis* (twisted head and neck), *opisthotonus* (tightness in the entire body with the head back and an arched neck), or *oculogyric crisis* (eyes rolled back in a locked position). Acute dystonic reactions can be painful and frightening for the client. Immediate treatment with anticholinergic drugs, such as intramuscular benzatropine usually brings rapid relief.

Table 3.4 lists the drugs, their routes and dosages, used to treat EPS. The addition of a regularly scheduled oral anticholinergic such as benzatropine may allow the client to continue taking the antipsychotic drug with no further dystonia. Recurrent dystonic reactions would necessitate a lower dosage or a change in the antipsychotic drug. Assessment of EPS using the Simpson–Angus rating scale is discussed further in Chapter 14.

Drug-induced parkinsonism, or **pseudoparkinsonism,** is often referred to by the generic label of EPS. Symptoms resemble those of Parkinson's disease and include a stiff,

Table 3.4	COMMONLY USED DRUGS USED TO TREAT EXTRAPYRAMIDAL SIDE-EFFECTS	
Generic (Trade) Name	**Oral Dosages (mg)**	**IM/IV Doses (mg)**
Benzatropine mesilate (Cogentin)	N/A	1–2 (max. 6)
Orphenadrine hydrochloride (Biorphen, Disipal)	150–300 (max. 400)	N/A
Procyclidine (Arpicolin, Kemadrin)	7.5–30 (max. 30)	5–10 in acute dystonia
Trihexyphenidyl (Artane, Broflex)	5–15 (max. 20)	N/A

N/A, not applicable.

Table adapted using British National Formulary (BNF) Online. (2008). http://www.bnf.org/bnf/bnf/55/

stooped posture; mask-like facies; decreased arm swing; a shuffling, festinating gait (with small steps); cogwheel rigidity (ratchet-like movements of joints); drooling; tremor; bradycardia; and coarse pill-rolling movements of the thumb and fingers while at rest. Parkinsonism is treated by changing to an antipsychotic medication that has a lower incidence of EPS or by adding an oral antimuscarinic agent.

Akathisia is reported by the client as an intense need to move about. The client appears restless or anxious and agitated, often with a rigid posture or gait and a lack of spontaneous gestures. This feeling of internal restlessness and the

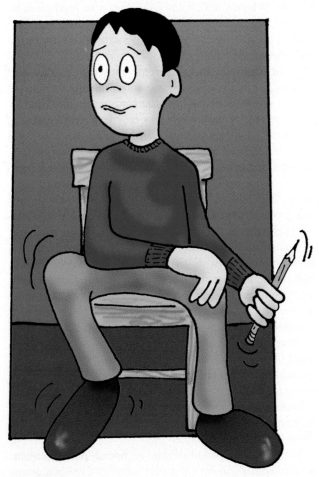

Akathisia

inability to sit still or rest often leads clients to discontinue their antipsychotic medication. Akathisia can be treated by a change in antipsychotic medication or by the addition of an oral agent such as a beta-blocker, anticholinergic or benzodiazepine.

Neuroleptic Malignant Syndrome. **Neuroleptic malignant syndrome (NMS)** is a potentially fatal idiosyncratic reaction to an antipsychotic (or neuroleptic) drug. Although the *DSM-IV-TR* (American Psychiatric Association, 2000) notes that the death rate from this syndrome has been reported at 10-20%, those figures may have resulted from biased reporting; the reported rates are now decreasing and, in the UK, while the exact incidence is difficult to calculate, it's estimated to range from 0.02 to 2.4% with conventional antipsychotics, with a much lower incidence for atypical antipsychotics (see http://www.patient.co.uk/ showdoc/40025090/). The major symptoms of NMS are rigidity; high fever; autonomic instability, such as unstable blood pressure, diaphoresis and pallor; delirium; and elevated levels of enzymes, particularly creatine phosphokinase. Clients with NMS usually are confused and often mute; they may fluctuate from agitation to stupor. All antipsychotics seem to have the potential to cause NMS, but high dosages of high-potency drugs increase the risk. NMS most often occurs in the first 2 weeks of therapy or after an increase in dosage, but it can occur at any time.

Dehydration, poor nutrition and concurrent medical illness all increase the risk for NMS. Treatment includes immediate discontinuation of all antipsychotic medications and the institution of supportive medical care to treat dehydration and hyperthermia until the client's physical condition stabilizes. After NMS, the decision to treat the client with other antipsychotic drugs requires full discussion between the client and the physician to weigh the relative risks against the potential benefits of therapy.

Tardive Dyskinesia. **Tardive dyskinesia (TD)**, a syndrome of permanent involuntary movements, is most commonly caused by the long-term use of conventional antipsychotic drugs. The pathophysiology is still not understood, and no effective treatment is available (Chouinard, 2004a). At least 20% of those treated with neuroleptics in the long term develop TD. The symptoms of TD include involuntary movements of the tongue, facial and neck muscles, upper and lower extremities, and truncal musculature. Tongue thrusting and protruding, lip smacking, blinking, grimacing and other excessive unnecessary facial movements are characteristic. After it has developed, TD is irreversible, although decreasing or discontinuing antipsychotic medications can arrest its progression. Unfortunately, antipsychotic medications can mask the beginning symptoms of TD, that is, increased dosages of the antipsychotic medication cause the initial symptoms to disappear temporarily. As the symptoms of TD worsen, however, they 'break through' the effect of the antipsychotic drug.

Preventing TD is one goal when administering antipsychotics. This can be done by keeping maintenance dosages as low as possible, changing medications and monitoring the client periodically for initial signs of TD using a standardized assessment tool such as the Abnormal Involuntary Movement Scale (see Chapter 14). Clients who have already developed signs of TD but still need to take an antipsychotic medication are often given one of the atypical antipsychotic drugs that have not yet been found to cause or, therefore, worsen TD.

Anticholinergic Side-effects. **Anticholinergic side-effects** often occur with the use of antipsychotics and include orthostatic hypotension, dry mouth, constipation, urinary hesitance or retention, blurred near vision, dry eyes, photophobia, nasal congestion and decreased memory. These side-effects usually decrease within 3 to 4 weeks but do not entirely remit. The client who is taking anticholinergic agents for EPS may have increased problems with anticholinergic side-effects. Using plenty of calorie-free drinks and fruit may alleviate dry mouth; stool softeners, adequate fluid intake, and the inclusion of grains and fruit in the diet may prevent constipation.

Other Side-effects. Antipsychotic drugs also increase blood prolactin levels. Elevated prolactin may cause breast enlargement and tenderness in men and women; diminished libido, erectile and orgasmic dysfunction, and menstrual irregularities; an increased risk for breast cancer; and may contribute to weight gain.

Weight gain can accompany most antipsychotic medications, but it is most likely with the atypical antipsychotic drugs. Weight increases are most significant with clozapine (Clozaril) and olanzapine (Zyprexa). Although the exact mechanism of this weight gain is unknown, it is associated with increased appetite, binge eating, carbohydrate craving, food preference changes and decreased satiety in some clients and a greater risk of hyperglycaemia and diabetes. In addition, clients with a genetic predisposition for weight gain seem to be at greater risk (Muller & Kennedy, 2006). Prolactin elevation may stimulate feeding centres, histamine antagonism stimulates appetite, and there may be an, as yet undetermined, interplay of multiple neurotransmitter and receptor interactions, with resultant changes in appetite, energy intake and feeding behaviour. Obesity is common in clients with schizophrenia, further increasing the risk for type 2 diabetes mellitus and cardiovascular disease (Newcomer & Haupt, 2006). In addition, clients with 'schizophrenia' are less likely to exercise or eat low-fat, nutritionally balanced diets; this pattern decreases the likelihood that they can minimize potential weight gain or lose excess weight. It is recommended that clients taking antipsychotics be involved in an educational programme to learn about healthy eating, exercise and maintaining the optimum weight for their individual circumstances.

Most antipsychotic drugs cause relatively minor cardiovascular adverse effects such as postural hypotension, palpitations and tachycardia. Some antipsychotic drugs, such as thioridazine (Melleril), have now been discontinued in the UK due to concerns over cardiac arrhythmias and the risk of sudden death.

Used with clients who have failed to respond to conventional antipsychotics, clozapine produces fewer traditional side-effects than do most antipsychotic drugs, but it has the potentially fatal side-effect of *agranulocytosis*. This develops suddenly and is characterized by fever, malaise, ulcerative sore throat and leucopenia. This side-effect may not be manifested immediately and can occur up to 24 weeks after the initiation of therapy. Leucocyte and differential blood counts must be normal before starting; monitor counts every week for 18 weeks then at least every 2 weeks and, if clozapine is continued and blood count stable after 1 year, at least every 4 weeks (and 4 weeks after discontinuation). If the leucocyte count is below 3000/mm³ or if the absolute neutrophil count is below 1500/mm³, Clozaril should be discontinued permanently and the client referred to a haematologist. Any interruption in therapy requires a return to more frequent monitoring for a specified period of time. Once clozapine has been discontinued, weekly monitoring of the white blood cell (WBC) count and absolute neutrophil count (ANC) is required for 4 weeks.

The educational and side-effect monitoring role of nurses is even more important with Clozaril than with other drugs.

WARNING ⬣ Clozapine

> May cause agranulocytosis, a potentially life-threatening event. Clients who are being treated with clozapine must have a baseline WBC count and differential before initiation of treatment and a WBC count every week throughout treatment and for 4 weeks after discontinuation of clozapine.

CLIENT INFORMATION

The nurse must inform clients taking antipsychotic medication about the intended benefits of the medication, the types of side-effect that may occur, weigh up with them possible benefits and problems and encourage clients to report any difficulties straight away, rather than discon-

Drug Alert!

PIMOZIDE

Following reports of sudden unexplained death, the Committee on Safety of Medicines (CSM) recommends electrocardiogram (ECG) before treatment. The CSM also recommends that patients on pimozide should have an annual ECG (if the QT interval is prolonged, treatment should be reviewed and either withdrawn or the dose reduced under close supervision) and that pimozide should not be given with other antipsychotic drugs (including depot preparations), tricyclic antidepressants or other drugs which prolong the QT interval, such as certain antimalarials, anti-arrhythmic drugs and certain antihistamines and should *not* be given with drugs that cause electrolyte disturbances (especially diuretics).

From British National Formulary (BNF) Online. (2008). http://www.bnf.org/bnf/bnf/56/3239.htm?q=%22pimozide%22#_hit

tinuing the medication. The nurse should teach the client methods of managing or avoiding unpleasant side-effects and maintaining the medication regime. Drinking sugar-free fluids and eating fruit can ease a dry mouth. The client should avoid calorie-laden drinks and sweets because they promote dental caries, contribute to weight gain and do little to relieve dry mouth. Methods to prevent or relieve constipation include exercising and increasing water and bulk-forming foods in the diet. Stool softeners are permissible, but the client should avoid laxatives. The use of sunscreen is recommended because photosensitivity can cause the client to sunburn easily.

Clients should monitor the amount of sleepiness or drowsiness they feel. They should avoid driving and performing other potentially dangerous activities until their response times and reflexes seem normal.

If the client forgets a dose of antipsychotic medication, he or she can take the missed dose if it is only 3 or 4 hours late. If the dose is more than 4 hours overdue or the next dose is due, the client can omit the forgotten dose. The nurse should encourage clients who have difficulty remembering to take their medication to use a chart and to record doses when taken or to use a 'Dossett box' or pillbox that can be prefilled with accurate doses for the day or week.

Antidepressant Drugs

Antidepressant drugs are primarily used in the treatment of major depressive illness, anxiety disorders, the depressed phase of bipolar disorder and psychotic depression. Off-label uses of antidepressants include the treatment of chronic pain, migraine headaches, peripheral and diabetic

neuropathies, sleep apnoea, dermatological disorders, panic disorder and eating disorders. Although the mechanism of action is not completely understood, antidepressants somehow interact with the two neurotransmitters, noradrenaline and serotonin, that regulate mood, arousal, attention, sensory processing and appetite.

In a large review of drug trial data, Kirsch *et al.* (2008) found little difference between placebos and selective serotonin reuptake inhibitor (SSRI) antidepressants in all but the most severely depressed patients: given these findings, health professionals need to be extremely wary about their use, given the possibilities of increased suicide risk and unpleasant side-effects. Nevertheless, many people believe that antidepressant medication has saved their lives and had a hugely positive outcome; nurses should stay aware of research and be prepared to support clients in understanding its implications (which include the inadvisability of rapidly coming off prescribed medication).

Antidepressants are divided into four groups:

1. *Tricyclic* and the related *cyclic* antidepressants, such as amitriptyline, clomipramine (Anafranil), dosulepin (Prothiaden), doxepin (Sinepin), imipramine, lofepramine, nortriptyline (Allegron), trimipramine (Surmontil), and trazadone (Molipaxin) and mianserin
2. *Selective serotonin reuptake inhibitors* (SSRIs) such as citalopram (Cipramil), escitalopram (Cipralex), fluoxetine (Prozac), fluvoxamine (Faverin), paroxetine (Seroxat) and sertraline (Lustral)
3. *MAO inhibitors* (MAOIs) such as phenelzine (Nardil), isocarboxazid, tranylcypromine and moclobamide (Manerix)
4. Other antidepressants such as duloxetine (Cymbalta), flupentixol (Fluanxol), mirtazapine (Zispin), reboxetine (Edronax), tryptophan (Optimax) and venlafaxine (Efexor).

Table 3.5 lists the usual daily dosages, and maximum daily dosages of the key antidepressants used in the UK.

The cyclic compounds became available in the 1950s and for years were the first choice of drugs to treat depression, even though they cause varying degrees of sedation, orthostatic hypotension (drop in blood pressure on rising) and anticholinergic side-effects. In addition, cyclic antidepressants are potentially lethal if taken in an overdose.

During that same period, the MAOIs were discovered to have positive effects for people with depression. Although the MAOIs have a low incidence of sedation and anticholinergic effects, and are particularly effective for people with phobias and depressed people with atypical, hypochondriacal or hysterical features, they must be used with extreme caution for several reasons:

• A life-threatening side-effect, hypertensive crisis, may occur if the client ingests foods containing tyramine (an amino acid) while taking MAOIs.

Table 3.5   ANTIDEPRESSANT DRUGS

Generic (Trade) Name	Usual Daily Dosages* (as antidepressant: doses different if used for anxiety)	Maximum Dosage (mg)
SSRIs		
Fluoxetine (Prozac)	20	20–60
Fluvoxamine (Faverin)	100	300
Paroxetine (Seroxat)	20	50
Sertraline (Lustral)	50	200
Citalopram (Cipramil)	20	60
Escitalopram (Cipralex)	10	20
Tricyclics		
Amitriptyline	75–100	150
Clomipramine (Anafranil)	30–150	250
Dosulepin (Prothiaden)	75	150
Doxepin (Sinepin)	30–300	300
Imipramine	150–200	200
Lofepramine	14–210	210
Nortriptyline (Allegron)	75–100	150
Trimipramine (Surmontil)	150–300	300
Tricyclic Related		
Mianserin	30–90	90
Trazodone (Molipaxin)	150	300
Other Antidepressants		
Venlafaxine (Efexor)	75–150	375
Reboxetine (Edronax)	8–10	12
Mirtazapine (Zispin)	15–45	45
Duloxetine (Cymbalta, Yentreve)	60	60
Tryptophan (Optimax)	3000	6000
MAOIs		
Phenelzine (Nardil)	45–60 (reduced gradually to lowest possible maintenance dose; 15 mg on alternate days may be adequate)	60 (reduced gradually to lowest possible maintenance dose; 15 mg on alternate days may be adequate)
Tranylcypromine	10	30
Isocarboxazid	10–20	40
Moclobamide	150–600	600

*Values are mg/day.

Table adapted using British National Formulary (BNF) Online. (2008). http://www.bnf.org/bnf/bnf/55/

- Because of the risk for potentially fatal drug interactions, MAOIs cannot be given in combination with other MAOIs, tricyclic antidepressants pethidine, CNS depressants, many antihypertensives or general anaesthetics.
- MAOIs are potentially lethal in overdose and pose a potential risk in clients with depression who may be considering suicide.

The SSRIs, first available in 1987 with the release of fluoxetine (Prozac), have replaced the cyclic drugs as the first choice in treating depression because they are equal in efficacy and produce fewer troublesome side-effects; the SSRIs are also less cardiotoxic in overdose. They are therefore preferred where there is a significant suicide risk. The SSRIs do, however, have significant side-effects of their own, which may cause people difficulty in continuing to take them: nausea and vomiting, in particular, are common. Venlafaxine, at a dose of at least 150 mg may also be more effective than SSRIs for major depression.

The **efficacy** of antidepressants is increasingly debated. Kirsch *et al.* (2008), in their groundbreaking meta-analysis, found that only in a very small group of severely depressed patients were SSRI antidepressants more effective than placebos, and that drug companies' interpretations of the results of clinical trials were distorted.

PREFERRED DRUGS FOR CLIENTS AT HIGH RISK FOR SUICIDE

Suicide is always a primary consideration when treating clients with depression. SSRIs, venlafaxine and bupropion may appear to be better choices for those who are potentially suicidal or highly impulsive, because they carry no risk of lethal overdose, in contrast to the cyclic compounds and the MAOIs. However, SSRIs are only effective for mild and moderate depression. Evaluation of the risk for suicide must continue even after treatment with antidepressants is initiated. The client may feel more energized but still have suicidal thoughts, which increase the likelihood of a suicide attempt. Also, because it often takes weeks before the medications have a full therapeutic effect, clients may become discouraged and tire of waiting to feel better, which can result in suicidal behaviour. In the US, there is an FDA-required warning for SSRIs.

MECHANISM OF ACTION

The precise mechanism by which antidepressants produce their therapeutic effects is not known, but much is known about their action on the CNS. The major interaction is with the monoamine neurotransmitter systems in the brain, particularly noradrenaline and serotonin. Both of these neurotransmitters are released throughout the brain and help to regulate arousal, vigilance, attention, mood, sensory processing and appetite. Noradrenaline, serotonin and dopamine are removed from the synapses after release, by reuptake into presynaptic neurons. After reuptake, these three neurotransmitters are reloaded for subsequent release or metabolized by the enzyme MAO. The SSRIs block the reuptake of serotonin; the cyclic antidepressants and venlafaxine block the reuptake of noradrenaline primarily and block serotonin to some degree; and the MAOIs interfere with enzyme metabolism. This is not the complete explanation, however; the blockade of serotonin and noradrenaline reuptake and the inhibition of MAO occur in a matter of hours, whereas antidepressants are rarely effective until taken for several weeks. The cyclic compounds may take 4 to 6 weeks to be effective; MAOIs need 2 to 4 weeks for effectiveness; and SSRIs may be effective in 2 to 3 weeks. Researchers believe that the actions of these drugs are an 'initiating event' and that eventual therapeutic effectiveness results when neurons respond more slowly, making serotonin available at the synapses (Lehne, 2006).

SIDE-EFFECTS OF SELECTIVE SEROTONIN REUPTAKE INHIBITORS

SSRIs have fewer side-effects compared with the cyclic compounds. Enhanced serotonin transmission can lead to several common side-effects such as anxiety, agitation, akathisia (motor restlessness), nausea, insomnia and sexual dysfunction, specifically diminished sexual drive or difficulty achieving an erection or orgasm. In addition, weight gain is both an initial and ongoing problem during antidepressant therapy, although SSRIs cause less weight gain than other

Drug Alert!

CSM WARNING

CSM advice: depressive illness in children and adolescents

The CSM has advised that the balance of risks and benefits for the treatment of depressive illness in individuals under 18 years of age is considered unfavourable for the SSRIs citalopram, escitalopram, paroxetine and sertraline, and for mirtazapine and venlafaxine. Clinical trials have failed to show efficacy and have shown an increase in harmful outcomes. However, it is recognized that specialists may sometimes decide to use these drugs in response to individual clinical need; children and adolescents should be monitored carefully for suicidal behaviour, self-harm or hostility, particularly at the beginning of treatment.

Only fluoxetine has been shown in clinical trials to be effective for treating depressive illness in children and adolescents. However, it is possible that, in common with the other SSRIs, it is associated with a small risk of self-harm and suicidal thoughts. Overall, the balance of risks and benefits for fluoxetine in the treatment of depressive illness in individuals under 18 years of age is considered favourable, but children and adolescents must be carefully monitored as above.

From British National Formulary (BNF) Online. (2008). http://www.bnf.org/bnf/bnf/55/3351.htm?q=%22ssri%22#_hit

antidepressants. Taking medications with food usually can minimize nausea. Akathisia is usually treated with a beta-blocker such as propranolol (Inderal) or a benzodiazepine. Insomnia may continue to be a problem even if the client takes the medication in the morning; a sedative-hypnotic or low-dosage trazodone may be needed.

Less common side-effects include sedation (particularly with paroxetine (Seroxat)), sweating, diarrhoea, hand tremor and headaches. Diarrhoea and headaches usually can be managed with symptomatic treatment. Sweating and continued sedation most likely indicate the need for a change to another antidepressant.

SIDE-EFFECTS OF CYCLIC ANTIDEPRESSANTS

Cyclic compounds have more side-effects than do SSRIs and the newer miscellaneous compounds. The individual medications in this category vary in terms of the intensity of side-effects, but generally side-effects fall into the same

Box 3.1   FOODS (CONTAINING TYRAMINE) TO AVOID WHEN TAKING MAOIs

- Mature or aged cheeses or dishes made with cheese, such as lasagna or pizza. All cheese is considered aged except cottage cheese, cream cheese, ricotta cheese and processed cheese slices
- Aged meats such as pepperoni, salami, mortadella, summer sausage, beef logs, meat extracts and similar products. Make sure meat and chicken are fresh and have been properly refrigerated
- Italian broad beans (fava), bean curd (tofu), banana peel, overripe fruit, avocado

- All tap beers and microbrewery beer. Drink no more than two cans or bottles of beer (including non-alcoholic beer) or 4 ounces of wine per day
- Sauerkraut, soy sauce or soybean condiments, or marmite (concentrated yeast)
- Yogurt, sour cream, peanuts, Brewer's yeast, monosodium glutamate (MSG)

categories. The cyclic antidepressants block cholinergic receptors, resulting in anticholinergic effects such as dry mouth, constipation, urinary hesitancy or retention, dry nasal passages and blurred near vision. More severe anticholinergic effects, such as agitation, delirium and ileus, may occur, particularly in older adults. Other common side-effects include orthostatic hypotension, sedation, weight gain and tachycardia. Clients may develop tolerance to anticholinergic effects, but these side-effects are common reasons why clients discontinue drug therapy. Clients taking cyclic compounds frequently report sexual dysfunction similar to problems experienced with SSRIs.

Weight gain, tiredness and sexual dysfunction are cited as common reasons for non-concordance, which is high – perhaps higher than 50% – in people who take antidepressants (Hitt, 2003; Ashton *et al.*, 2005). It also seems essential that prescribers and other professionals understand and explore people's expectations, fears and hopes from the prescription (Ashton *et al.*, 2005).

SIDE-EFFECTS OF MONOAMINE OXIDASE INHIBITORS

The most common side-effects of MAOIs include daytime sedation, insomnia, weight gain, dry mouth, orthostatic hypotension and sexual dysfunction. The sedation and insomnia are difficult to treat and may necessitate a change in medication. Of particular concern with MAOIs is the potential for a life-threatening hypertensive crisis if the client ingests food that contains tyramine or takes sympathomimetic drugs. Because the enzyme MAO is necessary to break down the tyramine in certain foods, its inhibition results in increased serum tyramine levels, causing severe hypertension, hyperpyrexia, tachycardia, diaphoresis, tremulousness and cardiac dysrhythmias. Drugs that may cause potentially fatal interactions with MAOIs include SSRIs, certain cyclic compounds, buspirone (Buspar), dextromethorphan and opiate derivatives such as pethidine. An early warning symptom of a harmful interaction may be a throbbing headache. The client must be able to follow a tyramine-free diet;

Box 3.1 lists the foods to avoid. Studies are currently under way to determine whether a selegiline transdermal patch would be effective in treating depression without the risks of dietary tyramine and orally ingested MAOIs.

SIDE-EFFECTS OF OTHER ANTIDEPRESSANTS

Of the other or novel antidepressant medications, trazodone and mirtazapine commonly cause sedation, and trazodone commonly causes headaches. Reboxetine and venlafaxine may cause loss of appetite, nausea, agitation and insomnia. Venlafaxine may also cause dizziness, sweating or sedation. Sexual dysfunction is much less common with the novel antidepressants, with one notable exception: Trazodone can cause priapism (a sustained and painful erection that necessitates immediate treatment and discontinuation of the drug). Priapism may also result in impotence.

DRUG INTERACTIONS

An uncommon but potentially serious drug interaction, called **serotonin** or serotonergic **syndrome**, can result from taking an MAOI and an SSRI at the same time. It also can occur if the client takes one of these drugs too close to the end of therapy with the other. In other words, one drug must clear the person's system before initiation of therapy with the other. Symptoms include agitation, sweating, fever, tachycardia, hypotension, rigidity, hyperreflexia and, in extreme reactions, even coma and death (Krishnan, 2006). These symptoms are similar to those seen with an SSRI overdose.

CLIENT INFORMATION

Clients should take SSRIs first thing in the morning unless sedation is a problem; generally paroxetine most often causes sedation. If the client forgets a dose of an SSRI, he or she can take it up to 8 hours after the missed dose. To minimize side-effects, clients generally should take cyclic compounds at night in a single daily dose when possible. If the client forgets a dose of a cyclic compound, he or she should take it within 3 hours of the missed dose or omit the dose for that day. Clients should exercise caution when driving or performing activities requiring sharp, alert reflexes until sedative effects can be determined.

Clients taking MAOIs need to be aware that a life-threatening hyperadrenergic crisis can occur if they do not observe certain dietary restrictions. They should receive a written list of foods to avoid while taking MAOIs. The nurse should make clients aware of the risk for serious or even fatal drug interactions when taking MAOIs and instruct them not to take any additional medication, including over-the-counter preparations, without checking with the physician or pharmacist.

Mood-Stabilizing Drugs

Mood-stabilizing drugs are used to treat bipolar disorder by stabilizing the client's mood, preventing or minimizing the highs and lows that characterize bipolar illness and treating acute episodes of mania. Lithium is the most established mood stabilizer; some anticonvulsant drugs, particularly carbamazepine (Tegretol) and valproic acid (Depakote, Depakene), are effective mood stabilizers.

MECHANISM OF ACTION

Although lithium has many neurobiological effects, its mechanism of action in bipolar illness is poorly understood. Lithium normalizes the reuptake of certain neurotransmitters such as serotonin, noradrenaline, acetylcholine and dopamine. It also reduces the release of noradrenaline through competition with calcium. Lithium produces its effects intracellularly rather than within neuronal synapses; it acts directly on G proteins and certain enzyme subsystems such as cyclic adenosine monophosphates and phosphatidylinositol. Lithium is considered a first-line agent in the treatment of bipolar disorder (Bauer & Mitchner, 2004).

The mechanism of action for anticonvulsants is not clear as it relates to their off-label use as mood stabilizers. Valproic acid and topiramate are known to increase levels of the inhibitory neurotransmitter GABA. Both valproic acid and carbamazepine are thought to stabilize mood by inhibiting the **kindling process**. This can be described as the snowball-like effect seen when minor seizure activity seems to build up into more frequent and severe seizures. In seizure management, anticonvulsants raise the level of the threshold to prevent these minor seizures. It is suspected that this same kindling process also may occur in the development of full-blown mania with stimulation by more frequent, minor episodes. This may explain why anticonvulsants are effective in the treatment and prevention of mania as well (Plata-Salaman *et al.*, 2005).

DOSAGE

Lithium is available in tablets, capsules, liquid and a sustained-released form; no parenteral forms are available. The effective dosage of lithium is determined by monitoring serum lithium levels and assessing the client's clinical response to the drug. Daily dosages generally range from 900 to 3600 mg; more importantly, the serum lithium level should be about 1.0 mmol/l. Serum lithium levels of less than 0.5 mmol/l are rarely therapeutic, and levels of more than 1.5 mmol/l are usually considered toxic. The lithium level should be monitored every 2 to 3 days while the therapeutic dosage is being determined; then, it should be monitored weekly. When the client's condition is stable, the level may need to be checked once a month or less frequently. Overdosage, usually with serum lithium concentration of over 1.5 mmol/l, may be fatal and toxic effects include tremor, ataxia, dysarthria, nystagmus, renal impairment and convulsions

WARNING ⬡ Lithium

> Toxicity is closely related to serum lithium levels and can occur at therapeutic doses. Facilities for serum lithium determinations are required to monitor therapy.

Carbamazepine is available in liquid, tablet and chewable tablet forms. Dosages usually range from 800 to 1200 mg/day; the extreme dosage range is 200 to 2000 mg/day. Valproic acid is available in liquid, tablet and capsule forms and as sprinkles, with dosages ranging from 1000 to 1500 mg/day; the extreme dosage range is 750 to 3000 mg/day. Serum drug levels, obtained 12 hours after the last dose of the medication, are monitored for therapeutic levels of both these anticonvulsants.

SIDE-EFFECTS

Common side-effects of lithium therapy include mild nausea or diarrhoea, anorexia, fine hand tremor, polydipsia, polyuria, a metallic taste in the mouth and fatigue or lethargy. Weight gain and acne are side-effects that occur later in lithium therapy; both are distressing for clients. Taking the medication with food may help with nausea, and the use of propranolol often improves the fine tremor. Lethargy and weight gain are difficult to manage or minimize, and frequently lead to non-concordance.

Toxic effects of lithium are severe diarrhoea, vomiting, drowsiness, muscle weakness and lack of co-ordination. Untreated, these symptoms worsen and can lead to renal failure, coma and death. When toxic signs occur, the drug should be discontinued immediately. If lithium levels exceed 3.0 mmol/l, dialysis may be indicated.

Side-effects of carbamazepine and valproic acid include drowsiness, sedation, dry mouth and blurred vision. In addition, carbamazepine may cause rashes and orthostatic hypotension, and valproic acid may cause weight gain, alopecia and hand tremor. Topiramate causes dizziness, sedation, weight loss (rather than gain) and increased incidence of renal calculi (Bauer & Mitchner, 2004).

WARNING ⬣ Valproic Acid and its Derivatives

Can cause hepatic failure, resulting in fatality. Liver function tests should be performed before therapy and at frequent intervals thereafter, especially for the first 6 months. Can produce teratogenic effects such as neural tube defects (e.g. spina bifida). Can cause life-threatening pancreatitis in both children and adults. Can occur shortly after initiation or after years of therapy.

WARNING ⬣ Carbamazepine

Can cause aplastic anaemia and agranulocytosis at a rate five to eight times greater than in the general population. Pretreatment haematological baseline data should be obtained and monitored periodically throughout therapy to discover lowered WBC or platelet counts.

WARNING ⬣ Lamotrigine

Can cause serious rashes requiring hospitalization, including Stevens-Johnson syndrome and, rarely, life-threatening toxic epidermal necrolysis. The risk for serious rashes is greater in children younger than 16 years.

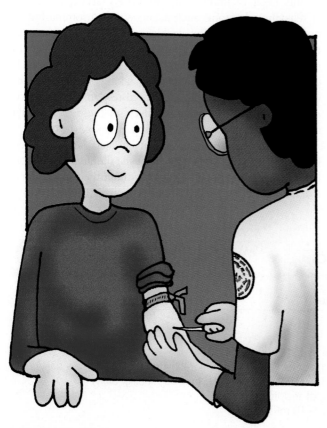

Periodic blood levels

CLIENT INFORMATION

For clients taking lithium and the anticonvulsants, monitoring blood levels periodically is important. The time of the last dose must be accurate so that plasma levels can be checked 12 hours after the last dose has been taken. Taking these medications with meals minimizes nausea. The client should not attempt to drive until dizziness, lethargy, fatigue or blurred vision has subsided.

Anti-anxiety Drugs (Anxiolytics)

Anti-anxiety drugs, or **anxiolytic drugs**, are used to treat anxiety and anxiety disorders, insomnia, OCD, depression, posttraumatic stress disorder (PTSD) and alcohol withdrawal. Anti-anxiety drugs are among the most widely prescribed medications today. A wide variety of drugs from different classifications have been used in the treatment of anxiety and insomnia. Benzodiazepines such as diazepam, alprazolam, chlordiazepoxide, lorazepam and oxazepam have proved to be the most effective in relieving anxiety and are the drugs most frequently prescribed, but should only be used for the short-term relief of moderate or severe (not mild) anxiety symptoms due to the risk of dependence and difficult withdrawal. They may also be prescribed for their anticonvulsant and muscle relaxant effects. Buspirone is a non-benzodiazepine often used for the relief of anxiety and therefore is included in this section.

MECHANISM OF ACTION

Benzodiazepines mediate the actions of the amino acid GABA, the major inhibitory neurotransmitter in the brain. Because GABA receptor channels selectively admit the anion chloride into neurons, activation of GABA receptors hyperpolarizes neurons and thus is inhibitory. Benzodiazepines produce their effects by binding to a specific site on the GABA receptor. Buspirone is believed to exert its anxiolytic effect by acting as a partial agonist at serotonin receptors, which decreases serotonin turnover (Chouinard, 2004b).

The benzodiazepines vary in terms of their half-lives, the means by which they are metabolized and their effectiveness in treating anxiety and insomnia. Table 3.6 lists dosages, half-lives and speed of onset after a single dose. Drugs with a longer **half-life** require less frequent dosing and produce fewer rebound effects between doses; however, they can accumulate in the body and produce 'next-day sedation' effects. Conversely, drugs with a shorter half-life do not accumulate in the body or cause next-day sedation, but they do have rebound effects and require more frequent dosing.

Benzodiazepines such as nitrazepam, flurazepam, loprazolam, lormetazepam and temazepam are also used as 'hypnotics', to help people sleep, though they should only be used once the cause of insomnia is clear and underlying factors (such as stress, alcohol, diet, unreasonable expectations of sleep) have been tackled. Other hypnotics include

Table 3.6 — ANTIANXIETY (ANXIOLYTIC) DRUGS

Generic (Trade) Name	Daily Dosage Range	Half-life (h)	Speed of Onset
Benzodiazepines			
Alprazolam (Xanax)	250–500 mcg (max. 3 mg)	12–15	Intermediate
Chlordiazepoxide (Librium)	30–100 mg (max. 100)	50–100	Intermediate
Diazepam (Valium)	6–30 mg (max. 30)	30–100	Very fast
Lorazepam (Ativan)	1–4 mg (max. 4)	10–20	Moderately slow
Oxazepam (Serax)	45–120 mg (max. 120)	3–21	Moderately slow
Non-benzodiazepine			
Buspirone (Buspar)	15–30 mg (max. 45)	3–11	Very slow

Table adapted using British National Formulary (BNF) Online. (2008). http://www.bnf.org/bnf/bnf/55/

zaleplon, zolpidem and zopiclone (see Table 3.7). Diazepam (Valium), chlordiazepoxide (Librium) and clonazepam are often used to manage alcohol withdrawal as well as to relieve anxiety.

SIDE-EFFECTS

Although not a side-effect in the true sense, one chief problem encountered with the use of benzodiazepines is their tendency to cause physical dependence. Significant discontinuation symptoms occur when the drug is stopped; these symptoms often resemble the original symptoms for which the client sought treatment. This is especially a problem for clients with long-term benzodiazepine use, such as those with panic disorder or generalized anxiety disorder. Psychological dependence on benzodiazepines is common: clients fear the return of anxiety symptoms or believe they are incapable of handling anxiety without the drugs. This can lead to overuse or abuse of these drugs. Buspirone does not cause this type of physical dependence.

The side-effects most commonly reported with benzodiazepines are those associated with CNS depression, such as drowsiness, sedation, poor co-ordination and impaired memory or clouded perceptions. When used for sleep, clients may complain of next-day sedation or a hangover effect. Clients often develop a tolerance to these symptoms, and they generally decrease in intensity. Common side-effects from buspirone include dizziness, sedation, nausea and headache (Chouinard, 2004b).

Elderly clients may have more difficulty managing the effects of CNS depression. They may be more prone to falls from the effects on co-ordination and sedation. They also may have more pronounced memory deficits and may have problems with urinary incontinence, particularly at night.

CLIENT INFORMATION

Clients need to know that anti-anxiety agents are aimed at relieving symptoms such as anxiety or insomnia but do not treat the underlying problems that cause the anxiety. Benzodiazepines strongly potentiate the effects of alcohol: one drink may have the effect of three drinks. Therefore, clients should not drink alcohol while taking benzodiazepines. Clients should be aware of decreased response time, slower reflexes and possible sedative effects of these drugs when attempting activities such as driving or going to work.

Benzodiazepine withdrawal can be fatal. After the client has started a course of therapy, he or she should never discontinue benzodiazepines abruptly or without the supervision of a doctor and other health-care professionals (Lehne, 2006).

Table 3.7 — NON-BENZODIAZEPINE HYPNOTICS

Generic (Trade) Name	Normal Dosage
Zolpidem tartrate (Stilnoct)	10 mg
Zopiclone (Zimovane)	7.5 mg
Chloral hydrate (as mixture)	5–20 ml (chloral hydrate 500 mg/5 ml)
Cloral betaine (as tablets: Welldorm)	1–2 tablets (each containing 414 mg chloral hydrate: max 5 tablets daily)
Cloral betaine (as Welldorm elixir)	15–45 ml (0.4–1.3 g of chloral hydrate: max 35 ml (1 g) daily)
Triclofos sodium (as elixir)	10–20 ml (1–2 g of triclofos sodium)
Clomethiazole (Heminevrin)	1–2 capsules (or 5–10 ml syrup)

Table adapted using British National Formulary (BNF) Online. (2008). http://www.bnf.org/bnf/bnf/55/

Stimulants

Stimulant drugs, specifically amphetamines, were first used for their pronounced effects of CNS stimulation to treat psychiatric disorders in the 1930s. In the past, they were used to treat depression and obesity, but those uses are uncommon in current practice. Dexamfetamine (Dexedrine) has been widely abused to produce a high or to remain awake for long periods. Today, the primary use of stimulants is for ADHD in children and adolescents, residual attention deficit disorder in adults, and narcolepsy (attacks of unwanted but irresistible daytime sleepiness that disrupt the person's life).

Methylphenidate and atomoxetine are used for the management of ADHD in children and adolescents as part of a comprehensive treatment programme. Growth is not generally affected but it is advisable to monitor growth during treatment. Dexamfetamine (dexamphetamine) is an alternative for children who do not respond to other drugs (British National Formulary, 2008)

MECHANISM OF ACTION

Amphetamines and methylphenidate are often termed *indirectly acting amines* because they act by causing release of the neurotransmitters (noradrenaline, dopamine and serotonin) from presynaptic nerve terminals, as opposed to having direct agonist effects on the postsynaptic receptors. They also block the reuptake of these neurotransmitters. Methylphenidate produces milder CNS stimulation than amphetamines. It was originally thought that the use of methylphenidate and amphetamines to treat ADHD in children produced the reverse effect of most stimulants – a calming or slowing of activity in the brain. However, this is not the case; the inhibitory centres in the brain are stimulated so the child has greater abilities to filter out distractions and manage his or her own behaviour. Atomoxetine helps to block the reuptake of noradrenaline into neurons, thereby leaving more of the neurotransmitter in the synapse to help convey electrical impulses to the brain.

WARNING ⬡ Amphetamines

Potential for abuse is high. Administration for prolonged periods may lead to drug dependence.

DOSAGE

For the treatment of narcolepsy in adults, both dexamfetamine and methylphenidate are given in divided doses totalling 20 to 200 mg/day. The higher dosages may be needed because adults with narcolepsy develop tolerance to the stimulants and so require more medication to sustain improvement. Stimulant medications are also available in sustained-release preparations so that once-a-day dosing is possible. Tolerance is not seen in people with ADHD.

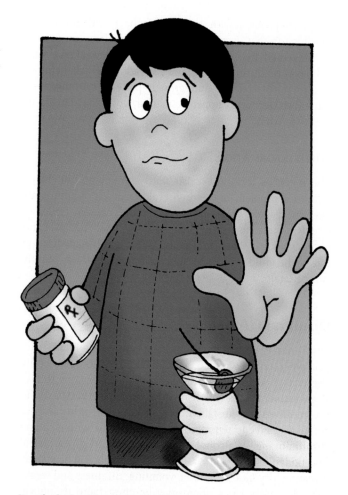

No alcohol with psychotropic drugs

WARNING ⬤ Methylphenidate

Use with caution in emotionally unstable clients, such as those with alcohol or drug dependence, because these clients may increase the dosage on their own. Chronic abuse can lead to marked tolerance and psychological dependence.

The dosages used to treat ADHD in children vary widely, depending on the physician; the age, weight and behaviour of the child; and the tolerance of the family for the child's behaviour. Table 20.1 lists the usual dosage ranges for these stimulants. Arrangements must be made for the school nurse or another authorized adult to administer the stimulants to the child at school. Sustained-released preparations eliminate the need for additional dosing at school.

SIDE-EFFECTS

The most common side-effects of stimulants are anorexia, weight loss, nausea and irritability. The client should avoid caffeine, sugar and chocolate, which may worsen these symptoms. Less common side-effects include dizziness, dry mouth, blurred vision and palpitations. The most common long-term problem with stimulants is the growth and weight suppression that occurs in some children. This can usually be prevented by taking 'drug holidays' on weekends and holidays, or during the summer vacation, which helps to restore normal eating and growth patterns. Atomoxetine can cause decreased appetite, nausea, vomiting, fatigue or upset stomach.

CLIENT INFORMATION

The potential for abuse exists with stimulants, but this is seldom a problem in children. Taking doses of stimulants after meals may minimize anorexia and nausea. Caffeine-free drinks are suggested; clients should avoid chocolate and excessive sugar. Most important is to keep the medication out of the child's reach because as little as a 10-day supply can be fatal.

Disulfiram (Antabuse)

Disulfiram is a sensitizing agent that causes an adverse reaction when mixed with alcohol in the body. This agent's only use is as a deterrent to drinking alcohol in persons receiving treatment for alcoholism. It is useful for persons who are motivated to abstain from drinking and who are not impulsive. Five to ten minutes after someone who is taking disulfiram ingests alcohol, symptoms begin to appear: facial and body flushing from vasodilation, a throbbing headache, sweating, dry mouth, nausea, vomiting, dizziness and weakness. In severe cases, there may be chest pain, dyspnoea, severe hypotension, confusion and even death. Symptoms progress rapidly and last from 30 minutes to 2 hours. Because the liver metabolizes disulfiram, it is most effective in persons whose liver enzyme levels are within or close to the normal range.

Disulfiram inhibits the enzyme aldehyde dehydrogenase, which is involved in the metabolism of ethanol. Acetaldehyde levels are then increased from 5 to 10 times higher than normal, resulting in the disulfiram-alcohol reaction. This reaction is potentiated by decreased levels of adrenaline and noradrenaline in the sympathetic nervous system, caused by inhibition of dopamine beta-hydroxylase (DBH) (Cornish et al., 2006).

Education is extremely important for the client taking disulfiram. Many common products, such as shaving cream, aftershave lotion, cologne and deodorant, and over-the-counter medications such as cough preparations, contain alcohol; when used by the client taking disulfiram, these products can produce the same reaction as drinking alcohol. The client must read product labels carefully and select items that are alcohol-free.

It seems likely that other, psychological, factors – in particular commitment to abstinence facilitated by group and individual support – are vital in enabling disulfiram to work (Neto et al., 2007)

WARNING ● Disulfiram

Never give disulfiram to a client in a state of alcohol intoxication or without the client's full knowledge. Instruct the client's relatives accordingly.

Other side-effects reported by people taking disulfiram include fatigue, drowsiness, halitosis, tremor and impotence. Disulfiram also can interfere with the metabolism of other drugs the client is taking, such as phenytoin (Epanutin), isoniazid, warfarin (Marevan), barbiturates and long-acting benzodiazepines, such as diazepam and chlordiazepoxide.

Acamprosate (Campral) is approved for people in recovery from alcohol abuse or dependence. It helps reduce the physical and emotional discomfort encountered during the first weeks or months of sobriety, such as sweating, anxiety and sleep disturbances. The dosage is two tablets (333 mg each) three times a day. Persons with renal impairments cannot take this drug. Side-effects are reported as mild and include diarrhoea, nausea, flatulence and pruritus.

CULTURAL CONSIDERATIONS

Studies in the US have shown that people from different ethnic backgrounds seem to respond differently to certain drugs used to treat mental disorders. The nurse should be familiar with these cultural differences.

Studies have shown that African–Americans respond more rapidly to antipsychotic medications and tricyclic antidepressants than do whites. In addition, African–Americans have a greater risk of developing side-effects from both these classes of drugs than do whites. Asian people metabolize antipsychotics and tricyclic antidepressants more slowly than do whites and therefore require lower dosages to achieve the same effects. Hispanic people also require lower dosages of antidepressants than do whites to achieve the desired results (Woods et al., 2003).

Asian people seem to respond therapeutically to lower dosages of lithium than do whites. African–Americans have higher blood levels of lithium than whites when given the same dosage, and they also experience more side-effects. This suggests that African–Americans require lower dosages of lithium than do whites to produce the desired effects (Chen et al., 2002).

While these results have not been replicated in the UK as yet, they certainly suggest that nurses need to be aware of the likelihood of similar findings.

HERBAL MEDICINES

Herbal medicines have been used for hundreds of years in many countries and are now being used with increasing frequency in the UK. St. John's Wort is used to treat depression but, according to the BNF, should *not* be used with antidepressants because of the potential for interaction. Kava is used to treat anxiety and can potentiate the effects of alcohol, benzodiazepines and other sedative-hypnotic agents. Valerian helps produce sleep and is sometimes used to relieve stress and anxiety. Ginkgo biloba is primarily used to improve memory, but is also taken for fatigue, anxiety and depression, though there is no clear evidence of its efficacy.

It is essential for the nurse to ask clients specifically if they use any herbal preparations. Clients may not consider these products as 'medicine' or may be reluctant to admit their use for fear of censure by health professionals. Herbal medicines are often chemically complex and not standardized or regulated for use in treating illnesses. Combining herbal preparations with other medicines can lead to unwanted interactions, so it is essential to assess a client's use of these products.

SELF-AWARENESS ISSUES

Nurses must examine their own beliefs and feelings about mental health problems as 'illnesses' and the role of drugs in treating mental disorders. Some nurses may be sceptical about some mental disorders and may believe that clients could gain control of their lives if they just put in enough effort; some may strip patients of all autonomy and responsibility for their actions by regarding them as 'ill'; some may feel actively antagonistic towards the 'medicalizing' of life-problems, or towards the sometimes sparse evidence for psychiatric diagnoses and interventions.

Nurses who work with people with mental disorders come to understand that many disorders seem similar to chronic physical illnesses, such as asthma or diabetes, which require lifelong medication to maintain health. Without proper medication management, some clients with certain mental disorders, such as the schizophrenias or bipolar affective disorder, seem to find it impossible to survive in, and to cope with, the world around them without significant input from professionals. The nurse must explain to the client and family that some mental disorders seem to require continuous medication management and follow-up, just as a chronic physical illness does. At the same time, people are always far more than the sum of their 'symptoms': no-one should ever be defined by or reduced to an 'illness' or a 'disease' and everyone should be regarded as an individual with strengths, resources, competencies and wisdom, able to live a meaningful and purposeful life. Social and psychological interventions based on principles of pragmatic optimism and respect are crucial to helping people achieve this.

There is much debate about the extent to which 'schizophrenia', for example, is an illness, many illnesses, a number of different disorders or simply a behavioural category. Nurses must be willing to engage with the research and form their own opinion, in line with the evidence and with principles of respect, optimism and curiosity. Yet it is crucial for the nurse to know about current biological theories and treatments, and to remain open to the evidence base as it develops. Many clients and their families will have questions about reports in the news about research or discoveries. The nurse can help them distinguish between what is factual and what is experimental or purely theoretical.

But clients and families need more than purely factual information to deal with mental health problems and its effect on their lives. Many clients do not understand the nature of their problem and ask, 'Why is this happening to me?' They need to be offered clear but thorough explanations – where possible – about the nature of the problem and how they can manage it. The nurse must learn to give out and exchange with clients information about any diagnosis, medication and side-effects, the psychotherapeutic treatments, the possible prognosis, while providing, alongside other professionals and non-professionals, the care and support needed both by those confronting mental health problems and their carers. They must suggest possible local and national resources for support, relevant websites, books and articles, and be prepared to be open and flexible in listening to and working with clients and carers. At the same time, they need to be sensitive to the effect that an overload of information may have.

Points to Consider When Working on Self-Awareness

- People with 'long-term' mental health problems may have periods of remission and exacerbation that appear similar to those with chronic physical illnesses. A recurrence of symptoms is not the client's fault, nor is it necessarily a failure of treatment or nursing care.
- Many people with apparently 'long-term' conditions lead a full, satisfying life, often 'symptom-free'.
- Research regarding the neurobiological causes of mental disorders is still in its infancy. Be sceptical, but willing to embrace new research and new ideas.
- Often, when clients stop taking medication or take medication improperly, it is not because they intend to; rather, it can be the result of faulty thinking and reasoning, stemming from psychotic symptomatology or the 'cognitive deficits' – in memory, attention processes and executive functioning – which can result from schizophrenia. It may also be the result of fear arising from lack of information or, commonly, as a result of unpleasant side-effects.

Critical Thinking Questions

1. It is possible to identify a gene associated with increased risk for the late onset of Alzheimer's disease. Should this test be available to anyone who requests it? Why or why not? What dilemmas might arise from having such knowledge?

2. What would be the implications for nursing if it became possible to predict certain illnesses such as schizophrenia through the identification of genes responsible for or linked to the disease? Should this influence whether people who carry such genes should have children? Who should make that decision?

3. It seems likely that there is no clear evidence for an SSRI being any more effective than a placebo in moderate depression. A client who previously took an SSRI and feels it helped is asking you if he should start on it again. How should you respond?

4. Drug companies research and develop new drugs. Much more money and effort are expended to produce new drugs for common disorders rather than drugs (often called 'orphan drugs') needed to treat rare disorders such as Tourette's syndrome. What are the ethical and financial dilemmas associated with research designed to produce new drugs?

KEY POINTS

- Neurobiological research is constantly expanding our knowledge in the field of psychiatric medicine and should be significantly affecting nursing practice.
- The cerebrum is the centre for co-ordination and integration of all information needed to interpret and respond to the environment.
- The cerebellum is the centre for co-ordination of movements and postural adjustments.
- The brain stem contains centres that control cardiovascular and respiratory functions, sleep, consciousness and impulses.

- The limbic system regulates body temperature, appetite, sensations, memory and emotional arousal.
- Neurotransmitters are the chemical substances manufactured in the neuron that aid in the transmission of information from the brain throughout the body. Several important neurotransmitters, including dopamine, noradrenaline, serotonin, histamine, acetylcholine, GABA and glutamate have been found to play a role in mental disorders and are targets of pharmacological treatment.
- Researchers continue to examine the roles of genetics, heredity and viruses in the development of 'mental illness'.
- Pharmacological treatment is based on the ability of medications to eliminate or minimize identified target symptoms.
- The following factors must be considered in the selection of medications to treat mental disorders: the efficacy, **potency** and half-life of the drug; the age and ethnicity of the client; other medications the client is taking; and the side-effects of the drugs.
- Antipsychotic drugs are the primary treatment for psychotic disorders such as schizophrenia, but they produce a host of side-effects that may themselves require pharmacological intervention. Neurological side-effects, which can be treated with anticholinergic medications, are called EPS and include acute dystonia, akathisia and pseudoparkinsonism. Some of the more serious neurological side-effects include tardive dyskinesia (permanent involuntary movements) and neuroleptic malignant syndrome, which can be fatal.
- Because of the serious side-effects of antipsychotic medications, clients must be well educated regarding their medications, medication concordance and side-effects. Health-care professionals must supervise the regime closely.
- Antidepressant medications include cyclic compounds, SSRIs, MAOIs and a group of newer drugs.
- The nurse must carefully and respectfully instruct clients receiving MAOIs to avoid foods containing tyramine because the combination produces a hypertensive crisis that can become life-threatening.
- The risk of suicide may increase as clients begin taking antidepressants. Although suicidal thoughts are still present, the medication may increase the client's energy, which may allow the client to carry out a suicide plan.

INTERNET RESOURCES

RESOURCES	INTERNET ADDRESS
British National Formulary 55 Online	http://www.bnf.org/bnf/bnf/55/
Mental Health Care	http://www.mentalhealthcare.org.uk/
Research Project Relating to DNA, Genetics, and Mental Disorders	http://www.nhgri.gov
US Food and Drug Administration	http://www.fda.gov

- Lithium and selected anticonvulsants are used to stabilize mood, particularly in bipolar affective disorder.
- The nurse must help monitor serum lithium levels regularly to ensure the level is in the therapeutic range and to avoid lithium toxicity. Symptoms of toxicity include severe diarrhoea and vomiting, drowsiness, muscle weakness and loss of co-ordination. Untreated, lithium toxicity leads to coma and death.
- Benzodiazepines are used to treat a wide variety of problems related to anxiety and insomnia. Clients taking them should avoid alcohol, which increases the effects of the benzodiazepines.
- The primary use of stimulants such as methylphenidate (Ritalin) is the treatment of children with ADHD. Methylphenidate has been proved successful in allowing these children to slow down their activity and focus on the tasks at hand and their schoolwork. Its exact mechanism of action is unknown.
- Clients from various cultures may metabolize medications at different rates and therefore require alterations in standard dosages.
- Assessing the use of herbal preparations is essential for all clients.

REFERENCES

American Psychiatric Association. (2000). *Diagnostic and statistical manual of mental disorders* (4th edn, text revision). Washington, DC: American Psychiatric Association.

Ashton, A., Jamerson, B., Weinstein, W., & Wagoner, C. (2005). Antidepressant-related adverse effects impacting treatment compliance: Results of a patient survey. *Current Therapeutic Research, 66*(2), 96–106.

Bauer, M. S. & Mitchner, L. (2004). What is a "mood stabilizer"? An evidence-based response. *American Journal of Psychiatry, 161*(1), 3–18.

British National Formulary Online (2008). Available: http://www.bnf.org/bnf/bnf/55/

Chen, J. P., Barron, C., Lin, K. M., et al. (2002). Prescribing medication for Asians with mental disorders. *Western Journal of Medicine, 176*(4), 271–275.

Chouinard, G. (2004a). New nomenclature for drug-induced movement disorders including tardive dyskinesia. *Journal of Clinical Psychiatry, 65*(Suppl. 9), 9–15.

Chouinard, G. (2004b). Issues in the clinical use of benzodiazepines: Potency, withdrawal, and rebound. *Journal of Clinical Psychiatry, 65*(Suppl. 5), 7–12.

Cornish, J. W., McNicholas, L. F., & O'Brien, C. P. (2006). Treatment of substance-related disorders. In A. F. Schatzberg & C. B. Nemeroff (Eds.), *Essentials of clinical pharmacology* (2nd edn, pp. 647–667). Washington, DC: American Psychiatric Publishing.

Daniel, D. G., Copeland, L. F., & Tamminga, C. (2006). Ziprasidone. In A. F. Schatzberg & C. B. Nemeroff (Eds.), *Essentials of clinical pharmacology* (2nd edn, pp. 297–305). Washington, DC: American Psychiatric Publishing.

Hitt, E. (2003). Managing weight gain as a side effect of antidepressant therapy. *Cleveland Clinical Journal, 70,* 614–623.

Kirsch, I., Deacon, B. J., Huedo-Medina, T. B., et al. (2008). Initial severity and antidepressant benefits: a meta-analysis of data submitted to the Food and Drug Administration. *PLoS Med, 5*(2): e45. doi:10.1371/journal.pmed.0050045.

Krishnan, K. R. R. (2006). Monoamine oxidase inhibitors. In A. F. Schatzberg & C. B. Nemeroff (Eds.), *Essentials of clinical pharmacology* (2nd edn, pp. 113-125). Washington, DC: American Psychiatric Publishing.

Lehne, R. A. (2006). *Pharmacology for nursing care* (6th edn). Philadelphia: W. B. Saunders.

MHRA. (2008). *Making regulatory decisions about medicines and medical devices.* Available: http://www.mhra.gov.uk/home/idcplg?IdcService=GET_FILE&dDocName=con2030689&RevisionSelectionMethod=Latest

Muller, D. J. & Kennedy, J. L. (2006). Genetics of antipsychotic treatment emergent weight gain in schizophrenia. *Pharmacogenomics, 7*(6), 863–887.

National Institutes of Health. (2007). *About ELSI.* Available: http://www.nhgri.nhi.gov/ELSI (retrieved 3 February 2002).

Neto, D., Lambaz, R., & Tavares, J. (2007). Compliance with aftercare treatment, including disulfiram, and effect on outcome in alcohol-dependent patients. *Alcohol & Alcoholism, 42*(6), 604–609.

Newcomer, J. & Haupt, D. (2006). The metabolic effects of antipsychotic medications. *Canadian Journal of Psychiatry 51*(8), 480–491.

Plata-Salaman, C. R., Shank, R. P., & Smith-Swintosky, V. L. (2005). Amino acid neurotransmitters. In B. J. Sadock & V. A. Sadock (Eds.), *Comprehensive textbook of psychiatry, Vol. 1* (8th edn, pp. 60–72). Philadelphia: Lippincott Williams & Wilkins.

Snowden, A. (2006). Exploring the impact of mental health nurse prescribing. *British Journal of Nursing, 15*(20), 1114–1118.

Swedo, S. E., Leonard, H. L., & Rapoport, J. L. (2004). The pediatric autoimmune neuropsychiatric disorders associated with streptococcal infection (PANDAS) subgroup: Separating fact from fiction. *Pediatrics, 113*(4), 907–911.

Tecott, L. H. & Smart, S. L. (2005). Monoamine transmitters. In B. J. Sadock & V. A. Sadock (Eds.), *Comprehensive textbook of psychiatry, Vol. 1* (8th edn, pp. 49-60). Philadelphia: Lippincott Williams & Wilkins.

Woods, S. W., Sullivan, M. C., Neuse, E. C., et al. (2003). Racial and ethnic effects on antipsychotic prescribing practices in a community mental health center. *Psychiatric Services, 54*(2), 177–179.

ADDITIONAL READING

Fujita, M., Kugaya, A., & Innis, R. B. (2005). Radiotracer imaging: Basic principles and exemplary findings in neuropsychiatric disorders. In B. J. Sadock & V. A. Sadock (Eds.), *Comprehensive textbook of psychiatry, Vol. 1* (8th edn, pp. 222–236). Philadelphia: Lippincott Williams & Wilkins.

Glassman, A. H. (2005). Schizophrenia, antipsychotic drugs, and cardiovascular disease. *Journal of Clinical Psychiatry, 66*(Suppl. 6), 5–10.

Kane, J. M., Eerdekens, M., Lindenmayer, J., et al. (2003). Long-acting injectable risperidone: Efficacy and safety for the first long-acting atypical antipsychotic. *American Journal of Psychiatry, 160*(6), 1125–1132.

Malaty, W. (2005). St. John's wort for depression. *American Family Physician, 71*(7), 1375–1376.

Vythilingam, M., Shen, J., Drevets, W. C., et al. (2005). Nuclear magnetic resonance imaging: Basic principles and recent findings in neuropsychiatric disorders. In B. J. Sadock & V. A. Sadock (Eds.), *Comprehensive textbook of psychiatry, Vol. 1* (8th edn, pp. 201–222). Philadelphia: Lippincott Williams & Wilkins.

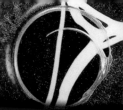

Chapter Study Guide

MULTIPLE-CHOICE QUESTIONS

Select the best answer for each of the following questions.

1. The signs of lithium toxicity include which of the following?
   a. Sedation, fever, restlessness
   b. Psychomotor agitation, insomnia, increased thirst
   c. Elevated white blood cell count, sweating, confusion
   d. Severe vomiting, diarrhoea, weakness

2. The nurse is teaching a client taking an MAOI about foods with tyramine that he or she should avoid. Which of the following statements indicates that there needs to be further discussion?
   a. 'I'm so glad I can have pizza as long as I don't order pepperoni.'
   b. 'I will be able to eat cottage cheese without worrying.'
   c. 'I will have to avoid drinking non-alcoholic beer.'
   d. 'I can eat green beans on this diet.'

3. A client who has been depressed and suicidal started taking a tricyclic antidepressant 2 weeks ago and is now ready to leave the hospital to go home. Which of the following is a concern for the nurse as discharge plans are finalized?

   a. The client may need a prescription for diphenhydramine (Benadryl) to use for side-effects.
   b. The nurse will need to evaluate the risk of suicide by overdose of the tricyclic antidepressant.
   c. The nurse will need to include teaching regarding the signs of neuroleptic malignant syndrome.
   d. The client will need regular laboratory work to monitor therapeutic drug levels.

4. Which of the following is a concern for children taking stimulants for ADHD for several years?
   a. Dependence on the drug
   b. Insomnia
   c. Growth suppression
   d. Weight gain

5. Clients taking which of the following types of psychotropic medications need close monitoring of their cardiac status?
   a. Antidepressants
   b. Antipsychotics
   c. Mood stabilizers
   d. Stimulants

FILL-IN-THE-BLANK QUESTIONS

Identify the drug classification for each of the following medications.

_____ 1. Clozapine (Clozaril)

_____ 2. Fluoxetine (Prozac)

_____ 3. Amitriptyline (Elavil)

_____ 4. Benzatropine (Cogentin)

_____ 5. Methylphenidate (Ritalin)

_____ 6. Carbamazepine (Tegretol)

_____ 7. Alprazolam (Xanax)

_____ 8. Quetiapine (Seroquel)

GROUP DISCUSSION TOPICS

1. What are the benefits and possible costs of SSRIs?
2. How should we approach working with someone who refuses to take an antipsychotic, despite being very distressed by accusatory voices?
3. If, as a nurse, we believe a psychiatrist is prescribing a dangerous level of lithium, how should we respond?

Care and Treatment Settings, the Multidisciplinary Team and Therapeutic Programmes

Key Terms

- **acute inpatient units**
- **assertive outreach**
- **care co-ordinator**
- **clubhouse model**
- **community mental health teams (CMHTs)**
- **crisis recovery and home treatment teams**
- **day treatment**
- **early intervention teams**
- **multidisciplinary teams**
- **recovery**
- **prison**
- **residential treatment settings**
- **homeless**

Learning Objectives

After reading this chapter, you should be able to:

1. Discuss traditional treatment settings.

2. Describe different types of residential and non-residential treatment settings and the services they provide.

3. Describe community care and treatment programmes that provide services to people with mental health problems.

4. Identify barriers to effective treatment for homeless people with mental health problems.

5. Discuss the issues related to people with mental health problems in the criminal justice system.

6. Describe the roles of different members of a multidisciplinary mental health-care team.

7. Identify the different roles of the nurse and other professionals in varied treatment settings and programmes.

As discussed in Chapter 1, mental health care has undergone profound changes in the past 50 years. Before the 1950s, treatment in large out-of-town asylums was usually the only available strategy for people with severe mental health problems: many of them stayed in such facilities for months or years, sometimes receiving humane, sensitive treatment and care, many times on the receiving end of abuse and neglect. The introduction of psychotropic medications in the 1950s offered hope of successfully treating the symptoms of 'mental illness' in a meaningful way, while social, political, ideological and economic changes led – haltingly and painfully – to a focus on 'community care' and a new era of care and treatment. Institutions could no longer hold clients with mental health problems indefinitely, and treatment in the 'least restrictive environment' became a guiding principle and right. Large state hospitals gradually closed. Treatment in the community was intended to replace much of state-hospital inpatient care. Adequate funding, however, has not always kept pace with the need for community programmes and treatment (see Chapter 1).

Today, people with mental health problems receive help in a variety of settings, the majority in the 'community'. This chapter describes the range of care and treatment settings available for those with mental health problems and the programmes that have been developed to meet their needs. Both of these sections discuss the challenges of integrating people with mental health problems with the community in which they live. The chapter also addresses two populations that are receiving inadequate treatment because they are not always directly connected with general services: those with mental health problems who are homeless and those in prison. Finally, the chapter describes the multidisciplinary team, including the crucial role of the nurse as a member of that team.

CARE AND TREATMENT SETTINGS

The division between inpatient settings and 'community' settings is intended to be far more fluid now than it has been historically. Nevertheless, services can still be broadly seen in terms of 'inpatient' settings and 'community' settings.

RESIDENTIAL AND INPATIENT SETTINGS

Acute Inpatient Settings

Since the closure of the asylums in the 1970s and 1980s, up until the present day, inpatient psychiatric care has remained a primary mode of treatment for people with 'mental illness'. Many **acute inpatient units** were built in the 1970s and 1980s in the grounds of district general hospitals. Even up until the past few years, 'acute' units frequently had patients who stayed many months or even years. Day hospitals or **day treatment** centres offered therapy and activity for inpatients and – sometimes – for outpatients.

A typical psychiatric unit emphasized – until very recently – medical treatment: drugs and electroconvulsive therapy (ECT), allied with some *talk therapy*, or focused

one-to-one interactions between 'patients' and staff, and – in rare settings – *milieu therapy*, the exploitation of the total environment and its possible beneficial effect on the client's treatment. Individual and group interactions focused in the main on psychodynamic and humanistic principles and nurses were often central to these processes (although in recent years this role has increasingly been handed to – or taken on by – occupational therapists and psychologists).

Today, a whole host of policy drivers are beginning to push inpatient units in a direction where they must provide rapid assessment, stabilization of 'symptoms', reduction of 'risk' and effective discharge planning and they must accomplish goals quickly, all – in theory – within a context of empowerment and '**recovery**' (Rae, 2007a). A client-centred multidisciplinary approach to a brief stay is essential and the role of the care programme approach and its care co-ordinator (a community clinician, usually a community psychiatric nurse or a social worker) is vital in bridging the gap between community and hospital. Once the client is 'safe' and feeling 'stable', the relevant clinicians, care co-ordinator and the client identify longer-term goals for the client to pursue in the community (CSIP/NIMHE, 2007).

Most areas now have developed **crisis recovery and home treatment teams** which 'gatekeep' a reducing number of inpatient beds and which are increasingly being seen as integral to acute care: the term 'transfer' (between, for example, inpatient unit and home treatment team) is increasingly being used rather than 'discharge' (National Audit Office, 2007). This process has led, in many areas, to patients who are admitted being more unwell and more disturbed than previously, necessitating a greater need for training and supervision for inpatient nurses. Nevertheless, the deliberate breaking down of boundaries between 'community care' and 'inpatient care', so that there is a 'seamless' acute service, often sharing staff across the settings, appears to be offering an exciting step forward, away from the sense of admission as 'failure', away from the sense that so many acute units had of being undervalued by the rest of the services, and away from the undoubted neglect and emotional abuse that so often characterized isolated acute inpatient units.

The increasing acuity of admitted patients and the increasing numbers of them who are formally detained patients (on a section of the Mental Health Act) has changed the nature of inpatient care and the demands on nursing and nurses. Increasing numbers of people on acute wards have major mental disorders and 'dual diagnoses'. In addition, there has been a growing emphasis from government – and society in general – on the management of 'risk' within mental health services: maintaining a therapeutic approach while working with very unwell people whose 'risk' is either very real or feared adds to the demands on inpatient nurses, as does the vast amount of (mostly justifiable) criticism of inpatient care in the UK over the past decade (Muijen, 2002; Mental Health Act Commission, 2005).

Some inpatient units have a locked entrance door, requiring staff with keys (or electronic cards) to let people in or out of the unit. This situation has both advantages and disadvantages, and exemplifies the tensions within inpatient care (Haglund *et al.*, 2006; Rae, 2007b). Nurses identify the *advantages* of providing protection against the 'outside world' (in particular threats from drug dealers) in a safe and secure environment as well as the primary *disadvantages* of making clients feel confined or dependent, and emphasizing the staff members' power over them.

Psychiatric Intensive Care Units

According to the 2002 National Minimum Standards, 'Psychiatric intensive care is for patients compulsorily detained, usually in secure conditions, who are in an acutely disturbed phase of a serious mental disorder. There is an associated loss of capacity for self-control, with a corresponding increase in risk, which does not enable their safe, therapeutic management and treatment in a general open acute ward' (NIMHE, 2002). There is much debate about the primary function and effectiveness of psychiatric intensive care units (PICUs) and their relationship with acute wards and the wider community, but they are increasing in number in the UK (along with 'low secure' units which tend to offer less intensive care to less 'disturbed' clients).

Special Hospitals

There are three high-security 'special hospitals' in England (Broadmoor, Rampton and Ashworth) and one in Scotland (Carstairs). Rampton has around 400 patients (many with learning disability), Broadmoor about 270 and Ashworth about 260. They care for people with mental disorders detained under the Mental Health Act (including those diagnosed with personality disorder) who need secure conditions due to a history of violence against themselves and/or others. Nurses play a vital role in the assessment, treatment and rehabilitation of people within these units.

COMMUNITY SETTINGS

An important concept in any treatment setting is, of course, discharge planning (or transfer planning), which needs to start from the very moment of admission. Environmental supports, such as housing and transportation, and access to community resources and services are crucial to successful discharge/transfer planning. In fact, the adequacy of discharge/transfer plans is a better predictor of how long the person could remain successfully in the community than are clinical indicators such as psychiatric diagnoses. As well as many other roles, the care coordinator (see below) plays a crucial part in planning a move from, say, an inpatient unit into the community.

Impediments to successful discharge/transfer planning can include alcohol and drug abuse, criminal or violent behaviour, non-concordance with medication regimens, and suicidal ideation. Decent housing is often not available to people with a recent history of drug or alcohol abuse or criminal behaviour, and clients who have suicidal ideas or a history

of aggression or 'non-compliance' with medication regimes may be ineligible for some treatment programmes or services. Clients with these impediments to successful discharge/transfer planning, therefore, may have a less-than-ideal plan in place because optimal services and supports are not available to them. Consequently, people discharged with these plans are readmitted more quickly and more frequently than those who have better discharge/transfer plans.

Clients do not keep follow-up appointments or referrals if they don't feel connected to services or if these services aren't perceived as helpful or valuable: attention to psychosocial factors that address the client's well-being, his or her preference for follow-up services, inclusion of friends and family, and familiarity with outpatient providers are critical to the success of a discharge plan (Williams, 2004).

Prince (2006) found that three types of intervention are significant in preventing rehospitalization for individuals with four or more prior inpatient stays. These interventions are symptom education, service continuity and establishment of daily structure. Clients who can recognize signs of impending relapse and seek help, participate in outpatient appointments and services, and have a daily plan of activities and responsibilities are least likely to require rehospitalization.

Creating successful discharge plans that offer optimal services and housing is essential if people with mental health problems are to be reintegrated into the community. An holistic approach to reintegration is the best way to prevent repeated hospital admissions and improve quality of life for clients. Community programmes after discharge from the hospital may need to include social services, day treatment and housing programmes, all geared toward survival in the community, empowered concordance with treatment recommendations, recovery and independent living. Crisis resolution/home treatment and assertive outreach team (AOT) programmes provide many of the services that are necessary to stop the revolving door of repeated hospital admissions punctuated by unsuccessful attempts at community living. AOT programmes are discussed in detail later in this chapter.

Crisis Recovery/Home Treatment Teams

As mentioned in the previous section, crisis recovery and home treatment teams have become increasingly important in their role as 'bridges' between acute inpatient settings and 'community' settings. They are multidisciplinary teams who often gatekeep beds and whose primary role is usually to provide – wherever possible – an alternative to admission.

Community Mental Health Teams

Community mental health teams (CMHTs) – sometimes now called primary care mental health teams – were traditionally (from the 1980s until the past few years) the main community resource for people across the whole range of mental health problems: the vast majority of people in mental health services were either cared for by a CMHT or within inpatient services. The main professional groupings within CMHTs were community psychiatric nurses (CPNs), with (more latterly) occupational therapists, social workers and other professionals joining them. Psychology and psychiatrist input was usually sessional rather than full time. As services developed around the turn of the century, the CMHT role became somewhat 'narrower', as much-criticized gaps in the service they provided were filled by new teams: crisis/home treatment teams began to take on some of the crisis intervention roles previously undertaken (often between 9 A.M. and 5 P.M.) by CMHTs; assertive outreach teams began actively to work with the more challenging longer-term clients (who had previously, on occasion, drifted between gaps in the service); **early intervention teams** began to work with young people who had previously fallen between child and adolescent services and the CMHTs.

The vast majority of care co-ordinators (usually, though not exclusively, CPNs/community mental health nurses (CMHNs) and social workers) work, still, within CMHTs and they remain the biggest provider of input across the system. CMHTs still undertake crisis work, early intervention work and some assertive outreach work (the degree dependent on local conditions/local politics), although alongside a renewed emphasis on work in primary care and with longer-term clients.

PRIMARY CARE LIAISON TEAMS/PRIMARY CARE MENTAL HEALTH WORKERS

There has been an increasing focus on the role of the GP and other primary-care professionals in helping to offer integrated care packages – covering both physical and mental health needs – to people with mental health problems. Increasingly, bridging the gap between the two parts of the service is carried out by specific teams or designated individuals: the often tense relationships between specialist services and primary care will also, it is hoped, be eased by the re-focusing of CMHTs on (and in) primary care.

Much more 'early intervention' work (with its advantages of having a preventive and health promotion role as well as one that de-stigmatizes and 'normalizes' by keeping people away from specialist services) is being carried out by GPs, by primary-care-based graduate mental health workers and by the newly developing roles of 'low-intensity' workers: focused CBT programmes are increasingly being offered in primary care settings.

Community Residential Settings

People with mental health problems may live in a variety of community **residential settings** that vary according to structure, level of supervision and services provided. Of course, the vast majority live in their own homes.

Some settings are designed as transitional housing, with the expectation that residents will progress to more independent living. Other residential programmes serve clients for as long as the need exists, sometimes years. 'Halfway houses' usually serve as temporary placements that provide support as clients prepare for independence. Group homes may house

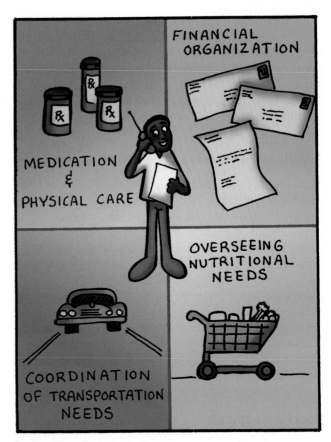

Case manager

six to ten residents who take turns cooking meals and sharing household chores under the supervision of one or two staff persons. Staff members are available for crisis intervention, transportation, assistance with daily living tasks and, sometimes, drug monitoring. In addition to on-site staff, many residential settings provide case management services for clients and put them in touch with other resources (e.g. vocational rehabilitation; medical, dental and psychiatric care; psychosocial rehabilitation programmes or services) as needed.

Sometimes termed 'seriously mentally ill' or 'SMI' clients, there are many people with severe and persistent mental health problems living in the community. The population includes people who were hospitalized before 'community care' and often remained hospitalized despite efforts at community placement; it also includes people who have been hospitalized consistently for long periods despite efforts to minimize their hospital stays. Community placement of clients with problematic behaviours (indeed, with any kind of mental health problem) still meets, on occasion, considerable resistance from the public, creating a barrier to successful living in community settings. One approach to working with longer-term clients has been a hostel, a unit within or outside hospital grounds that is designed to be more 'home-like' and less institutional. Many hostel projects have been established that provide access to community facilities and on normal expectations such as cooking, cleaning and doing housework.

Some agencies provide respite housing, or crisis housing services, for clients in need of short-term temporary shelter.

These clients may live in group homes or independently most of the time but have a need for 'respite' from their usual residences. This usually occurs when clients experience a crisis, feel overwhelmed or cannot cope with problems or emotions. Respite services often provide increased emotional support and assistance with problem solving in a setting away from the source of the clients' distress. The concept of a crisis hostel or 'crisis house' has recently grown in popularity. The criterion for using many of these services – in line with recovery principles – is, frequently, the client's own perception of being in crisis and needing a more structured environment.

Someone's living environment obviously affects his or her level of functioning, rate of 'relapse' and ability to remain in a community setting. In fact, someone's living environment is often more predictive of their ability to live a satisfying, meaningful and purposeful life than the characteristics of his or her 'illness'. Finding quality living situations for people with mental health problems is a difficult task and many still live in poorer, high-crime or commercial, rather than more affluent, residential areas (Segal & Riley, 2003). Reynolds (2005) found clear links between overcrowded family housing and depression, anxiety and relationship problems.

Frequently, residents oppose plans to establish a group home or residential facility in their neighbourhood. They argue that having a group home will decrease their property values, and they may believe that people with mental illness are violent, will act bizarrely in public or will be a menace to their children. These people have strongly ingrained stereotypes and a great deal of misinformation. Local residents must be given the facts so that safe, affordable and desirable housing can be established for persons needing residential care. Nurses are in an ideal position to advocate for clients by providing education to members of the community.

Clubhouse Model

In 1948, Fountain House pioneered the **clubhouse model** of community-based rehabilitation in New York City. Currently, more than 400 such clubhouses have been established in 27 countries throughout the world (Ferguson, 2004). Many clubhouses are 'intentional communities' based on the belief that men and women with serious and persistent psychiatric disabilities can, and will, achieve normal life goals when given the opportunity, time, support and fellowship. The essence of membership in the clubhouse is based on the four guaranteed rights of members:

- A place to come to
- Meaningful work
- Meaningful relationships
- A place to return to (lifetime membership).

The clubhouse model provides members with many opportunities, including daytime work activities focused on the care, maintenance and productivity of the clubhouse; evening, weekend and holiday leisure activities; transitional and independent employment support and efforts; and housing options. Members are encouraged and assisted to use community mental health services.

The clubhouse model recognizes the professional–client relationship as a key to successful treatment and rehabilitation while acknowledging that brief encounters that focus on symptom management are not sufficient to promote recovery efforts. The clubhouse model exists to promote the rehabilitation alliance as a positive force in the members' lives.

The clubhouse focus is on health, not illness. Taking prescribed drugs, for example, is not a condition of participation in the clubhouse. Members, not staff, must ultimately make decisions about treatment, such as whether or not they need hospital admission. Clubhouse staff supports members, helps them to obtain needed assistance and, most of all, allows them to make the decisions that ultimately affect all aspects of their lives. This approach to recovery is the cornerstone and the strength of the clubhouse model.

Assertive Outreach Programmes

One of the newer approaches to community-based treatment for people with mental health problems in the UK is **assertive outreach** (Box 4.1). Marx *et al.* (1973) conceived this idea in Madison, Wisconsin in the US. They believed that skills training, support and teaching should be done in the community – where it is needed – rather than in the

---

Box 4.1 ASSERTIVE OUTREACH TEAM FEATURES

- Delivery by a discrete multidisciplinary team able to provide a full range of interventions
- Most services provided directly by team, not brokered out
- Low staff-to-client ratios (maximum 1:12)
- Most interventions provided in community settings
- Emphasis on engagement and maintaining contact with clients
- Caseloads shared across clinicians, staff know and work with the entire caseload, although a CPA care co-ordinator is allocated and responsible
- Highly co-ordinated, intensive service with brief daily handover meetings and weekly clinical review meetings
- Availability out-of-hours and seven days a week, with capacity to manage crises and increase contact to daily according to need
- Time-unlimited service while there is evidence of benefit, or continuity of care according to need

From National Forum for Assertive Outreach. (2005). *http://nfao.co.uk/Annual%20Report/Annual_report_2005_06.pdf*

hospital. Their programme was first known as the Madison model, then 'training in community living', then AOT or the programme for assertive treatment. Assertive outreach programmes in the UK have their roots in the Madison model.

AOTs in the UK offer help to those people that traditional mental health services have found difficult to engage: these tend to be people who have a number of complex needs, a history of frequent inpatient admission, chaotic lifestyles and a reluctance to connect with conventional services. An AOT programme has a problem-solving orientation: staff members attend to specific life issues, no matter how mundane. AOT programmes provide most services directly rather than relying on referrals to other programmes or agencies, and they implement the services in the clients' homes or communities, not in offices. The AOT services are also intense; as many face-to-face contacts as necessary with clients are tailored to meet clients' needs. A team approach allows all staff to be equally familiar with all clients, so clients do not have to wait for an assigned person. AOT programmes also make a long-term commitment to clients, providing services for as long as the need persists and with no time constraints (Redko *et al.*, 2004).

AOT programmes have also been successful in the US, Canada and Australia (Latimer, 2005; Udechuku *et al.*, 2005) in decreasing hospital admissions and fostering community integration for persons with mental health problems. Research in the UK is just beginning to be undertaken.

SPECIAL POPULATIONS OF CLIENTS WITH MENTAL HEALTH PROBLEMS

The Homeless

Homeless people with mental health problems have become – belatedly – the focus of some studies and some government investment (Croft-White & Parry-Crooke, 2004; Desai & Rosenheck, 2005). Many nurses work in the statutory and non-statutory sectors providing care and treatment for this vulnerable group of people. Frequent shifts between the street, mental health services and institutions worsen the marginal existence of such homeless people, as do the high levels of alcohol and drug misuse. Compared with homeless people without mental health problems, the homeless *with* such problems are homeless longer, spend more time in shelters, have fewer contacts with family, spend more time in jail and face greater barriers to employment. They are significantly more likely to commit suicide and to be suffering from major mental health problems such as bipolar disorder, schizophrenia or depression than the general population. For them, shelters, rehabilitation programmes and prisons may serve as makeshift alternatives to decent inpatient care or supportive housing, and professionals and voluntary workers usually supersede families as the primary source of help.

In addition, Dean and Craig's (1999) survey suggested that 94% of homeless men and 90% of homeless women developed mental health problems before they became homeless. MIND's findings (2006) suggest that 1 in 5 people identify mental health problems as a reason for becoming homeless. According to the Office of the Deputy Prime Minister (2004, p. 10):

- Only a quarter of rough sleepers are registered with a GP, and homeless people are 40 times more likely not to be registered with a GP relative to the rest of the population.
- Many homeless people have difficulties registering with a GP (which is often the first step to getting help for mental as well as physical health problems) because there is a commonly held belief that they might be difficult or that they need a permanent address to register. Primary care registration rates vary between 24% and 92% for homeless people, the former described in a study of rough sleepers and the latter in families in bed and breakfast accommodation.
- Homeless people are four times more likely than the general public to turn to A&E services if they cannot access a GP.
- Some homeless people face difficulties in accessing integrated care, which can mean they present late in the pattern of illness with problems that could have been prevented or treated by early intervention through accessing the services of a GP, dentist or health visitor.

Providing housing alone does not significantly alter the prognosis of homelessness for people with mental health problems. In a study conducted in the US, Min *et al.* (2004) found that psychosocial rehabilitation services, peer support, vocational training and daily living skill training were effective in decreasing the number of days the clients stayed at shelters. In the UK, voluntary services for the homeless such as Crisis and Shelter do brilliant work but often struggle to provide help that links appropriately with mental health services. Lack of flexibility of mental health services, overt and covert discrimination against the homeless, lack of information, structural hurdles, lack of resources and resistance to change within the existing services all contribute to difficulties offering care to this group of people, many of whom also have significant physical problems and misuse drugs and alcohol.

Prisoners

The UK has one of the highest rates of incarceration in Europe. There was one **prison** suicide every 4 days between 1999 and 2003 and this appears to be increasing. Rates of severe mental illness, such as schizophrenia, are more than ten times higher among male inmates than the general population, according to the Prison Reform Trust; 72% of male and 70% of female sentenced prisoners suffer from two or more mental health disorders. Research shows that suicide among male prisoners is five times that of the general population (Fazel *et al.*, 2005) Some two-thirds of female prisoners in the UK are suffering from a mental disorder and a third of them harm themselves. Factors cited as reasons why mentally disordered people end up in the criminal justice system include lack of adequate community support and the attitudes of police, the courts, the mental health system and society generally (Konrad, 2002). Poor health promotion and the complex, interweaving relationships between homelessness, social deprivation, substance misuse, crime, relationship breakdown and mental distress are undoubtedly key contributors.

Public concern about the potential danger of people with 'mental illness' is fuelled by the media attention that surrounds any violent criminal act committed by a mentally ill person. Although it is true that people with some specific untreated major mental illnesses may be at increased risk of being violent, most people with mental health problems do not – and never will – represent a significant danger to others. This fact, however, does not keep people from clinging to stereotypes of 'the mad' as people to be feared, avoided and institutionalized. If such people cannot be confined in mental hospitals for any period, there seems to be tacit public and governmental support for arresting and incarcerating them instead.

People with mental health problems who are in the criminal justice system face several barriers to successful community reintegration (McCoy *et al.*, 2004):

- Poverty
- Homelessness
- Substance use
- Violence
- Victimization, rape and trauma
- Self-harm.

Frequently, the individual with mental health problems can be diverted to community mental health services or to inpatient units, if needed, instead of being arrested and going through the criminal justice system. Community mental health teams and mentally disordered offender/forensic teams provide assessment and treatment services and education to police and probation officers to help them recognize mental health problems and help change their attitude about offenders with such problems.

MULTIDISCIPLINARY TEAM

Regardless of the treatment setting, recovery programme, or population, a **multidisciplinary** (or **interdisciplinary**) **team** (MDT) approach is essential in dealing with the multifaceted problems of clients with mental health problems. Different members of the team have expertise in specific areas. By collaborating, they can (and should) meet clients' needs more effectively. Members of the multidisciplinary team may be psychiatrists, psychologists, mental health nurses, social workers, occupational therapists, support workers and others. Not all settings have a full-time member from each discipline on their team; the programmes and services that the team offers determine its composition in any setting.

- **Occupational Therapy**: Occupational therapists (OTs) work in psychiatric units, day hospitals and in the community. OTs are employed by health authorities, social services departments, social care trusts and voluntary organizations. Their role is to help people with mental, physical and social problems to build up the confidence and skills needed for personal, social, domestic, leisure or work activities. They focus on the active learning of specific skills and techniques for coping more effectively. This may involve the use of arts, crafts, group work (such as anxiety management and assertiveness training), individual counselling and training in the activities of daily living, such as self-care, shopping, cooking and budgeting.
- **Psychiatrists.** Psychiatrists are qualified doctors who take postgraduate training in psychiatry after completion of a general medical training, and specialize in the treatment of mentally distressed people. Psychiatrists are not only hospital-based; in some areas they have close links with GPs' surgeries. Others work in community mental health centres or in multidisciplinary teams. They work closely with a number of different mental health professionals. Consultant psychiatrists often (though not always) lead the multidisciplinary team.
- **Community Mental Health Nurses.** Community mental health nurses (CMHNs) (formerly community psychiatric nurses or CPNs) have been at the forefront of community care for people with mental health problems for some four decades now, working in the community to undertake key mental health promotion, psychotherapeutic, monitoring and assessment, and care co-ordination roles. The clinical practice of CMHNs includes caring for clients and families struggling with issues such as schizophrenia, bipolar disorder, depression, anxiety, eating disorders, postnatal disorders, substance misuse, domestic violence, child abuse and grief. They work in community mental health teams, primary care mental health teams, crisis and home treatment teams, forensic teams, drug and alcohol and assertive outreach teams among others.
- **Inpatient Mental Health Nurses.** Nurses in inpatient units work therapeutically with clients, ensure safety, work towards recovery and manage inpatient environments.
- **Social Workers.** A mental health social worker is a specialist mental health worker who works closely with individuals and families to support them through crises or in the longer term. If unit-based, their role may also involve helping people prepare for leaving the hospital.
- **Approved Mental Health Practitioner.** An approved mental health practitioner (AMHP) is a qualified practitioner – usually a social worker, nurse, OT or psychologist who has undergone additional training and been approved by the local authority to carry out various designated functions under the Mental Health Act 2007. An AMHP has a role in mental health assessment to be undertaken jointly with medical professionals in order to ascertain whether compulsory admission to hospital

Box 4.2 THE MENTAL HEALTH NURSE AS CARE CO-ORDINATOR

- Undertakes – with appropriate others – an assessment of need.
- Oversees care-planning and resource allocation.
- Keeps in close contact with the user and significant others.
- Advises other members of the care team about changes in a user's circumstances that may warrant a review.
- Evaluates the impact of interventions and updates the user's care plan and any crisis plan.

Adapted from Callaghan, P. (2006). Discharge planning. In P. Callaghan & H. Waldock (Eds.), *Oxford handbook of mental health nursing* (p. 96). Oxford: Oxford University Press.

is necessary. AMHPs have a particular responsibility to examine alternatives to hospitalization.

- **Psychologists.** Clinical and counselling psychologists are specialists trained in psychological assessments and treatments. They frequently lead in the provision of therapies such as CBT, undertake psychometric testing and employ other measurement/assessment tools. They may – along with other professionals – undertake research and conduct clinical supervision.

(Adapted from MIND, 2008; Royal College of Psychiatrists, 2008.)

Other possible members of an MDT include Support, Time and Recovery (STR) workers, outreach workers, mental health workers, housing officers, employment officers, support workers, vocational therapists, art therapists and psychotherapists. Professionals such as GPs, health visitors, district nurses, midwives, practice nurses, speech therapists, pharmacists and physiotherapists also contribute to MDT work.

It is important to bear in mind that roles are not (and should not be) set in stone: the work undertaken by different professions changes from society to society, from year to year and from setting to setting. Overlaps between the professions are huge, although their attempts at maintaining their own distinct identity often lead to territorial and political tensions which can be detrimental to holistic, collaborative and empowering care.

Functioning as an effective team member requires the development and practice of several core skill areas (White & Brooker, 2001):

- Interpersonal skills, such as tolerance, patience and understanding
- Humanity, such as warmth, acceptance, empathy, genuineness and non-judgemental attitude
- Knowledge base about mental disorders, symptoms and behaviour
- Communication skills
- Personal qualities such as consistency, assertiveness and problem-solving abilities

- Teamwork skills, such as collaborating, sharing and integrating
- Risk assessment/risk management skills.

The role of the case manager/**care co-ordinator** (Box 4.2) has become increasingly important. No standard formal educational programme to become a case manager or care co-ordinator exists, however, and people from many different backgrounds may fill this role. In most settings, a social worker or psychiatric nurse is the case manager. Liberman *et al.* (2001) identified three distinct sets of competencies necessary for effective 'case managers': clinical skills, relationship skills and liaison and advocacy skills. Clinical skills include treatment planning, symptom and functional assessment and skills training. Relationship skills include the ability to establish and maintain collaborative, respectful and therapeutic alliances with a wide variety of clients. Liaison and advocacy skills are necessary to develop and maintain effective interagency contacts for housing, financial entitlements and vocational rehabilitation.

As clients' needs become more varied and complex, the MHN has traditionally led the care co-odination process and is in an ideal position to fulfil the role of care co-ordinator.

SELF-AWARENESS ISSUES

Mental health nursing is evolving as changes continue in health care. Since the 1960s, the focus had shifted from traditional hospital-based goals of symptom and medication management to more client-centred goals, which included working collaboratively toward an improved quality of life and recovery from mental health problems for service users. Nevertheless, with political and ideological changes and an increasing focus on risk since the 1990s, there remains a tension between this empowering model (deepened by the emphasis on 'recovery') and a more rigid, 'old-fashioned' view that demands nurses act in a more traditionally controlling and custodial way.

Critical Thinking Questions

1. Discuss the role of the nurse in advocating for social or legislative policy changes needed to provide recovery-focused services for clients in all settings.
2. When should programmes for special populations, such as teenagers with mental health problems who are offenders, or the elderly homeless, be considered successful?
3. How can the nurse reconcile the trend for short-term 'crisis' inpatient hospitalization with the long-term needs of some clients with severe and persistent mental health problems?

There are, seemingly, ever-increasing demands on the nurse to be forever expanding and developing his or her repertoire of personal qualities, experiences, knowledge, skills and abilities in order to help clients (and other professionals) effectively. It is hugely difficult – but an absolute prerequisite – for the nurse to be actively supportive of the client even when he or she believes the client has made choices that are less than ideal. The requirement for the nurse to practise in an autonomous and independent way (though within a panoply of local and national guidance, monitoring and the meeting of targets) can feel both unsettling and liberating.

These challenges may overwhelm the nurse at times, and he or she may feel under-prepared or ill-equipped to meet them. Support, both formal (in the form of clinical supervision, good leadership and management, appropriate training and opportunities for reflection) and informal (intra- and interdisciplinary discussion and the involvement of friends and family) is crucial.

In whatever setting, the nurse may experience frustration when working with adults with mental health problems, often potentially feeling rejected or inadequate when clients choose not to engage.

Points to Consider when Working in Community-based Settings

• The client (and the nurse!) can make mistakes, survive them, and learn from them. Mistakes are a part of normal life for everyone, and it is not the nurse's role to protect clients from such experiences.
• The nurse will not always have the answer to solve a client's problems or resolve a difficult situation.
• As clients move toward recovery, they need support to make decisions and follow a course of action, even if the nurse thinks the client is making decisions that are unlikely to be successful.

• Working with clients in community settings demands an even more collaborative relationship than the traditional role of caring for the client in an inpatient setting. The nurse may be more familiar and comfortable with the latter.

KEY POINTS

• People with mental health problems are treated in a variety of settings, and some are not in touch with needed services at all.
• Shortened inpatient hospital stays necessitate changes in the ways Trusts deliver services to clients.
• Planned, thoughtful, collaborative discharge/transfer planning is a good indicator of how successful the client's community reintegration will be.
• Impediments to successful discharge/transfer planning include alcohol and drug abuse, criminal or violent behaviour, non-concordance with medication and suicidal ideation.
• Community residential settings vary in terms of structure, level of supervision and services provided. Some residential settings are transitional, with the expectation that clients will progress to independent living; others serve the client for as long as he or she needs.
• Types of residential settings include board and care homes, adult foster homes, halfway houses, group homes and independent-living programmes.
• A client's ability to remain in the community is closely related to the quality and adequacy of his or her living environment.
• Poverty among people with mental health problems is a significant barrier to maintaining housing in the community and is seldom adequately addressed in rehabilitation programmes.
• Rehabilitation refers to services designed to promote a process for clients with 'mental illness' to return to the community after hospitalization. 'Recovery' goes far beyond this narrow definition and beyond symptom control and medication management to include personal growth, reintegration into the community, empowerment, finding meaning, purpose and hope, increased independence and improved quality of life.
• The clubhouse model of psychosocial rehabilitation/recovery is an intentional community based on the belief that men and women with mental health problems can and will achieve normal life goals when provided time, opportunity, support and fellowship.
• AOT may be one of the most effective approaches to community-based treatment. It includes 24-hour-a-day services, low staff-to-client ratios, in-home or community services, intense and frequent contact and unlimited duration of input.

INTERNET RESOURCES

RESOURCES	INTERNET ADDRESS
• CRISIS	http://www.crisis.org.uk
• Fountain House (clubhouse model)	http://www.fountainhouse.org
• National Association of Psychiatric Intensive Care Units	www.napicu.org.uk/
• National Forum for Assertive Outreach	http://nfao.co.uk/
• National Institute for Mental Health in England	www.nimhe.csip.org.uk
• Prison Reform Trust	www.prisonreformtrust.org.uk
• Sainsbury Centre For Mental Health	http://www.scmh.org.uk
• SHELTER	http://www.shelter.org.uk/

- Services such as AOT must be provided along with stable housing and adequate employment to produce positive outcomes for adults with mental health problems who are homeless.

- Adults with mental health problems may end up in the criminal justice system more frequently because of lack of adequate community support and the attitudes of the criminal justice system and society as a whole, as well as because of the interrelationships between deprivation, homelessness, poor self-esteem, relationship breakdown and substance/alcohol misuse.

- Barriers to community reintegration for people with mental health problems who have been incarcerated include poverty, homelessness, substance abuse, violence, victimization, rape, trauma and self-harm.

- The multidisciplinary team can include the psychiatrist, psychologist, nurse, social worker, occupational therapist and many others.

- The mental health nurse is in an ideal position to fulfil the role of care co-ordinator. The nurse can offer evidence-based psychotherapeutic interventions; assess, monitor and refer clients for general medical and mental health problems; administer drugs; monitor for drug side-effects; provide drug and patient and family health education; monitor for general medical disorders that have psychological and physiological components.

- Empowering clients to pursue full recovery requires collaborative working relationships with clients rather than the traditional approach of caring for clients.

REFERENCES

Callaghan, P. (2006). Discharge planning. In P. Callaghan & H. Waldock (Eds.), *Oxford handbook of mental health nursing.* Oxford: Oxford University Press.

Croft-White, G. & Parry-Crooke, G. (2004). Hidden homelessness: Lost voices. The invisibility of homeless people with multiple needs. Available: http://www.crisis.org.uk/publications/LostVoices.pdf

CSIP/NIMHE. (2007). A positive outlook. *A good practice toolkit to improve discharge from inpatient mental health care.* Available: http://www.cat.csip.org.uk/_library/A%20Positive%20Outlook.pdf

Dean, R. & Craig, T. (1999). *Pressure points: Why people with mental health problems become homeless.* London: CRISIS

Desai, M. M. & Rosenheck, R. A. (2005). Unmet need for medical care among homeless adults with serious mental illness. *General Hospital Psychiatry, 27*(6), 418–425.

Fazel, S., Benning, R., & Danesh, J. (2005). Suicides in male prisoners in England and Wales, 1978–2003. *Lancet, 366*(9493), 1301–1302.

Ferguson, A. (2004). Clubhouse: The recovery model. *Mental Health Practice, 7*(9), 22–23.

Haglund, K., von Knorring, L., & von Essen, L. (2006). Psychiatric wards with locked doors: advantages and disadvantages according to nurses and mental health assistants. *Journal of Clinical Nursing, 15*(4), 387–394.

Konrad, N. (2002). Prisons as new asylums. *Current Opinions in Psychiatry, 15*(6), 583–587.

Latimer, E. (2005). Economic considerations associated with assertive community treatment and supported employment for people with severe mental illness. *Journal of Psychiatry & Neuroscience, 30*(5), 355–359.

Liberman, R. P., Hilty, D. M., Drake, R. E., *et al.* (2001). Requirements for multidisciplinary teamwork in psychiatric rehabilitation. *Psychiatric Services, 52*(10), 1331–1342.

Marx, A. J., Test, M. A., & Stein, L. I. (1973). Extrahospital management of severe mental illness: feasibility and effects of social functioning. *Archives of General Psychiatry, 29*(4), 505–511.

McCoy, M. L., Roberts, D. L., Hanrahan, P., *et al.* (2004). Jail linkage assertive community treatment services for individuals with mental illnesses. *Psychiatric Rehabilitation Journal, 27*(3), 243–250.

Mental Health Act (as amended). (2007). London: OPSI. Available: http://www.dh.gov.uk/en/Healthcare/NationalServiceFrameworks/Mentalhealth/DH_089882

Mental Health Act Commission. (2005). *In place of fear.* Available: http://www.psychminded.co.uk/news/news2006/jan06/MHAC11thannualreport.pdf

Min, S., Wong, Y. L. I., & Rothbard, A. B. (2004). Outcomes of shelter use among homeless persons with serious mental illness. *Psychiatric Services, 55*(3), 284–289.

MIND. (2008). *A brief guide to who's who in mental health.* Available: http://www.mind.org.uk/Information/Factsheets/History+of+mental+health/A+brief+guide+to+whos+who+in+mental+health.htm

MIND Statistics. (2006). *The social context of mental distress.* Available: http://www.mind.org.uk/Information/Factsheets/Statistics/Statistics+6.htm

Muijen, M. (2002). Acute wards: problems and solutions. *Psychiatric Bulletin, 26,* 342–343.

National Audit Office. (2007). *Helping people through crisis – report on Crisis Resolution and Home Treatment services.* Available: http://www.nao.org.uk/publications/nao_reports/07-08/crisis_rept_survey.pdf

NIMHE. (2002). *Minimum standards for general adult services in PICU's and low secure environments – policy implementation guidance.* Available: http://www.napicu.org.uk/standards.pdf

Office of the Deputy Prime Minister. (2004). Homelessness statistics December 2003 and addressing the health needs of homeless people – policy briefing 7. Available: http://www.communities.gov.uk/documents/housing/pdf/137779.pdf

Prince, J. D. (2006). Practices preventing rehospitalization of individuals with schizophrenia. *Journal of Nervous and Mental Disease, 194*(6), 397–403.

Rae, G. M. (2007a). Acute in-patient psychiatry: service improvement – the time is now. *Psychiatric Bulletin, 31,* 259–261.

Rae, M. (2007b). Review of open doors in acute inpatient units: discussion paper CSIP/NIMHE. Available: www.nimhe.csip.org.uk/silo/files/reviewofopendoorsfinalapril20072doc.doc

Redko, C., Durbin, J., Waysylenki, D., *et al.* (2004). Participant perspectives on satisfaction with assertive community treatment. *Psychiatric Rehabilitation Journal, 27*(3), 283–286.

Reynolds, L. (2005). *Full house? How overcrowded housing affects families.* London: Shelter.

Royal College of Psychiatrists. (2008). *Mental health information: the mental health team.* Available: http://www.rcpsych.ac.uk/pdf/Mental%20Health%20Team%20PDF.pdf

Segal, S. P. & Riley, S. (2003). Caring for persons with serious mental illness: policy and practice suggestions. *Social Work in Mental Health, 1*(3), 1–17.

Udechuku, A., Oliver, J., Hallam, K., *et al.* (2005). Assertive community treatment of the mentally ill: service model and effectiveness. *Australasian Psychiatry, 13*(2), 129–134.

White, L. & Brooker, C. (2001). Working with a multidisciplinary team in a secure psychiatric environment. *Journal of Psychosocial Nursing, 39*(9), 26–31.

Williams, C. C. (2004). Discharge planning process on a general psychiatry unit. *Social Work in Mental Health, 2*(1), 17–31.

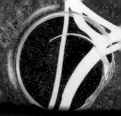

Chapter Study Guide

MULTIPLE-CHOICE QUESTIONS

Select the best answer for each of the following questions.

1. All the following are characteristics of assertive outreach programmes except
   a. Services are provided in the home or community.
   b. Services are provided by a multidisciplinary team.
   c. Services have high staff–client ratios.
   d. Services are delivered between nine and five on weekdays.

2. Recovery principles incorporate all but one of the following:
   a. Optimism
   b. Collaboration
   c. A focus on strengths
   d. Strict diagnostic criteria

3. The primary purpose of rehabilitation/recovery should be to
   a. Control psychiatric symptoms
   b. Manage clients' medications
   c. Develop a life of meaning and purpose
   d. Reduce hospital readmissions

4. Homeless people with mental health problems would benefit most from:
   a. Case management services
   b. Outpatient psychiatric care to manage psychiatric symptoms
   c. Stable housing in a residential neighbourhood
   d. A combination of stable housing, focused care and treatment, and community support

FILL-IN-THE-BLANK QUESTIONS

Identify the multidisciplinary team member responsible for the functions listed below.

_____ Assesses, makes diagnoses and prescribes treatment

_____ Focuses on functional abilities and work, incorporating arts, crafts and a range of problem-solving approaches

_____ Assesses, plans, implements and evaluates health care of people in the community, frequently acting as care co-ordinator

_____ Offers focused psychological treatment programmes and psychometric testing

GROUP DISCUSSION TOPICS

1. Identify the barriers to community reintegration faced by prisoners with mental health problems.

2. Discuss the advantages and disadvantages of maintaining distinct professional roles.

3. Explore factors that have caused an increased number of people with mental health problems to end up in prison.

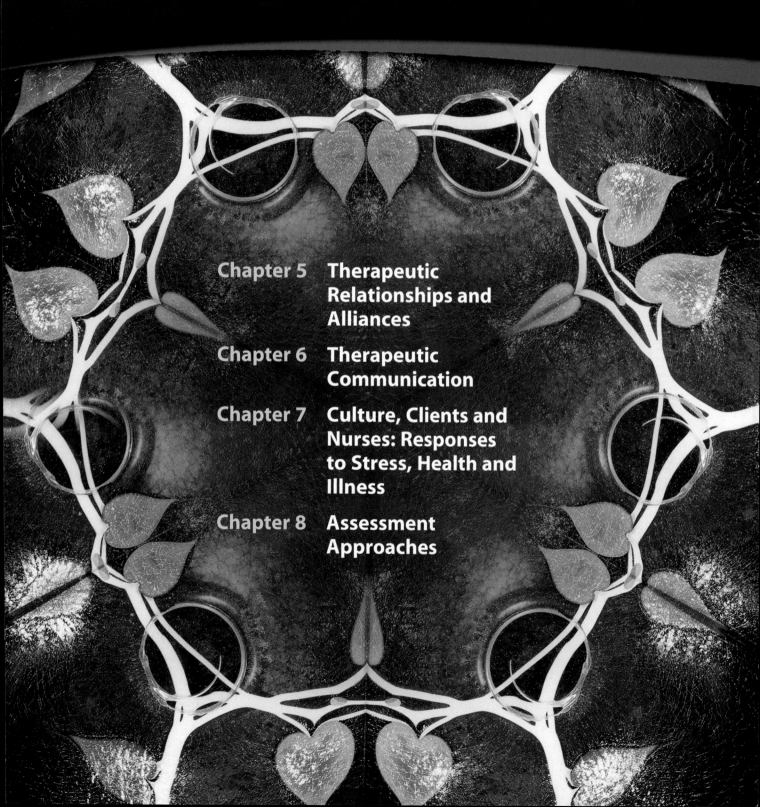

Unit

2

Building the Nurse–Client Relationship

Therapeutic Relationships and Alliances

Key Terms

- acceptance
- advocacy
- attitudes
- beliefs
- confidentiality
- congruence
- countertransference
- empathy
- exploitation
- genuine interest
- intimate relationship
- orientation phase
- patterns of knowing
- positive regard
- preconceptions
- problem identification
- self-awareness
- self-disclosure
- social relationship
- termination or resolution phase
- therapeutic alliance
- therapeutic use of self
- transference
- unknowing
- values
- working phase

Learning Objectives

After reading this chapter, you should be able to:

1. Describe how the nurse uses the necessary components involved in building and enhancing the nurse–client alliance (focus, concreteness, trust, genuine interest, empathy, acceptance and positive regard).

2. Explain the importance of values, beliefs and attitudes in the development of the nurse–client relationship.

3. Describe the importance of self-awareness and therapeutic use of self in the nurse–client relationship.

4. Identify self-awareness issues that can enhance or hinder the nurse–client relationship.

5. Define Carper's four patterns of knowing and give examples of each.

6. Describe the differences between social, intimate and therapeutic relationships.

7. Describe and implement the phases of the nurse–client relationship as outlined by Hildegard Peplau.

8. Explain the negative behaviours that can hinder or diminish the nurse–client relationship.

9. Explain the various possible roles of the nurse (teacher, carer, advocate and parent surrogate) in the nurse–client relationship.

The ability to establish therapeutic relationships (sometimes termed a therapeutic alliance) with clients is one of the most important skills a nurse can develop: without it, nothing else really matters! Although important in all nursing specialties, the therapeutic relationship is especially crucial to the success of interventions with clients requiring mental health care, because the therapeutic relationship and the communication within it serve as the foundation for treatment and success.

This chapter examines the crucial components involved in establishing appropriate therapeutic nurse–client relationships: focus and concreteness, trust, genuine interest, acceptance, positive regard, self-awareness and therapeutic use of self. It explores the tasks that should be accomplished in each phase of the nurse–client relationship and the techniques the nurse can use to help achieve them. It also discusses each of the therapeutic roles of the nurse: teacher, carer, advocate and parent surrogate.

A 'relationship' does not have to be long term, or be developed over a considerable period of time: a helpful, trusting alliance can be built rapidly as long as – at its heart – is the nurse's compassion and desire for effectiveness.

COMPONENTS OF A THERAPEUTIC RELATIONSHIP

Many factors can enhance the nurse–client relationship, and it is the nurse's responsibility to develop them. They promote trusting communication and enhance relationships in all aspects of the nurse's life.

Focus, Purpose and Concreteness

The nurse needs to be clear that his or her role is to have purposeful, transparent conversations with people that are founded on establishing rapport and connecting, exchanging information and agreeing, wherever appropriate, an action plan with the client. He or she must be aware of using language appropriately, of being clear about what he or she, and what the client, is saying, and of knowing what the desired goal of the conversation is.

Box 5.1

Make the care of people your first concern, treating them as individuals and respecting their dignity.

From NMC. (2008). *The Code: Standards of conduct, performance and ethics for nurses and midwives*. Available: *http://www.nmc-uk.org/aArticle.aspx?ArticleID=3236*

Box 5.2   TRUSTING BEHAVIOURS

Trust is built in the nurse–client relationship when the nurse exhibits the following behaviours:

- Treating the client as a human being
- Friendliness
- Caring
- Interest
- Understanding
- Consistency
- Suggesting without telling
- Approachability
- Listening
- Keeping promises
- Providing schedules of activities
- Honesty

From *http://www.mentalhealth.org.uk/information/mental-health-overview/mental-illness.* Copyright © Mental Health Foundation.

Trust

The nurse–client relationship requires trust. Trust builds when the client is confident in the nurse and when the nurse's presence and actions convey integrity and reliability. It develops when the client believes that the nurse will be consistent in his or her words and actions and can be relied on to do what he or she says. Some behaviours that the nurse can exhibit to help build the client's trust include being friendly, caring, interested, understanding and consistent; keeping promises; and listening to and being honest with the client (Box 5.2).

Congruence occurs when words and actions match. For example, the nurse says to the client, 'I have to leave now to go to a clinical conference, but I'll be back at 2 PM' and indeed returns at 2 PM to see the client. The nurse needs to exhibit congruent behaviours to have any chance of building a trusting alliance with the client. Trust erodes when a client sees inconsistency between what the nurse says and does: inconsistent or incongruent behaviours include making verbal commitments and not following them through. For example, the nurse tells the client she will come and see him at home every Tuesday at 10 AM, but the very next week she has to attend a meeting and doesn't show up. Another example of incongruent behaviour is when the nurse's voice or body language is inconsistent with the words he or she speaks. For example, an angry client confronts a nurse and accuses her of not liking her. The nurse responds by saying, 'Of course I like you, Nancy! I am here to help you.' But as she says these words, the nurse backs away from Nancy and looks over her shoulder: the verbal and non-verbal components of the message do not match.

When working with a client with mental health problems, some of the elements of the disorder, such as paranoia, low self-esteem and anxiety, may make trust difficult to establish. For example, a client with depression may have little energy to listen to or to comprehend what the nurse is saying; similarly, a client with panic disorder may be too anxious to focus on the nurse's communication. Although clients with mental disorders frequently give incongruent messages because of their illness, the nurse must continue to provide consistent congruent messages. Examining one's own behaviour, and doing one's best to make messages clear, simple and congruent, help to facilitate trust between the nurse and the client.

Genuine Interest and Curiosity

When the nurse is comfortable with himself or herself, aware of his or her strengths and limitations and clearly focused, the client perceives a genuine person showing **genuine interest**. A client with mental health problems can detect when someone is exhibiting dishonest or artificial behaviour, such as asking a question and then not waiting for the answer, talking over him or her, or assuring him or her everything will be all right. The nurse should be open and honest and display congruent behaviour. Sometimes, however, responding with truth and honesty alone does not provide the best professional response. In such cases, the nurse may choose to disclose to the client a personal experience related to the client's current concerns. Doing so helps to develop trust and allows the client to see the nurse as a real person with perhaps similar problems. The client may then choose to reveal more information to the nurse. This self-disclosure, revealing personal information (e.g. biographical data, ideas, thoughts, feelings), can enhance openness and honesty. Nevertheless, the nurse must *not* shift emphasis to his or her own problems rather than the client's.

Empathy

Imagining what it is like to be someone other than yourself is at the core of our humanity. It is the essence of compassion, and it is the beginning of morality.

Ian McEwan (2001)

Empathy is the attempt of the nurse to perceive – as far as is ever possible – the thoughts, meanings and feelings of the client and to communicate that understanding back to the client. It is considered one of the essential skills a nurse must develop – it is also one of the most complex and challenging. Empathy has been shown to influence positively client outcomes: clients tend to feel better about themselves and more understood when the nurse seems to be empathic (Welch, 2005). Being able to put himself or herself in the client's shoes does *not* mean, though, that the nurse has had the same exact experiences as the client, nor does it mean the nurse 'knows what it's like' for the client. Nevertheless, by active, focused listening and consciously, deliberately attempting to sense the meaning of a situation for the client, the nurse can begin to help clarify the client's thoughts and feelings about the experience. Both the client and the nurse give a 'gift of self' when empathy occurs – the client by feeling safe enough to share feelings and the nurse by listening closely enough to understand. A new, rich 'story' – a fresh, less distressing 'take' on reality – can begin to be co-constructed during a therapeutic conversation or across a series of conversations.

Several therapeutic communication techniques, such as reflection, restatement and clarification, help the nurse to send empathic messages to the client. For example, a client says,

'I'm so confused! My son just visited and wants to know where the locker key is.'

Using *reflection*, the nurse might respond,

'You're confused because your son asked for the locker key?'

The nurse, using *clarification*, could reply,

'Are you confused about why your son visited?'

From these empathic moments, a bond can be established that can serve as the foundation for an effective nurse–client relationship. More examples of therapeutic communication techniques are found in Chapter 6.

CLINICAL VIGNETTE: THERAPEUTIC RELATIONSHIPS

Two mental health students have arrived for their first day on an inpatient unit. They are apprehensive, uncertain what to expect and standing next to each other in the lounge. They are not at all sure how to react to the people around them and are fearful of what to say. Suddenly they hear one of the clients shout, 'Oh look, the students are here. Now we can have some fun!' Another client replies, 'Not me, I just want to be left alone.' A third client says, 'I want to talk to the good-looking one . . .'

The nurse must understand the difference between empathy and *sympathy* (feelings of concern or sadness or outrage one feels for another, that arise – seemingly spontaneously – in the nurse), while appreciating the complex overlap between the two. If empathy is viewed merely as an intellectual exercise, then the alliance is likely to remain superficial and unhelpful; at the same time, if the conversation stays at a level of emotion exchange then it may well reinforce a sense of 'stuckness' and militate against the development of trust. By remaining satisfied with a feeling of sympathy and by merely expressing that sympathy, the nurse may end up invalidating or inhibiting the client's own thoughts and feelings. In the above example, the nurse talking from a position of sympathy might have responded, 'I know how confusing sons can be. My son confuses me, too, and I know how bad that makes you feel.' The nurse's own feelings of sadness or even pity could influence the relationship and hinder the nurse's abilities to focus on the client's needs and desires. Sympathy often shifts the emphasis to the nurse's feelings, hindering the nurse's ability to view the client's needs objectively and blocking a conversation from becoming focused on both the acknowledgement of distress and the need for change.

Acceptance

The nurse who does not become upset or respond negatively to a client's emotions conveys **acceptance** to the client. Avoiding judgements of the person, no matter what their behaviour, is, in this sense, acceptance. This does not mean acceptance of inappropriate or damaging behaviour, but rather acceptance of the person as worthwhile. The nurse must negotiate boundaries for behaviour in the nurse–client relationship and, by being clear and firm without anger or judgement, the nurse allows the client to feel intact while still conveying that he or she feels certain behaviour is unacceptable. As an example, a client puts his arm around the nurse's waist. An appropriate response might be for the nurse to remove his hand and say,

'John, don't put your hand on me. We were talking about your relationship with your girlfriend and that doesn't mean you need to touch me. Shall we carry on?'

An inappropriate response might be,

'John, stop that! What's got into you? I'm leaving, and I might come back tomorrow'

Leaving and threatening not to return punishes and rejects the client while failing to clearly address the inappropriate behaviour.

Positive Regard

The nurse who appreciates the client as a unique, worthwhile human being can respect the client regardless of his or her behaviour, background or lifestyle. This unconditional, non-judgemental attitude is known as **positive regard** and implies respect. Calling the client by name, spending time with the client and listening and responding openly are measures by which the nurse conveys respect and positive regard to the client. The nurse also conveys positive regard by allowing the client's ideas and preferences to drive the planning of care. Doing so shows that the nurse believes the client has the ability to make positive and meaningful contributions to his or her own plan of care.

The nurse relies on presence, or *attending,* using non-verbal and verbal communication techniques to make the client aware that he or she is receiving full attention. Non-verbal techniques that create an atmosphere of presence include leaning toward the client, maintaining eye contact, being relaxed, having arms resting at the sides and having an interested but neutral attitude. Verbally attending means that the nurse avoids communicating value judgements about the client's behaviour. For example, the client may say, 'I was so mad, I yelled and screamed at my mother for an hour.' If the nurse responds with, 'Well, that didn't help, did it?' or 'I can't believe you did that', the nurse is communicating a value judgement that the client was 'wrong' or 'bad'. A better response would be 'What happened then?' or 'You must have been really upset.' The nurse maintains attention on the client and avoids communicating negative opinions or value judgements about the client's behaviour.

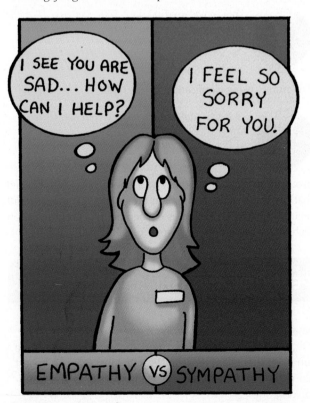

Empathy vs. sympathy

Self-Awareness and Therapeutic Use of Self

Before he or she can begin to understand clients, the nurse must first be working to know himself or herself better. **Self-awareness** is a never-ending process of developing an understanding of one's own values, beliefs, thoughts, feelings, attitudes, motivations, prejudices, strengths and limitations and how these qualities affect others. Self-awareness allows the nurse to observe, pay attention to, and try to understand the subtle responses and reactions of clients when interacting with them.

Values are abstract standards that give a person a sense of right and wrong and establish a code of conduct for living. To gain insight into oneself and personal values, the values clarification process is helpful.

The values clarification process has three steps: choosing, prizing and acting. *Choosing* is when the person considers a range of possibilities and freely chooses the value that feels right. *Prizing* is when the person considers the value, cherishes it and publicly attaches it to himself or herself. *Acting* is when the person puts the value into action. For example, a clean and orderly student has been assigned to live with another student who leaves clothes and food all over their room. At first the orderly student is unsure why she hesitates to return to the room and feels tense around her roommate. As she examines the situation, she realizes that they view the use of personal space differently (choosing). Next she discusses her conflict and choices with her adviser and friends (prizing). Finally, she decides to negotiate with her roommate for a compromise (acting).

Beliefs are ideas that one holds to be true, for example, 'All old people have poor memories', 'If the sun is shining, it will be a good day', or 'All doctors are arrogant'. Some beliefs have objective evidence to substantiate them. For example, people who believe in evolution have accepted the evidence that supports this explanation for the origins of life. Other beliefs are irrational and may persist, despite these beliefs having no supportive evidence or the existence of contradictory empirical evidence. For example, many people harbour irrational beliefs about cultures different from their own that they developed simply from others' comments or fear of the unknown, not from any evidence to support such beliefs.

Attitudes are general feelings or a frame of reference around which a person organizes knowledge about the world. Attitudes such as being hopeful, optimistic, pessimistic, positive or negative, colour how we look at ourselves, the world and other people. A positive mental attitude, for example, occurs when a person chooses to put a positive spin on an experience, comment or judgement. For example, in a crowded supermarket, the person at the front is paying with change, slowly counting it out. The person waiting in line who has a positive attitude might be thankful for the extra minutes and might begin to use them to do deep-breathing exercises and to relax. A negative attitude also colours how one views the world and other people. For example, a person who has had an unpleasant experience with a rude waiter may develop a negative attitude toward all waiters. Such a negative attitude might cause the person to behave impolitely and unpleasantly with every waiter he or she encounters (and thus invite more rudeness). The nurse should re-evaluate and readjust beliefs and attitudes periodically as he or she gains experience and wisdom. Ongoing challenges to self-awareness allow the nurse to accept values, attitudes and beliefs of others that may differ from his or her own:

Box 5.3 lists questions designed to increase the nurse's cultural awareness. A person who does not assess personal attitudes and beliefs may hold a prejudice (hostile attitude) toward a group of people because of preconceived ideas or stereotypical images of that group. For example, a nursing student comes from a white, Protestant, middle-class environment; until beginning university in a multicultural urban environment, she had little experience with cultures other than her own. She came with an ethnocentric attitude of believing that her culture was superior to all others. Once she became friends with students from Zimbabwe, she began to realize that each culture has its own beauty and style, its own myriad beliefs, contradictions, certainties and uncertainties, its own intrinsic worth. By letting her new experiences and friends become part of her view of the world, the student has revised her beliefs and attitudes and expanded her understanding of herself, other people and the world. Box 5.4 provides an example of a values clarification exercise that can assist nurses to become aware of their own beliefs and thoughts about other cultures.

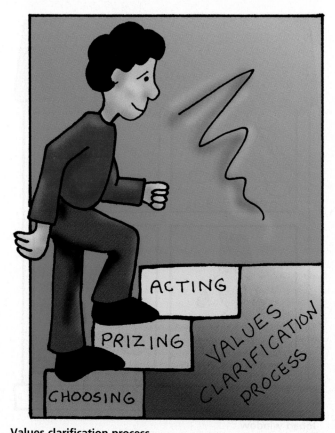

Values clarification process

Box 5.3   CULTURAL AWARENESS QUESTIONS

ACKNOWLEDGING YOUR CULTURAL HERITAGE

- Which ethnic group, socioeconomic class, religion, age group and community do you belong to?
- What experiences have you had with people from ethnic groups, socioeconomic classes, religions, age groups or communities different from your own?
- What were those experiences like? How did you feel about them?
- When you were growing up, what did your parents and significant others say about people who were different from your family?

- What aspects of your ethnic group, socioeconomic class, religion, age, gender or community do you find embarrassing or wish you could change? Why?
- What socio-cultural factors in your background might contribute to being rejected by members of other cultures?
- What personal qualities do you have that will help you establish interpersonal relationships with people from other cultural groups? What personal qualities may be detrimental?

THERAPEUTIC USE OF SELF

By developing self-awareness and beginning to understand his or her attitudes, the nurse can begin to use aspects of his or her personality, experiences, values, feelings, intelligence, needs, coping skills and perceptions to establish compassionate and effective relationships with clients. This process is sometimes called the '**therapeutic use of self**'. Nurses can use themselves as a therapeutic tool to establish therapeutic alliances with clients and help them grow, change and heal. Peplau (1952), who first described this therapeutic use of self in the nurse–client relationship, believed that nurses must clearly understand themselves to promote their clients' growth and to avoid limiting clients' choices to those that nurses value.

Our actions arise from conscious and unconscious responses that are formed by genetic factors, our biology and chemistry, by our life experiences and our educational, spiritual and cultural values. We tend to employ automatic responses or behaviours because they are familiar: we need, continually, to examine these ritualized ways of responding or behaving and evaluate how they help or hinder the therapeutic relationship.

One tool that is useful in learning more about oneself is the Johari window (Luft, 1970), which creates a 'word portrait' of a person in four areas and indicates how well that person knows himself or herself and communicates with others. The four areas evaluated are as follows:

- Quadrant 1: Open/public self – qualities one knows about oneself and others also know
- Quadrant 2: Blind/unaware self – qualities known only to others
- Quadrant 3: Hidden/private self – qualities known only to oneself

- Quadrant 4: Unknown – an empty quadrant to symbolize qualities as yet undiscovered by oneself or others

In creating a Johari window, the first step is for the nurse to appraise his or her own qualities by creating a list of them: values, attitudes, feelings, strengths, behaviours, accomplishments, needs, desires and thoughts. The second

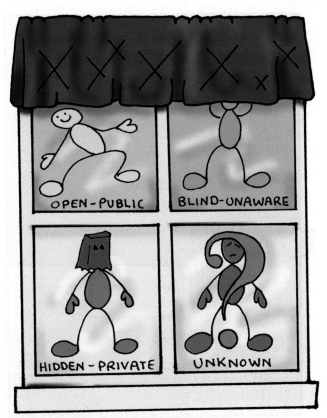

Johari window

step is to find out the perceptions of others by interviewing them and asking them to identify qualities, both positive and negative, they see in the nurse. To learn from this exercise, the opinions given must be honest; there must be no sanctions taken against those who list negative qualities. The third step is to compare lists and to assign qualities to the appropriate quadrant.

If quadrant 1 is the longest list, this indicates that the nurse is open to others; a smaller quadrant 1 means that the nurse shares little about himself or herself with others. If quadrants 1 and 3 are both small, the person demonstrates little insight. Any change in one quadrant is reflected by changes in other quadrants. The goal is to work toward moving qualities from quadrants 2, 3 and 4 into quadrant 1

Box 5.4   **VALUES CLARIFICATION EXERCISE**

VALUES CLARIFICATION

Your values are your ideas about what is most important to you in your life – what you want to live by and live for. They are the silent forces behind many of your actions and decisions. The goal of 'values clarification' is for their influence to become fully conscious, for you to explore and honestly acknowledge what you truly value at this time. You can be more self-directed and effective when you know which values you really choose to keep and live by as an adult and which ones will get priority over others. Identify your values first, and then rank your top three or five.

- ☐ Being with people
- ☐ Being loved
- ☐ Being married
- ☐ Having a special partner
- ☐ Having companionship
- ☐ Loving someone
- ☐ Taking care of others
- ☐ Having someone's help
- ☐ Having a close family
- ☐ Having good friends
- ☐ Being liked
- ☐ Being popular
- ☐ Getting someone's approval
- ☐ Being appreciated
- ☐ Being treated fairly
- ☐ Being admired
- ☐ Being independent
- ☐ Being courageous
- ☐ Having things in control
- ☐ Having self-control
- ☐ Being emotionally stable
- ☐ Having self-acceptance
- ☐ Having pride or dignity
- ☐ Being well organized
- ☐ Being competent

- ☐ Learning and knowing a lot
- ☐ Achieving highly
- ☐ Being productively busy
- ☐ Having enjoyable work
- ☐ Having an important position
- ☐ Making money
- ☐ Striving for perfection
- ☐ Making a contribution to the world
- ☐ Fighting injustice
- ☐ Living ethically
- ☐ Being a good parent (or child)
- ☐ Being a spiritual person
- ☐ Having a relationship with God
- ☐ Having peace and quiet
- ☐ Making a home
- ☐ Preserving your roots
- ☐ Having financial security
- ☐ Holding on to what you have
- ☐ Being safe physically
- ☐ Being free from pain
- ☐ Not getting taken advantage of
- ☐ Having it easy
- ☐ Being comfortable
- ☐ Avoiding boredom
- ☐ Having fun
- ☐ Enjoying sensual pleasures
- ☐ Looking good
- ☐ Being physically fit
- ☐ Being healthy
- ☐ Having prized possessions
- ☐ Being a creative person
- ☐ Having deep feelings
- ☐ Growing as a person
- ☐ Living fully
- ☐ 'Smelling the flowers'
- ☐ Having a purpose

By Joyce Sichel. From Bernard, M. E. & Wolfe, J. L. (Eds.). (2000). *The RET resource book for practitioners*. New York: Albert Ellis Institute.

(qualities known to self and others). Doing so indicates that the nurse is gaining self-knowledge and awareness. See the accompanying figure for an example of a Johari window.

PATTERNS OF KNOWING

Peplau (1952) identified **preconceptions**, or ways one person expects another to behave or speak, as a roadblock to the formation of an authentic relationship. Preconceptions often prevent people from getting to know one another. Preconceptions and different or conflicting personal beliefs and values may prevent the nurse from developing a therapeutic relationship with a client. Here is an example of preconceptions that interfere with a therapeutic relationship: Mr Jones, a client, has the preconceived stereotypical idea that all male nurses are gay and refuses to have Samuel, a male nurse, take care of him. Samuel, meanwhile, has a preconceived stereotypical notion that all Welshmen are aggressive, so he is relieved that Mr Jones has refused to work with him. Both men are missing the opportunity to do some important work together . . .

Carper (1978) identified four **patterns of knowing** in nursing: empirical knowing (derived from the science of nursing), personal knowing (derived from life experiences), ethical knowing (derived from moral knowledge of nursing) and aesthetic knowing (derived from the art of nursing). These patterns provide the nurse with a clear method of observing and understanding every client interaction. Understanding where knowledge comes from and how it affects behaviour helps the nurse become more self-aware (Table 5.1). Munhall (1993) added another pattern that she called **unknowing**: for the nurse to admit he or she does not know the client or the client's subjective world opens the way for a truly authentic encounter. The nurse in a state of unknowing is open to seeing and hearing the client's views without imposing any of his or her values or viewpoints. In mental health nursing, negative preconceptions on the nurse's part can adversely affect the therapeutic relationship and client outcomes; thus, it is especially important for the nurse to work on developing

this openness and acceptance toward the client. Holding on to uncertainty – often incredibly anxiety-provoking – can be a crucial element in a successful nurse–client relationship.

MINDFULNESS

Mindfulness is an approach to the self, other people and the world that can help form the basis of satisfying relationships; the skills and attitudes embedded in a mindful approach to life can help the nurse develop as a professional and can be invaluable in helping clients to cope with their problems and move towards a life full of purpose and meaning.

Mindfulness is, in essence, about being aware, being awake: noticing what's going on, internally and externally, without judgement. It incorporates more formal practices such as meditation and less formal aspects such as noticing: noticing sensations, thoughts, feelings, states of mind, comfort, discomfort: again, without judgement or criticism or a desire to change. It is about learning to be grounded, centred in the here and now, accepting the way things actually are – not blinding ourselves with attempts to avoid reality.

Mindfulness is an approach that stems, originally, from Buddhist practices but which is increasingly used in conjunction with cognitive therapies such as dialectical behaviour therapy and mindfulness-based cognitive therapy. Its principles also often form part of other approaches such as psychodynamic, humanistic and gestalt therapies (see Chapter 2).

TYPES OF RELATIONSHIPS

Each relationship is of course unique because of the various combinations of traits and characteristics of and circumstances related to the people involved. Although every relationship is different, all relationships can be categorized into three major types: social, intimate and therapeutic.

Table 5.1	CARPER'S PATTERNS OF NURSING KNOWLEDGE	
Pattern	**Example**
Empirical knowing (obtained from the science of nursing)	Client with panic disorder begins to have an attack. Panic attack will raise pulse rate
Personal knowing (obtained from life experience)	Client's face shows the panic
Ethical knowing (obtained from the moral knowledge of nursing)	Although the nurse's shift has ended, she remains with the client
Aesthetic knowing (obtained from the art of nursing)	Although the client shows outward signals now, the nurse has sensed previously the client's jumpiness and subtle differences in the client's demeanor and behaviour

Adapted from Carper, B. (1978). Fundamental patterns of knowing in nursing. *Advances in Nursing Sciences, 1*(1), 13–23.

Social Relationship

A **social relationship** is primarily initiated for the purpose of friendship, socialization, companionship or accomplishment of a task. Communication, which may be superficial, usually focuses on sharing ideas, feelings and experiences and meets the basic need for people to interact. Advice is often given. Roles may shift during social interactions. Outcomes of this kind of relationship are rarely assessed. When a nurse greets a client and chats about the weather or a sports event or engages in small talk or socializing, this is a social interaction. This is acceptable in nursing, indeed a vital part of establishing rapport and initially connecting with someone and of giving a message that the client is far more than the sum of his 'problems', but for the nurse–client relationship to be effective, social interaction must be limited. If the relationship becomes more social than therapeutic, serious work that helps the client move forward will not be done.

Intimate Relationship

A healthy **intimate relationship** involves two people who are emotionally committed to each other. Both parties are concerned about having their individual needs met and helping each other to meet needs as well. The relationship may include sexual or emotional intimacy as well as sharing of mutual goals. Evaluation of the interaction may be ongoing or not. The intimate relationship, in this sense (of course!) has no place in a healthy, effective nurse–client interaction, though commitment and sharing in themselves can be essential and it would be naïve to see nurses as not themselves benefiting from therapeutic conversations.

Therapeutic Relationship

The **therapeutic relationship** differs from the social or intimate relationship in many ways because it directly focuses on the needs, experiences, feelings and ideas of the client only. The nurse and client agree about the areas to work on, the environment in which this work will take place and jointly evaluate the outcomes. The nurse uses communication skills, personal strengths and experiences and understanding of human behaviour to interact purposefully with the client. In the therapeutic relationship, the parameters are clear: the focus is the client's needs, not the nurse's. The nurse should not necessarily be concerned about whether or not the client likes him or her or is grateful (unless this is information that can be used openly to aid the development of the alliance and help the client move towards his or her goals). Such concern is often a signal that the nurse is focusing on a personal need to be liked or needed. The nurse must guard against allowing the therapeutic relationship to slip into a more social relationship. The nurse must constantly focus on the client's needs, not his or her own: this one-way focus is why many clinicians and writers prefer the term '**therapeutic alliance**' to 'therapeutic relationship'.

The nurse's level of self-awareness can either benefit or hamper the therapeutic relationship. For example, if the nurse is nervous around the client, the relationship is more apt to stay social because superficiality is safer. If the nurse is aware of his or her fears, he or she can discuss them with a supervisor or colleague, paving the way for a more genuinely therapeutic relationship to develop.

Relationships are, of course, rarely straightforward and there will almost certainly be 'social' and 'intimate' elements to a therapeutic relationship: the nurse's job is to be aware of these and their impact on the primary task: to help the client.

ESTABLISHING THE THERAPEUTIC RELATIONSHIP

The nurse who has self-confidence rooted in self-awareness is ready to establish effective therapeutic alliances with clients. Because personal growth is ongoing over one's lifetime, the nurse cannot expect to have complete self-knowledge. Awareness of his or her strengths and limitations at any particular moment, however, is a good start.

Phases

Peplau studied and wrote about the interpersonal processes and the phases of the nurse–client relationship for 35 years. Her work provides the nursing profession with a model that can be used to understand and document progress with interpersonal interactions. Peplau's model (1952) has three phases: orientation, working and resolution or termination (Table 5.2). In real life, these phases are not, of course, that clear-cut; they overlap and interlock.

1. ORIENTATION

The **orientation phase** begins when the nurse and client meet and ends when the client begins to identify problems to examine. During the orientation phase, the nurse establishes roles, the purpose of meeting and the parameters of subsequent meetings; identifies the client's problems; and clarifies expectations.

Before meeting the client, the nurse has important work to do. He or she may need to read background materials available on the client, become familiar with any medications the client is taking, gather necessary paperwork and arrange for a quiet, private comfortable setting. This is a time for self-assessment. The nurse should consider his or her personal strengths and limitations in working with this client. Are there any areas that might signal difficulty because of past experiences? For example, if this client had been violent towards his children and the nurse's father had also been violent, the nurse needs to consider the situation: how does it make me feel? What memories does it prompt, and can I work with the client without these memories interfering? The nurse must

Table 5.2   PHASES OF THE NURSE–CLIENT RELATIONSHIP

Orientation	Working		Termination
	Identification	Exploitation	
Client			
• Seeks assistance • Conveys needs • Asks questions • Shares preconceptions and expectations of nurse based on past experience	• Participates in identifying problems • Begins to be aware of time • Responds to help • Identifies with nurse • Recognizes nurse as a person • Explores feelings • Fluctuates dependence, independence and inter-dependence in relationship with nurse • Increases focal attention • Changes appearance (for better or worse) • Understands continuity between sessions (process and content) • Testing manoeuvres decrease	• Makes full use of services • Identifies new goals • Attempts to attain new goals • Rapid shifts in behaviour: dependent, independent • Exploitative behaviour • Self-directing • Develops skill in inter-personal relationships and problem solving • Displays changes in manner of communication (more open, flexible)	• Abandons old needs • Aspires to new goals • Becomes independent of helping person • Applies new problem-solving skills • Maintains changes in style of communication and interaction • Shows positive changes in view of self • Integrates illness • Exhibits ability to stand alone
Nurse			
• Responds to client • Gives parameters of meetings • Explains roles • Gathers data • Helps client identify problem and solution • Helps client plan use of community resources and services • Reduces anxiety and tension • Practises active listening • Focuses client's energies • Clarifies preconceptions and expectations of nurse	• Maintains separate identity • Exhibits ability to edit speech or control focal attention • Shows unconditional acceptance • Helps express needs, feelings • Assesses and adjusts to needs • Provides information • Provides experiences that diminish feelings of helplessness • Does not allow anxiety to overwhelm client • Helps client focus on cues • Helps client develop responses to cues • Uses word stimuli	• Continues assessment • Meets needs as they emerge • Understands reason for shifts in behaviour • Initiates rehabilitative plans • Reduces anxiety • Identifies positive factors • Helps plan for total needs • Facilitates forward movement of personality • Deals with therapeutic impasse	• Sustains relationship as long as client feels necessary • Promotes family interaction to assist with goal planning • Teaches preventive measures • Uses community agencies • Teaches self-care • Terminates nurse–client relationship

Adapted from Forchuck, C. & Brown, B. (1989). Establishing a nurse–client relationship. *Journal of Psychosocial Nursing*, 27(2), 30–34.

examine preconceptions about the client and ensure that he or she can put them aside and get to know the real person. The nurse must come to each client without preconceptions or prejudices. It may be useful for the nurse to discuss all potential problem areas with a supervisor or colleague.

During the orientation phase, the nurse begins to build trust with the client. It is the nurse's responsibility to establish a therapeutic environment that fosters trust and understanding

(Table 5.3). The nurse should share appropriate information about himself or herself at this time, including name and role: for example, 'Hello, James. My name is Miss Ames and I'll be visiting you for the next six weeks, if that's OK. I'm a third year nursing student at the University of Surrey.'

The nurse needs to listen closely to the client's history, perceptions and misconceptions. He or she needs to convey empathy and understanding, acknowledging clearly the client's

| **Table 5.3** | **COMMUNICATION DURING THE PHASES OF THE NURSE–CLIENT RELATIONSHIP** |

Phase of Relationship	Sample Conversation	Communication Skill
Orientation	**Nurse:** 'Hello, Mr O'Hare. I'm Sally Fourth, a nursing student from Surrey University. I'll be coming to the hospital for the next 6 Mondays. I'd like to meet with you each time I am here to work with you on your goals. What do you think would be most helpful for us to talk about?'	Establishing trust; placing boundaries on the relationship and first mention of termination in 6 weeks. Agreeing focus
Orientation	**Nurse:** 'Mr O'Hare, if it's OK with you, we'll meet every Monday from June 1 to July 15 at 11 AM in conference room 2. We can use that time to work on your thoughts and feelings since the death of your twin sister.'	Establishing specifics of the relationship; time, date, place and duration of meetings (can be written as a formal contract or stated as an informal contract)
Orientation	**Nurse:** 'Mr O'Hare, it's important that I tell you I'll be sharing some of what we talk about with my mentor and other staff at the clinical conference. I won't be sharing any information with your wife or children without your permission. If I feel a piece of information may be helpful, I will ask you first if I may share it with your wife. Is that OK?'	Establishing confidentiality
Working	**Client:** 'Sally, I miss my sister Eileen so much.' **Nurse:** 'How long have you been without your sister, Brian – can I call you Brian?'	Gathering data; establishing level of informality
Working	**Client:** 'Without my twin, I'm not half the person I was.' **Nurse:** 'It sounds such a hard experience to have been through, Brian. Maybe if we look at the strengths you feel you do have still.'	Promoting self-esteem
Working	**Client:** 'Oh, why talk about me. I'm nothing without my twin.' **Nurse:** 'Brian, I feel you're a person in your own right. I think working together we can identify the strengths you have. Will you try with me?'	Overcoming resistance
Termination	**Nurse:** 'Well, Brian, as you know I only have 1 week left to meet with you.' **Client:** 'I am going to miss you. I feel better when you are here.' **Nurse:** 'I'll miss you as well, Brian. I've learnt a lot from working with you.'	Sharing of the termination experience with the client demonstrates the partnership and the caring of the relationship

current concerns and fears (Forchuk, 2002). If the relationship gets off to a positive start, it is more likely to succeed and to meet established goals.

At the first meeting, the client may be distrustful if previous relationships with professionals have been unsatisfactory. The client may use rambling or superficial speech, or exaggerate episodes as ploys to avoid discussing the real problems. It may take several sessions until the client believes that he or she can trust the nurse enough to work effectively and collaboratively with him or her.

Nurse–client Contracts. Although many clients have had prior experiences in the mental health system, the nurse must always outline the responsibilities of each person. At the outset, both nurse and client should agree on these responsibilities in an informal or verbal contract. In some instances, a formal or written contract may also be appropriate; examples include if a written contract has been necessary in the past with the client or if the client feels a need for the boundaries and containment that might be offered by something written down.

A contract might state the following:

- Time, place and length of sessions
- When sessions will terminate
- Who will be involved in the treatment plan (family members, health team members)
- Client responsibilities (e.g. arrive on time, end on time)
- Nurse's responsibilities (arrive on time, end on time, maintain confidentiality at all times, evaluate progress with client, document sessions)

Confidentiality. **Confidentiality** means respecting the client's right to keep private any information about his or her mental and physical health and related care. Confidentiality means allowing only those dealing with the client's care to have access to the information that the client divulges. Only under precisely defined conditions can third parties have access to this information; for example, child protection, the protection of vulnerable adults and major crime-risks, such as terrorism, may all necessitate a considered breach of confidentiality (Box 5.5).

Adult clients can decide which family members, if any, may be involved in treatment and may have access to clinical information. Ideally, the people close to the client and responsible for his or her care are involved. The client must decide, however, who will be included. For the client to feel safe, boundaries must be clear. The nurse must clearly state information about who will have access to client assessment data and progress evaluations. He or she should tell the client that members of the mental health team share appropriate information among themselves to provide consistent care, and that only with the client's permission will they include a family member. If the client has an appointed guardian, that person can review client information and make treatment decisions that are in the client's best interest. For a child, the parent or appointed guardian is allowed access to information and can make treatment decisions as outlined by the health-care team.

The nurse must be alert if a client asks him or her to keep a secret, because this information may relate to the client potentially harming himself or herself or others and/or may be an attempt to alter the relationship with the nurse in a damaging way. The nurse must avoid any promises to keep secrets. If the nurse has promised not to tell before hearing the message, he or she could be jeopardizing the client's trust. In most cases, even when the nurse refuses to agree to keep information secret, the client continues to relate issues anyway. The following is an example of a good response to a client who is suicidal but requests secrecy:

Client: *'I'm going to jump off the car park tonight, but please don't tell anyone.'*
Nurse: *'I really can't keep a promise like that, especially if it involves your safety. It sounds like you're feeling frightened, though. What do you think the staff and I can do to help you to feel safer?'*

The nurse documents the client's problems with planned interventions. The client must understand that the nurse will collect data about him or her that helps in developing a formulation, planning health care (including medications) and protecting the client's human and civil rights. The client needs to know the limits of confidentiality in nurse–client interactions and how the nurse will use and share this information with professionals involved in client care.

Self-disclosure. **Self-disclosure** means revealing personal information such as biographical information and personal ideas, thoughts and feelings about oneself to clients. Traditionally, conventional wisdom held that nurses should share only their name, marital status and number of children and perhaps should give a general idea about their residence, such as 'I live in Enfield.' Now, however, it is believed that conscious, thoughtful self-disclosure can improve rapport between the nurse and client. The nurse can use self-disclosure to convey shared humanity, support, educate clients, demonstrate that a client's anxiety is normal and even facilitate emotional healing (Ashmore & Banks, 2003a).

Nurses should remember these therapeutic goals of self-disclosure and use disclosure to help the client feel more comfortable and more willing to share thoughts and feelings. Sharing may help the client gain insight about his or her situation or encourage him or her to resolve concerns. The nurse should not use self-disclosure to meet personal needs.

When using self-disclosure, the nurse must consider cultural factors. For example, if the client is from a culture that demands men be stoic and non-communicative, he or she may deem self-disclosure inappropriate. The nurse should keep self-disclosure brief and comfortable, respect the client's privacy by making sure the discussion takes place away from others and understand that each experience is different. The nurse must monitor his or her own comfort level. If the nurse has unresolved feelings about the issue, he or she should not share personal experiences.

Disclosing personal information can be harmful and inappropriate for a client, so the nurse must give it careful thought. For example, when working with a client whose parents are getting a divorce, the nurse says, 'My parents got a divorce when I was 12 and it was a horrible time for me.' The nurse has shifted the focus away from the client and has given the client the idea that this experience will be horrible for the client. Although the nurse may have meant to communicate empathy, the result can be quite the opposite. If the client does not seem ready to deal with the issue, or if the conversation is purely social, it is not a

Box 5.5   RESPECT PEOPLE'S CONFIDENTIALITY

- You must respect people's right to confidentiality
- You must ensure that people are informed about how and why information is shared by those who will be providing their care
- You must disclose information if you believe someone may be at risk of harm, in line with the law of the country in which you are practising

From NMC. (2008). *The Code: Standards of conduct, performance and ethics for nurses and midwives.* Available: *http://www.nmc-uk.org/a Article.aspx?ArticleID=3236*

good time to disclose information about oneself (Ashmore & Banks, 2003b).

2. WORKING

The **working phase** of the nurse–client relationship is usually divided into two sub-phases. During **problem identification**, the client identifies the issues or concerns causing problems. During **exploitation**, the nurse guides the client to examine feelings and responses and to develop better coping skills and a more positive self-image; this encourages behaviour change and develops independence. (Note that Peplau's use of the word *exploitation* had a very different meaning than current usage, which involves unfairly using or taking advantage of a person or situation. For that reason, this phase is better conceptualized as intense exploration and elaboration on earlier themes that the client discussed.) The trust established between nurse and client at this point allows them to examine the problems and to work on them within the security of the relationship. The client must believe that the nurse will not turn away or be upset when the client reveals experiences, issues, behaviours and problems. Very occasionally, the client might use outrageous stories or 'acting-out' behaviours to test the nurse. Testing behaviour challenges the nurse to stay focused and not to react or to be distracted. Sometimes when the client becomes uncomfortable, because he or she is getting too close to an uncomfortable or distressing realization, he or she will use testing behaviours to avoid the subject. The nurse may respond by saying, 'It seems as if we've hit an uncomfortable point for you. Would you like to let it go for now?' This statement focuses on the issue at hand and diverts attention from the testing behaviour.

The nurse must remember that it is the client who examines and explores problem situations and relationships. The nurse should remain non-judgemental; he or she should allow the client to analyse situations but offer alternative views if appropriate.

The specific tasks of the working phase include the following:

- Maintaining the relationship
- Gathering more data
- Exploring perceptions of reality
- Developing positive coping mechanisms
- Promoting a positive self-concept
- Encouraging verbalization of feelings
- Facilitating behaviour change
- Working through resistance
- Evaluating progress and redefining goals as appropriate
- Providing opportunities for the client to practise new behaviours
- Promoting independence.

As the nurse and client work together, it is common for the client unconsciously to transfer to the nurse feelings he or she has for significant others. This is called **transference**. For example, if the client has had negative experiences with authority figures, such as a parent or teachers or principals, he or she may display similar reactions of negativity and resistance to the nurse, who also is viewed as an authority. A similar process can occur when the nurse responds to the client based on personal unconscious needs and conflicts; this is called **countertransference**. For example, if the nurse is the youngest in her family and often felt as if no one listened to her when she was a child, she may respond with anger to a client who does not listen or resists her help. Again, self-awareness is important so that the nurse can identify when transference and countertransference might occur. By being aware of such 'hot spots', the nurse has a better chance of responding appropriately rather than letting old unresolved conflicts interfere with the relationship.

3. TERMINATION

The **termination or resolution phase** is the final stage in the nurse–client relationship. It begins when the problems are resolved, and it ends when the relationship is ended. Both nurse and client usually have feelings about ending the relationship; the client especially may feel the termination as an impending loss. Often clients try to avoid termination by acting angrily or aggressively

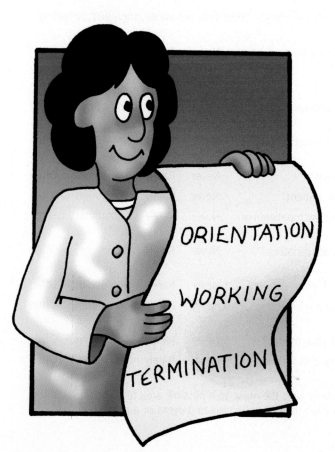

Phases of nurse–client relationship

or as if the problem has not been resolved. The nurse can acknowledge the client's angry feelings and assure the client that this response is normal to ending a relationship. If the client tries to reopen and discuss old resolved issues, the nurse must avoid feeling as if the sessions were unsuccessful; instead, he or she should identify the client's stalling manoeuvres and refocus the client on newly learned behaviours and skills to handle the problem. It is appropriate to tell the client that the nurse enjoyed the time spent with the client and will remember him or her, but it is inappropriate for the nurse to agree to see the client outside the therapeutic relationship.

Katrina sees Mrs O'Shea for the last time at the CMHT office. Mrs O'Shea is sobbing quietly.

Mrs O'Shea: 'Oh, Katrina, you've been so helpful to me. I just know I will go back to my old self without you here to help me.'

Katrina: 'Mrs O'Shea, I think we've had a really productive time together. You seem to have learned so many new ways to have better relationships with your children, and I'm sure you'll go home and be able to use those skills.'

AVOIDING BEHAVIOURS THAT DIMINISH THE THERAPEUTIC RELATIONSHIP

The nurse has power over the client by virtue of his or her professional role. That power can be abused if excessive familiarity occurs, a cold, aloof distance is maintained, an intimate relationship develops or if confidentiality is breached.

Inappropriate Boundaries

All staff members, whether new or experienced, are at risk of allowing a therapeutic relationship to expand into an inappropriate relationship. Self-awareness and honest reflection are extremely important: the nurse who is in touch with his or her feelings and aware of his or her influence over others can help maintain the boundaries of the professional relationship. The nurse must maintain professional boundaries to ensure the best therapeutic outcomes. It is the nurse's responsibility to define the boundaries of the relationship clearly in the orientation phase and to ensure that those boundaries are maintained throughout the relationship. The nurse must act warmly and empathetically, but must not try

Table 5.4 NURSING BOUNDARY INDEX				
Please rate yourself according to the frequency that the following statements reflect your behaviour, thoughts, or feelings within the past 2 years while providing patient care.				
1. Have you ever received any feedback about your behaviour for being overly intrusive with patients or their families?	Never	Rarely	Sometimes	Often
2. Do you ever have difficulty setting limits with patients?	Never	Rarely	Sometimes	Often
3. Do you arrive early or stay late to be with your patient for a longer period of time?	Never	Rarely	Sometimes	Often
4. Do you ever find yourself relating to patients or peers as you might a family member?	Never	Rarely	Sometimes	Often
5. Have you ever acted on sexual feelings you have for a patient?	Never	Rarely	Sometimes	Often
6. Do you feel that you are the only one who understands the patient?	Never	Rarely	Sometimes	Often
7. Have you ever received feedback that you get 'too involved' with patients or families?	Never	Rarely	Sometimes	Often
8. Do you derive conscious satisfaction from patients' praise, appreciation or affection?	Never	Rarely	Sometimes	Often
9. Do you ever feel that other staff members are too critical of 'your' patient?	Never	Rarely	Sometimes	Often
10. Do you ever feel that other staff members are jealous of your relationship with a patient?	Never	Rarely	Sometimes	Often
11. Have you ever tried to 'match-make' a patient with one of your friends?	Never	Rarely	Sometimes	Often
12. Do you find it difficult to handle patients' unreasonable requests for assistance, verbal abuse or sexual language?	Never	Rarely	Sometimes	Often
Any item that is responded to with a 'sometimes' or 'often' should alert the nurse to a possible area of vulnerability. If the item is responded to with a 'rarely', the nurse should determine whether it was an isolated event or a possible pattern of behaviour.				

*Pilette, P., Berck, C., & Achber, L. (1995). Therapeutic management. *Journal of Psychosocial Nursing, 33*(1), 45

to be friends with the client. Social interactions that continue beyond the first few minutes of a meeting contribute to the conversation staying on the surface. This lack of focus on the problems that have been agreed on for discussion erodes the professional relationship.

If a client is attracted to a nurse or vice versa, it is up to the nurse to maintain professional boundaries. Accepting gifts or giving a client one's home address or phone number would be considered a breach of ethical conduct and exceptionally damaging to both parties. Nurses must continually assess themselves and ensure they keep their feelings in check and focus on the clients' interests and needs. Nurses can assess their behaviour by using the Nursing Boundary Index in Table 5.4. Clinical supervision, as ever, can be a vital tool here: the ability to discuss, either individually or in groups, issues with and about clients is essential at times. A full discussion of ethical dilemmas encountered in relationships is found in Chapter 9.

Feelings of Sympathy and Encouraging Client Dependency

The nurse must not let attempts at empathy turn into an unhelpful sympathy for the client. Unlike the therapeutic use of empathy, the nurse who merely feels sorry for the client often tries to compensate by trying to please him or her. When the nurse's behaviour is rooted only in sympathy, the client finds it easier to manipulate, or to be uncertain of, the nurse's feelings. This discourages the client from exploring his or her problems, thoughts and feelings; discourages client growth; and often leads to client dependency.

The client may make increased requests of the nurse for help and assistance or may appear to regress and act as if he or she cannot carry out tasks previously done. These can be signals that the nurse has been 'overdoing' for the client and may be contributing to the client's dependency. Clients sometimes test the nurse to see how much the nurse is willing to do. If the client co-operates only when the nurse is in attendance and does not carry out agreed-on behaviour in the nurse's absence, the client has become too dependent. In any of these instances, the nurse needs to reassess his or her professional behaviour and refocus on the client's needs and therapeutic goals.

Non-acceptance and Avoidance

The nurse–client relationship can be jeopardized if the nurse finds the client's behaviour unacceptable or distasteful and allows those feelings to show by avoiding the client or making verbal responses or facial expressions of annoyance or turning away from the client. The nurse should be aware of the client's behaviour and background before beginning the relationship; if the nurse believes there may be conflict, he or she must explore this possibility with a colleague. If the nurse is aware of a prejudice that would place the client in an unfavourable light, he or she must explore this issue as well. Sometimes by talking about and confronting these feelings, the nurse can accept the client and not let a prejudice hinder the relationship. If the nurse cannot resolve such negative feelings, however, he or she should consider requesting the client see someone else. It is the nurse's responsibility to treat each client with acceptance and positive regard, regardless of the client's history. Part of the nurse's responsibility is to continue to become more self-aware and to confront and resolve any prejudices that threaten to hinder the nurse–client relationship (Box 5.6).

ROLES OF THE NURSE IN A THERAPEUTIC RELATIONSHIP

The mental health nurse needs to adopt various roles in order to provide effective care. We need to understand the importance of assuming the appropriate role for the work that we're doing at a particular time with a particular client.

Teacher/Learner

The teaching role is inherent in many aspects of client care. During the working phase of the nurse–client relationship, the nurse may teach the client ways to try out new methods of coping and solving problems. He or she may offer

---

Box 5.6   **POSSIBLE WARNINGS OR SIGNALS OF ABUSE OF THE NURSE–CLIENT RELATIONSHIP**

- Secrets, reluctance to talk to others about the work being done with clients
- Sudden increase in phone calls between nurse and client, or calls outside clinical hours
- Nurse making more exceptions for client than normal
- Inappropriate gift-giving between client and nurse
- Loaning, trading or selling goods or possessions

- Nurse disclosure of personal issues or information
- Inappropriate touching, comforting or physical contact
- Overdoing, over-protecting or over-identifying with client
- Change in nurse's body language, dress or appearance (with no other satisfactory explanation)
- Extended one-on-one sessions or home visits

information about the medication regime and available community resources. To be a good teacher, the nurse must feel confident about the knowledge he or she has – and must know the limitations of that knowledge base. The nurse should be familiar with the resources in the health-care setting and community and on the Internet, which can provide needed information for clients. The nurse must be honest about what information he or she can provide and when and where to refer clients for further information. This behaviour and honesty builds trust in clients. It is crucial, always, for the nurse not to consider himself or herself an 'expert' on someone else's life: the client is always the expert on his or her own life. Nurses need to be humble enough and confident enough to ask clients to teach them what it's like to be experiencing their life at that moment in time, to teach them what it feels like for that person to be 'depressed', to teach them what it feels like to experience the voices.

Carer

The primary care-giving role in mental health settings is the implementation of the therapeutic relationship to build trust, explore feelings, assist the client in problem solving and help the client meet psychosocial needs. If the client also requires physical nursing care, the nurse may need to explain to the client the need for touch while performing physical care. Some clients may confuse physical care with intimacy and sexual interest, which can erode the therapeutic relationship. The nurse must consider the relationship boundaries and parameters that have been established and must re-emphasize as necessary the goals that were established together at the beginning of the relationship.

Advocate

Advocacy is the process of acting on the client's behalf when he or she cannot do so. This includes ensuring privacy and dignity, promoting informed consent, preventing unnecessary examinations and procedures, accessing necessary services and benefits and ensuring safety from abuse and exploitation by any health professional or authority figure.

Being an advocate involves risk-taking: more senior clinicians may (very occasionally) attempt to embarrass, intimidate or humiliate, and the nurse needs to stay focused on the appropriateness of his or her behaviour and not be intimidated.

The role of advocate requires the nurse to be observant of other health-care professionals. At times, staff members may be reluctant to see what is happening or become involved when a colleague violates the boundaries of a professional relationship. Nurses must take action by talking to the colleague or a supervisor when they observe boundary violations. The NMC Code of Professional Conduct (2008) highlights the nurse's legal responsibility to report

boundary violations and unethical conduct on the part of other professionals. There is a full discussion of ethical conduct in Chapter 9.

There is debate about the role of nurse as advocate. There are times when the nurse may choose not to advocate for the client's autonomy or right to self-determination, such as by supporting involuntary hospitalization for a suicidal client. At these times, acting in the client's 'best interest' (keeping them safe) is in direct opposition to the client's wishes. Some critics view this as paternalistic and controlling and interference with the true role of advocacy.

Parent Surrogate

When a client exhibits child-like behaviour or when a nurse is required to provide personal care such as feeding or bathing, the nurse may be tempted to assume the parental role (as evidenced in choice of words and non-verbal communication). The nurse may begin to sound authoritative, with an attitude of 'I know what's best for you' and the client may respond by acting more child-like and stubborn. Neither party realizes they have fallen – in transactional analysis terms – from adult–adult communication to critical parent-adapted child communication. It is easy for the client to view the nurse in such circumstances as a parent surrogate and for the relationship to become destructive. In such situations, the nurse must be clear, respectful and take his or her own behaviour back to an adult position. By retaining an open, easygoing, non-judgemental attitude, the nurse can continue to nurture the client while establishing boundaries. The nurse must ensure the relationship remains therapeutic and does not become social or intimate (Box 5.7).

SELF-AWARENESS ISSUES

Self-awareness is critical in establishing effective therapeutic nurse–client relationships. For example, a nurse who is prejudiced against people from a certain culture or religion but is not consciously aware of it may have difficulty relating to a client from that culture or religion. If the nurse is aware of, acknowledges, and is open to reassessing the prejudice, the relationship has a better chance of being authentic. If the nurse has certain beliefs and attitudes that he or she will not change, it may be best for another nurse to care for the client. Examining personal strengths and weaknesses helps one gain a strong sense of self. Understanding oneself helps one understand and accept others who may have different ideas and values. The nurse must continue on a path of self-discovery to become more self-aware and more effective in caring for clients.

Nurses also need to learn to 'care for themselves'. This means balancing work with leisure time, building satisfying personal relationships with friends and taking time to relax and pamper oneself. Nurses who are overly committed to

Box 5.7   METHODS TO AVOID INAPPROPRIATE RELATIONSHIPS BETWEEN NURSES AND CLIENTS

- Accept that *all* staff members, whether male or female, junior or senior or from any discipline, are at risk of over-involvement and loss of boundaries
- Assume that boundary violations will occur. Supervisors should recognize potential 'problem' clients and regularly raise the issue of sexual feelings or boundary loss with staff members
- Provide opportunities for staff members to discuss their dilemmas and effective ways of dealing with them, for example in 1:1 and group clinical supervision
- Service areas should develop orientation programmes to include how to set limits, how to recognize clues that the relationship is losing boundaries, what the institu-
tion expects of the professional, clearly defined consequences, case studies, how to develop skills to maintain boundaries and recommended reading
- Provide resources for confidential and non-judgemental assistance
- Hold regular meetings to discuss inappropriate relationships and feelings toward clients
- Provide senior staff to lead groups and model effective therapeutic interventions with difficult clients
- Use clinical vignettes for training
- Use situations that reflect not only sexual dilemmas but also other boundary violations, including problems with abuse of authority and power

work can become burnt-out, rarely finding time to relax or see friends, and sacrificing their own personal lives in the process. When this happens, the nurse is more prone to boundary violations with clients (e.g. sharing frustrations, responding to the client's personal interest in the nurse). In addition, the nurse who is stressed or overwhelmed tends to lose the objectivity that comes with self-awareness and personal growth activities. In the end, nurses who fail to take good care of themselves also cannot take good care of clients and families.

Points to Consider When Building Therapeutic Relationships

- Attend teaching and training workshops about values clarification, beliefs and attitudes to help you assess and learn about yourself.
- Keep a journal of thoughts, feelings and lessons learned to provide self-insight.
- Encourage feedback from colleagues about your relationships with clients.
- Develop a continually changing 'care plan' for self-growth.
- Read books on topics that support the strengths you have identified and help to develop your areas of weakness.

KEY POINTS

- Factors that enhance the nurse–client relationship include trust and congruence, genuine interest, empathy, acceptance and positive regard.
- Self-awareness is crucial in the therapeutic relationship. The nurse's values, beliefs and attitudes all come into play as he or she forms a relationship with a client.

- Carper identified four patterns of knowing: empirical, aesthetic, personal and ethical.
- Munhall established the pattern of unknowing as an openness that the nurse brings to the relationship that prevents preconceptions from clouding his or her view of the client.
- The three types of relationships are social, intimate and therapeutic. The nurse–client relationship should be therapeutic, not social or intimate.
- Nurse theorist Hildegard Peplau developed the phases of the nurse–client relationship: orientation, working (with subphases of problem identification and exploitation) and termination or resolution. These phases are ongoing and overlapping.
- The orientation phase begins when the nurse and client meet and ends when the client begins to identify problems to examine.

Critical Thinking Questions

1. When is it appropriate to accept a gift from a client? What types of gifts are acceptable? Under what circumstances should the nurse accept a gift from a client?
2. What relationship-building behaviours might the nurse use with a client who is very distrustful of the healthcare system?
3. What would you do if you found yourself attracted to a client?
4. What would you do if you really disliked a client?
5. What preconceptions do *you* have about mental health clients? Are there some types of people or problem you find particularly difficult to work with?

- Tasks of the working phase include maintaining the relationship, gathering more data, exploring perceptions of reality, developing positive coping mechanisms, promoting a positive self-concept, encouraging verbalization of feelings that facilitate behaviour change, working through resistance, evaluating progress and redefining goals as appropriate, providing opportunities for the client to practise new behaviours and promoting independence.
- Termination begins when the problems are resolved and ends when the relationship is ended.
- Factors that diminish the nurse–client relationship include loss of, or unclear, boundaries, intimacy and abuse of power.
- Therapeutic roles of the nurse in the nurse–client relationship include teacher, carer, advocate and parent surrogate.

REFERENCES

Ashmore, R. & Banks, D. (2003a). Mental health nursing students' rationales for self-disclosure. 1. *British Journal of Nursing, 12*(20), 1220–1227.

Ashmore, R. & Banks, D. (2003b). Mental health nursing students' rationales for self-disclosure. 2. *British Journal of Nursing, 12*(21), 1274–1280.

Carper, B. (1978). Fundamental patterns of knowing in nursing. *Advances in Nursing Science, 1*(1), 13–23.

Forchuk, C. (2002). People with enduring mental health problems described the importance of communication, continuity of care, and stigma. *Evidence–Based Nursing, 5*(3), 93–99.

Luft, J. (1970). *Group processes: An introduction in group dynamics.* Palo Alto, CA: National Press Books.

McEwan, I. (2001). Only love and then oblivion. Love was all they had to set against their murderers. *The Guardian* 15 September 2001.

Munhall, P. (1993). Unknowing: toward another pattern of knowing in nursing. *Nursing Outlook, 41*(3), 125–128.

NMC. (2008). *The Code: Standards of conduct, performance and ethics for nurses and midwives.* Available: http://www.nmc-uk.org/aArticle. aspx?ArticleID=3236

Peplau, H. E. (1952). *Interpersonal relations in nursing.* New York: G. P. Putnam's Sons.

Welch, M. (2005). Pivotal moments in the therapeutic relationship. *International Journal of Mental Health Nursing, 14*(3), 161–165.

ADDITIONAL READING

Baer, R.A., Smith, G.T., & Allen, K.B. (2004). Assessment of mindfulness by self-report: The Kentucky Inventory of Mindfulness Skills. *Assessment, 11*, 191–206.

Barker, P. (2001). The Tidal Model: the lived-experience in person-centred mental health nursing care. *Nursing Philosophy, 2*(3), 213–223.

Barker, P. (Ed.). (2003). *Psychiatric and mental health nursing: The craft of caring.* London: Arnold.

Beeber, L. S. (2000). Hildahood: taking the interpersonal theory of nursing to the neighborhood. *Journal of the American Psychiatric Nurses Association, 6*(2), 49–55.

Cameron, D., Kapur , R., & Campbell, P. (2005). Releasing the therapeutic potential of the psychiatric nurse: a human relations perspective of the nurse-patient relationship. *Journal of Psychiatric and Mental Health Nursing, 12*, 64–74.

Edd, J. R., Fox, P. G., & Burns, K. (2005). Advocating for the rights of the mentally ill: a global issue. *International Journal of Psychiatric Nursing Research, 11*(1), 1211–1217.

Hanson, B. & Taylor, M. F. (2000). Being-with, doing-with: a model of the nurse–client relationship in mental health nursing. *Journal of Psychiatric and Mental Health Nursing, 7*, 417–423.

Junghan, U., Leese, M., Priebe, S., & Slade, M. (2007). Staff and patient perspectives on unmet need and therapeutic alliance in community mental health services. *British Journal of Psychiatry, 191*, 543–547.

Kabat-Zinn, J. (2004). *Wherever you go, there you are.* London: Piatkus

Kabat-Zinn, J. (2005). *Coming to our senses: Healing ourselves and the world through mindfulness.* London: Piatkus

Maatta, S. (2006). Closeness and distance in the nurse-patient relation. The relevance of Edith Stein's concept of empathy. *Nursing Philosophy, 7*, 3–10.

McCabe, C. (2004). Nurse-patient communication: an exploration of patients' experiences. *Journal of Clinical Nursing, 13*(1), 41–49.

McCabe, R. & Priebe, S. (2004). The therapeutic relationship in the treatment of severe mental illness: a review of methods and findings. *International Journal of Social Psychiatry, 50*(2), 115–128.

Mead, N. & Bower, P. (2000). Patient-centredness: a conceptual framework and review of the empirical literature. *Social Science and Medicine, 51*, 1087–1110.

O'Brien, L. (2000). Nurse–client relationships: The experience of community psychiatric nurses. *Australian and New Zealand Journal of Mental Health Nursing, 9*, 184–194.

Vatne, S. & Hoem, E. (2008). Acknowledging communication: a milieu-therapeutic approach in mental health care. *Journal of Advanced Nursing, 61*(6), 690–698.

INTERNET RESOURCES

RESOURCE	INTERNET ADDRESS
• Practitioner–client relationships and the prevention of abuse (Nursing and Midwifery Council)	http://www.positive-options.com/news/downloads/ NMC_-_Practitioner-Client_relationships_and_Abuse_- _2002.pdf
• Psychminded	http://www.psychminded.co.uk
• Summary of the Work of Hildegard Peplau	http://www.enursescribe.com/Peplau.htm
• The Tidal Model	http://www.tidal-model.co.uk

Chapter Study Guide

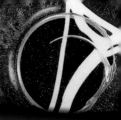

MULTIPLE CHOICE QUESTIONS

Select the best answer for each of the following questions.

1. Building trust is important in
   a. The orientation phase of the relationship
   b. The problem identification subphase of the relationship
   c. All phases of the relationship
   d. The exploitation subphase of the relationship

2. Abstract standards that provide a person with his or her code of conduct are
   a. Values
   b. Attitudes
   c. Beliefs
   d. Personal philosophy

3. Ideas that one holds as true are
   a. Values
   b. Attitudes
   c. Beliefs
   d. Personal philosophy

4. The emotional frame of reference by which one sees the world is created by
   a. Values
   b. Attitudes
   c. Beliefs
   d. Personal philosophy

FILL-IN-THE-BLANK QUESTIONS

Identify the pattern of knowing as described by Carper.

_____ The nurse reviews the client's medication regime.

_____ The nurse notices that the client is in a dark cluttered room. Knowing the importance of environment, the nurse begins to open the curtains.

_____ The nurse's grandmother also suffered from dementia, so the client's behaviour does not surprise her.

_____ As the report is given, the nurse realizes that client confidentiality has been breached.

GROUP DISCUSSION TOPICS

1. Construct dialogue examples of each of the following:

   Congruence

   Positive regard

   Acceptance

2. Explore occasions when you have felt no empathy for someone.
3. Discuss the concept of 'difficult' clients: are some people harder to engage with than others?

CLINICAL EXAMPLE

Mr V., 56 years of age, came to the UK 25 years ago. He has seen many groups of student nurses come and go on his unit. He looks over the newest group and points at one nurse. 'I'll take the cute little thing over there', he announces to the Ward Manager and students. He sidles up to the chosen student and puts his arm around her. You are the nurse he has chosen. Create a dialogue that indicates an orientation phase with evidence of trust-building and relationship-enhancing behaviours for working with this client.

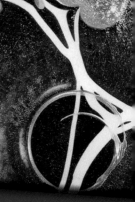

Chapter 6

Therapeutic Communication

Key Terms

- abstract messages
- active listening
- active observation
- body language
- circumstantiality
- closed body positions
- communication
- concrete message
- congruent message
- content
- context
- contract
- cues (overt and covert)
- culture
- directive role
- distance zones
- eye contact
- incongruent message
- intimate zone
- metaphor
- non-directive role
- non-verbal communication
- personal zone
- process

Listening with empathy means you listen in such a way that the other person feels you are really listening, really understanding, hearing with your whole being – with your heart. But how many of us can listen like that? We agree in principle that we should listen with our heart, so that we can really hear what the other is saying. We agree that we should give the speaker the feeling that he is being listened to and being understood: only that can give him a feeling of relief. But, in fact, how many of us can listen like that?

(Thich Nhat Hanh, 2001, p. 92)

Learning Objectives

After reading this chapter, you should be able to:

1. Describe the goals of therapeutic communication.

2. Identify therapeutic and non-therapeutic verbal communication skills.

3. Discuss non-verbal communication skills such as facial expression, body language, vocal cues, eye contact, and understanding of levels of meaning and context.

4. Discuss boundaries in therapeutic communication with respect to distance and use of touch.

5. Distinguish between concrete and abstract messages.

6. Given a hypothetical situation, select an effective therapeutic response to the client.

- proverbs
- proxemics
- public zone
- religion
- social zone
- spirituality
- therapeutic communication
- verbal communication

Communication is the process that people use to exchange information. Messages are simultaneously sent and received on two levels: verbally through the use of words and non-verbally by behaviours that accompany the words (DeVito, 2004).

Verbal communication consists of the words a person uses to speak to one or more listeners. Words are symbols that represent the objects and concepts being discussed. Placement of words into phrases and sentences that are understandable to both speaker and listeners gives an order and a meaning to these symbols. In verbal communication, **content** is the literal words that a person speaks. **Context** is the environment in which communication occurs, and can include the time and the physical, social, emotional and cultural environments. Context includes the circumstances or parts that clarify the meaning of the content of the message (Greene & Burleson, 2003). It is discussed in more detail throughout this chapter.

Non-verbal communication is the behaviour that accompanies verbal content, such as body language, eye contact, facial expression, tone of voice, speed and hesitations in speech, grunts and groans and distance from the listeners. Non-verbal communication can indicate the speaker's thoughts, feelings, needs and values that he or she acts out mostly unconsciously.

Process denotes all non-verbal messages that the speaker uses to give meaning and context to the message. The process component of communication requires the listeners to observe the behaviours and sounds that accent the words and to interpret the speaker's non-verbal behaviours to assess whether they agree or disagree with the verbal content. A **congruent message** is when content and process agree. For example, a client says, 'I know I haven't been myself. I need help.' She has a sad facial expression and a genuine and sincere tone of voice. The process validates the content as being true. But when the content and process disagree – when what the speaker says and what he or she does do not agree – the speaker is giving an **incongruent message**. For example, if the client says, 'I'm here to get help', but has a rigid posture, clenched fists, an agitated and frowning facial expression and snarls the words through clenched teeth, the message is incongruent. The process or observed behaviour invalidates what the speaker says (content).

Non-verbal process represents a more accurate message than does verbal content. 'I'm sorry I yelled and screamed at you' is readily believable when the speaker has a slumped posture, a resigned voice tone, downcast eyes and a shameful facial expression, because the content and process are congruent. The same sentence said in a loud voice and with raised eyebrows, a piercing gaze, an insulted facial expression, hands on hips and outraged body language invalidates the words (incongruent message). The message conveyed is 'I'm apologizing because I think I have to. I'm not really sorry.'

WHAT IS THERAPEUTIC COMMUNICATION?

Therapeutic communication is an interpersonal interaction between the nurse and client during which the nurse focuses on the client's specific needs to promote an effective exchange of information. Skilled use of therapeutic communication techniques helps the nurse understand and empathize with the client's experience and begin moving with them towards change.

Therapeutic communication can help nurses to accomplish many goals alongside their clients:

- Establish an effective therapeutic nurse–client alliance
- Identify the most important client concern at that moment (the client's primary short-term goal)
- Identify the client's overall dreams, wishes, desires and hopes
- Assess the client's perception of the problem – and of possible solutions – as they unfold. This includes detailed actions (behaviours and messages) of the people involved and the client's thoughts and feelings about the situation, others and self
- Facilitate the client's expression of emotions
- 'Teach' the client, friends and family necessary self-care skills
- Recognize and clarify the client's needs
- Implement collaborative, agreed interventions designed to address the client's needs
- Guide the client toward identifying a plan of action to a satisfying, ethical and socially acceptable resolution.

Establishing a therapeutic relationship is one of the most important responsibilities of the nurse when working with clients. Communication is the means by which a therapeutic relationship is initiated, maintained and terminated. The therapeutic relationship is discussed in depth in Chapter 5 and comprises elements such as confidentiality, self-disclosure and therapeutic use of self. To have effective therapeutic communication, the nurse also must consider privacy and respect of boundaries, use of touch and active listening and observation.

Privacy and Respecting Boundaries

Privacy is desirable but not always possible in therapeutic communication. In clients' own homes, issues of privacy – and a respect for boundaries – are complex: dogs, TVs, children, neighbours and phones may all make communication problematic. Clients may feel more comfortable and relaxed – nurses may not! Nurses need to develop the skills necessary to work openly and collaboratively with people in their own homes in order to ensure the flow of conversation is honest, clear and constructive – and to build on the unique opportunities working with someone in such a setting offers in terms of engagement, exchanging information and action planning.

Being in someone's home is, of course, a privilege, not a right; offering care to someone in an alien environment such as a hospital, day centre, CMHT or GP surgery or residential unit is, similarly, a privilege, but brings with it a variety of different challenges. In these settings, an interview or conference room may be ideal if the nurse believes the room is not too isolated for the interaction. The nurse can, of course, also talk with the client at the end of a hall or in a quiet corner of a day room or lobby, depending on the physical layout of the setting. In hospital, talking in the client's room or in a dormitory may offer a little of the sense of security someone could have in their own home.

In all settings, a balance between privacy and safety is paramount. Privacy is essential in order to engender trust; at the same time, nurses need to be sure that conversations are undertaken without undue risk to themselves or their clients. If, for example, a client in hospital has difficulty maintaining boundaries or is at risk of sexually disinhibited or aggressive behaviour, then his or her own room may not be the best setting: a more formal setting would be desirable. Equally, expecting someone to 'open up' in a room full of people is inconsiderate at best, abusive at worst.

Proxemics is the study of the space between people during communication. People feel more comfortable with smaller distances when communicating with someone they know rather than with strangers (DeVito, 2004). People from the UK, Ireland, Australia, New Zealand, United States, Canada and many Eastern European nations generally seem to observe four **distance zones**:

- **Intimate zone** (0 to 18 inches between people): this amount of space is comfortable for parents with young children, people who mutually desire personal contact or people whispering. Invasion of this intimate zone by anyone else can be threatening and produces anxiety.
- **Personal zone** (18 to 36 inches): this distance is comfortable between family and friends who are talking.

- **Social zone** (4 to 12 feet): this distance is acceptable for communication in social, work and business settings.
- **Public zone** (12 to 25 feet): this is an acceptable distance between a speaker and an audience, small groups and other informal functions (Hall, 1963).

People from some cultures (e.g. Mediterranean, East Indian, Asian, Middle Eastern) are more comfortable with less than 4 to 12 feet of space between them while talking. The nurse born and bred in the UK may feel uncomfortable if people from these cultures stand close when talking. Conversely, clients from these backgrounds may perceive the nurse as remote and indifferent (Andrews & Boyle, 2003).

Both the client and the nurse can feel threatened if one invades the other's personal or intimate zone, which can result in tension, irritability, fidgeting or even flight from the situation. When the nurse must invade the intimate or personal zone, he or she always should ask the client's permission. For example, if a nurse performing an assessment in a community setting needs to take the client's blood pressure, he or she should say something like, 'Mr Smith, to take your blood pressure I'll need to put this cuff around your arm and listen with my stethoscope. Are you OK with this?' He or she should ask permission in a yes/no format so the client's response is clear. This is one of the times when yes/no questions are appropriate.

Communication with someone may be most comfortable – and thus effective – when the nurse and client are roughly 3 to 6 feet apart. If a client invades the nurse's intimate space (0 to 18 inches), the nurse should set limits gradually, depending on how often the client has invaded the nurse's space and the perceived safety and comfort of the situation.

CLINICAL VIGNETTE: PERSONAL BOUNDARIES BETWEEN NURSE AND CLIENT

Saying he wanted to discuss his wife's condition, a man accompanied the nurse down the narrow hallway of his house but did not move away when they reached the kitchen. He was 12 inches from the nurse. The nurse was uncomfortable with his closeness, but she did not perceive any physical threat from him. Because this was the first visit to this house, the nurse indicated two armchairs and said, 'Let's sit over here, Mr Barrett' (offering collaboration). If sitting down were not an option and Mr Barrett 'moved in' to compensate for the nurse's backing up, the nurse could neutrally say, 'I feel a bit uncomfortable when anyone gets too close to me, Mr Barrett. Would you mind moving back a bit?' (setting limits). In this message, the nurse has taken the blame instead of shaming the other person and has gently given an order for distance between herself and Mr Barrett. If Mr Barrett were to move closer to the nurse again,

the nurse could note the behaviour and ask the client about it – for example, 'You've moved in again very close to me, Mr Barrett. What's that about?' (encouraging evaluation). The use of an open-ended question provides an opportunity for the client to address his behaviour. He may have difficulty hearing the nurse, want to keep this discussion confidential so his wife will not hear it, come from a culture in which 12 inches is an appropriate distance for a conversation or be using his closeness as a manipulative behaviour (ensure attention, threat or sexual invitation). After discussing Mr Barrett's response and understanding that he can hear adequately, the nurse can add, 'We can talk OK from 2 or 3 feet apart, Mr Barrett. Otherwise, I'll have to leave or we can continue this discussion in your wife's room' (setting limits). If Mr Barrett again moves closer, the nurse will leave or move to the wife's room to continue the interview.

Touch

As intimacy increases, the need for distance decreases. Knapp (1980) identified five types of touch:

- *Functional–professional* touch is used in examinations or procedures such as when the nurse touches a client to give an injection or a masseuse performs a massage.
- *Social–polite* touch is used in greeting, such as a handshake and the 'air kisses' some women use to greet acquaintances, or when a gentle hand guides someone in the correct direction.
- *Friendship–warmth* touch involves a hug in greeting, an arm thrown around the shoulder of a good friend or the back slapping some men use to greet friends and relatives.
- *Love–intimacy* touch involves tight hugs and kisses between lovers or close relatives.
- *Sexual-arousal* touch is used by lovers.

Touching a client can be comforting and supportive when it is welcome and permitted. The nurse should observe the client for cues that show if touch is desired or indicated. For example, holding the hand of a sobbing mother whose child is ill may be appropriate and therapeutic. If the mother pulls her hand away, however, she could be signalling to the nurse that she feels uncomfortable being touched. The nurse can also ask the client about touching (e.g. 'Would it help you to squeeze my hand?').

Although touch can be comforting and therapeutic, it is a potentially invasive move into intimate and personal space. Some clients with mental health problems have difficulty understanding the concept of personal boundaries or knowing when touch is or is not appropriate. Equally, someone who is already feeling particularly anxious or under attack may interpret being touched as a threat, and may attempt to protect himself or herself by hitting out. Unless they need to get close to a client to perform a specific nursing intervention, in a residential setting nurses should serve as role models and refrain from invading clients' personal and intimate space.

Active Listening and Observation

To receive the sender's simultaneous 'messages', the nurse must employ active listening and active observation. **Active listening** (a concept first explored by Gerard Egan in 1975 (2006) means attempting to minimize other internal mental activities and to concentrate exclusively on what the client says (nearly always a challenging and complex process!). **Active observation** means ensuring awareness of the speaker's non-verbal actions as he or she communicates (challenging, also, in the midst of the complexities of human interaction).

Peplau (1952) talked of observation as the first step in the therapeutic interaction. The nurse observes the client's behaviour and guides him or her in giving detailed descriptions of that behaviour. The nurse (and/or the client) may also document these details (though rarely without allowing the client to be aware of what she's writing). To help the client develop more awareness of his or her interpersonal skills, the nurse analyses with him or her the information discussed, offers possibilities about the underlying needs that may relate to the behaviour and connects pieces of information (making links between various sections of the conversation).

A common misconception by people learning the art of therapeutic communication is that they must always be ready with questions the instant the client has finished speaking. Hence, they are constantly thinking ahead regarding the next question rather than actively listening to what the client is saying. The result can be that the nurse does not understand the client's concerns, and the conversation is vague, superficial and frustrating to both participants. When a superficial conversation occurs, the nurse may complain that the client is not co-operating, is repeating things or is not taking responsibility for getting better. Superficiality, however, can be the result of the nurse's failure to listen to cues in the client's responses and repeatedly asking the same question. In this case, the nurse cannot even begin to understand the client's experiences and is working from his or her assumptions rather than from the client's true situation.

While listening to a client's story, it is almost impossible for the nurse not to make assumptions. A person's life experiences, knowledge base, values and prejudices often colour the interpretation of a message. In therapeutic communication, the nurse must ask specific questions to get the entire story from the client's perspective, to clarify assumptions and to develop empathy with the client. Empathy is the

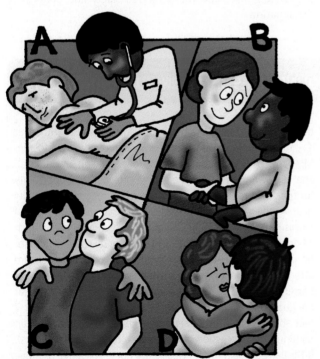

Four types of touch: A, functional–professional touch; B, social–polite touch; C, friendship–warmth touch; D, love–intimacy touch

ability to fully understand the experience of another for a moment in time. Nurses develop empathy in part by gathering as much information about an issue as possible directly from the client to avoid interjecting their personal experiences and interpretations of the situation. The nurse asks as many questions as needed to gain a clear understanding of the client's perceptions of an event or issue.

Active listening and observation help the nurse to:

- Recognize the issue that is most important to the client at this time
- Know what further questions to ask the client
- Use additional therapeutic communication techniques to guide the client to describe his or her perceptions fully
- Understand the client's perceptions of the issue instead of jumping to conclusions
- Interpret and respond to the message objectively.

VERBAL COMMUNICATION SKILLS

Using Concrete Messages

The nurse should use words that are as clear as possible when speaking to the client so that the client can understand the message. Anxious people lose cognitive processing skills – the higher the anxiety, the less ability to process concepts – so concrete messages are important for accurate information exchange. In a **concrete message**, the words are explicit and need no interpretation; the speaker uses nouns instead of pronouns – for example, 'What physical symptoms caused you to come to the hospital today?' or 'When was the last time you took your Seroxat?' Concrete questions are clear, direct and easy to understand. They elicit more accurate responses and avoid the need to go back and rephrase unclear questions, which interrupts the flow of a therapeutic interaction.

Abstract messages, in contrast, are unclear patterns of words that often contain figures of speech that are difficult to interpret. They require the listener to interpret what the speaker is asking. For example, a nurse who wants to know why a client was admitted to the unit asks, 'How did you get here?' This is an abstract message: the terms *how* and *here* are vague. An anxious client might not be aware of where he or she is and reply, 'Where am I?' or might interpret this as a question about how he or she was conveyed to the hospital and respond, 'The ambulance brought me'. Clients who are anxious, from different cultures, cognitively impaired or suffering from some mental disorders often function at a concrete level of comprehension and have difficulty answering abstract questions. The nurse must be sure that statements and questions are clear and concrete.

The following are examples of abstract and concrete messages:

Abstract (unclear): 'Get the stuff from him.'
Concrete (clear): 'John will be home today at 5 p.m., and you can pick up your clothes at that time.'

Abstract (unclear): 'Your performance really has to improve.'
Concrete (clear): 'To be allowed to give out medication, you'll have to be able to calculate dosages correctly by the end of this week.'

Using Therapeutic Communication Techniques

The nurse can use many therapeutic communication techniques to interact with clients. The choice of technique depends on the intent of the interaction and the client's ability to communicate verbally. Overall, the nurse selects techniques that facilitate the interaction and enhance communication between client and nurse. Table 6.1 lists these techniques and gives examples. Techniques such as exploring, focusing, restating, and reflecting encourage the client to discuss his or her feelings or concerns in more depth. Other techniques help focus or clarify what is being said. The nurse may give the client feedback using techniques such as making an observation or presenting reality.

Avoiding Non-therapeutic Communication

In contrast, there are many non-therapeutic techniques that nurses should avoid (Table 6.2). These responses cut off communication and make it more difficult for the interaction to continue. Responses such as 'Everything will work out' or 'Maybe tomorrow will be a better day' may be intended to comfort the client, but instead may impede the communication process. Asking 'Why' questions (in an effort to gain information) may be perceived as criticism by the client, conveying a negative judgement from the nurse. Many of these responses are common in social interaction. Therefore, it takes practice for the nurse to avoid making these types of comments.

Interpreting Signals or Cues

To try and understand what a client means, the nurse watches and listens carefully for **cues**. These may be verbal or non-verbal messages that signal key words or issues for the client. Finding cues is a function of active listening. Cues can be buried in what a client says or can be acted out in the process of communication. Often, cue words introduced by the client can help the nurse to know what to ask next or how to respond to the client. The nurse might build his or her responses on these cue words or concepts. Understanding this can relieve pressure on us if we're anxious about 'what to ask next'. The following example illustrates questions the nurse might ask when responding to a client's cue:

Client: 'I had a boyfriend when I was younger.'
Nurse: 'You had a boyfriend?' (reflecting) 'Tell me about you and your boyfriend.'
(encouraging description)
'How old were you when you had this boyfriend?'
(placing events in time or sequence)

Table 6.1   THERAPEUTIC COMMUNICATION TECHNIQUES

Therapeutic Communication Technique	Examples	Rationale
Accepting – indicating reception	'Yes.' 'I follow what you said.' Nodding	An accepting response indicates the nurse has heard and followed the train of thought. It does not indicate agreement but is non-judgemental. Facial expression, tone of voice, and so forth also must convey acceptance or the words lose their meaning
Broad openings – allowing the client to take the initiative in introducing the topic	'Is there something you'd like to talk about?' 'Where would you like to begin?' 'What would tell you, in half-hour's time, that this conversation has been helpful?'	Broad openings make explicit that the client has the lead in the interaction. For the client who is hesitant about talking, broad openings may stimulate him or her to take the initiative
Consensual validation – searching for mutual understanding, for accord in the meaning of the words	'Tell me whether my understanding of it agrees with yours.' 'Are you using this word to convey that . . . ?'	For verbal communication to be meaningful, it is essential that the words being used have the same meaning for both (all) participants. Sometimes, words, phrases or slang terms have different meanings and can be easily misunderstood
Encouraging comparison – asking that similarities and differences be noted	'Was it something like . . . ?' 'Have you had similar experiences?'	Comparing ideas, experiences or relationships brings out many recurring themes. The client benefits from making these comparisons because he or she might recall past coping strategies that were effective or remember that he or she has survived a similar situation
Encouraging description of perceptions – asking the client to verbalize what he or she perceives	'Tell me when you feel anxious.' 'What is happening?' 'What does the voice seem to be saying?'	To understand the client, the nurse must see things from his or her perspective. Encouraging the client to describe ideas fully may relieve the tension the client is feeling, and he or she might be less likely to take action on ideas that are harmful or frightening
Encouraging expression – asking the client to appraise the quality of his or her experiences	'What are your feelings about . . . ?' 'Does this make things worse?'	The nurse asks the client to consider people and events in light of his or her own values. Doing so encourages the client to make his or her own appraisal rather than to accept the opinion of others
Exploring – delving further into a subject or idea	'Tell me more about that.' 'Would you describe it more fully?' 'What kind of work?'	When clients deal with topics superficially, exploring can help them examine the issue more fully. Any problem or concern can be better understood if explored in depth. If the client expresses an unwillingness to explore a subject, however, the nurse must respect his or her wishes
Focusing – concentrating on a single point	'This point seems worth looking at more closely—do you agree?' 'Of all the concerns you've mentioned, which is most troublesome?'	The nurse encourages the client to concentrate his or her energies on a single point, which may prevent a multitude of factors or problems from overwhelming the client. It is also a useful technique when a client jumps from one topic to another

Table 6.1   THERAPEUTIC COMMUNICATION TECHNIQUES (*Continued*)

Therapeutic Communication Technique	Examples	Rationale
Formulating a plan of action – asking the client to consider kinds of behaviour likely to be appropriate in future situations	'What could you do to let your anger out harmlessly?' 'Next time this comes up, what might you do to handle it?'	It may be helpful for the client to plan in advance what he or she might do in future similar situations. Making definite plans increases the likelihood that the client will cope more effectively in a similar situation
General leads – giving encouragement to continue	'Go on.' 'And then?' 'Tell me about it.'	General leads indicate that the nurse is listening and following what the client is saying without taking away the initiative for the interaction. They also encourage the client to continue if he or she is hesitant or uncomfortable about the topic
Giving information – making available the facts that the client needs	'My name is . . .' 'Visiting hours are ...' 'The reason I'm here is . . .'	Informing the client of facts increases his or her knowledge about a topic or lets the client know what to expect. The nurse is functioning as a resource person. Giving information also builds trust with the client
Giving recognition – acknowledging, indicating awareness	'Good morning, Mr S. . . .' 'You've finished your list of things to do.' 'I notice that you've combed your hair.'	Greeting the client by name, indicating awareness of change, or noting efforts the client has made all show that the nurse recognizes the client as a person, as an individual. Such recognition does not carry the notion of value, that is, of being 'good' or 'bad'
Making observations – verbalizing what the nurse perceives	'You seem tense.' 'Are you uncomfortable when ...?' 'I notice that you're biting your lip.'	Sometimes clients cannot verbalize or make themselves understood. Or the client may not be ready to talk
Offering self – making oneself available	'I'll sit with you awhile.' 'I'll stay here with you.' 'I'm interested in what you think.'	The nurse can offer his or her presence, interest and desire to understand. It is important that this offer is unconditional, that is, the client does not have to respond verbally to get the nurse's attention
Placing event in time or sequence – clarifying the relationship of events in time	'What seemed to lead up to . . . ?' 'Was this before or after . . . ?' 'When did this happen?'	Putting events in proper sequence helps both the nurse and client to see them in perspective. The client may gain insight into cause-and-effect behaviour and consequences, or the client may be able to see that perhaps some things are not related. The nurse may gain information about recurrent patterns or themes in the client's behaviour or relationships
Presenting reality – offering for consideration that which is real	'I can't see anyone else in the room.' 'That sound was a car backfiring.' 'Your mother isn't here, John; I'm a nurse.'	When it seems obvious that the client is misinterpreting reality, the nurse can indicate what is real. The nurse does this by calmly and quietly expressing the nurse's perceptions or the facts, not by way of arguing with the client or belittling his or her experience. The intent is to indicate an alternative line of thought for the client to consider, not to 'convince' the client that he or she is wrong

(continued)

Table 6.1 THERAPEUTIC COMMUNICATION TECHNIQUES (*Continued*)

Therapeutic Communication Technique	Examples	Rationale
Reflecting – directing client actions, thoughts and feelings back to client	*Client:* 'Do you think I should tell the doctor . . . ?' *Nurse:* 'Do you think you should?' *Client:* 'My brother spends all my money and then has the nerve to ask for more.' *Nurse:* 'This causes you to feel angry?'	Reflection encourages the client to recognize and accept his or her own feelings. The nurse indicates that the client's point of view has value, and that the client has the right to have opinions, make decisions and think independently
Restating – repeating the main idea expressed	*Client:* 'I can't sleep. I stay awake all night.' *Nurse:* 'You have difficulty sleeping.' *Client:* 'I'm really angry, I'm really upset.' *Nurse:* 'You're really angry and upset.'	The nurse repeats what the client has said in approximately or nearly the same words the client has used. This restatement lets the client know that he or she communicated the idea effectively. This encourages the client to continue. Or if the client has been misunderstood, he or she can clarify his or her thoughts
Seeking information – seeking to make clear that which is not meaningful or that which is vague	'I'm not sure that I follow.' 'Have I heard you correctly?'	The nurse should seek clarification throughout interactions with clients. Doing so can help the nurse to avoid making assumptions that understanding has occurred when it has not. It helps the client to articulate thoughts, feelings and ideas more clearly
Silence – absence of verbal communication, which provides time for the client to put thoughts or feelings into words, to regain composure or to continue talking	Nurse says nothing but continues to maintain eye contact and conveys interest	Silence often encourages the client to verbalize, provided that it is interested and expectant. Silence gives the client time to organize thoughts, direct the topic of interaction or focus on issues that are most important. Much non-verbal behaviour takes place during silence, and the nurse needs to be aware of the client and his or her own non-verbal behaviour
Suggesting collaboration – offering to share, to strive, to work with the client for his or her benefit	'Perhaps you and I can discuss and discover the triggers for your anxiety.' 'Let's go to your room, and I'll help you find what you're looking for.'	The nurse seeks to offer a relationship in which the client can identify problems in living with others, grow emotionally and improve the ability to form satisfactory relationships. The nurse offers to do things with, rather than for, the client
Summarizing – organizing and summing up that which has gone before	'Have I got this straight?' 'You've said that . . .' 'During the past hour, you and I have discussed . . .'	Summarization seeks to bring out the important points of the discussion and to increase the awareness and understanding of both participants. It omits the irrelevant and organizes the pertinent aspects of the interaction. It allows both client and nurse to depart with the same ideas and provides a sense of closure at the completion of each discussion
Translating into feelings – seeking to verbalize client's feelings that he or she expresses only indirectly	*Client:* 'I'm dead.' *Nurse:* 'Are you suggesting that you feel lifeless?' *Client:* 'I'm way out in the ocean.' *Nurse:* 'You seem to feel lonely or deserted.'	Often what the client says, when taken literally, seems meaningless or far removed from reality. To understand, the nurse must concentrate on what the client might be feeling to express himself or herself this way

Table 6.1	THERAPEUTIC COMMUNICATION TECHNIQUES (*Continued*)	
Therapeutic Communication Technique	**Examples**	**Rationale**
Verbalizing the implied – voicing what the client has hinted at or suggested	Client: 'I can't talk to you or anyone. It's a waste of time.' Nurse: 'Do you feel that no one understands?'	Putting into words what the client has implied or said indirectly tends to make the discussion less obscure. The nurse should be as direct as possible without being unfeelingly blunt or obtuse. The client may have difficulty communicating directly. The nurse should take care to express only what is fairly obvious; otherwise, the nurse may be jumping to conclusions or interpreting the client's communication.
Voicing doubt – expressing uncertainty about the reality of the client's perceptions	'Isn't that unusual?' 'Really?' 'That's hard to believe.'	Another means of responding to distortions of reality is to express doubt. Such expression permits the client to become aware that others do not necessarily perceive events in the same way or draw the same conclusions. This does not mean the client will alter his or her point of view, but at least the nurse will encourage the client to reconsider or re-evaluate what has happened. The nurse neither agreed nor disagreed; however, he or she has not let the misperceptions and distortions pass without comment

Adapted from Hays, J. S. & Larson, K. (1963). *Interaction with patients.* New York: Macmillan Press.

If a client has difficulty attending to a conversation and drifts into a rambling discussion or a flight of ideas, the nurse listens carefully for a theme, or a topic around which the client composes his or her words. Using the theme, the nurse can assess the non-verbal behaviours that accompany the client's words and build responses based on these cues. In the following examples, the underlined words are themes and cues to help the nurse formulate further communication

Theme of sadness:

> *Client:* 'Oh, hi, nurse.' (face is sad; eyes look teary; voice is low, with little inflection)
> *Nurse:* 'You seem sad today, Mrs Venezia.'
> *Client:* 'Yes, it is the <u>anniversary</u> of my <u>husband's death</u>.'

Nurse: '<u>How long ago</u> did your husband die?' (Or the nurse can use the other cue:

Nurse: 'Tell me about your <u>husband's death</u>, Mrs Venezia.')

Theme of loss of control:

> *Client:* 'I had an accident in the car this morning. I'm okay. I lost my wallet, and I have to go to the bank to cover a cheque I wrote last night. I can't get in contact with my husband at work. <u>I don't know where to start.</u>'

Nurse: 'I'm getting the impression you feel out of control.' (translating into feelings)

Clients may use many word patterns to 'cue' the listener to their intent. **Overt cues** are clear statements of intent, such as 'I want to die'. The message is clear that the client is thinking of suicide or self-harm. **Covert cues** are vague or hidden messages that need interpretation and exploration – for example, if a client says, 'Nothing can help me'. The nurse is unsure, but it sounds as if the client might be saying he feels so hopeless and helpless that he plans to commit suicide. The nurse can explore this covert cue to clarify the client's intent and to protect the client. Most suicidal people are ambivalent about whether to live or die and often admit their plan when directly asked about it. When the nurse suspects self-harm or suicide, he or she can use a yes/no question to elicit a clear response.

Theme of hopelessness and suicidal ideation:

> *Client:* 'Life is hard. I want it to be done. There's no rest. Sleep, sleep is good . . . forever.'
> *Nurse:* 'I can hear you saying things seem hopeless. Would you feel OK talking a bit more about that?'
> *Nurse* (perhaps later, after more opportunity for client to talk about feelings): 'I'm wondering if you are planning to kill yourself?' (verbalizing the implied)

Other word patterns that need further clarification for meaning include metaphors and proverbs. When a client uses these figures of speech, the nurse must follow up with questions to clarify what the client is trying to say.

Table 6.2 THERAPEUTIC COMMUNICATION TECHNIQUES

Techniques	Examples	Rationale
Advising – telling the client what to do	'I think you should . . .' 'Why don't you . . .'	Giving advice implies that only the nurse knows what is best for the client
Agreeing – indicating accord with the client	'That's right' 'I agree.'	Approval indicates the client is 'right' rather than 'wrong'. This gives the client the impression that he or she is 'right' because of agreement with the nurse. Opinions and conclusions should be exclusively the client's. When the nurse agrees with the client, there is no opportunity for the client to change his or her mind without being 'wrong'
Belittling feelings expressed – misjudging the degree of the client's discomfort	Client: 'I have nothing to live for . . . I wish I was dead.' Nurse: 'Everybody gets down in the dumps', or 'I've felt that way myself.'	When the nurse tries to equate the intense and overwhelming feelings the client has expressed to 'everybody' or to the nurse's own feelings, the nurse implies that the discomfort is temporary, mild, self-limiting or not very important. The client is focused on his or her own worries and feelings; hearing the problems or feelings of others is not helpful
Challenging – demanding proof from the client	'But how can you be Prime Minister?' 'If you're dead, why is your heart beating?'	Often the nurse believes that if he or she can challenge the client to prove unrealistic ideas, the client will realize there is no 'proof' and then will recognize reality. Actually, challenging causes the client to defend the delusions or misperceptions more strongly than before
Defending – attempting to protect someone or something from verbal attack	'This hospital has an excellent reputation.' 'I'm sure your doctor has your best interests in mind.'	Defending what the client has criticized implies that he or she has no right to express impressions, opinions or feelings. Telling the client that his or her criticism is unjust or unfounded does not change the client's feelings but only serves to block further communication
Disagreeing – opposing the client's ideas	'That's wrong.' 'I definitely disagree with . . .' 'I don't believe that.'	Disagreeing implies the client is 'wrong'. Consequently, the client feels defensive about his or her point of view or ideas
Disapproving – denouncing the client's behaviour or ideas	'That's bad.' 'I'd rather you wouldn't . . .'	Disapproval implies that the nurse has the right to pass judgement on the client's thoughts or actions. It further implies that the client is expected to please the nurse
Giving approval – sanctioning the client's behaviour or ideas	'That's good.' 'I'm glad that ...'	Saying what the client thinks or feels is 'good' implies that the opposite is 'bad'. Approval, then, tends to limit the client's freedom to think, speak or act in a certain way. This can lead to the client's acting in a particular way just to please the nurse
Giving literal responses – responding to a figurative comment as though it were a statement of fact	*Client:* 'They're looking in my head with a television camera.' *Nurse:* 'Try not to watch television', or 'What channel?'	Often the client is at a loss to describe his or her feelings, so such comments are the best he or she can do. Usually, it is helpful for the nurse to focus on the client's feelings in response to such statements

Table 6.2	THERAPEUTIC COMMUNICATION TECHNIQUES (*Continued*)	
Techniques	**Examples**	**Rationale**
Indicating the existence of an external source – attributing the source of thoughts, feelings and behaviour to others or to outside influences	'What makes you say that?' 'What made you do that?' 'Who told you that you were a prophet?'	The nurse can ask, 'What happened?' or 'What events led you to draw such a conclusion?', but to question, 'What made you think that?' implies that the client was made or compelled to think in a certain way. Usually, the nurse does not intend to suggest that the source is external, but that is often what the client thinks
Interpreting – asking to make conscious that which is unconscious; telling the client the meaning of his or her experience	'What you really mean is . . .' 'Unconsciously you're saying . . .'	The client's thoughts and feelings are his or her own, not to be interpreted by the nurse for hidden meaning. Only the client can identify or confirm the presence of feelings
Introducing an unrelated topic – changing the subject	*Client:* 'I'd like to die.' *Nurse:* 'Did you have visitors last evening?'	The nurse takes the initiative for the interaction away from the client. This usually happens because the nurse is uncomfortable, doesn't know how to respond or has a topic he or she would rather discuss
Making stereotyped comments – offering meaningless clichés or trite comments	'It's for your own good.' 'Keep your chin up.' 'Just have a positive attitude and you'll be better in no time.'	Social conversation contains many clichés and much meaningless chitchat. Such comments are of no value in the nurse–client relationship. Any automatic responses lack the nurse's consideration or thoughtfulness
Probing – persistent questioning of the client	'Now tell me about this problem. You know I have to find out.' 'Tell me your psychiatric history.'	Probing tends to make the client feel used or invaded. Clients have the right not to talk about issues or concerns if they choose. Pushing and probing by the nurse will not encourage the client to talk
Reassuring – indicating there is no reason for anxiety or other feelings of discomfort	'I wouldn't worry about that.' 'Everything will be all right.' 'You're coming along just fine.'	Attempts to dispel the client's anxiety by implying that there is not sufficient reason for concern completely devalue the client's feelings. Vague reassurances with out accompanying facts are meaningless to the client
Rejecting – refusing to consider or showing contempt for the client's ideas or behaviours	'Let's not discuss . . .' 'I don't want to hear about . . .'	When the nurse rejects any topic, he or she closes it off from exploration. In turn, the client may feel personally rejected along with his or her ideas
Requesting an explanation – asking the client to provide reasons for thoughts, feelings, behaviours, events	'Why do you think that?' 'Why do you feel that way?'	There is a difference between asking the client to describe what is occurring or has taken place and asking him to explain why. Usually, a 'why' question is intimidating. In addition, the client is unlikely to know 'why' and may become defensive trying to explain himself or herself
Testing – appraising the client's degree of insight	'Do you know what kind of hospital this is?' 'Do you still have the idea that . . . ?'	These types of questions force the client to try to recognize his or her problems. The client's acknowledgement that he or she doesn't know these things may meet the nurse's needs but is not helpful for the client
Using denial – refusing to admit that a problem exists	*Client:* 'I'm nothing.' *Nurse:* 'Of course you're something—everybody's something.' *Client:* 'I'm dead.' *Nurse:* 'Don't be silly.'	The nurse denies the client's feelings or the seriousness of the situation by dismissing his or her comments without attempting to discover the feelings or meaning behind them

Adapted from Hays, J. S. & Larson, K. (1963). *Interaction with patients.* New York: Macmillan Press.

A **metaphor** is a phrase that describes an object or situation by comparing it to something else familiar.

> **Client:** *'My son's bedroom looks like a bomb went off in it.'*
> **Nurse:** *'You're saying your son is really messy?'* (verbalizing the implied)
> **Client:** *'My mind is like mashed potatoes.'*
> **Nurse:** *'I get the idea you find it difficult to put thoughts together.'* (translating into feelings)

Proverbs are old accepted sayings with generally accepted meanings.

> **Client:** *'People who live in glass houses shouldn't throw stones.'*
> **Nurse:** *'Who do you think is criticizing you but actually has similar problems?'* (encouraging description of perception)

NON-VERBAL COMMUNICATION SKILLS

Non-verbal communication includes facial expression, eye contact, space, time, boundaries and body movements. It is as important, if not more so, than verbal communication in engaging with, exchanging information with and planning with clients. It is estimated that one-third of meaning is transmitted by words and two-thirds is communicated non-verbally. The speaker may verbalize what he or she believes the listener wants to hear, whereas non-verbal communication conveys the speaker's actual meaning. Non-verbal communication involves the unconscious mind acting out emotions related to the verbal content, the situation, the environment and the relationship between the speaker and the listener.

Knapp and Hall (2002) listed the ways in which non-verbal messages accompany verbal messages:

- Accent: using flashing eyes or hand movements
- Complement: giving quizzical looks, nodding
- Contradict: rolling eyes to demonstrate that the meaning is the opposite of what one is saying
- Regulate: taking a deep breath to demonstrate readiness to speak, using 'and uh' to signal the wish to continue speaking
- Repeat: using non-verbal behaviours to augment the verbal message, such as shrugging after saying 'Who knows?'
- Substitute: using culturally determined body movements that stand in for words, such as pumping the arm up and down with a closed fist to indicate success.

Facial Expression

The human face produces the most visible, complex and sometimes confusing non-verbal messages. Facial movements connect with words to illustrate meaning; this connection demonstrates the speaker's internal dialogue (Greene & Burleson, 2003). Facial expressions can be categorized into expressive, impassive and confusing:

- An *expressive* face portrays the person's moment-by-moment thoughts, feelings and needs. These expressions may be evident even when the person does not want to reveal his or her emotions.
- An *impassive* face is frozen into an emotionless deadpan expression similar to a mask.
- A *confusing* facial expression is one that is the opposite of what the person wants to convey. A person who is verbally expressing sad or angry feelings while smiling is exhibiting a confusing facial expression.

Facial expressions often can affect the listener's response. Strong and emotional facial expressions can persuade the listener to believe the message. For example, by appearing perplexed and confused, a client could manipulate the nurse into staying longer than scheduled. Facial expressions such as happy, sad, embarrassed or angry usually have the same meaning across cultures, but the nurse should identify the facial expression and ask the client to validate the nurse's interpretation of it – for instance, 'You're smiling, but I get the feeling you're very angry' (Sheldon, 2004).

Frowns, smiles, puzzlement, relief, fear, surprise and anger are common facial communication signals. Looking away, not meeting the speaker's eyes and yawning indicate that the listener is disinterested, lying or bored. To ensure the accuracy of information, the nurse identifies the non-verbal communication and checks its congruency with the content (Sheldon, 2004). An example is 'Mr Jones, you said everything's fine today, but you were frowning when you said it. I get the idea maybe everything isn't really fine?' (verbalizing the implied).

Body Language

Body language (gestures, postures, movements and body positions) is a non-verbal form of communication. **Closed body positions,** such as crossed legs or arms folded across the chest, indicate that the interaction might threaten the listener, who is defensive or not accepting. A better, more accepting body position may be to sit facing the client with both feet on the floor, knees parallel, hands at the side of the body and legs uncrossed or crossed only at the ankle. This open posture can demonstrate unconditional positive regard, trust, care and acceptance. The nurse indicates interest in and acceptance of the client by facing and slightly leaning toward him or her while maintaining non-threatening eye contact.

Hand gestures add meaning to the content. A slight lift of the hand from the arm of a chair can punctuate or strengthen the meaning of words. Holding both hands with palms up while shrugging the shoulders often means 'I don't know'. Some people use many hand gestures to demonstrate or act out what they are saying, whereas others use very few gestures.

each other is also important. Sitting beside or across from the client can put the client at ease, whereas sitting behind a desk (creating a physical barrier) can increase the formality of the setting and may decrease the client's willingness to open

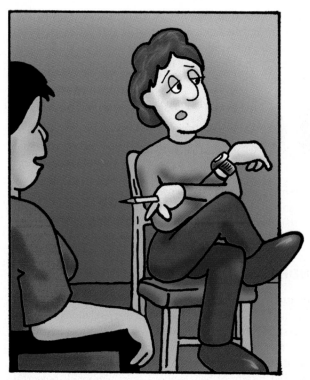

Closed body position

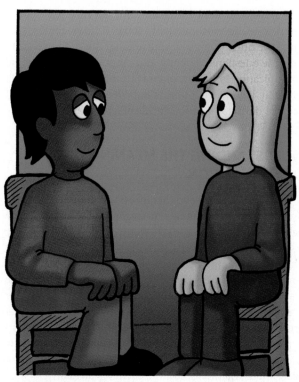

Accepting body position

up and communicate freely. The nurse may, rarely, wish to create a more formal setting with some clients, such as those who have difficulty maintaining boundaries.

There can, however, be no absolute rules about how to sit, stand or gesture when with a client: we need to ensure there is a connection between us, and sitting awkwardly or in an 'over-professional' way can be counter-productive. Sometimes, matching someone's posture (at least initially) can help generate rapport; sitting in a similarly closed position to a client and then gradually opening up one's own posture can help relax the person.

Vocal Cues

Vocal cues are non-verbal sound signals transmitted along with the content: voice volume, tone, pitch, intensity, emphasis, speed and pauses augment the sender's message. Volume, the loudness of the voice, can indicate anger, fear, happiness or deafness. Tone can indicate whether someone is relaxed, agitated or bored. Pitch varies from shrill and high to low and threatening. Intensity is the power, severity and strength behind the words, indicating the importance of the message. Emphasis refers to accents on words or phrases that highlight the subject or give insight on the topic. Speed is the number of words spoken per minute. Pauses also contribute to the message, often adding emphasis or feeling.

The high-pitched rapid delivery of a message often indicates anxiety. The use of extraneous words with long tedious descriptions is called **circumstantiality**.

Circumstantiality can indicate that the client (or the nurse!) is confused about what is important, or is a poor historian.

Slow, hesitant responses may indicate that the person is depressed, confused and searching for the correct words, having difficulty finding the right words to describe an incident, or reminiscing. It is important for the nurse to validate these non-verbal indicators rather than to assume that he or she knows what the client is thinking or feeling (e.g. 'Mr Smith, you sound anxious. Is that how you're feeling?').

Eye Contact

We can understand so much from each other's eyes. Messages that the eyes offer can include humour, interest, puzzlement, hatred, happiness, sadness, horror, warning and pleading. **Eye contact**, looking into the other person's eyes during communication, is used to assess the other person and the environment, and to indicate whose turn it is to speak; it increases during listening but decreases while speaking (DeVito, 2004). Although maintaining good eye contact is usually desirable, it is important that the nurse doesn't 'stare' at the client and remembers that the length of time that each individual (and each culture) feels comfortable maintaining eye-contact differs.

Silence

Silence or long pauses in communication may indicate many different things. The client may be depressed and struggling to find the energy to talk. Sometimes pauses indicate the client is thoughtfully considering the question before responding. At times, the client may seem to be 'lost in his or her own thoughts' and not paying attention to the nurse.

It is important to allow the client sufficient time to respond, even if it seems uncomfortably long. It may confuse the client if the nurse 'jumps in' with another question or tries to restate the question differently. Also, in some cultures, verbal communication is slower, often with many pauses, and the client may believe the nurse is impatient or disrespectful if he or she does not wait for the client's response.

UNDERSTANDING THE MEANING OF COMMUNICATION

Few messages in social and therapeutic communication have only one level of meaning; messages often contain more meaning than just the spoken words (DeVito, 2004). The nurse must try to discover – with the client – all the meaning in his or her communication. For example, the depressed client might say, 'I'm so tired that I just can't go on.' If the nurse considers only the literal meaning of the words, he or she might assume the client is experiencing the fatigue that often accompanies depression. However, statements such as the previous example often mean the client wishes to die. The nurse would need to further assess the client's statement to determine whether or not the client is suicidal.

It is sometimes easier for clients to 'act out' their emotions than to organize their thoughts and feelings into words to describe feelings and needs. For example, people who outwardly appear dominating and strong and often manipulate and criticize others, in reality may have low self-esteem and feel insecure. They do not verbalize their true feelings but act them out behaviourally toward others. Insecurity and low self-esteem often translate into jealousy and mistrust of others and attempts to feel more important and strong by dominating or criticizing them.

We need to be exceptionally wary of words like 'depressed', 'anxious' or 'paranoid', whether we're using them or a client is using them: in themselves, they have no meaning until we've clarified what they mean for each individual:

'How does your depression affect you?'
'When you're paranoid, what are you thinking and feeling?'
'What happens when you get anxious?'

UNDERSTANDING CONTEXT

Understanding the context of communication is extremely important in accurately identifying the meaning of a message. Think of the difference in the meaning of 'I'm going to kill you!' when stated in two different contexts: anger during an argument and when one friend discovers another is planning a surprise party for him or her. Understanding the context of a situation gives the nurse more information and reduces the risk for assumptions.

To clarify context, the nurse must gather information from verbal and non-verbal sources and validate findings with the client. For example, if a client says, 'I collapsed', she may mean she fainted or felt weak and had to sit down. Or she could mean she was tired and went to bed. To clarify these terms and view them in the context of the action, the nurse could say

'What do you mean collapsed?' (seeking clarification) or
'If you don't mind, tell me where you were and what you were doing when you collapsed.' (placing events in time and sequence)

Assessment of context focuses on *who* was there, *what* happened, *when* it occurred, *how* the event progressed and *why* the client believes it happened as it did.

UNDERSTANDING SPIRITUALITY

Spirituality is a concept that encompasses a client's belief about life, health, illness, death and one's relationship to the universe: it's about what provides – or could provide – meaning to the client. Spirituality (which can include humanistic and scientific ideas) differs from **religion**, which is an organized system of beliefs about one or more all-powerful, all-knowing forces that are seen as governing the universe, and offers guidelines for living in harmony with the universe and others (Andrews & Boyle, 2003). Spiritual and religious beliefs are usually supported by others who share them and follow the same rules and rituals for daily living. Spirituality and religion often provide comfort and hope to people and can greatly affect a person's health and health-care practices.

The nurse must first assess his or her own spiritual and religious beliefs. Religion and spirituality are highly subjective and can be vastly different among people. The nurse must remain objective and non-judgemental regarding the client's beliefs and must not allow them to alter nursing care. The nurse must assess the client's spiritual and religious needs and guard against imposing his or her own on the client. The nurse must ensure that the client is not ignored or ridiculed because his or her beliefs and values differ from those of the staff (Chant *et al.*, 2002).

As the therapeutic relationship develops, the nurse must be aware of, and respect, the client's religious and spiritual beliefs. Ignoring or being judgemental will quickly erode trust and could stall the relationship. Chapter 7 gives a more detailed discussion on spirituality.

CULTURAL CONSIDERATIONS

Culture is all the socially learned behaviours, values, beliefs and customs transmitted down to each generation. The rules about the way in which to conduct communication vary because they arise from each culture's specific social relationship patterns (Sheldon, 2004). Each culture has its own rules governing verbal and non-verbal communication (though increasingly these are becoming more complex and overlapping, shaped by historical forces and dependent upon gender, class, age, ethnicity and many other factors). In Western cultures, the handshake is – traditionally – a non-verbal greeting used primarily by men, often to size up or judge someone they have just met. For women, a polite 'hello' has long been an accepted form of greeting. In some Asian cultures, bowing is the accepted form of greeting and departing, and a method of designating social status.

Because of these differences, cultural assessment is necessary when establishing a therapeutic relationship. The nurse must assess the client's emotional expression, beliefs, values and behaviours; modes of emotional expression; and views about mental health and illness – if at all possible, by asking directly.

When caring for people who do not speak English, the services of a qualified translator who is skilled at obtaining accurate data are necessary. He or she should be able to translate technical words into another language while retaining the original intent of the message and not injecting his or her own biases. The nurse is responsible for knowing how to contact a translator, regardless of the setting.

The nurse must understand the differences in how various cultures communicate. It helps to see how a person from another culture acts toward and speaks with others. Indigenous British cultures are, essentially, still individualistic; they value self-reliance and independence, and focus on individual goals and achievements. Others, such as many Asian cultures, are more collectivistic, valuing the group and observing obligations that enhance the security of the group. Persons from these cultures can be more private and guarded when speaking to members outside the group and sometimes may even ignore outsiders until they are formally introduced to the group. Cultural differences in greetings, personal space, eye contact, touch and beliefs about health and illness are discussed in depth in Chapter 7.

THE THERAPEUTIC COMMUNICATION SESSION

Goals

The nurse uses all the therapeutic communication techniques and skills previously described to help achieve the following goals and to help make the phases of rapport-building and engagement, information-exchange and action planning as effective as possible:

- Establish rapport with the client by being empathetic, genuine, caring and unconditionally accepting of the client regardless of his or her behaviour or beliefs.
- Actively listen to the client to identify the issues of concern and to formulate a client-centred goal for the interaction.
- Gain an in-depth understanding of the client's perception of the issue, and foster empathy in the nurse–client relationship.
- Explore the client's thoughts and feelings.
- Facilitate the client's expression of thoughts and feelings.

- Guide the client to develop new skills in problem solving.
- Promote the client's evaluation of solutions.

Often the nurse – particularly in community settings – can plan the time and setting for therapeutic communication, such as having an in-depth, one-on-one interaction with an assigned client. The nurse has time to think about where to meet and what to say, and will have a general idea of the topic, such as finding out what the client sees as his or her major concern or following up on interaction from a previous encounter. At times, however, a client may approach the nurse saying, 'Can I talk to you right now?' Or the nurse may see a client sitting alone, crying and decide to approach the client for an interaction. In these situations, the nurse may know that he or she will be trying to find out what is happening with the client at that moment in time.

When meeting the client for the first time, introducing oneself and establishing a contract for the relationship is an appropriate start for therapeutic communication. The nurse can ask the client how he or she prefers to be addressed. A **contract** for the relationship may include outlining the care the nurse will give, the times the nurse will be with the client and acceptance of these conditions by the client.

Nurse: 'Hello, Mr Kirk. My name is Joan, and I'll be working with you today. I'm here from 7 AM to 3.30 PM. Right now I've got about 10 minutes, and I see you're dressed and ready for the day. I'd really like to spend some time talking to you if it's convenient.' (giving recognition and introducing self, setting limits of contract)

After making the introduction and establishing the contract, the nurse can engage in 'small talk' to break the ice and to help get acquainted with the client if they have not met before. This 'social' chat – or (in solution-focused terms), 'problem-free talk'– can also help identify client strengths and resources and begin the relationship by treating them as 'person first, client second'. The nurse might then use a broad opening question to guide the client toward identifying the major topic of concern. Broad opening questions are helpful to begin the therapeutic communication session because they allow the client to focus on what he or she considers important. The following is a good example of how to begin the therapeutic communication:

Nurse: 'Hello, Mrs Nagy. My name's John, and I'll be working with you today and tomorrow from 7 AM to 3 PM. What would you like me to call you?' (introducing self, establishing limits of relationship)

Client: 'Hi, John. You can call me Peggy.'

Nurse: 'The rain today's a bit of a relief from all that heat, isn't it?'

Client: 'Really? It's hard to tell what it's doing outside. Still seems hot in here to me.'

Nurse: 'Yeah. It does get stuffy here sometimes. So tell me, how are you doing today?' (broad opening)

NON-DIRECTIVE ROLE

When beginning therapeutic interaction with a client, it should usually be the client (not the nurse) who identifies the focus of the conversation. The nurse uses active listening skills to identify the topic of concern. The client identifies the goal, and information-exchange about this topic focuses on the client. The nurse acts as a guide in this conversation. The therapeutic communication centres on achieving the goal within the time limits of the conversation.

The following are examples of client-centred goals:

- Client will discuss her concerns about her 16-year-old daughter, who is having trouble in school.
- Client will describe the difficulty she has with side-effects of her medication.
- Client will share his distress about son's drug abuse.
- Client will identify the greatest concerns he has about being a single parent.

The nurse is assuming a **non-directive role** in this type of therapeutic communication, using broad openings and open-ended questions to collect information and help the client to identify and discuss the topic of concern. The client does most of the talking. The nurse guides the client through the interaction, facilitating the client's expression of feelings and identification of issues. The following is an example of the nurse's non-directive role:

Client: 'I'm so upset about my family.'
Nurse: 'You're upset?' (reflecting)
Client: 'Yeah, I am. I can't sleep. My appetite's completely gone. I just don't know what to do.'
Nurse: 'Go on.' (using a general lead)
Client: 'Well, my husband works long hours and is very tired when he gets home. He barely sees the children before their bedtime.'
Nurse: 'I see.' (accepting)
Client: 'I'm busy trying to fix dinner, trying to keep an eye on the children, but I also want to talk to my husband.'
Nurse: 'How do you feel when all this is happening?' (encouraging expression)
Client: 'Like I'm torn in several directions at once. Nothing seems to go right, and I can't straighten everything out.'
Nurse: 'It sounds like you're feeling overwhelmed.' (translating into feelings)
Client: 'Yes, I am. I can't do everything at once all by myself. I think we have to make some changes.'
Nurse: 'Perhaps you and I can discuss some potential changes you'd like to make.' (suggesting collaboration)

In some therapeutic interactions, the client wants only to talk to an interested listener and feel like he or she has been heard. Often just sharing a distressing event can allow the client to express thoughts and emotions that he or she has been holding back. It serves as a way to lighten the emotional load and release feelings without a need to alter the situation. Other times, the client may need to reminisce and share pleasant memories of past events. Older adults often find great solace in reminiscing about events in their lives, such as what was happening in the world when they were growing up, how they met and when they married their spouses, and so forth. Reminiscence is discussed further in Chapter 21.

DIRECTIVE ROLE

When the client is suicidal, experiencing a crisis or seems out of touch with reality, the nurse often needs to use a more **directive role**, asking direct yes/no questions and using direct problem solving to help the client develop new coping mechanisms to deal with present here-and-now issues. The following is an example of therapeutic communication using a more directive role:

Nurse: 'I see you've been sitting here in the corner of the room away from everyone else this morning.' (making observation)
Client: 'Yeah, what's the point?'
Nurse: 'What's the point of what?' (seeking clarification)
Client: 'Of anything.'
Nurse: 'You sound like you're feeling pretty hopeless.' (verbalizing the implied) *'Are you thinking about suicide?'* (seeking information)
Client: 'I have been thinking I'd be better off dead.'

The nurse uses a very direct role in this example because the client's safety is at stake.

As the nurse–client relationship progresses, the nurse uses therapeutic communication to implement many interventions in the client's plan of care. In Unit 4, specific mental health problems and disorders are discussed, as are specific therapeutic communication interventions and examples of how to use the techniques effectively.

How to Phrase Questions

The manner in which the nurse phrases questions is important. Open-ended questions elicit more descriptive information; yes/no questions yield just an answer. The nurse asks different types of questions based on the information he or she wishes to obtain or on his or her assessment of where in the therapeutic relationship things have got to. The nurse uses active listening to build questions based on the cues the client has given in his or her responses.

In English, people frequently substitute the word *feel* for the word *think*. Emotions differ from the cognitive process of thinking, so using the appropriate term is important. For example, 'What do you feel about that test?' is a vague question that could elicit several types of answers. A more specific question is, 'How well do you think you did on the test?' The nurse should ask, 'What did you think about . . . ?' when discussing cognitive issues and 'How did you feel about . . . ?' when trying to elicit the client's emotions and feelings. Box 6.1 lists

Box 6.1 'FEELING' WORDS

Afraid	Hopeless
Alarmed	Horrified
Angry	Impatient
Anxious	Irritated
Ashamed	Jealous
Bewildered	Joyful
Calm	Lonely
Carefree	Pleased
Confused	Powerless
Depressed	Relaxed
Ecstatic	Resentful
Embarrassed	Sad
Enraged	Scared
Envious	Surprised
Excited	Tense
Fearful	Terrified
Frustrated	Threatened
Guilty	Thrilled
Happy	Uptight
Hopeful	

'feeling' words that are commonly used to express or describe emotions. The following are examples of different responses that clients could give to questions using 'think' and 'feel':

> **Nurse:** 'What did you think about your daughter's role in her accident?'
> **Client:** 'She's just not a careful driver. She drives too fast.'
> **Nurse:** 'How did you feel when you heard about your daughter's car accident?'
> **Client:** 'Relieved that neither she nor anyone else was injured.'

Using active listening skills, asking many open-ended questions and building on the client's responses help the nurse obtain a complete description of an issue or an event and understand the client's experience. Some clients do not have the skill or patience to describe how an event unfolded over time without assistance from the nurse. Clients tend to recount the beginning and the end of a story, leaving out crucial information about their own behaviour. The nurse can help the client by using techniques such as clarification and placing an event in time or sequence.

ASKING FOR CLARIFICATION

Nurses often believe they should always be able to understand what the client is saying. This is not the case: the client's thoughts and communications may be unclear, and the nurse's abilities to listen and understand may be compromised by poor listening, distraction or lack of experience. The nurse should never assume that he or she understands; rather, he or she should ask for clarification if there is doubt – even (especially!) if there is no doubt! Asking for clarification to confirm the nurse's understanding of what the client intends to convey is paramount to accurate 'data collection' (Summers, 2002) and, more importantly, offers respect and humanity.

If the nurse feels that he or she needs more information or clarification on a previously discussed issue, he or she may need to return to that issue. The nurse also may need to ask questions in some areas to clarify information. The nurse then can use the therapeutic technique of consensual validation, or repeating his or her understanding of the event that the client just described to see whether their perceptions agree. It is important to go back and clarify rather than to work from assumptions.

The following is an example of clarifying and focusing techniques:

> **Client:** 'I saw it coming. No one else had a clue this would happen.'
> **Nurse:** 'What was it you saw coming?' (seeking information)
> **Client:** 'We were doing well, and then the floor dropped out from under us. There was little anyone could do but hope for the best.'
> **Nurse:** 'Help me understand by describing what you mean by "doing well".' (seeking information)
> 'Who are the "we" you refer to?' (focusing)
> 'How did the floor drop out from under you?' (encouraging description of perceptions)
> 'What did you hope would happen when you "hoped for the best"?' (seeking information)

CLIENT'S AVOIDANCE OF THE ANXIETY-PRODUCING TOPIC

Sometimes clients begin discussing a topic of minimal importance because it is less threatening than the issue that is increasing the client's anxiety. The client is discussing a topic but seems to be focused elsewhere. Active listening and observing changes in the intensity of the non-verbal process help to give the nurse a sense of what is going on. Many options can help the nurse to determine which topic is more important:

1. Ask the client which issue is more important at this time.
2. Go with the new topic because the client has given non-verbal messages that this is the issue that needs to be discussed.
3. Reflect the client's behaviour signalling there is a more important issue to be discussed.
4. Mentally file the other topic away for later exploration.
5. Ignore the new topic because it seems that the client is trying to avoid the original topic.

The following example shows how the nurse can try to identify which issue is most important to the client:

Client: *'I don't know whether it is better to tell or not tell my husband that I won't be able to work anymore. He gets so upset whenever he hears bad news. He has an ulcer, and bad news seems to set off a new bout of bleeding and pain.'*

Nurse: *'Which issue is more difficult for you to confront right now: your bad news or your husband's ulcer?'* (encouraging expression)

Guiding the Client in Problem Solving and Empowering the Client to Change

Many therapeutic situations involve problem solving. The nurse is not expected to be an expert or to tell the client what to do to fix his or her problem: as previously mentioned, the client is always the expert in his or her life. Rather, the nurse should help the client explore possibilities and find solutions to his or her problem. Often, just helping the client to discuss and explore his or her perceptions of a problem stimulates potential solutions in the client's mind (Adkins, 2003). The nurse should introduce the concept of problem solving and solution finding and offer himself or herself in this process.

Virginia Satir (1967) explained how important the client's participation is to finding effective and meaningful solutions to problems. If someone else tells the client how to solve his or her problems and does not allow the client to participate and develop problem-solving skills and paths for change, the client may fear growth and change. The nurse who gives advice or directions about the way to fix a problem does not allow the client to play a role in the process and implies that the client is less than competent. This process makes the client feel helpless and not in control, and lowers self-esteem. The client may even (understandably) resist the directives in an attempt to regain a sense of control.

When a client is more involved in the solution-finding/problem-solving process, he or she is more likely to follow through on agreed solutions. The nurse who empowers the client to solve his or her own problems helps the client to develop new coping strategies, maintains or increases the client's self-esteem and demonstrates the belief that the client is capable of change. These goals encourage the client to expand his or her repertoire of skills and to feel competent; feeling effective and in control is a far more comfortable state for any client than a desperate battle to respond appropriately to an all-knowing nurse.

Problem solving is frequently used in crisis intervention but is equally effective for general use. The problem-solving process is used when the client has difficulty finding ways to solve the problem or when working with a group of people whose divergent viewpoints hinder finding solutions. It involves several steps:

1. Identify the problem
2. Brainstorm all possible solutions
3. Select the best alternative
4. Implement the selected alternative
5. Evaluate the situation
6. If dissatisfied with results, select another alternative and continue the process.

Identifying the problem involves (obviously) engaging the client in therapeutic communication. The client tells the nurse the problem and what he or she has tried to do to solve it:

Nurse: *'I see you're frowning. What's going on?'* (making observation; broad opening)

Client: *'I've tried to get my husband more involved with the children rather than just yelling at them when he comes in from work, but I haven't got anywhere.'*

Nurse: *'What have you tried that hasn't worked?'* (encouraging expression)

Client: *'Before my surgery, I tried to involve him in their homework. My husband is a math whiz. Then I tried TV time together, but the kids like cartoons and he wants to watch stuff about history, natural science or travel.'*

Nurse: *'How have you involved your husband in this plan for him to get more involved with the children?'* (seeking information)

Client: *'Uh, I haven't. I mean, he always says he wants to spend more quality time with the kids, but he doesn't. Do you mean it would be better for him to decide how he wants to do this – I mean, spend quality time with the kids?'*

Nurse: *'That sounds like it might be a good place to start. Perhaps you and your husband could discuss this when he comes to visit and decide what would work for both of you.'* (formulating a plan of action)

It is important to remember that the nurse is facilitating the client's problem-solving abilities. The nurse may not believe the client is choosing the best or most effective solution, but it is essential that the nurse supports the client's choice and assists him or her to implement the chosen alternative. If the client makes a mistake or the selected alternative isn't successful, the nurse can support the client's efforts and assist the client to try again. Effective problem solving involves helping the client to resolve his or her own problems as independently as possible.

THERAPEUTIC COMMUNICATION IN THE CLIENT'S HOME

The nurse may well be the major carer and resource for increasingly high-risk clients treated in the home. Effective, compassionate therapeutic communication techniques and skills are essential to successful collaborative work with clients and their carers in the community.

Working with several people at one time, rather than just with the client, is the standard in community care. Self-awareness and sensitivity to the beliefs, behaviours and feelings of others are paramount in successful communication with people in the community.

As just one example, caring for older adults in the family unit and in communities today is a major mental health nursing concern and responsibility. It is important to assess the relationships of family members; identifying their areas of agreement and conflict can greatly affect the care of clients. To be responsive to the needs of these clients and their families for support and caring, the nurse must communicate and relate to clients and carers and establish a therapeutic relationship.

When practising in the community, the nurse needs self-awareness and knowledge about cultural differences. When the nurse enters the home of a client, the nurse is the outsider and must learn to negotiate the cultural context of each family by understanding their beliefs, customs and practices, and not judging them according to his or her own cultural context. Asking the family for help in learning about their culture demonstrates the nurse's unconditional positive regard and genuineness. Families from other cultural backgrounds will usually be patient and forgiving of any cultural mistakes that nurses might make as they learn different customs and behaviours.

The nurse also needs to understand the health-care practices of various cultures in order to make sure that these practices do not hinder or alter the prescribed therapeutic regimes. Very occasionally, cultural healing practices, remedies and even dietary practices may alter the client's immune system and may enhance or interfere with prescribed medications.

 SELF-AWARENESS ISSUES

Therapeutic communication is the primary vehicle that nurses use to help people in mental health settings. The nurse's skill in therapeutic communication influences the effectiveness of many interventions and, therefore, the nurse must evaluate and improve his or her communication skills on an ongoing basis. When the nurse examines his or her personal beliefs, attitudes and values as they relate to communication, or directly asks for feedback from colleagues, supervisors or clients themselves, he or she should be gaining awareness of the factors influencing communication.

The nurse will experience many different emotional reactions to clients, such as sadness, anger, frustration and discomfort. The nurse must reflect on these experiences to determine how emotional responses affect both verbal and non-verbal communication. When working with clients from different cultural or ethnic backgrounds, the nurse needs to know, or to find out, what communication styles are comfortable for the client in terms of eye contact, touch, proximity and so forth. The nurse can then adapt his or her communication style in ways that are beneficial to the nurse–client relationship.

Points to Consider When Working on Therapeutic Communication Skills

- Remember that non-verbal communication is just as important as the words you speak. Be mindful of your facial expression, body posture and other non-verbal aspects of communication as you work with clients.

- Ask colleagues for feedback about your communication style. Ask them how they communicate with clients in difficult or uncomfortable situations.
- Examine your communication by asking questions such as 'How do I relate to men? To women? To authority figures? To elderly people? To people from cultures different from my own?' 'What types of clients or situations make me uncomfortable? Sad? Angry? Frustrated?' Use these self-assessment data to improve your communication skills.

Critical Thinking Questions

1. Explain why the nurse's attempt to solve the client's problem is less effective than guiding the client to identify his or her own ways to resolve the issue.
2. The nurse is working with a client whose culture includes honouring one's parents and being obedient, keeping 'private' matters within the family only, and not talking with strangers about family matters. Given this client's belief system, how might the nurse use therapeutic communication effectively?

KEY POINTS

- Communication is the process people use to exchange information through verbal and non-verbal messages. It is composed of both the literal words or content and all the non-verbal messages (process), including body language, eye contact, facial expression, tone of voice, rate of speech, context and hesitations that accompany the words. To communicate effectively, the nurse must be skilled in the analysis of both content and process.
- Therapeutic communication is an interpersonal interaction between the nurse and client during which the nurse focuses on the needs of the client to promote an effective exchange of information between the nurse and client.
- Goals of therapeutic communication include establishing rapport, actively listening, gaining the client's perspective, exploring the client's thoughts and feelings and guiding the client in problem solving.
- The crucial components of therapeutic communication are confidentiality, privacy, respect for boundaries, self-disclosure, use of touch and active listening and observation skills.
- Proxemics is concerned with the distance zones between people when they communicate: intimate, personal, social and public.
- Active listening involves refraining from other internal mental activities and trying to concentrate exclusively on what the client is saying.

INTERNET RESOURCES

RESOURCES	INTERNET ADDRESS
• Brief Therapy Practice	http://www.brieftherapy.org.uk/
• Mental Health Recovery Resources	http://www.namiscc.org/MentalHealthRecovery.htm
• Psychnet-UK	http://www.psychnet-uk.com/
• Resources for Listening and Communicating	http://www.allaboutcounseling.com
• Tidal Model	http://www.tidal-model.co.uk

- Verbal messages need to be clear and concrete rather than vague and abstract. Abstract messages requiring the client to make assumptions can be misleading and confusing. The nurse needs to clarify any areas of confusion so that he or she does not make assumptions based on his or her own experiences.
- Non-verbal communication includes facial expressions, body language, eye contact, proxemics (environmental distance), touch and vocal cues. All are important in understanding the speaker's message.
- Understanding the context is important to the accuracy of the message. Assessment of context focuses on the who, what, when, how and why of an event.
- Spirituality and religion can greatly affect a client's health and health care. These beliefs vary widely and are highly subjective. The nurse must be careful not to impose his or her beliefs on the client or to allow differences to erode trust.
- Cultural differences can greatly affect the therapeutic communication process.
- When guiding a client in the problem-solving process, it is important that the client (not the nurse) chooses and implements solutions.
- Therapeutic communication techniques and skills are essential to successful management of clients in the community.
- The greater the nurse's understanding of his or her own feelings and responses, the better the nurse can communicate and understand others.

REFERENCES

Adkins, E. (2003). The first day of the rest of their lives. *Journal of Psychosocial Nursing and Mental Services, 41*(7), 28–32.

Andrews, M. & Boyle, J. (2003). *Transcultural concepts in nursing care* (4th edn). Philadelphia: Lippincott Williams & Wilkins.

Chant, S., Jenkinson, T., Randle, J., *et al.* (2002). Communication skills: Some problems in nursing education and practice. *Journal of Clinical Nursing, 11*(1), 12–21.

DeVito, J. A. (2004). *The interpersonal communication handbook* (10th edn). Boston: Pearson Education.

Egan, G. (2006). The skilled helper: *A problem-management and opportunity-development approach to helping* (international edn). London: Thomson Learning.

Greene, J. O. & Burleson, B. R. (Eds.). (2003). *Handbook of communication and social interaction skills*. Mahwah, NJ: Erlbaum Associates.

Hall, E. (1963). Proxemics: The study of man's spatial relationships. In J. Gladstone (Ed.), *Man's image in medicine and anthropology* (pp. 109–120). Philadelphia: Mosby.

Knapp, M. L. (1980). *Essentials of nonverbal communication*. New York: Holt, Rinehart & Winston.

Knapp, M. L. & Hall, J. (2002). Nonverbal behaviour in human interaction (5th edn). New York: Wadsworth.

Peplau, H. (1952). Interpersonal relations in nursing. New York: G. P. Putnam.

Satir, V. (1967). Conjoint family therapy: A guide to theory and technique (rev. edn). Palo Alto, California: Science and Behaviour Books, Inc.

Sheldon, L. K. (2004). Communication for nurses: Talking with patients. Thorofare, New Jersey: SLACK, Inc.

Summers, L. C. (2002). Mutual timing: an essential component of provider/patient communication. *Journal of the American Academy of Nurse Practitioners, 14*(1), 19–25.

Thich Nhat Hanh. (2001). *Anger: Wisdom For Cooling The Flames* (p. 92). London: Rider.

ADDITIONAL READING

Burnard, P. (2002). *Learning human skills: An experiential and reflective guide for nurses and health care professionals*. Cheltenham: Butterworth-Heinemann.

Burnard, P. (2006). *Counselling skills for health professionals*. Oxford: Nelson Thornes.

Moss, B. (2007). *Communication skills for health and social care*. London: Sage.

Robb, M., Barrett, S., & Komaromy, C. (2003). *Communication, relationships and care: A reader*. Abingdon: Routledge.

Chapter Study Guide

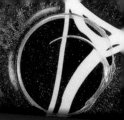

MULTIPLE-CHOICE QUESTIONS

Select the best answer for each of the following questions.

1. **Client:** 'I had an accident.'

   Nurse: 'Tell me about your accident.'

   This is an example of which therapeutic communication technique?
   a. Making observations
   b. Offering self
   c. General lead
   d. Reflection

2. 'Earlier today you said you were concerned that your son was still upset with you. When I stopped by your room about an hour ago, you and your son seemed relaxed and smiling as you spoke to each other. How did things go between the two of you?'

   This is an example of which therapeutic communication technique?
   a. Consensual validation
   b. Encouraging comparison
   c. Accepting
   d. General lead

3. 'Why do you always complain about the night nurse? She is a nice woman and a fine nurse and has five kids to support. You're wrong when you say she is noisy and uncaring.'

   This example reflects which non-therapeutic technique?
   a. Requesting an explanation
   b. Defending
   c. Disagreeing
   d. Advising

4. 'How does Jerry make you upset?' is a non-therapeutic communication technique because it
   a. Gives a literal response
   b. Indicates an external source of the emotion
   c. Interprets what the client is saying
   d. Is just another stereotyped comment

5. **Client:** 'I was so upset about my sister ignoring my pain when I broke my leg.'

   Nurse: 'When are you going to your next diabetes education programme?'

   This is a non-therapeutic response because the nurse has
   a. Used testing to evaluate the client's insight
   b. Changed the topic
   c. Exhibited an egocentric focus
   d. Advised the client what to do

6. When the client says, 'I met Joe at the dance last week', what is the best way for the nurse to ask the client to describe her relationship with Joe?
   a. 'Joe who?'
   b. 'Tell me about Joe.'
   c. 'Tell me about you and Joe.'
   d. 'Joe, you mean that blond guy with the dark blue eyes?'

7. Which of the following is a concrete message?
   a. 'Help me put this pile of books on Marsha's desk.'
   b. 'Get this out of here.'
   c. 'When is she coming home?'
   d. 'They said it is too early to get in.'

GROUP DISCUSSION TOPICS

Define and discuss the relevance of the following.

1. Culture

2. Proxemics

3. Incongruent messages

4. Spirituality

5. Non-verbal communication

6. Metaphor

7. Therapeutic use of self

SHORT-ANSWER QUESTIONS

In the following client statements, underline the cues (words, phrases or issues) that should be followed up with therapeutic communication interventions. Then, write a therapeutic response.

1. 'I feel good.'

2. 'I can't take it anymore.'

3. 'I have two children, one from my wife and one from my girlfriend.'

4. 'We were standing on the corner.'

5. 'My son is never going to understand the way his wife is ruining them.'

Culture, Clients and Nurses: Responses to Stress, Health and Illness

Key Terms

- cultural diversity
- culturally competent
- culture
- environmental control
- ethnicity
- hardiness
- race
- resilience
- resourcefulness
- selfefficacy
- sense of belonging
- social network
- social organization
- social support
- socioeconomic status
- spirituality
- time orientation

Learning Objectives

After reading this chapter, you should be able to:

1. Discuss the influences of age, growth and development on people's responses to stress.

2. Identify the roles that physical health and biological make-up play in someone's emotional responses.

3. Explain the importance of personal characteristics, such as self-efficacy, hardiness, resilience, resourcefulness and spirituality, in a person's response to stressors.

4. Explain the influence of interpersonal factors, such as sense of belonging, social networks and family support, on someone's response to stress.

5. Describe various cultural beliefs and practices that can affect mental health.

6. Explain the cultural factors that the nurse must consider when working with people from different cultural backgrounds.

7. Explain the nurse's role in assessing and working with people from different cultural backgrounds.

Nursing philosophies often describe the person or individual as a 'biopsychosocial' being who possesses unique characteristics and responds to others and the world in various and diverse ways. This view of the individual as unique requires nurses to assess each person and his or her responses in order to plan and provide nursing care that is personally meaningful. This uniqueness of response may also partially explain why some people become 'ill' and others do not. Understanding why two people raised in a similarly stressful environment (for example one with neglect or abuse) turn out differently is difficult: one person may become reasonably successful and maintain a satisfying marriage and family, whereas the other may feel chronically isolated, depressed and lonely. Although we do not know exactly what makes the difference, studies have begun to show that an interplay between personal, interpersonal and cultural factors seem to influence a person's response.

This chapter examines some of the personal, interpersonal and cultural factors that create the unique individual response to stress and ill-health, and to care and treatment. In determining how a person copes with these things, we cannot single out one or two aspects. Rather, we must consider each person as a combination of all these overlapping and interacting factors.

INDIVIDUAL FACTORS

Age, Growth and Development

A person's age seems to affect how he or she copes with ill-health. For instance, the age at onset of schizophrenia seems to be a strong predictor of prognosis (Buchanan & Carpenter, 2005). People with a younger age at onset have poorer outcomes, such as more negative signs (apathy, social isolation, lack of volition) and less-effective coping skills, than do people with a later age at onset. A possible reason for this difference is that younger clients have not had experiences of successful independent living or the opportunity to work and be self-sufficient, and have a less well-developed sense of personal identity than older clients.

Someone's age can also influence how he or she expresses his or her experience of overwhelming stress or 'ill-health'. A young child diagnosed with ADHD may lack the understanding and ability to describe his or her feelings, which may make management of the disorder more challenging. In this instance, nurses must be aware of the child's level of language and work to understand the experience as he or she describes it.

Erik Erikson described psychosocial development across the life span in terms of developmental tasks to accomplish at each stage (Table 7.1). Each stage of development depends on the successful completion of the previous stage. In each stage, the person must complete a critical life task that is essential to well-being and mental health. Failure to complete the critical task results in a negative outcome for that stage of development and impedes completion of future tasks. For example, the infancy stage (birth to 18 months) is the stage of 'trust versus mistrust', when infants must learn to develop basic trust that their parents or guardians will take care of them, feed them, change their nappies, love them and keep them safe. If the infant does not develop trust in this stage, he or she may be unable to love and trust others later in life because the ability to trust others is essential to establishing good relationships. Specific developmental tasks for adults are summarized in Table 7.2.

According to Erikson's theory, people may get 'stuck' at any stage of development. For example, a person who never completed the developmental task of autonomy may become overly dependent on others. Failure to develop identity can result in role confusion or an unclear idea about who one

Table 7.1	ERIKSON'S STAGES OF PSYCHOSOCIAL DEVELOPMENT
Stage	**Tasks**
Trust vs. mistrust (infant)	Viewing the world as safe and reliable
	Viewing relationships as nurturing, stable and dependable
Autonomy vs. shame and doubt (toddler)	Achieving a sense of control and free will
Initiative vs. guilt (preschool)	Beginning to develop a conscience
	Learning to manage conflict and anxiety
Industry vs. inferiority (school age)	Building confidence in own abilities
	Taking pleasure in accomplishments
Identity vs. role diffusion (adolescence)	Formulating a sense of self and belonging
Intimacy vs. isolation (young adult)	Forming adult, loving relationships and meaningful attachment to others
	Being creative and productive
Generativity vs. stagnation (middle adult)	Establishing the next generation
Ego integrity vs. despair (maturity)	Accepting responsibility for one's self and life

Table 7.2	ADULT GROWTH AND DEVELOPMENT TASKS

Stage	Tasks
Young adult (25–45 years of age)	Accept self
	Stabilize self-image
	Establish independence from parental home and financial independence
	Establish a career or vocation
	Form an intimate bond with another person
	Build a congenial social and friendship group
	Become an involved citizen
	Establish and maintain a home
Middle adult (45–65 years of age)	Express love through more than sexual contacts
	Maintain healthy life patterns
	Develop sense of unity with mate
	Help growing and grown children to be responsible adults
	Relinquish central role in lives of grown children
	Accept children's mates and friends
	Create a comfortable home
	Be proud of accomplishments of self and mate/spouse
	Reverse roles with aging parents
	Achieve mature civic and social responsibility
	Adjust to physical changes of middle age
	Use leisure time creatively
	Cherish old friends and make new ones
Older adult (65 years of age and older)	Prepare for retirement
	Recognize the aging process and its limitations
	Adjust to health changes
	Decide where to live out remaining years
	Continue warm relationship with mate/spouse
	Adjust living standards to retirement income
	Maintain maximum level of health
	Care for self physically and emotionally
	Maintain contact with children and relatives
	Maintain interest in people outside the family
	Find meaning in life after retirement
	Adjust to the death of mate/spouse or other loved ones

is as a person. Negotiating these developmental tasks affects how the person responds to stress and ill-health. Lack of success may result in feelings of inferiority, doubt, lack of confidence and isolation – all of which can affect how a person responds to stress and ill-health.

Genetics and Biological Factors

Heredity and biological factors are not under voluntary control. We cannot – at the present level of scientific knowledge – change these factors. Research has identified genetic links to several disorders. For example, some people are born with a gene associated with one type of Alzheimer's disease. Although specific genetic links have not been identified for several mental disorders (e.g. bipolar disorder, major depression, alcoholism), research has shown that these disorders tend to appear more frequently in particular families. Genetic make-up influences tremendously a

person's response to stress, to ill-health and perhaps even to treatment. This is one reason why family history and background are essential parts of any nursing assessment; perhaps more importantly, knowledge both of previous mental health problems within the family and of the resources and strengths the family has been/is able to bring to life challenges is vital in working effectively with people and helping them find solutions.

Physical Health and Health Practices

Physical health can also influence how a person responds to psychosocial stress or ill-health. The healthier a person is, the better, potentially, he or she can cope with stress or ill-health. Poor nutritional status, lack of sleep or a chronic physical illness or disability may impair a person's capacity to cope. Unlike the case of genetic factors, a person is, with appropriate information, support and collaborative care, able to tackle issues of nutrition, sleep, weight and exercise, and thus influence his or her ability to deal effectively with mental health problems; partly for this reason (and partly because of the fact that mental health problems can lead to deleterious physical consequences) nurses *must* assess the client's physical health even when the client is apparently seeking help for purely mental health problems.

Exercise

The Mental Health Foundation (2005) and many others have shown that walking and stretching exercises diminished the negative effects of depression and anxiety. It is suggested that continued participation in exercise is a positive indicator of improved health, while cessation from participation in exercise might indicate declining mental health.

Response to Drugs

Biological differences can affect a client's response to treatment, specifically to psychotropic drugs. Ethnic groups differ in the metabolism and efficacy of psychoactive compounds. Some ethnic groups metabolize drugs more slowly (meaning that the serum level of the drug remains higher), which increases the frequency and severity of side-effects. Clients who metabolize drugs more slowly generally need

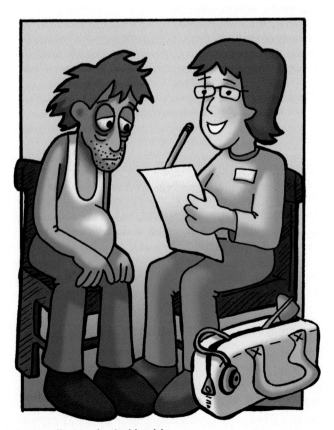

Assess client's physical health

lower doses of a drug to produce the desired effect (Purnell & Paulanka, 2003). In general, people from non-white backgrounds treated with Western dosing protocols have higher serum levels per dose and suffer more side-effects. Although many non-Western countries report successful treatment with lower dosages of psychotropic drugs, Western dosage protocols frequently continue to drive prescribing practices in the UK. When evaluating the efficacy of psychotropic medications, the nurse *must* be alert to side-effects and serum drug levels in clients from different ethnic backgrounds.

Self-efficacy

Self-efficacy is a belief that personal abilities and efforts can affect the events in our lives. A person who believes that his or her behaviour makes a real difference is more likely to take action. People with high self-efficacy set personal goals, are self-motivated, cope effectively with stress and request support from others when needed. People with low self-efficacy have low aspirations, experience much self-doubt and may be plagued by anxiety and depression. Bandura (2004) suggested that, rather than focusing on solving specific problems, care and treatment should focus on developing a client's skills to take control of his or her life (i.e. develop self-efficacy) so that he or she can make life changes. The four main ways to do so are as follows:

- Experience of success or mastery in overcoming obstacles
- Social modelling (observing successful people instills the idea that one can also succeed)
- Social persuasion (persuading people to believe in themselves)
- Reducing stress, building physical strength and learning how to interpret physical sensations positively (e.g. viewing fatigue as a sign that one has accomplished something rather than as a lack of stamina).

Cutler (2005) reports a relationship between self-efficacy and the client's motivation for self-care and follow-up after discharge from inpatient treatment. Clients returning to the community with higher self-efficacy were more confident and had positive expectations about their personal success. She suggests that therapeutic interventions designed to promote the client's self-efficacy can have positive effects on interpersonal relationships and coping upon return to the community.

The concept of self-efficacy is an interpersonal one, of course: if mental health professionals feel – and give a strong conscious or unconscious message – that someone is unable to change, to take control of his or her life, then he or she is less likely to do so. Equally, an expectation that someone is capable of taking control when he or she clearly isn't yet ready to do so, can be equally harmful.

Hardiness

Hardiness is the ability to resist a move into 'disorder' or 'illness' when under stress. First described by Kobasa (1979), hardiness has three components:

1. Commitment: active involvement in life activities
2. Control: ability to make appropriate decisions in life activities
3. Challenge: ability to perceive change as beneficial rather than just stressful.

Hardiness has been found to have a moderating or buffering effect on people experiencing stress. Kobasa (1979) found that male executives who had high stress but low occurrence of ill-health scored higher on the hardiness scale than executives with high stress and high occurrence of ill-health. Study findings suggested that stressful life events caused more harm to people with low hardiness than with high hardiness.

Personal hardiness is often described as a pattern of attitudes and actions that helps the person turn stressful circumstances into opportunities for growth. Maddi (2005) found that persons with high hardiness perceived stressors more accurately and were able to problem solve in the situation more effectively. Hardiness has been identified as an important resilience factor for families coping with the mental health problems of one of their members (Greeff *et al.*, 2006).

We need – as we do with so many areas of psychology – to exercise some caution and scepticism when considering the concept of hardiness. Some believe that the concept – like so many in psychology –can be used in a vague and indistinct way, and may not be helpful to everyone. Some research on hardiness suggests that its effects are not the same for men and women. In addition, hardiness may be useful only to those who value individualism, such as people from some Western cultures. For people and cultures who value relationships over individual achievement, hardiness may not be beneficial or, indeed, make much sense as a concept (Brooks, 2003).

Resilience and Resourcefulness

Two closely related concepts, resilience and resourcefulness, help people to cope with stress and to minimize the effects of disorder and 'illness' (Edward & Warelow, 2005).

Resilience can be defined as a quality whereby a person has healthy responses to stressful circumstances or risky situations, and is intended to help explain why, for example, one person reacts to a slightly stressful event with severe anxiety, whereas another person does not experience distress even when confronting a major disruption. Studies on resilience first focused on factors that resulted in positive outcomes for children who were at risk because their parents had alcohol or mental health problems. The factors that seemed to enhance outcomes were children's abilities to develop self-esteem and self-efficacy through relationships with others, have new experiences and obtain assistance with life transitions as they matured (Krafcik, 2002).

Studies found that families who draw on and use their strengths show improved resilience and more positive outcomes than families who view themselves as victims of multiple problems, such as poverty, unemployment and low socioeconomic status. Family protective mechanisms that improve the resilience of children include instilling positive family values, promoting positive communication and social interaction, maintaining flexible family roles, exercising control over children and providing academic support to children. Family protective factors that improve the resilience of adolescents include caring and supportive relationships with adults; high expectations for good 'citizenship', academic achievement and spiritual involvement; and encouragement to participate in caring for siblings, household chores, part-time work and carefully selected safe activities outside the home

Resourcefulness involves using problem-solving abilities and believing that one can cope with adverse or novel situations. People develop resourcefulness through interactions with others, that is, through successfully coping with life experiences (Krafcik, 2002). Examples of resourcefulness include performing health-seeking behaviours, learning self-care, monitoring one's thoughts and feelings about stressful situations and taking action to deal with stressful circumstances.

Spirituality

Spirituality involves the essence of a person's being and his or her beliefs about the meaning of life and the purpose for living. It may include belief in God or a higher power, the practice of a theistic or non-theistic religion, humanism, a belief in the fundamental need for discovering truth in scientific endeavour, cultural, political and/or philosophical beliefs and practices and a focused relationship with the Earth and the environment. Although, of course, some people with mental health problems have disturbing religious delusions and some religious belief systems are actively opposed to contemporary mental health care, for many religion and spirituality are a source of comfort and help in times of stress or trauma. Studies have shown that a deep sense of spirituality can be a genuine help to many adults with mental health problems, serving as a primary coping device and a source of meaning and coherence in their lives, often, at the same time, helping to provide a social network (Sageman, 2004).

Spiritual beliefs and activities and the associated social support have been shown to be very important for many people, and seem to be linked with better health and a sense of well-being. These activities have also been found to help people cope with poor physical or mental health. Hope and faith have been identified as critical factors in both psychiatric and physical rehabilitation (Baetz *et al.*, 2002).

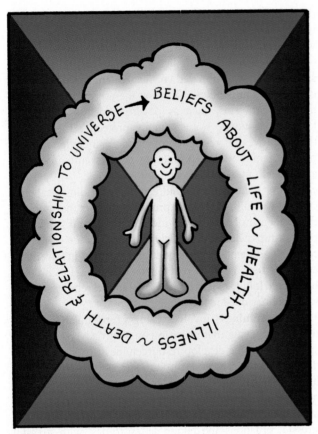

Spirituality

Studies have shown that religion and spirituality can be helpful to families who have a relative with mental health problems. Religion has been found to play an important role in providing support to carers and often as a major source of solace (Longo & Peterson, 2002).

Because spiritual or religious beliefs and practices help many clients to cope with stress and ill-health, the nurse must be particularly sensitive to, and accepting of, such beliefs and practices. Incorporating those practices into the care of clients can help them cope with ill-health and find meaning and purpose in the situation. Doing so can also offer a strong source of support (Huguelet *et al.*, 2006).

INTERPERSONAL FACTORS

Sense of Belonging

A **sense of belonging** is the feeling of 'connectedness' with or involvement in a social system or environment of which a person feels an integral part (Ross, 2002). Abraham Maslow described a sense of belonging as a basic human psychosocial need that involves both feelings of 'value' and 'fit'. *Value* refers to feeling needed and accepted. *Fit* refers to feeling that one meshes or fits in with the system or environment. This means that when a person belongs to a system or group, he or she feels valued and

worthwhile within that support system. Examples of support systems include family, friends, co-workers, clubs or social groups, and, on occasion, health and social care workers.

A person's sense of belonging is closely related to his or her social and psychological functioning. A sense of belonging has been found to promote health, a lack of belonging to impair it. An increased sense of belonging has also been associated with decreased levels of anxiety. People with a sense of belonging are less alienated and isolated, have a sense of purpose, believe they are needed by others and feel productive socially. Hence, it is vital that the nurse should focus on interventions that help increase a client's sense of belonging (Granerud & Severinsson, 2006).

Social Networks and Social Support

Social networks are groups of people whom one knows and with whom one feels connected. Studies have found that having a social network can help reduce stress, diminish ill-health and positively influence the ability to cope and to adapt (Chanokruthai *et al.*, 2005). **Social support** is emotional and practical sustenance that comes from friends, family members and, sometimes, health-care professionals, who help a person when a problem arises. It is different from social contact, which does not always directly provide emotional support.

People who are supported emotionally and functionally have been found to be healthier than those who are not supported (Vanderhorst & McLaren, 2005). Meaningful social relationships with family or friends have been found to improve the health and well-being outcomes for older adults. An essential element of improved outcomes is that family or friends respond with support when it is requested. In other words, the person must be able to count on these friends or family to help or support him or her by visiting, by talking on the phone, by e-mail or text messaging. The primary components of satisfactory support, then, are the person's ability and willingness to request support when needed *and* the ability and willingness of the support system to respond.

So, two key components are necessary for a support system to be effective: the client's perception of the support system and the responsiveness of that support system. The client must perceive that the social support system bolsters his or her confidence and self-esteem and provides stress-related interpersonal help, such as offering assistance in solving a problem. The client must also perceive that the actions of the support system are consistent with the client's desires and expectations – in other words, the support provided is what the client wants, *not what the 'supporter' believes would be good for the client*. Also, the support system must be able to provide direct help or material aid (e.g. providing transportation, making a follow-up appointment). Some people have the capacity to seek help when needed, whereas a lack of well-being may cause others to withdraw from potential providers of support. The nurse can help the client to find support people who will be available and helpful and can work with the client on ways to request – and accept – support when needed.

Family Support

Family as a source of social support can be a key factor in the recovery of clients with mental health problems. Although family members are not always a positive resource in mental health, they are most often an important part of recovery. Health-care professionals cannot – and should not – totally replace family members. The nurse must encourage family members to continue to support the client even while he or she is in the hospital, and should identify family strengths, such as love and caring, as a resource for the client (Reid *et al.*, 2005).

HIGH AND LOW EXPRESSED EMOTION

The idea of 'expressed emotion' has been around for some four decades and offers an interesting insight (with a fair body of research underpinning it) into the role that families and other key individuals can play in maintaining, improving or worsening psychosis, depression and other mental health problems. 'High expressed emotion' involves three elements that seem to be contributory to a drop in a mood or to the development of psychosis: hostility, emotional over-involvement and criticism

'Low expressed emotion' incorporates warmth and positive remarks towards the client: it is thought that these help reduce stress vulnerability and the likelihood of a worsening in mental state.

By being aware of the presence or absence of these factors, and working collaboratively with families and clients together, the nurse can help improve the quality of life for all involved. Box 7.1 demonstrates key aspects to consider when working with families.

CULTURAL FACTORS

Culture can be defined as all the socially learned behaviours, values, beliefs, customs and ways of thinking of a population that guide its members' views of themselves and the world. These affect all aspects of the person's being, including health, illness, care and treatment.

Burnard (2005, p. 1) says that 'We all live within and are influenced by our culture. Most of the time, our own is taken-for-granted. We only 'notice culture' when we see someone else's and when it is markedly different to our own. We are probably hardly aware of our own culture, until faced with another.' It is at this point – when 'faced with another' – that nurses often fail to give effective and compassionate care. **Cultural diversity** refers to the vast

---

Box 7.1   FAMILY INTERVENTION

In family interventions, clinicians should take the following family characteristics into consideration:

- Structure, e.g. nuclear or extended
- Significant members
- Cultural and social norms
- Expectations of the patient
- Knowledge of the illness
- Acceptance of medical or psychological intervention
- Gender-role expectations
- External support systems

From Bhugra, D. & McKenzie, K. (2003). Expressed emotion across cultures. *Advances in Psychiatric Treatment*, 9, 342–348, with permission. © 2009 The Royal College of Psychiatrists.

---

array of differences that exist among populations, and among groups and individuals within populations: coming to terms with – and embracing – that increasing diversity within the wider population and within mental health populations is vital.

According to the UK Office for National Statistics (2002), 4.6 million people (7.9%) of people came from ethnic groups other than 'white': 'Indians were the largest of these groups, followed by Pakistanis, those of Mixed ethnic backgrounds, Black Caribbeans, Black Africans and Bangladeshis'. In the UK the number of people who came from an ethnic group other than 'white' grew by 53% between 1991 and 2001, from 3.0 million in 1991 to 4.6 million in 2001. Since 2002, changes in migration and employment patterns within Europe have meant an increasing population of people coming from Eastern Europe, in particular Romania and Poland. According to the Office for National Statistics (ONS), 'Taking 2005 and 2006 together, Poland overtook India to become the second most common citizenship of immigrants to Britain with 124,000 Polish citizens arriving in the UK for at least a year during that period.'

This changing composition of society has massive implications for health-care professionals, who are still, despite recent shifts, predominantly drawn from 'indigenous', white ethnic groups and are often unfamiliar with the cultural beliefs and practices of people from other countries (Purnell & Paulanka, 2003).

Nurses and other health and social care workers must learn about other cultures and become skilled at providing care to people with cultural backgrounds that are different from their own. Finding out about another's cultural beliefs and practices, and attempting to understand their

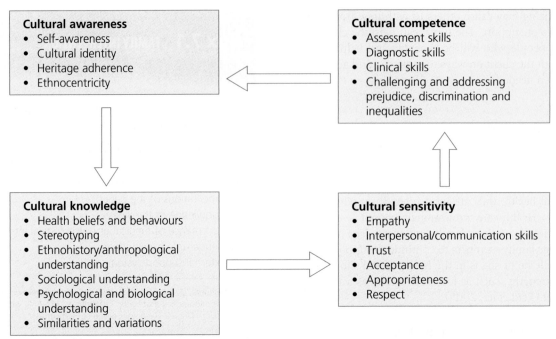

Figure 7.1. The Papadopoulos, Tilki and Taylor model for developing cultural competence. From Papadopoulos, I., Tilki, M., & Taylor, S. (2004). Promoting cultural competence in health care through a research-based intervention in the UK. *Diversity in Health and Social Care, 1*(2), 107–115. Reproduced with permission.

meaning, is essential in providing holistic and meaningful care to the client. Factors such as cultural awareness, cultural sensitivity, cultural competence and cultural knowledge need to be embedded in nurses' training and professional and personal development (Papadopoulos *et al.*, 2004) (Figure 7.1).

Additionally, it is vital for nurses from other cultures to attempt to understand the cultural factors that influence people from white indigenous populations.

Culturally competent nursing care, though, doesn't just demand that nurses are sensitive to 'culture' when it relates to ethnicity or **race**. It means being sensitive to the complex, interweaving issues of ethnicity, culture, race, age, gender, sexual orientation, social class, sub-culture and economic situation in a society that is itself struggling to cope effectively with these issues.

Refugees and Asylum Seekers

People who are refugees and/or seeking asylum often present with a bewildering number of complex difficulties. Traditionally, this increasingly important group is not cared for particularly well by mainstream mental health services. The combination of post-traumatic issues, the stresses of cultural adjustment in a hostile society and the possibility of pre-existing mental health problems, alongside social deprivation and personal and institutional racism (Box 7.2), often conspires to cause high levels of distress – and high levels of risk of self-harm, suicide and (occasionally) violence in members of this group. Nurses need a high level of knowledge and skill, and a clear,

open and tolerant set of values (as well as good clinical supervision), to ensure effective and compassionate care (Box 7.3).

Factors in Cultural Assessment

Giger and Davidhizar (2003) recommend a model for assessing and working with clients, using six cultural phenomena: communication, physical distance or space, social organization, time orientation, environmental control and biological variations (Box 7.4). Each phenomenon is discussed in more detail below.

COMMUNICATION

Verbal communication can, obviously, be difficult when the client and nurse do not speak the same language (Box 7.5). The need for skilled, experienced help from an interpreter must be considered, though this in itself can raise further problems: access to professional interpreters can be difficult (and expensive) and there can be a temptation to use family members as cheap alternatives – a temptation that can lead (in rare instances) to deliberate misinformation or partial information being communicated or obtained. There is no reason why nurses shouldn't learn a few words of a client's language and bilingual cards and other pictorial resources can aid communication.

Accent and dialect can also hamper understanding, even among people from broadly similar backgrounds. Content, tone, volume and speed of verbal communication can vary across and within cultures: some people (e.g. older white

Box 7.2 POSSIBLE ISSUES FACED BY REFUGEES

Causes
  War
  Human rights abuses
  Persecution on grounds of politics, religion, gender
  or ethnicity
Resultant losses
  Country
  Culture
  Family
  Profession
  Language
  Friends
  Plans for future

Issues in country of asylum
  Multiple changes
  Psychological and practical adjustment
  Uncertain future
  Traumatic life events
  Hardship
  Racism
  Stereotyping by host community
  Unknown cultural traditions

From Tribe, R. (2002). Mental health of refugees and asylum-seekers. *Advances in Psychiatric Treatment*, 8, 240–247, with permission. © 2009 The Royal College of Psychiatrists.

Box 7.3 POINTS TO CONSIDER WHEN TREATING ASYLUMSEEKERS OR REFUGEES

- Bear in mind that the patient may be extremely anxious about the security of personal information
- Issues of trust may be problematic
- Never contact the local embassy of their country of origin for information; instead, use organizations such as:
  - Human Rights Watch (33 Islington High Street, London N1 9LH. Tel.: 020 7713 1995; fax: 020 7713 1800; http://www.hrw.org)
  - Amnesty International (99–119 Rosebery Avenue, London EC1R 4RE. Tel.: 020 7814 6200)
- It is usually unwise to put patients from the same country in the same therapeutic group

From Tribe, R. (2002). Mental health of refugees and asylum-seekers. *Advances in Psychiatric Treatment*, 8, 240–247, with permission. © The Royal College of Psychiatrists.

louder and use hand gestures more frequently than northern Europeans.

The nurse should also be aware that non-verbal communication has different meanings in various cultures. For example, some people in some cultures welcome touch and consider it supportive, whereas other cultures find touch offensive. Some Asian women avoid shaking hands with one another or with men. Some Native American tribes believe that vigorous handshaking is aggressive, whereas people from Spain and France may consider a firm handshake a sign of strength and good character.

Box 7.4 IMPORTANT FACTORS IN CULTURAL ASSESSMENT

Communication
Physical distance or space
Social organization
Time orientation
Environmental control
Biological variations

From Giger, J. N. & Davidhizar, R. E. (2003). *Transcultural nursing: Assessment and intervention* (4th edn). St. Louis: Mosby.

English men) are notoriously reticent; some older South Asian women can be softly spoken and reluctant to express direct opinions; Mediterranean people may often appear

Box 7.5 SOME ISSUES TO CONSIDER WHEN A LANGUAGE AND CULTURE ARE NOT SHARED

- Spend a few minutes with the interpreter before and after the session to clarify objectives, and review the meeting afterwards
- Try to use the same interpreter for all the meetings with each individual or family; it is important to consider matching on age, gender and religious issues
- Using an interpreter may mean that more time should be allocated for the meeting.
- Avoid specialist terminology
- Use trained and experienced interpreters whenever possible; remember that they are part of the consultation and respect their contribution and different training
- Always remain aware that you are interviewing someone from a different culture, who therefore may put different interpretations on events or feelings
- Health beliefs about many aspects of psychiatry may be different across cultures
- Remember that words may not translate exactly across languages

From Tribe, R. (2002). Mental health of refugees and asylum-seekers. *Advances in Psychiatric Treatment, 8,* 240–247, with permission. © The Royal College of Psychiatrists.

Although Western cultures view direct eye contact as positive, Asian cultures may find it rude, and people from these backgrounds may avoid looking strangers in the eye when talking to them. People from Middle Eastern cultures may maintain very intense eye contact, which may appear to be glaring to those from different cultures. These differences are important to note because many people make inferences about a person's behaviour based on the frequency or duration of eye contact. Chapter 6 provides a detailed discussion of communication techniques.

PHYSICAL DISTANCE OR SPACE

Various cultures have different perspectives on what they consider a comfortable physical distance from another person during communication. In the UK and many other Western cultures, 2 to 3 feet is, for many, a comfortable distance. Latin Americans and people from the Middle East tend to stand closer to one another than do people in Western cultures. People from Asian cultures are usually more comfortable with distances greater than 2 or 3 feet. The nurse should be conscious of these cultural differences in space and should allow enough room for clients to be comfortable (Giger & Davidhizar, 2003).

SOCIAL ORGANIZATION

Social organization refers to family structure and organization, religious values and beliefs, ethnicity and culture, all of which affect a person's role and, therefore, his or her health and illness behaviour. In Western cultures, people may seek the advice of a friend or family member or may make most decisions independently. Many Asian

people strongly value the role of family in making healthcare decisions. People from these backgrounds may delay making decisions until they can consult appropriate family members. Autonomy in health-care decisions may be an unfamiliar and undesirable concept because the cultures consider the collective to be greater than the individual.

TIME ORIENTATION

Time orientation, or whether one views time as precise or approximate, differs among cultures. Many people from Western countries focus on the urgency of time, valuing punctuality and precise schedules. Clients from other cultures may not perceive the importance of adhering to specific follow-up appointments or procedures or time-related treatment regimens. Nurses can become resentful and angry when these clients miss appointments or fail to follow specific treatment regimens, such as taking medications at prescribed times. Nurses should not label such clients as 'non-compliant' or 'difficult to engage' when their behaviour may be related to a different cultural orientation to the meaning of time. When possible, the nurse should be sensitive to the client's time orientation, as with follow-up appointments. When timing is essential, as with some medications, the nurse should explain the importance of more precise timing.

ENVIRONMENTAL CONTROL

Environmental control refers to a client's ability to control the surroundings or to direct factors in the environment (Giger & Davidhizar, 2003). People who believe they have control of their health are more likely to seek care, to change their behaviour and to follow care and treatment recommendations. Those who believe that 'illness' is a result of nature or natural causes (taking a 'personalistic' or 'naturalistic' view) are less likely to seek traditional health care because they do not believe it can help them.

BIOLOGICAL VARIATIONS

Biological variations exist among people from different cultural backgrounds, and research is just beginning to help us understand these variations. For example, we now know that differences related to **ethnicity**/cultural origins cause variations in response to some psychotropic drugs (discussed earlier).

Socioeconomic Status and Social Class

Socioeconomic status refers to one's income, education and occupation. It strongly influences a person's health, including whether or not the person has adequate access to health care or can afford prescribed treatment. People who live in poverty are also at risk for threats to health, such as inadequate housing, lead paint, violence, drug and alcohol misuse or sub-standard schooling.

Social class may have a less overt influence in the UK now than in much of the 20th century: barriers among the social classes are looser and mobility a little more common. Nevertheless, class – still often 'betrayed' by language, accent, attitude and belief and lifestyle – remains a strong determinant of the likelihood of developing both physical and mental health problems and a potential barrier to equitable access to care and treatment. In addition, the wealth gap between rich and poor has actually increased in the past 20 years, and there remains – across the UK – many examples of the persistence of the 'postcode lottery' in health care.

In many other countries, social class may have an even more powerful influence on social relationships and can determine how people relate to one another, even in a health-care setting. For example, the caste system still exists in India, and people from a lower caste may feel unworthy or undeserving of the same level of health care as people in higher castes.

The nurse must determine the degree to which social class is a factor in how clients relate to health-care professionals and the health-care system as a whole – and, of course, how his or her own social class affects his or her attitude to clients.

Nurse's Role when Working with Clients of Various Cultures

It is vital to understand that variations among people from any culture are wide: few fit perfectly a general 'textbook' pattern of behaviour and belief. In addition, there is really no such thing as 'Asian culture' or 'working-class culture', or 'gay culture': ethnicity, nationality, class, age, sexuality, geography, history, politics, gender, religion, sub-culture, genetics and individual and family experiences can all filter, and be filtered by, more generalized 'cultural' beliefs. Individual assessment of each person and family – as well as a genuine desire to try to understand other cultures and their beliefs and practices – is necessary to the provision of culturally competent care.

To provide culturally competent care, then, the nurse must find out as much as possible about a client's cultural values, beliefs and health practices. Often, of course, the client is the best source for that information, so the nurse must ask the client what is important to him or her – for instance, 'How would you like to be cared for?' or 'What do you expect (or want) me to do for you?' (Andrews & Boyle, 2003). Asking questions for strengths and resources – people, practices, places, beliefs – that lie within the person's culture (or sub-culture) is essential.

At an initial meeting, the nurse may have to rely on what he or she knows (if anything) about a client's particular cultural group, such as preferences for greeting, eye contact and physical distance. Based on the client's behaviour, the nurse can alter that approach as needed. For example, if a client from a culture that, as far as the nurse knows, does not usually shake hands offers the nurse his or her hand, the nurse should return the handshake. Variation among members of the same cultural group is wide, and the nurse must remain alert for these individual differences.

A client's health practices and religious beliefs are other important areas to assess. The nurse might ask, 'Do you have any preferences for particular food or is there anything you can't eat?' or 'How can we help you in practising your religious or spiritual beliefs?' The nurse can also gain an understanding of the client's health and illness beliefs by asking, 'How do you think this problem came about?', 'What do your family and friends think about it?' and 'What kinds of treatment have you already tried?'

An open and objective approach to the client is essential. Clients will be more likely to share personal and cultural information if the nurse is genuinely interested in knowing and does not appear sceptical or judgemental; as ever in nursing, a respectful curiosity is vital.

The nurse should ask these same questions even to clients from his or her own cultural background. Again, people in a cultural group vary widely, so the nurse should not assume that he or she knows what a client believes or practises just because the nurse shares the same culture.

SELF-AWARENESS ISSUES

The nurse must be aware of the factors that influence a client's response to stress and ill-health, including individual, interpersonal and cultural factors discussed earlier.

Assessment of these factors can help guide the planning and implementation of nursing care. Biological and hereditary factors cannot, as we saw before, be changed. Others, such as interpersonal factors, *can* be changed but only with difficulty. For instance, helping a client to develop a social support system requires more than simply giving him or her a list of community contacts. The client needs to feel that these resources are valuable to him or her; must perceive them as helpful, responsive and supportive; and must be willing to engage with them and to use them.

Nurses with limited experience in working with various ethnic or other cultural groups may feel anxious when encountering someone from a different cultural background and worry about saying 'the wrong thing' or doing something offensive or disrespectful to the client or family. Nurses may have stereotypical concepts about some cultural groups and be unaware of them until they encounter a client from that group. It is a constant challenge – and an obligation – to remain aware of one's feelings and to handle them effectively.

Training should always be accessed (where provided) and nurses must remain cognizant at all times of cultural contexts; consideration of cultural contexts should be an integral part of a clinical supervision process.

Points to Consider When Working with Individual Responses to Stress and Ill-health

- Approach every client with openness, genuineness and caring.
- Maintain curiosity: never think you know everything!
- Ask the client at the beginning of the interview how he or she prefers to be addressed and ways the nurse can promote any spiritual, religious and health practices.
- Ask clients about their own attitude – and those of their friends and family – to 'mental health' and 'mental illness'.
- Recognize any negative feelings or stereotypes and discuss them with an appropriate colleague or others to dispel myths and misconceptions.
- Remember that a wide variety of factors influence the client's complex response to stress and ill-health.

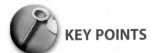 **KEY POINTS**

- Each client is unique, with different biological, psychological and social factors that influence his or her response to stress and ill-health.
- Individual factors that influence a client's response to illness include age, growth and development; biological and genetic factors; hardiness, resilience and resourcefulness; and self-efficacy and spirituality.

Critical Thinking Questions

1. What is the cultural and ethnic background of your family? How does that influence your beliefs about mental health and mental illness?
2. How would you describe yourself in terms of the individual characteristics that affect one's response to illness, such as growth and development, biological factors, self-efficacy, hardiness, resilience and resourcefulness and spirituality?
3. Which of the categories of factors that influence the client's response to illness – individual, interpersonal and cultural – do you think is most influential? Why?

- Biological make-up includes the person's heredity and physical health.
- Younger clients may have difficulty expressing their thoughts and feelings, so they often have poorer outcomes when experiencing stress or illness at an early age.
- People who have difficulty negotiating the tasks of psychosocial development have less effective skills to cope with ill-health.
- There are cultural/ethnic differences in how people respond to certain psychotropic drugs; these differences can affect dosage and side-effects. Nurses must be aware of these cultural differences when treating clients. Clients from non-Western countries generally require lower doses of psychotropic drugs to produce desired effects.
- Self-efficacy is a belief that a person's abilities and efforts can influence the events in her or his life. A person's sense of self-efficacy is an important factor in coping with stress and illness.
- Hardiness is a person's ability to resist illness when under stress.
- Resilience is a person's ability to respond in a healthy manner to stressful circumstances or risky situations.
- Resourcefulness is demonstrated in one's ability to manage daily activities and is a personal characteristic acquired through interactions with others.
- Spirituality involves the inner core of a person's being and his or her beliefs about the meaning of life and the purpose for living. It may or may not include belief in God or a higher power.
- Interpersonal factors that influence the client's response to ill-health include a sense of belonging, or personal involvement in a system or environment, and social networks, which provide social support or emotional sustenance.
- The increasing social and cultural diversity in the UK makes it essential for nurses to be knowledgeable about the health and cultural practices of various ethnic or racial groups. To provide competent nursing care, nurses

must be sensitive to, and knowledgeable about, factors that influence the care of clients, including issues related to culture, race, gender, sexual orientation and social and economic situations.

- Culture often has the most influence on a person's health beliefs and behaviours.
- A model for assessing clients from various ethnic backgrounds includes six cultural phenomena: communication techniques and style, physical distance and space, social organization, time orientation, environmental control and biological variations. The nurse must bear these six phenomena in mind when working with people.
- Socioeconomic status and class have a strong influence on a person's health, in terms of belief and lifestyle and in terms of access to services.
- Knowledge of various cultural patterns and differences helps the nurse begin to relate to persons of different ethnic and cultural backgrounds.
- Nurses who are unsure of a person's social or cultural preferences need to ask the client directly during the initial encounter about preferred terms of address and ways the nurse can help support the client's spiritual, religious or health practices.

REFERENCES

Andrews, M. M. & Boyle, J. S. (2003). *Transcultural concepts in nursing care* (4th edn). Philadelphia: Lippincott Williams & Wilkins.

Baetz, M., Larson, D. B., Marcoux, G., *et al.* (2002). Canadian psychiatric inpatient religious commitment: an association with mental health. *Canadian Journal of Psychiatry, 47*(2), 159–166.

Bandura, A. (2004). Health promotion by social cognitive means. *Health Education and Behaviour, 31*(2), 143–164.

Bhugra, D. & McKenzie, K. (2003). Expressed emotion across cultures. *Advances in Psychiatric Treatment, 9*, 342–348.

Brooks, M. V. (2003). Health-related hardiness and chronic illness: a synthesis of current research. *Nursing Forum, 38*(3), 11–20.

Buchanan, B. W. & Carpenter, W. T. (2005). Concept of schizophrenia. In B. J. Sadock & V. A. Sadock (Eds.), *Comprehensive textbook of psychiatry, Vol. 1* (8th edn, pp. 1329–1345). Philadelphia: Lippincott Williams & Wilkins.

Burnard, P. (2005) .Cultural sensitivity in community nursing. *Journal of Community Care, 19*, 10.

Chanokruthai, C., Williams, R. A., & Hagerty, B. M. (2005). The role of sense of belonging and social support on stress and depression, in individuals with depression. *Archives of Psychiatric Nursing, 19*(1), 18–29.

Cutler, C. G. (2005). Self-efficacy and social adjustment of patients with mood disorder. *Journal of the American Psychiatric Nurses Association, 11*(5), 283–289.

Edward, K. & Warelow, P. (2005). Resilience: when coping is emotionally intelligent. *Journal of the American Psychiatric Nurses Association, 11*(2), 101–102.

Giger, J. N. & Davidhizar, R. E. (2003). *Transcultural nursing: Assessment and intervention* (4th edn). St. Louis: Mosby.

Granerud, A. & Severinsson, E. (2006). The struggle for social integration in the community: the experiences of people with mental health problems. *Journal of Psychiatric and Mental Health Nursing, 13*(3), 288–293.

Greeff, A. P., Vansteenween, A., & Mieke, I. (2006). Resiliency in families with a member with a psychological disorder. *American Journal of Family Therapy, 34*(4), 285–300.

Huguelet, P., Mohr, S., Borras, L., Gillieron, C., & Brandt, P. (2006). Spirituality and religious practices among outpatients with schizophrenia and their clinicians. *Psychiatric Services, 57*(3), 366–372.

Kobasa, S. C. (1979). Stressful life events, personality, and health: an inquiry into hardiness. *Journal of Personality & Social Psychology, 37*(1), 1–11.

Krafcik, K. A. (2002). Predictors of resourcefulness in school aged children. *Issues in Mental Health Nursing, 23*(4), 385–407.

Longo, D. A. & Peterson, S. A. (2002). The role of spirituality in psychosocial rehabilitation. *Psychiatric Rehabilitation Journal, 25*(4), 333–340.

Maddi, S. R. (2005). On hardiness and other pathways to resilience. *American Psychologist, 60*(3), 261–262.

Mental Health Foundation (2005). *Up and Running report.* Available at: http://www.mentalhealth.org.uk/publications/?EntryId5=4

Office for National Statistics (2002). *Minority ethnic groups in the UK.* Available: http://www.statistics.gov.uk/pdfdir/meg1202.pdf

Papadopoulos, I., Tilki, M., & Taylor, S. (2004). Promoting cultural competence in healthcare through a research-based intervention in the UK. *Diversity in Health and Social Care, 1*, 107–115.

Purnell, L. D. & Paulanka, B. J. (Eds.). (2003). *Transcultural healthcare: A culturally competent approach* (2nd edn). Philadelphia: F. A. Davis.

INTERNET RESOURCES

RESOURCES	INTERNET ADDRESS
Black and Minority Ethnic Mental Health (DOH)	http://www.dh.gov.uk/en/Healthcare/NationalService-Frameworks /Mentalhealth/BMEmentalhealth/index.htm
Black Mental Health UK	http://blackmentalhealth.org.uk/
Culture Med™ (extensive bibliography of transcultural nursing articles)	http://www.sunyit.edu/library/html/culturemed/bib/
Health for Asylum Seekers and Refugees Portal	http://www.harpweb.org.uk/
National BME Mental Health Network	http://www.bmementalhealth.org.uk/
Research Centre for Transcultural Studies in Health	http://www.mdx.ac.uk/www/rctsh/

Reid, J., Lloyd, C., & de Groot, L. (2005). The psychoeducation needs of parents who have an adult son or daughter with a mental illness. *Australian e-Journal for the Advancement of Mental Health, 4*(2), 1–13.

Ross, N. (2002). Community belonging and health. *Health Reports, 13*(3), 33–40.

Sageman, S. (2004). Breaking through the despair: spiritually oriented group therapy as a means of healing women with severe mental illness. *Journal of the American Academy of Psychoanalysis and Dynamic Psychiatry, 32*(1), 125–141.

Tribe, R. (2002). Mental health of refugees and asylum-seekers. *Advances in Psychiatric Treatment, 8,* 240–247.

Vanderhorst, R. K. & McLaren, S. (2005). Social relationships as predictors of depression and suicidal ideation in older adults. *Aging and Mental Health, 9*(6), 517–525.

ADDITIONAL READING

Campinha-Bacote, J. (2002). The process of cultural competence in the delivery of health care services: a model of care. *Journal of Transcultural Nursing, 13*(3), 181–184.

Chady, S. (2001). The NSF for mental health from a transcultural perspective. *British Journal of Nursing, 10*(15), 830–835.

Chin, P. (2005). Chinese. In J. G. Lipson & S. L. Dibble (Eds.), *Culture and clinical care* (pp. 98–108). San Francisco: UCSF Nursing Press.

Coles, R. (Ed.) (2001). *The Erik Erikson reader*. London: Norton.

Leighton, K. (2005). Transcultural nursing: the relationship between individualist ideology and individualized mental health care. *Journal of Psychiatric & Mental Health Nursing, 12*(1), 85–94.

Maslow, A. (1954). *Motivation and personality*. New York: Harper.

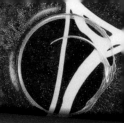

Chapter Study Guide

MULTIPLE-CHOICE QUESTIONS

Select the best answer for each of the following questions.

1. Which of the following is important for nurses to remember when administering psychotropic drugs to people from a non-white background?
   a. Lower doses may be used to produce desired effects.
   b. Fewer side-effects occur with non-white clients.
   c. Response to the drug is similar to that in whites.
   d. No generalization can be made.

2. Which of the following states the 'naturalistic' view of what causes ill-health?
   a. Illness is a natural part of life and therefore unavoidable.
   b. Illness is caused by cold, heat, wind and dampness.
   c. Only natural agents are effective in treating illness.
   d. Outside agents, such as evil spirits, upset the body's natural balance.

3. Which of the following is most influential in determining health beliefs and practices?
   a. Cultural factors
   b. Individual factors
   c. Interpersonal factors
   d. All the above are equally influential

4. Which of the following assessments most indicates positive growth and development for a 30-year-old adult?
   a. Is dissatisfied with body image
   b. Enjoys social activities with three or four close friends
   c. Frequently changes jobs to 'find the right one'
   d. Plans to move from parental home in near future

5. Which of the following statements would cause concern for the achievement of developmental tasks of a 55-year-old woman?
   a. 'I feel like I'm taking care of my parents now.'
   b. 'I really enjoy just sitting around visiting friends.'
   c. 'My children need me now just as much as when they were small.'
   d. 'When I retire, I want a smaller house to take care of.'

6. Which of the following client statements would most indicate self-efficacy?
   a. 'I like to get several opinions before deciding a course of action.'
   b. 'I know if I can learn to relax, I will feel better.'
   c. 'I'm never sure if I'm making the right decision.'
   d. 'No matter how hard I try to relax, something always comes up.'

FILL-IN-THE-BLANK QUESTIONS

Identify the developmental task that corresponds to the following age groups, according to Erik Erikson.

_____ Infant

_____ School age

_____ Adolescence

_____ Young adult

_____ Maturity

GROUP DISCUSSION TOPICS

1. Try to come to an agreement about what culturally competent nursing care consists of.

2. What might be the result of achieving or failing to achieve a psychosocial developmental task, according to Erik Erikson?

3. What is the essential difference between hardiness and resilience? How 'hardy' and 'resilient' do the members of the group feel they are?

Assessment Approaches

Key Terms

- abstract thinking
- affect
- automatisms
- blunted affect
- broad affect
- circumstantial thinking
- collaboration
- concrete thinking
- delusion
- flat affect
- flight of ideas
- hallucinations
- ideas of reference
- inappropriate affect
- insight
- judgement
- labile
- loose associations
- mood
- neologisms
- obliged to warn
- psychomotor retardation
- restricted affect
- self-concept
- tangential thinking
- thought blocking

- thought broadcasting
- thought content
- thought insertion
- thought process

- thought withdrawal
- waxy flexibility
- word salad

Learning Objectives

After reading this chapter, you should be able to:

1. Outline the principles underpinning effective collaborative assessment.

2. Identify categories that can be used to assess the client's mental health status in an initial psychosocial assessment.

3. Formulate questions and conversational styles to establish rapport and exchange meaningful information in each category.

4. Describe the client's functioning in terms of self-concept, roles and relationships.

5. Recognize key physiological functions that may be impaired in people with mental disorders.

6. Link psychosocial assessment data to formulation and care planning stages of the nursing process.

7. Examine one's own feelings and any discomfort discussing suicide, homicide or self-harm behaviours with a client.

For the purposes of this book, we are suggesting a flexible nursing process that encompasses four overlapping, cyclical stages: assessment/formulation, planning, intervention and evaluation.

'Assessment' is, traditionally, the first step of the 'nursing process' (the others, in the UK, being planning, intervention and evaluation). It involves rapport-building and engagement, information exchange and the analysis of that information in order to develop a plan of care that meets a clients' needs. In mental health nursing, the process will usually include some form of 'risk assessment' that is either integrated into, or additional to, the rest of the process. Assessment is, in practice, often – though not always – based on an existing model of nursing and should have structured documentation intended to aid the process and to ensure that key areas are not missed.

The first purpose of assessment is to *engage* with someone, establish rapport, to help reduce someone's anxiety, to offer reassurance, information and explanation. The second purpose is to ascertain past '*history*' – both long- and short-term – with a view to informing the client's present care and to identifying strengths, resources and perceived deficits. The third purpose of assessment is to construct a comprehensive picture of the client's *current* emotional state and cognitive and behavioural functioning that can act as a baseline to evaluate the effectiveness of treatment and interventions or a measure of the client's progress. The fourth purpose of a good assessment is to develop a tentative *formulation* that will inform a plan for future care.

Several key issues need to be borne in mind when considering the processes of 'assessment' in modern mental health nursing:

1. Assessment is never a completely separate process to care and treatment.
2. Assessment can be therapeutic – or counter-therapeutic – in itself.
3. Assessment is 'done with', not 'done to', someone.
4. Assessment is not merely the completion of documentation.
5. Assessment is about the *exchange* of information; it is not a one-way process.
6. Assessment is a transparent, open, interactive process, a key part of which involves two or more people having purposeful conversations.
7. Assessment is both a 'formal' and an informal process.
8. Assessment should not be purely deficit- or symptom-driven; it should be a process whereby a rich, complex narrative is developed.
9. Assessment is collaborative, tentative, ongoing and ever-changing; it is neither 'scientific' nor fixed.
10. Assessment must interact primarily with the views and assessments of the client themselves, with other professionals and with those of carers, friends and family as appropriate.

FACTORS INFLUENCING ASSESSMENT

Client Participation/Feedback

A thorough assessment requires active client participation. If the client is unable or unwilling to participate, some areas of the assessment will be incomplete or vague. For example, the person who is extremely depressed may not have the energy to answer questions or complete the assessment. People exhibiting psychotic thought processes or impaired cognition may have an insufficient attention span or may be unable to comprehend the questions being asked. The nurse may need to have several contacts with such clients to complete the assessment or gather further information as his or her condition permits.

Client's Health Status

The client's health status can, obviously, also affect a specific assessment. If the person is anxious, tired or in pain, the nurse may have difficulty eliciting the client's full participation in the assessment. The information that the nurse obtains – and provides – may reflect the client's pain or anxiety rather than an accurate assessment of the client's situation. The nurse needs to recognize these situations and deal with them before continuing the full assessment. The client may need to rest, receive medication to alleviate pain or become calmer before the assessment can continue.

Client's Previous Experiences/ Misconceptions About Health Care

The client's perception of his or her circumstances can elicit emotions that interfere with developing an accurate assessment. If the client is reluctant to seek treatment or has had previous unsatisfactory experiences with the health-care system, he or she may have difficulty answering questions directly. The client may minimize or maximize symptoms or problems, or may refuse to provide information in some areas. The nurse must address the client's feelings and perceptions to establish a trusting working relationship before proceeding with the assessment.

Client's Ability to Understand

The nurse must also determine the client's ability to hear, read and understand the language being used in the assessment process. If the client's primary language differs from that of the nurse, the client may misunderstand or misinterpret what the nurse is saying, which results in inaccurate information being exchanged. A client with impaired hearing may also fail to understand what the nurse is asking. Many clients find it impossible to understand jargon such as 'suicidal ideation' or 'hallucinosis' or 'the CPA'; most don't think in terms of 'risk'. It is important that the information in the assessment reflects the client's health status: it should not be a result of poor communication skills on the part of the nurse.

Nurse's Attitude and Approach

The nurse's attitude and approach can influence the assessment. If the client perceives the nurse's questions to be short and curt, or feels rushed or pressured to complete a particular assessment, he or she may provide only superficial information or omit discussing problems in some areas altogether. The client may also refrain from offering sensitive information if he or she perceives the nurse as non-accepting, defensive or judgemental. For example, a client may be reluctant to relate instances of child abuse or domestic violence if the nurse seems uncomfortable or non-accepting. The nurse must be aware of his or her own feelings and responses and approach the assessment matter-of-factly.

TYPES OF ASSESSMENT

As mentioned before, assessment is an ongoing, tentative and transparent process. It may consist of one or more purposeful 'formal' assessments, undertaken with the support of documentation which has been developed for that purpose by the service, and during which the nurse engages collaboratively and therapeutically in the process, exchanges 'information' with the client and works with him or her to develop an agreed plan of care. One such formal assessment may be undertaken when, for example, someone is first admitted to an inpatient unit or is seen for the first time at a health centre or in the person's own home. We will concentrate here on this initial 'psychosocial assessment' but the principles are relevant to all types of assessment.

Conducting an Initial Psychosocial Assessment Interview

According to Barker (2003, p. 61), the 'key assessment questions' are:

- What is the person's problem?
- To what extent does it distress the person?
- To what extent does it interfere, in what way, with everyday living?
- To what extent is the person able to exercise any kind of control over the problem?

These seemingly straightforward questions entail a great deal of skill and interpersonal capability to answer; they also require a conversational, respectful and focused approach.

ASSESSMENT PHASE 1: RAPPORT/ ENGAGEMENT

Establishing as much rapport and trust as early as possible in an assessment interview, and maintaining it, is vital.

The first aspect of establishing engagement and trust involves a conscious use of the environment. The nurse should conduct an assessment interview in an environment that is comfortable, private and safe for both the client and the nurse. A room that is fairly quiet with few distractions allows the client to give his or her full attention to the interview, though obviously this may prove more problematic in someone's own home. In an inpatient setting, conducting the interview in a place such as a conference room ensures the client that no one will overhear what is being discussed. Seating needs to be well placed – with chairs neither too close nor too far from each other. Tea, coffee or cold drinks should be offered.

The nurse should not choose an isolated location for the interview, particularly if the client is unknown to the nurse or has a history of any threatening behaviour. The nurse must ensure the safety of self and client even if that means another person is present during the assessment: this may be particularly important in a community setting.

The second aspect of engagement is the conscious and deliberate use of the nurse's own interpersonal skills. The most useful assessment interviews are conversational and interactive, and frequently start with 'problem-free talk' – talking about areas of the person's life that may not be directly connected with problems, such as – in an inpatient setting – how the person got here, or – in a community setting – paintings on the wall or books or CDs that may be visible. 'Problem-free talk' helps engagement, emphasizes to the client (and to the nurse) that the client lives a rich, complex life that is not just defined by mental health problems, *and* begins an exploration of aspects of someone's life – strengths and resources – that may offer clues towards ways to find solutions.

Alongside these initial engagement processes, agreement about the purpose of the interview should be established, the time available ascertained and issues of confidentiality made clear. Any documentation to be used by the nurse should be shown and explained to the client.

ASSESSMENT PHASE 2: INFORMATION EXCHANGE

The nurse must offer an opportunity for someone to express any fears they may have and to ask any questions they may want. It must be emphasized that this is a collaborative process.

The nurse may use open-ended questions to start the assessment process (see Chapter 6). Doing so allows the client to begin as he or she feels comfortable, and also gives the nurse an idea about the client's perception of his or her situation. Examples of open-ended questions are:

- What brings you here today?
- Tell me what's been happening to you?
- Why do you think your GP referred you?
- How do you think I can help you?

If the client cannot organize his or her thoughts, or has difficulty answering open-ended questions, the nurse may need to use more direct questions to obtain information. Questions need to be clear, simple and focused on one specific area of someone's life; they should not cause the client to remember several things at once. Questions regarding several different behaviours – 'How are your eating and sleeping habits and have you been taking any over-the-counter medications that affect your eating and sleeping?' – can be confusing to the client. The following are examples of focused or closed-ended questions:

- How many hours did you sleep last night?
- Have you been thinking about suicide?
- How much alcohol have you been drinking?
- How well have you been sleeping?
- How many meals a day do you eat?
- What over-the-counter medications are you taking?

The nurse should use a non-judgemental tone and language, particularly when asking about sensitive information such as drug or alcohol use, sexual behaviour, abuse or violence or childrearing practices. Using non-judgemental language and a matter-of-fact tone avoids giving the client verbal cues to become defensive or to not tell the truth. For example, when asking a client about his or her parenting role, the nurse might ask, 'What types of discipline do you use?' rather than, 'How often do you hit your child?' The first question is more likely to elicit honest and accurate information; the second question gives the impression that physical discipline is wrong, and it may cause the client to respond dishonestly.

If family members, friends or other carers are with the client, the nurse should, if possible, obtain their perceptions of the client's behaviour and emotional state. How this is accomplished depends on the situation. Sometimes the client may not give permission for the nurse to conduct separate interviews with family members. The nurse should be aware that friends or family may not feel comfortable talking about the client in his or her presence and may provide limited information. Or the client may not feel comfortable participating in the assessment without family or friends and this, too, may limit the amount or type of information the nurse obtains. It is always desirable to conduct at least part of the assessment without others, especially in cases of suspected abuse or intimidation. The nurse should make every effort to assess the client in privacy in cases of suspected abuse.

CONTENT OF THE ASSESSMENT

The information gathered in a psychosocial assessment can be organized in many different ways. Most assessment tools or conceptual frameworks contain similar categories with some variety in arrangement or order. The nurse should use some kind of organizing framework so that he or she can assess the client in a thorough and systematic way that lends itself to analysis and serves as a basis for the client's care. It must be remembered that sensitivity needs to inform the whole process: some areas of questioning can be seen as patronizing or irrelevant, and the individual client's situation may well need to take precedence over any mechanized completion of documentation.

The framework for psychosocial assessment discussed here and used throughout this book contains the following components:

- History
- General appearance and motor behaviour
- Mood and affect
- Thought process and content
- Sensory and intellectual processes
- Judgement and insight
- Self-concept
- Roles and relationships
- Physiological and self-care concerns.

Box 8.1 lists the factors the nurse should include in each of these areas of the psychosocial assessment.

Goal-setting

The initial part of the information-exchange phase of a thorough psychosocial assessment – indeed one that runs from beginning to end of any assessment – is that of helping a client identify his or her goals. Not only does this help clarify for both nurse and client where he or she wants to get to, it also offers both client and nurse valuable information about where things are now. Example questions that can be used are:

- How will you know you're no longer 'depressed'?
- How will your wife know things are OK now?
- What will you be doing differently when you're not feeling anxious?
- What will tell you that you've taken the very first step to getting better?
- How will you know you don't need to be in hospital any longer?
- What would a video of 'a good day' look like?

These questions can be incorporated into the assessment process at any point.

History

Background assessments include the client's history, age and developmental stage, cultural and spiritual beliefs, and beliefs about health and illness. The history of the client, as well as his or her family, may provide some insight into the client's current situation. For example, has the client experienced similar difficulties in the past? How did they cope then? Has the client been admitted to the hospital, and, if so, what was that experience like? A family history that is positive for alcoholism, bipolar disorder or suicide is significant because it increases the client's risk for these problems.

Box 8.1 PSYCHOSOCIAL ASSESSMENT COMPONENTS

Goal-setting
  What the person wants
  What others want
History
  Age
  Developmental stage
  Cultural considerations
  Spiritual beliefs
  Previous history
General assessment and motor behaviour
  Hygiene and grooming
  Appropriate dress
  Posture
  Eye contact
  Unusual movements or mannerisms
  Speech
Mood and affect
  Expressed emotions
  Facial expressions
Thought process and content
  Content (what client is thinking)
  Process (how client is thinking)
  Clarity of ideas
  Self-harm or suicidal thoughts, feelings or urges
Sensory and intellectual processes
  Orientation

Confusion
Memory
Abnormal sensory experiences or misperceptions
Concentration
Abstract thinking abilities
Judgement and insight
  Judgement (interpretation of environment)
  Decision-making ability
  Insight (understanding one's own part in current situation)
Self-concept
  Personal view of self
  Description of physical self
  Personal qualities or attributes
Roles and relationships
  Current roles
  Satisfaction with roles
  Success at roles
  Significant relationships
  Support systems
Physiological and self-care considerations
  Eating habits
  Sleep patterns
  Health problems
  Compliance with prescribed medications
  Ability to perform activities of daily living

The client's chronological age and developmental stage are important factors in the psychosocial assessment. The nurse evaluates the client's age and developmental level for congruence with expected norms. For example, a client may be struggling with personal identity and attempting to achieve independence from his or her parents. If the client is 17 years old, these struggles are normal and anticipated because these are two of the primary developmental tasks for the adolescent. If the client is 35 years old and still struggling with these issues of self-identity and independence, the nurse may need to explore the situation further. The client's age and developmental level may also be incongruent with expected norms if the client has a developmental delay or learning disability.

The nurse must be sensitive to the client's cultural and spiritual beliefs to avoid making inaccurate assumptions about his or her psychosocial functioning (Schultz & Videbeck, 2005). Many cultures have beliefs and values about a person's role in society or acceptable social or personal behaviour that may differ from those of the nurse. Western cultures generally expect that as a person reaches adulthood, he or she becomes financially independent, leaves home and makes his or her own life decisions. In contrast, in parts of some cultures, three generations may live in one household, and elders of the family make major life decisions for all. Another example is the assessment of eye contact. Western cultures consider good eye contact to be a positive characteristic indicating self-esteem and paying attention. People from other cultures, such as India or Pakistan, might consider such eye contact to be a sign of disrespect.

As has been mentioned before, the nurse must not stereotype clients. Just because a person's physical characteristics seem to the nurse to be consistent with a particular ethnic group, he or she may not have the attitudes, beliefs and behaviours stereotypically attributed to that group. For example, many people of Asian ancestry have beliefs and values that are more consistent with 'Western' beliefs and values than with those typically associated with Asian countries. To avoid making inaccurate assumptions, the nurse must ask clients about the beliefs or health practices that are important to them, or how they view themselves in the context of society or relationships (see Nurse's Role when Working with Clients of Various Cultures, in Chapter 7).

The nurse must also consider the client's beliefs about health and illness when assessing the client's psychosocial

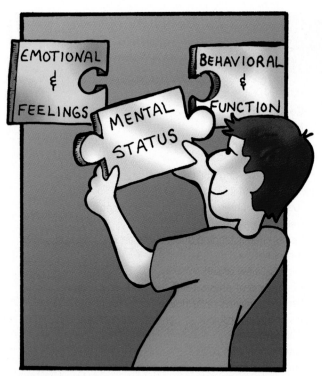

Building a picture of your client through psychosocial assessment

functioning. Some people view emotional or mental health problems as family concerns to be handled only among family members. They may view seeking outside or professional help as a sign of individual weakness. Others may believe that their problems can be solved only with the right medication, and they will not accept other forms of therapy. Another common problem is the misconception that one should take medication only when feeling sick. Many mental disorders, like some medical conditions, may require clients to take medications on a long-term basis, perhaps even for a lifetime.

General Appearance and Motor Behaviour

The nurse assesses the client's overall appearance, including dress, hygiene and grooming. Does the client seem to be appropriately dressed for his or her age and the weather? Is the client unkempt or dishevelled? Does the client appear to be his or her stated age? The nurse also observes the client's posture, eye contact, facial expression and any unusual tics or tremors. He or she documents observations and examples of behaviours to avoid excessive subjectivity or misinterpretation. Specific terms used in making assessments of general appearance and motor behaviour include the following:

- **Automatisms:** repeated purposeless behaviours often indicative of anxiety, such as drumming fingers, twisting locks of hair or tapping the foot
- **Psychomotor retardation:** overall slowed movements
- **Waxy flexibility:** maintenance of posture or position over time even when it is awkward or uncomfortable.

The nurse assesses the client's speech for quantity, quality and any abnormalities. Does the client talk non-stop? Does the client perseverate (seem to be stuck on one topic and unable to move to another idea)? Are responses a minimal 'yes' or 'no' without elaboration? Is the content of the client's speech relevant to the question being asked? Is the rate of speech fast or slow? Is the tone audible or loud? Does the client speak in a rhyming manner? Does the client use **neologisms** (invented words that have meaning only for the client)? The nurse notes any speech difficulties such as stuttering or lisping and discusses them, if appropriate, with the person.

Mood and Affect

Mood refers to the client's pervasive and enduring emotional state. **Affect** is the outward expression of the client's emotional state. The client may make statements about feelings, such as 'I'm depressed' or 'I'm high', or the nurse may infer the client's mood from data such as posture, gestures, tone of voice and facial expression. The nurse also assesses for consistency among the client's mood, affect and situation. For instance, the client may have an angry facial expression but deny feeling angry or upset in any way. Or the client may be talking about the recent loss of a family member while laughing and smiling. The nurse must note such inconsistencies and – wherever appropriate – check them out with the person.

Common terms used in assessing affect include the following:

- **Blunted affect:** showing little, or a slow-to-respond, facial expression
- **Broad affect:** displaying a full range of emotional expressions
- **Flat affect:** showing no facial expression
- **Inappropriate affect:** displaying a facial expression that is incongruent with mood or situation; often silly or giddy regardless of circumstances
- **Restricted affect:** displaying one type of expression, usually serious or somber.

The client's mood may be described as happy, sad, depressed, euphoric, anxious or angry. When the client exhibits unpredictable and rapid mood swings from depressed and crying to euphoria with no apparent stimuli, the mood is called **labile** (rapidly changing).

The nurse may find it helpful to ask the client to estimate the intensity of his or her mood. The nurse can do so by asking the client to rate his or her mood on a scale of 0 to 10. For example, if the client reports being depressed, the nurse might ask, 'On a scale of 0 to 10, with 0 being least depressed and 10 being most depressed, where would you place yourself right now?'

Thought Process and Content

Thought process refers to how the client thinks. The nurse can infer a client's thought processes from speech and speech patterns. **Thought content** is what the client actually says, or rather can be inferred from what the client says. The nurse assesses whether or not the client's verbalizations seem to make sense; that is, if ideas are related and flow logically from one to the next. The nurse also must determine whether the client seems preoccupied, as if talking or paying attention to someone or something else. When the nurse encounters clients with marked difficulties in thought process and content, he or she may find it helpful to ask focused questions requiring short answers. Common terms related to the assessment of thought process and content include the following (American Psychiatric Association, 2000):

- **Circumstantial thinking:** a client eventually answers a question but only after giving excessive unnecessary detail
- **Delusion:** a fixed false belief not apparently based in reality
- **Flight of ideas:** excessive amount and rate of speech composed of fragmented or unrelated ideas
- **Ideas of reference:** client's inaccurate interpretation that general events are personally directed to him or her, such as hearing a speech on the news and believing the message had personal meaning
- **Loose associations:** disorganized thinking that jumps from one idea to another with little or no evident relation between the thoughts
- **Tangential thinking:** wandering off the topic and never providing the information requested
- **Thought blocking:** stopping abruptly in the middle of a sentence or train of thought; sometimes unable to continue the idea
- **Thought broadcasting:** a delusional belief that others can hear or know what the client is thinking
- **Thought insertion:** a delusional belief that others are putting ideas or thoughts into the client's head – that is, the ideas are not those of the client
- **Thought withdrawal:** a delusional belief that others are taking the client's thoughts away and the client is powerless to stop it
- **Word salad:** flow of unconnected words that convey no meaning to the listener.

ASSESSMENT OF SUICIDE OR HARM TOWARD OTHERS

The nurse must determine whether the depressed or hopeless client has suicidal ideation or a clear, potentially lethal plan. The nurse does so by asking the client directly 'Do you have thoughts of suicide?' or 'What thoughts of suicide have you had?' Box 8.2 lists assessment questions the nurse should ask any client who has suicidal ideas.

Likewise, if the client is angry, hostile or making threatening remarks about a family member, spouse or anyone else, the nurse must ask if the client has thoughts or plans about hurting that person. The nurse does so by questioning the client directly:

- What thoughts have you had about hurting [person's name]?
- What is your plan?
- What do you want to do to [person's name]?

Box 8.2   SUICIDE ASSESSMENT QUESTIONS

Ideation: 'Are you thinking about killing yourself?'
Plan: 'Do you have a plan to kill yourself?'
Method: 'How do you plan to kill yourself?'
Access: 'How would you carry out this plan? Do you have access to the means to carry out the plan?'
Where: 'Where would you kill yourself?'
When: 'When do you plan to kill yourself?'
Timing: 'What day or time of day do you plan to kill yourself?'

When a client makes specific threats or has a plan to harm another person, the team is legally **obliged to warn** the person who is the target of the threats or plan. This is one situation in which the nurse must breach a client's confidentiality to protect the threatened person.

Sensory and Intellectual Processes

ORIENTATION

Orientation refers to the client's recognition of person, place, and time – that is, knowing who and where he or she is and the correct day, date and year. Occasionally, a fourth sphere situation is added (whether or not the client accurately perceives his or her current circumstances). Absence of correct information about person, place and time is referred to as disorientation. The order of person, place and time is significant. When a person is disoriented, he or she frequently first loses track of time, then place and finally person. Orientation may return in the reverse order: first, the person knows who he or she is, then realizes place and finally time.

Disorientation is not synonymous with confusion. A confused person cannot make sense of his or her surroundings or figure things out even though he or she may be fully oriented.

MEMORY

The nurse directly assesses memory, both recent and longer-term, by asking questions with verifiable answers. For example, if the nurse asks, 'Do you have any memory problems?' the client may inaccurately respond 'no', and the nurse cannot verify that. Similarly, if the nurse asks 'What did you do yesterday?' the nurse may be unable to verify the accuracy of the client's responses. Hence, questions to assess memory, where this may seem to be a possible problem area, may include the following:

- What is the name of the Prime Minister?
- Who was the Prime Minister before that?

- What road do you live in?
- What's your phone number?

ABILITY TO CONCENTRATE

If it appears to be necessary, the nurse may assess the client's ability to concentrate by asking the client to perform certain tasks, such as:

- Spell the word *world* backward.
- Begin with the number 100, subtract 7, subtract 7 again, and so on. This is called 'serial sevens'.
- Repeat the days of the week backward.
- Perform a three-part task, such as 'Take a piece of paper in your right hand, fold it in half, and put it on the floor' (the nurse should give all the instructions at one time).

ABSTRACT THINKING AND INTELLECTUAL ABILITIES

When assessing intellectual functioning, the nurse must consider the client's level of formal education. Lack of formal education could hinder performance in many tasks in this section.

The nurse assesses the client's ability to use ***abstract thinking***, which is to make associations or interpretations about a situation or comment. The nurse can usually do so by asking the client to interpret a common proverb such as 'a stitch in time saves nine'. If the client can explain the proverb correctly, his or her abstract thinking abilities may well be intact. If the client provides a literal explanation of the proverb and cannot interpret its meaning, abstract thinking abilities may be lacking. When the client continually gives literal translations, this is evidence of ***concrete thinking***. For instance,

- *Proverb:* A stitch in time saves nine.
    Abstract meaning: If you take the time to fix something now, you'll avoid bigger problems in the future.
    Literal translation: Don't forget to sew up holes in your clothes (concrete thinking).
- *Proverb:* People who live in glass houses shouldn't throw stones.
    Abstract meaning: Don't criticize others for things you may also be guilty of doing.
    Literal translation: If you throw a stone at a glass house, the glass will break (concrete thinking).

The nurse also may assess the client's intellectual functioning by asking him or her to identify the similarities between pairs of objects; for example, 'What is similar about an apple and an orange?' or 'What do the newspaper and the television have in common?'

Sensory-Perceptual Alterations

Some clients experience **hallucinations** (false sensory perceptions or perceptual experiences that do not really exist). Hallucinations can involve the five senses and bodily sensations.

Auditory hallucinations (hearing voices) are the most common; visual hallucinations (seeing things that don't really exist) are the second most common. Initially, clients perceive hallucinations as real experiences, but, later on, they may recognize them as hallucinations.

Judgement and Insight

Judgement refers to the ability to interpret one's environment and situation correctly and to adapt one's behaviour and decisions accordingly. Problems with judgement may be evidenced as the client describes recent behaviour and activities that reflect a lack of reasonable care for self or others. For example, the client may spend large sums of money on frivolous items when he or she cannot afford basic necessities such as food or clothing. Risky behaviours such as picking up strangers in bars or engaging in unprotected sexual activity also may indicate poor judgement. The nurse also may assess a client's judgement by asking the client hypothetical questions, such as 'If you found a stamped addressed envelope on the ground, what would you do?'

Insight is the ability to understand the true nature of one's situation and accept some personal responsibility for that situation. The nurse frequently can infer insight from the client's ability to describe realistically the strengths and weaknesses of his or her behaviour. An example of poor insight would be a client who places all blame on others for his own behaviour, saying 'It's my wife's fault that I drink and get into fights, because she nags me all the time.' This client is not accepting responsibility for his drinking and fighting. Another example of poor insight would be the client who expects all problems to be solved with little or no personal effort: 'The problem is my medication. As soon as the doctor gets the medication right, I'll be just fine.' 'Insight' can, of course, be subjective and the nurse needs to be wary of dismissing someone who disagrees with her or other professionals as having 'lack of insight'. It is always important to see 'insight' as relative and interpersonal (and to remember none of us has complete 'insight'!)

Self-concept

Self-concept is the way one views oneself in terms of personal worth and dignity. To assess a client's self-concept, the nurse can ask the client to describe himself or herself and what characteristics he or she likes and what he or she would change. The client's description of self in terms of physical characteristics gives the nurse information about the client's body image, which is also part of self-concept.

Also included in an assessment of self-concept are the emotions that the client frequently experiences, such as sadness or anger, and whether or not the client is comfortable with those emotions. The nurse also must assess the client's

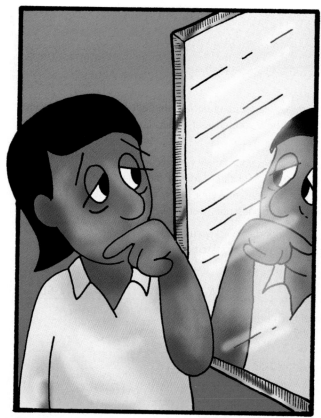

Self-concept

coping strategies. He or she can do so by asking, 'What do you do when you have a problem? How do you solve it? What usually works to deal with anger or disappointment?'

Roles and Relationships

People function in their community through various roles, such as mother, wife, son, daughter, teacher, secretary or volunteer. The nurse assesses the roles the client occupies, client satisfaction with those roles, and whether the client believes he or she is fulfilling the roles adequately (Hanna & Roy, 2001). The number and type of roles may vary, but they usually include family, occupation and hobbies or activities. Family roles include son or daughter, sibling, parent, child and spouse or partner. Occupation roles can be related to a career, school or both. The ability to fulfil a role, or the lack of a desired role, is often central to the client's psychosocial functioning. Changes in roles may also be part of the client's difficulty.

Relationships with other people are essential to one's social and emotional health. Relationships vary, of course, in terms of significance, level of intimacy or closeness and intensity. The inability to sustain satisfying relationships can result from mental health problems or can contribute to the worsening of some problems. The nurse must assess the relationships in the client's life, the client's satisfaction with those relationships or any loss of relationships. Common questions include the following:

- Do you feel close to your family?
- Do you have or want a relationship with one particular, significant person?
- Do your relationships give you enough companionship or intimacy?
- Do you feel your relationships satisfy you sexually?
- Do you have any/many close friends?
- Have you been involved in any abusive relationships?

If the client's family relationships seem to be a significant source of stress, or if the client is closely involved with his or her family, a more in-depth assessment of this area may be useful. Box 8.3 is the McMaster Family Assessment Device, an example of such an in-depth family assessment.

Physiological and Self-care Considerations

When doing a psychosocial assessment, the nurse must include physiological functioning. Although a full physical health assessment may not be indicated, emotional problems often affect some areas of physiological function. Emotional problems can greatly affect eating and sleeping patterns: under stress, people may eat excessively or not at all and may sleep up to 20 hours a day or be unable to sleep more than 2 or 3 hours a night. Clients with bipolar disorder may not eat or sleep for days. Clients with major depression may not be able to get out of bed. Therefore, the nurse *must* assess the client's usual patterns of eating and sleeping and then determine how those patterns have changed.

The nurse also asks the client if he or she has any major or chronic health problems and if he or she takes prescribed medications as ordered and follows dietary recommendations. The nurse also explores the client's use of alcohol and over-the-counter or illicit drugs. Such questions require non-judgemental phrasing and tone; the nurse must reassure the client that truthful information is crucial in determining the client's plan of care.

Non-concordance with prescribed medications is an important area. If the client has stopped taking medication or is taking medication other than as prescribed, the nurse must help the client feel comfortable enough to reveal this information. The nurse should explore with the client any barriers to taking the medication. Is the client choosing non-concordance because of undesirable side-effects? Has the medication failed to produce the desired results? Does the client have difficulty obtaining the medication? Does the client feel the medication might be too expensive?

Short Assessments and Risk Assessments

Many local services have developed their own 'short' screening and assessment tools, many of them multidisciplinary rather than specific to nursing. More generic ones include the Camberwell Assessment of Need Short Appraisal Schedule (CANSAS) (Royal College of Psychiatrists, 1999).

Box 8.3   McMASTER FAMILY ASSESSMENT DEVICE

Instructions: The following are a number of statements about families. Please read each statement carefully, and decide how well it describes your own family. You should answer according to how you see your family. For each statement, there are four possible responses:

Strongly Agree (SA)   Check SA if you believe the statement describes your family very accurately.
Agree (A)   Check A if you believe the statement describes your family for the most part.
Disagree (D)   Check D if you believe the statement does not describe your family for the most part.
Strongly Disagree (SD)   Check SD if you believe the statement does not describe your family at all.

Try not to spend too much time thinking about each statement, but respond as quickly and honestly as you can. If you have trouble with one, answer with your first reaction. Please be sure to answer every statement, and mark all your answers in the space provided next to each statement.

Statements	SA	A	D	SD
1. Planning family activities is difficult because we misunderstand each other.	____	____	____	____
2. We resolve most everyday problems around the house.	____	____	____	____
3. When someone is upset the others know why.	____	____	____	____
4. When you ask someone to do something, you have to check that they did it.	____	____	____	____
5. If someone is in trouble, the others become too involved.	____	____	____	____
6. In times of crisis we can turn to each other for support.	____	____	____	____
7. We don't know what to do when an emergency comes up.	____	____	____	____
8. We sometimes run out of things that we need.	____	____	____	____
9. We are reluctant to show our affection to each other.	____	____	____	____
10. We make sure members meet their family responsibilities.	____	____	____	____
11. We cannot talk to each other about the sadness we feel.	____	____	____	____
12. We usually act on our decisions regarding problems.	____	____	____	____
13. You only get the interest of others when something is important to them.	____	____	____	____
14. You can't tell how a person is feeling from what they are saying.	____	____	____	____
15. Family tasks don't get spread around enough.	____	____	____	____
16. Individuals are accepted for what they are.	____	____	____	____
17. You can easily get away with breaking the rules.	____	____	____	____
18. People come right out and say things instead of hinting at them.	____	____	____	____
19. Some of us just don't respond emotionally.	____	____	____	____
20. We know what to do in an emergency.	____	____	____	____
21. We avoid discussing our fears and concerns.	____	____	____	____
22. It is difficult to talk to each other about tender feelings.	____	____	____	____
23. We have trouble meeting our bills.	____	____	____	____
24. After our family tries to solve a problem, we usually discuss whether it worked or not.	____	____	____	____
25. We are too self-centred.	____	____	____	____
26. We can express our feelings to each other.	____	____	____	____
27. We have no clear expectations about toilet habits.	____	____	____	____
28. We do not show our love for each other.	____	____	____	____
29. We talk to people directly rather than through go-betweens.	____	____	____	____
30. Each of us has particular duties and responsibilities.	____	____	____	____
31. There are lots of bad feelings in the family.	____	____	____	____
32. We have rules about hitting people.	____	____	____	____
33. We get involved with each other only when something interests us.	____	____	____	____
34. There's little time to explore personal interests.	____	____	____	____
35. We often don't say what we mean.	____	____	____	____
36. We feel accepted for what we are.	____	____	____	____

continued ⋯⟶

Box 8.3 McMaster Family Assessment Device, cont.

Statements	SA	A	D	SD
37. We show interest in each other when we can get something out of it personally.	___	___	___	___
38. We resolve most emotional upsets that come up.	___	___	___	___
39. Tenderness takes second place to other things in our family.	___	___	___	___
40. We discuss who is to do household jobs.	___	___	___	___
41. Making decisions is a problem for our family.	___	___	___	___
42. Our family shows interest in each other only when they can get something out of it.	___	___	___	___
43. We are frank with each other.	___	___	___	___
44. We don't hold to any rules or standards.	___	___	___	___
45. If people are asked to do something, they need reminding.	___	___	___	___
46. We are able to make decisions about how to solve problems.	___	___	___	___
47. If the rules are broken, we don't know what to expect.	___	___	___	___
48. Anything goes in our family.	___	___	___	___
49. We express tenderness.	___	___	___	___
50. We control problems involving feelings.	___	___	___	___
51. We don't get along well together.	___	___	___	___
52. We don't talk to each other when we are angry.	___	___	___	___
53. We are generally dissatisfied with the family duties assigned to us.	___	___	___	___
54. Even though we mean well, we intrude too much into each other's lives.	___	___	___	___
55. There are rules about dangerous situations.	___	___	___	___
56. We confide in each other.	___	___	___	___
57. We cry openly.	___	___	___	___
58. We don't have reasonable transport.	___	___	___	___
59. When we don't like what someone has done, we tell them.	___	___	___	___
60. We try to think of different ways to solve problems.	___	___	___	___

From Schutle, N. S., & Malouff, J. M. (1995). Sourcebook of adult assessment strategies. New York: Plenum Press, Brown University/ Butler Hospital Family Research Program. © 1982.

There are a whole host of risk assessment/screening tools in use, many of which are reviewed by the Department of Health (2007) and many of which have undergone local adaptation. The philosophy underpinning what is seen as best practice incorporates five points (Department of Health, 2007, p.4):

- The need to balance care needs against risk needs, and an emphasis on
- Positive risk management
- **Collaboration** with the service user and others involved in care
- The importance of recognizing and building on the service user's strengths
- The organization's role in risk management alongside the individual practitioner's.

The assessment of 'risk' is not scientific; accurate prediction is impossible. The best way to reduce the risk of self-harm, suicide, neglect, abuse by others and violence is to engage actively and respectfully with clients, to be focused and concrete in exchanging information and to incorporate safety issues into a negotiated care plan. Risk assessment is *not* the completion of a form in an office away from the client (Figure 8.1).

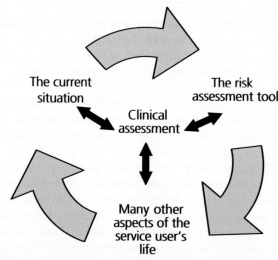

Figure 8.1. Risk assessment tools as one part of the overall clinical assessment process. From Department of Health. (2007). Best practice in managing risk: principles and guidance for best practice in the assessment and management of risk to self and others in mental health services. Available: http://www.dh.gov.uk/en/Publicationsandstatistics/Publications/PublicationsPolicyAndGuidance/DH_076511

Table 8.1	'OBJECTIVE' MEASURES OF PERSONALITY

Test	Description
Minnesota Multiphasic Personality Inventory (MMPI)	566 multiple-choice items; provides scores on 10 clinical scales such as hypochondriasis, depression, hysteria, paranoia; 4 special scales such as anxiety and alcoholism; 3 validity scales to evaluate the truth and accuracy of responses
MMPI-2	Revised version of MMPI with 567 multiple-choice items; provides scores on same areas as MMPI
Milton Clinical Multiaxial Inventory (MCMI) and MCMI-II (revised version)	175 true-false items; provides scores on various personality traits and personality disorders
Psychological Screening Inventory (PSI)	103 true-false items; used to screen for the need for psychological help
Beck Depression Inventory (BDI)	21 items rated on scale of 0–3 to indicate level of depression
Tennessee Self-Concept Scale (TSCS)	100 true-false items; provides information on 14 scales related to self-concept

Adams, R. L. & Culbertson, J. L. (2005). Personality assessment: adults and children. In B. J. Sadock & V. A. Sadock (Eds.), *Comprehensive textbook of psychiatry, Vol. 1* (8th edn, pp. 874–895). Philadelphia: Lippincott Williams & Wilkins

Table 8.2	PROJECTIVE MEASURES OF PERSONALITY

Test	Description
Rorschach test	10 stimulus cards of ink blots; client describes perceptions of ink blots; narrative interpretation discusses areas such as coping styles, interpersonal attitudes, characteristics of ideation
Thematic Apperception Test (TAT)	20 stimulus cards with pictures; client tells a story about the picture; narrative interpretation discusses themes about mood state, conflict, quality of interpersonal relationships
Sentence completion test	Client completes a sentence from beginnings such as 'I often wish', 'Most people', and 'When I was young'

Adams, R. L. & Culbertson, J. L. (2005). Personality assessment: adults and children. In B. J. Sadock & V. A. Sadock (Eds.), *Comprehensive textbook of psychiatry, Vol. 1* (8th edn, pp. 874–895). Philadelphia: Lippincott Williams & Wilkins.

Psychological Tests

Psychological tests are another source of data for the nurse to use in planning care for the client. Two basic types of tests are *intelligence tests* and personality tests. Intelligence tests are designed to evaluate the client's cognitive abilities and intellectual functioning. Personality tests reflect the client's *personality* in areas such as self-concept, impulse control, reality testing and major defences (Adams & Culbertson, 2005). Personality tests may be objective (constructed of true and false, or multiple-choice, questions). Table 8.1 describes selected objective personality tests. The nurse compares the client's answers with standard answers or criteria and obtains a score.

Other personality tests, called projective tests, are unstructured and are usually conducted by the interview method. The stimuli for these tests, such as pictures or Rorschach's ink blots, are standard, but clients may respond with answers that are very different. The evaluator analyses the client's responses and gives a narrative result of the testing. Table 8.2 lists commonly used projective personality tests.

Both intelligence tests and personality tests are frequently criticized as being culturally biased and are rarely used now by nurses in the UK

ASSESSMENT PHASE 3: ANALYSIS AND FORMULATION

After completing a formal psychosocial assessment, the nurse analyses – with the client and possibly with others – all the data that he or she has collected. Data analysis involves thinking about the overall assessment rather than focusing on isolated bits of information and – crucially – checking out hunches and hypotheses with the client. The nurse looks for patterns or themes in the data that lead to conclusions about the client's strengths and needs, and to a particular formulation. No one statement or behaviour is adequate to reach such a conclusion. The nurse must also consider the congruence of all information provided by the client, family or carers, as well as his or her own observations. It is not uncommon for the client's perception of his or her behaviour and situation to differ from that of others.

Formulation and Care Planning

In the US, traditionally, data analysis led to the formulation of 'nursing diagnoses' as a basis for the client's plan of care. Nursing diagnoses – an attempt at making the art and craft of nursing more 'scientific' – have been an integral part of the nursing process there for many years. Diagnoses have never really 'taken-off' in the UK and, with the sweeping changes occurring here in mental health care, the nurse needs to articulate the client's apparent needs in ways that are clear to herself, to professionals in other disciplines, as well as to families and carers, *and* to give voice to the person's own perceptions and experiences. This process involves what we will term a 'Formulation', the second phase of assessment and one that acts as a bridge between assessment and care plan. The care programme approach, a multidisciplinary treatment plan or critical pathway, may be the vehicle for the next stage of the nursing process – the planning of care. The nurse must describe and document goals and interventions that the client and many others, not just professional nurses, can understand. Formulations, care plans and interventions used in this book will be based on those found in Schultz, JM and Videbeck, SL (2002) and will retain much of the wording found there, though in clinical settings, the descriptions … The descriptions should contain no jargon or terms that are unclear to the client, family or other providers of care.

Psychiatric Diagnoses

As mentioned in Chapter 1, medical diagnoses of 'psychiatric illness' are found in the World Health Organization's *ICD-10* and the American Psychiatric Association's *DSM-IV-TR*. These taxonomies are used by psychiatrists and by some psychologists in diagnosis and treatment. Although neither *ICD-10* nor the *DSM-IV-TR* is a substitute for a thorough psychosocial nursing assessment, the descriptions of disorders and related behaviours can be a valuable resource for the nurse to use as a reference.

Axis V of *DSM-IV-TR*, the Global Assessment of Functioning (GAF), may be particularly helpful. The GAF is used to make a judgement about the client's overall level of functioning (Box 8.4). The GAF score given to the client may describe his or her current level of functioning as well as the highest level of functioning in the past year or 6 months. This information may be useful in helping to set appropriate goals for the client's care.

ASSESSMENT PHASE 4: CHECKING OUT/NEXT STEPS

The final phase of a psychosocial assessment is that of planning next steps. This may include:

- Checking if the client, his or her carers or family have anything they want to know or if there is anything that frightens or confuses them
- Checking if the assessment process has been useful and if anything new has arisen that the client, carers or family were previously unaware of
- Agreeing the need for any further assessments
- Ensuring that the client feels safe
- Summarizing and agreeing a formulation
- Agreeing next steps in terms of what the nurse will do now and what the client will do now: planning and intervention stages.

SELF-AWARENESS ISSUES

Self-awareness is, as ever, crucial when a nurse is trying to obtain and provide accurate and complete information from the client during the assessment process. The nurse must be aware of any feelings, biases and values that could interfere with the psychosocial assessment of a client, particularly someone with different beliefs, values and behaviours. The nurse cannot let personal feelings and beliefs influence the client's treatment. Self-awareness does not mean that the nurse's beliefs are wrong or must necessarily change, but it does help the nurse to be open and accepting of others' beliefs and behaviours, even when the nurse does not agree with them.

Two areas that may be uncomfortable or difficult for the nurse to assess are sexuality and self-harm behaviours. The unexperienced nurse may feel uncomfortable, as if prying into personal matters, when asking questions about a client's intimate relationships and behaviour, and any self-harm behaviours or thoughts of suicide. Asking such questions, however, is essential to obtaining a thorough and complete assessment. The nurse needs to remember that it may be uncomfortable for the client to discuss these topics as well.

The nurse may hold beliefs that differ from the client's, but he or she must not make judgements about the client's practices. For example, the nurse may believe that abortion is a sin, but the client might have had several elective abortions. Or the nurse may believe that adultery is wrong, but, during the course of an assessment, he or she may discover that a client has had several extramarital affairs.

Being able to listen to the client without judgement and to support the discussion of personal topics takes practice and usually gets easier with experience. Talking to more experienced colleagues about such discomfort and methods to alleviate it often helps. It may also help for the nurse to preface uncomfortable questions by saying to the client, 'I'd like to ask you some personal questions. Hopefully, what you say will help us understand each other better and it will help the staff provide better care for you.'

The nurse must assess the client for suicidal thoughts. Some nurses feel uncomfortable discussing suicide, or believe that asking about suicide might suggest it to a client who had not previously thought about it. This is not the case. It has been shown that the safest way to assess a client with suspected mental disorders is to ask him or her clearly and directly about suicidal ideas. It is the nurse's professional responsibility to keep the client's safety needs first and foremost, and this includes overcoming any personal discomfort in talking about suicide (Schultz & Videbeck, 2005).

Points to Consider When Doing a Psychosocial Assessment

- The nurse is trying to gain – and provide – all the information needed to help the client. Judgements are not part of the assessment process.

Box 8.4   GLOBAL ASSESSMENT OF FUNCTIONING (GAF) SCALE

Consider psychological, social and occupational functioning on a hypothetical continuum of mental health to illness. Do not include impairment in functioning due to physical (or environmental) limitations. (Note: Use intermediate codes when appropriate, e.g. 45, 68, 72.)

CODE

100 | 91	Superior functioning in a wide range of activities; life's problems never seem to get out of hand; is sought out by others because of his or her many positive qualities. No symptoms
90 | 81	Absent or minimal symptoms (e.g. mild anxiety before an exam), good functioning in all areas, interested and involved in a wide range of activities, socially effective, generally satisfied with life; no more than everyday problems or concerns (e.g. an occasional argument with family members)
80 | 71	If symptoms are present, they are transient and expectable reactions to psychosocial stressors (e.g. difficulty concentrating after family argument); no more than slight impairment in social, occupational or school functioning (e.g. temporarily falling behind in schoolwork)
70 | 61	Some mild symptoms (e.g. depressed mood and mild insomnia) OR some difficulty in social, occupational or school functioning (e.g. occasional truancy, or theft within the household), but generally functioning pretty well; has some meaningful interpersonal relationships
60 | 51	Moderate symptoms (e.g. flat affect and circumstantial speech, occasional panic attacks) OR moderate difficulty in social, occupational or school functioning (e.g. few friends, conflicts with peers or co-workers).
50 | 41	Serious symptoms (e.g. suicidal ideation, severe obsessional rituals, frequent shoplifting) OR any serious impairment in social, occupational or school functioning (e.g. no friends, unable to keep a job)
40 | 31	Some impairment in reality testing or communication (e.g. speech is at times illogical, obscure or irrelevant) OR major impairment in several areas such as work or school, family relations, judgement, thinking or mood (e.g. depressed man avoids friends, neglects family and is unable to work; child frequently beats up younger children, is defiant at home and is failing at school).
30 | 21	Behaviour is considerably influenced by delusions or hallucinations OR serious impairment in communication or judgement (e.g. sometimes incoherent, acts grossly inappropriately, suicidal preoccupation) OR inability to function in almost all areas (e.g. stays in bed all day; no job, home or friends)
20 | 11	Some danger of hurting self or others (e.g. suicide attempts without clear expectation of death; frequently violent; manic excitement) OR occasionally fails to maintain minimal personal hygiene (e.g. smears faeces) OR gross impairment in communication (e.g. largely incoherent or mute)
10 | 1	Persistent danger of severely hurting self or others (e.g. recurrent violence) OR persistent inability to maintain minimal personal hygiene OR serious suicidal act with clear expectation of death
0	Inadequate information

The rating of overall psychological functioning on a scale of 0–100 was operationalized by Luborsky in the Health-Sickness Rating Scale (Luborsky, L. (1962). Clinicians' judgements of mental health. *Archives of General Psychiatry*, 7, 407–417). Spitzer and colleagues developed a revision of the Health-Sickness Rating Scale called the Global Assessment Scale (GAS) (Endicott, J., Spitzer R. L., Fleiss, J. L., & Cohen, J.(1976). The Global Assessment Scale: a procedure for measuring overall severity of psychiatric disturbance. *Archives of General Psychiatry*, 33, 766–771). A modified version of the GAS was included in DSM-III-R as the Global Assessment of Functioning (GAF) Scale.

- Being open, clear and direct when asking about personal or uncomfortable topics helps to alleviate the client's anxiety or hesitancy about discussing the topic.
- Examining one's own beliefs and gaining self-awareness is a growth-producing experience for the nurse.
- If the nurse's beliefs differ strongly from those of the client, the nurse should express his or her feelings to colleagues or discuss the differences with them. The nurse must not allow personal beliefs to interfere with the nurse–client relationship and the assessment process.

Critical Thinking Questions

1. The nurse is preparing to do a psychosocial assessment for a client who is seeking help because she has been physically abusive to her children. What feelings might the nurse experience? How might the nurse view this client?
2. The nurse has discovered through the assessment process that the client drinks a bottle of vodka every 2 days. The client states this is not a problem. How does the nurse proceed? What could the nurse say to this client?
3. The nurse is assessing a client who is illiterate. How will the nurse assess the intellectual functioning of this client? What other areas of a psychosocial assessment might be impaired by the client's inability to read or write?

 KEY POINTS

- The nursing process consists of overlapping stages: assessment/formulation, care planning, intervention and evaluation.
- The purpose of an initial psychosocial assessment is to construct a picture of the client's current emotional state and cognitive and behavioural function. This baseline clinical picture serves as the basis for developing a plan of care to meet the client's needs.
- Assessment involves four overlapping phases: 'rapport and engagement', 'information-exchange', 'analysis and formulation' and 'checking out/next steps'.
- Assessment should be focused on strengths, resources, achievements, exceptions to the problem and possible solutions, as well as on deficits, problems and 'symptoms'.
- The components of a thorough psychosocial assessment include the client's history, general appearance and motor behaviour, mood and affect, thought process and content, sensory and intellectual process, judgement and insight, self-concept, roles and relationships and physiological and self-care considerations.
- The nurse must remain aware that the assessment is always partial and that it is 'true' only for the point in time that it is undertaken.

- Several important factors in the client can influence the psychosocial assessment: ability to participate and give feedback (both on the part of the nurse and the client!), physical health status, emotional well-being and perception of the situation and ability to communicate.
- The environment and the nurse's attitude and approach can greatly influence the psychosocial assessment. The nurse must conduct the assessment professionally, nonjudgementally and matter-of-factly, while not allowing personal feelings to influence the interview.
- To avoid making inaccurate assumptions about the client's psychosocial functioning, the nurse must be sensitive to the client's cultural and spiritual beliefs. Many cultures have values and beliefs about a person's role in society or acceptable social or personal behaviour that may differ from the beliefs and values of the nurse.
- Accurate analysis of assessment data involves considering the entire assessment and identifying patterns of behaviour as well as congruence among components and sources of information.
- Self-awareness on the nurse's part is crucial to obtain an accurate, objective and thorough psychosocial assessment.
- Areas that are often difficult for nurses to assess include sexuality and self-harm behaviours and suicidality. Discussion with colleagues and experience with clients can help the nurse to deal with uncomfortable feelings.
- The client's safety is a priority; therefore, asking clients clearly and directly about suicidal ideation is essential.
- Assessment can in itself be therapeutic – the nurse should see each engagement with a client as potentially helpful.

REFERENCES

Adams, R. L. & Culbertson, J. L. (2005). Personality assessment: adults and children. In B. J. Sadock & V. A. Sadock (Eds.), *Comprehensive textbook of psychiatry Vol. 1* (8th edn, pp. 874–895). Philadelphia: Lippincott Williams & Wilkins.

American Psychiatric Association. (2000). *Diagnostic and statistical manual of mental disorders* (4th edn, text revision). Washington, DC: American Psychiatric Association.

Barker, P. (Ed.). (2003). *Assessment – the foundation of practice in psychiatric and mental health nursing.* London: Arnold.

Department of Health. (2007). *Best practice in managing risk: principles and guidance for best practice in the assessment and management of risk to self and others in mental health services.* Available: http://www.dh.gov.uk/en/Publicationsandstatistics/Publications/PublicationsPolicyAndGuidance/DH_076511

Hanna, D. R. & Roy, C. Sr. (2001). Roy adaptation model and perspectives on family. *Nursing Science Quarterly*, 14(1), 9–13.

Royal College of Psychiatrists. (1999). *Camberwell Assessment of Need Short Appraisal Schedule (CANSAS).* Available: http://www.iop.kcl.ac.uk/virtual/?path=/hsr/prism/can/adultcan/cansas/

Schultz, J. M. & Videbeck, S. (2005). *Lippincott's manual of psychiatric nursing care plans* (7th edn). Philadelphia: Lippincott Williams & Wilkins.

ADDITIONAL READING

Barker, P. (2004). *Assessment in psychiatric and mental health nursing: In search of the whole person.* Cheltenham: Nelson Thornes.

Department of Health. (2006). *From values to action: The Chief Nursing Officer's review of mental health nursing.* Available: http://www.dh.gov.uk/en/Publicationsandstatistics/Publications/PublicationsPolicyAndGuidance/DH_4133839

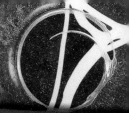

Chapter Study Guide

MULTIPLE-CHOICE QUESTIONS

Select the best answer for each of the following questions.

1. Which of the following is an example of an open-ended question?
   a. Who is the Prime Minister?
   b. What concerns you most about your health?
   c. What is your address?
   d. Have you lost any weight recently?

2. Which of the following is an example of a closed question?
   a. How have you been feeling lately?
   b. How is your relationship with your wife?
   c. Have you had any health problems recently?
   d. Where are you employed?

3. Which of the following is not included in the assessment of sensory and intellectual processes?
   a. Concentration
   b. Memory
   c. Judgement
   d. Orientation

4. Assessment data about the client's speech patterns are categorized in which of the following areas?
   a. History
   b. General appearance and motor behaviour
   c. Sensory and intellectual processes
   d. Self-concept

5. When the nurse is assessing whether or not the client's ideas seem logical and make sense, the nurse is examining which of the following?
   a. Thought content
   b. Thought process
   c. Memory
   d. Sensory

6. The client's belief that a news broadcast has special meaning for him or her is an example of
   a. Abstract thinking
   b. Flight of ideas
   c. Ideas of reference
   d. Thought broadcasting

7. The client who believes everyone is out to get him or her is experiencing a(n)
   a. Delusion
   b. Hallucination
   c. Idea of reference
   d. Loose association

8. To assess the client's ability to concentrate, the nurse could ask the client to do which of the following?
   a. Explain what 'a rolling stone gathers no moss' means
   b. Name the last three Prime Ministers
   c. Repeat the days of the week backward
   d. Tell what a typical day is like

FILL-IN-THE-BLANK QUESTIONS

Identify each of the following terms being described.

_____ 1. Repeated purposeless behaviours often indicating anxiety

_____ 2. The belief that others can read one's thoughts

_____ 3. Generally slowed body movements

_____ 4. Flow of unconnected words that have no meaning

GROUP DISCUSSION TOPICS

Identify questions that the nurse might ask to assess each of the following.

1. Abstract thinking ability

2. Insight

3. Self-concept

4. Judgement

5. Mood

6. Orientation

CLINICAL EXAMPLE

The nurse at a CMHT is meeting a new client for the first time and plans to do a psychosocial assessment. When the client arrives, the nurse finds a young woman who looks somewhat apprehensive and is crying and twisting tissues in her hands. The client can tell the nurse her name and age, but begins crying before she can provide any other information. The nurse knows it is essential to obtain information from this young woman, but it is clear she will have trouble answering all interview questions at this time.

1. How should the nurse approach the crying client? What should the nurse say and do?

2. Identify five questions that the nurse could choose to ask this client initially. Give a rationale for the chosen questions.

3. What, if any, assumptions might the nurse make about this client and her situation?

4. If the client decided to leave the clinic before the assessment formally began, what would the nurse need to do?

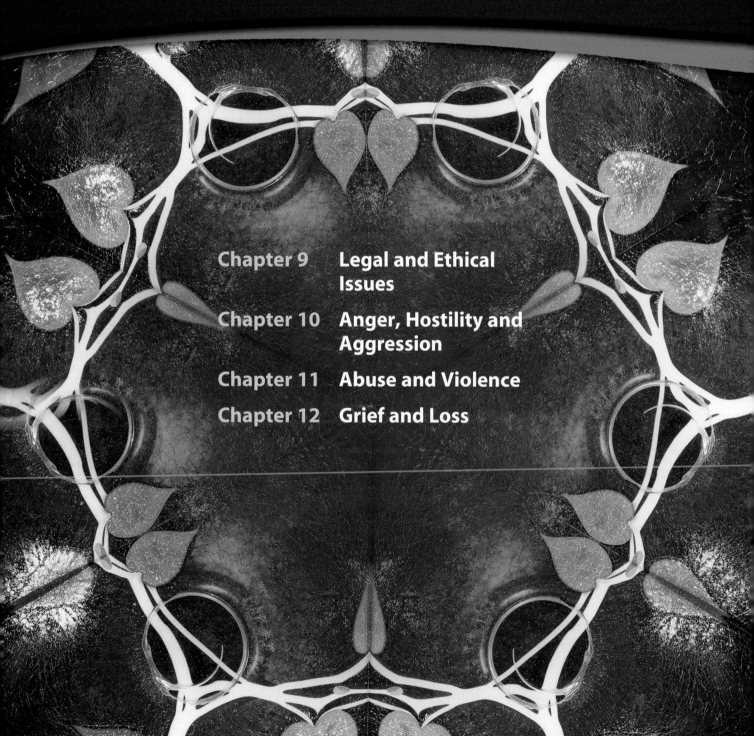

3 Key Social, Cultural and Psychological Issues

unit 3

Legal and Ethical Issues

Key Terms

- assault
- autonomy
- battery
- beneficence
- breach of duty
- community treatment orders
- deontology
- duty
- duty to warn
- ethical dilemma
- ethics
- false imprisonment
- fidelity
- injury or damage
- justice
- least restrictive environment
- negligence
- non-maleficence
- restraint
- seclusion
- standards of care
- tort
- utilitarianism
- veracity

Learning Objectives

After reading this chapter, you should be able to:

1. Describe the rights of the client in inpatient and community settings.

2. Discuss the legal and ethical issues related to seclusion and restraint.

3. Identify pertinent ethical issues in the practice of mental health nursing.

4. Describe the most common types of torts in the mental health setting.

Historically, people seen as 'mad' or as suffering from some form of mental disorder or disability had few rights and were frequently subjected to forcible institutionalization, 'warehousing' and inhumane treatments (see Chapter 1). From the late 1950s onward, ideological shifts and consequent recognition of patients' rights, and changes in laws governing voluntary and involuntary admission and treatment, improved the rights of people being cared for within the mental health system. This chapter discusses the legal considerations related to mental health care and treatment (largely, but not exclusively, involving the 1983 Mental Health Act and its 2007 amendments) and ethical issues that commonly arise in mental health settings. The law in this chapter is that which applies in England; other parts of the UK have their own similar, but not identical, provisions (see Appendix B, which outlines some key elements in Scottish law). Ethical thinking and reasoning, of course, are informed by similar principles across borders (see Box 9.2 which sets out the principles underpinning Scottish practice).

LEGAL CONSIDERATIONS

Rights of Clients and Related Issues

People receiving mental health care retain all civil rights afforded to all citizens – except the right to leave the hospital in the case of compulsory detention (discussed later). They have the right to refuse treatment, to send and to receive sealed mail and to have or to refuse visitors. Any restrictions (e.g. mail visitors, clothing) must be made for a verifiable, documented reason. Examples include the following:

- A suicidal client may not be permitted to keep a belt, shoelaces or scissors, because he or she may use these items for self-harm.
- A client who becomes aggressive after having a particular visitor may have that person restricted from visiting for a period of time.
- A client making threatening phone calls to others outside the hospital may be permitted only supervised phone calls until his or her condition improves.

LEAST RESTRICTIVE ENVIRONMENT AND CODE OF PRACTICE

Clients must be treated in the **least restrictive environment** appropriate to meet their needs. This requirement is one of the reasons for the very detailed Code of Practice (2008) for the Mental Health Act. Professionals must 'have regard' to the Code (s.118(2D) Mental Health Act 1983). The Code must be followed unless there is good reason for not doing so: '. . . reasons for not following the Code must be spelled out clearly, logically and convincingly' (per Lord Hope in R (Munjaz) v. Mersey Care NHS Trust [2006] 2AC 148 para. 69; cited in Bowen, 2007, p. 59).

Box 9.1   FUNDAMENTAL PRINCIPLES OF THE MENTAL HEALTH ACT 1983

The following issues must be addressed:

- Respect for patients' past and present wishes and feelings
- Respect for diversity, generally including, in particular, diversity of religion, culture and sexual orientation
- Minimizing restrictions on liberty
- Involvement of patients in planning, developing and delivering care and treatment appropriate to them
- Avoidance of unlawful discrimination
- Effectiveness of treatment
- Views of carers and other interested parties
- Patient well-being and safety
- Public safety

The Code is not a 'Bill of Rights' for patients but must be drafted in such a way as to satisfy the fundamental principles set out in s.118(2B) of the Mental Health Act 1983 (Box 9.1).

COMPULSORY DETENTION AND TREATMENT

Most clients are admitted to inpatient settings on a *voluntary* basis, which means they are willing to seek treatment and agree to be hospitalized. Some clients, however, do not wish to be hospitalized and treated. Health-care professionals must respect these wishes unless the criteria set out in the Mental Health Act 1983, as amended by the Mental Health Act 2007, are satisfied. A patient may be detained for assessment under Section 2 of the Act if suffering from mental disorder of a nature or degree which warrants hospitalization for assessment and he or she needs to be detained in his or her own interests or to protect others. Admission for treatment under Section 3 may only occur when the patient is suffering from mental disorder of a nature or degree making it appropriate to treat him in hospital, that such treatment is necessary for the patient's own protection or the protection of others and that it cannot be provided unless the patient is detained and appropriate treatment is available. Clients hospitalized against their will under these conditions may only be detained for as long as the criteria are met. Compulsory detention curtails the client's right to freedom (the ability to leave the hospital when he or she wishes). All other client rights, however, remain intact.

A person can be detained under Section 4 for up to 72 hours on an emergency basis if the formalities required under Section 2 would mean undesirable delay, provided at least one of the criteria in Section 2 is met.

Box 9.2 MILLAN PRINCIPLES

1. **Non-discrimination:** People with mental disorder should, wherever possible, retain the same rights and entitlements as those with other health needs.

2. **Equality:** All powers under the 2003 Act should be exercised without any direct or indirect discrimination on the grounds of physical disability, age, gender, sexual orientation, language, religion or national, ethnic or social origin.

3. **Respect for diversity:** Service users should receive care, treatment and support in a manner that affords respect for their individual qualities, abilities and diverse backgrounds, and properly takes into account their age, gender, sexual orientation, ethnic group and social, cultural and religious background.

4. **Reciprocity:** Where society imposes an obligation on an individual to comply with a programme of treatment or care, it should impose a parallel obligation on the health and social care authorities to provide safe and appropriate services, including ongoing care following discharge from compulsion.

5. **Informal care:** Whenever possible, care, treatment and support should be provided to people with mental disorder without the use of compulsory powers.

6. **Participation:** Service users should be fully involved, so far as they are able to be, in all aspects of their assessment, care, treatment and support. Their past and present wishes should be taken into account. They should be provided with all the information and support necessary to enable them to participate fully. Information should be presented in an understandable format.

7. **Respect for carers:** Those who provide care to service users on an informal basis should be respected for their role and experience, receive appropriate information and advice and have their views and needs taken into account.

8. **Least restrictive alternative:** Service users should be provided with any necessary care, treatment and support in the least invasive manner, and in the least restrictive manner and environment, compatible with the delivery of safe and effective care, taking account, where appropriate, of the safety of others.

9. **Benefit:** Any intervention under the 2003 Act should be likely to produce for the service user a benefit that cannot reasonably be achieved other than by the intervention.

10. **Child welfare:** The welfare of a child with mental disorder should be paramount in any interventions imposed on the child under the 2003 Act.

The Millan principles lead to another set of underpinning factors to be taken into consideration when implementing the provisions of the 2003 Act. Practitioners must:

- Take into account the past and present wishes of the patient
- Take into account the views of the named person, carer or guardian
- Consider the range of treatment options available
- Provide maximum benefit with minimum restriction to the patient
- Ensure the patient does not face any kind of discrimination on the grounds of age, gender, religion, sexual orientation or ethnicity
- Inform the carer about intended actions and take into account his or her needs

Restraint is the use of physical force to a person, without his or her permission, to restrict his or her freedom of movement in order to minimize unacceptable behaviour. Force should only be used as a last resort and only by appropriately trained staff. Provided the restraint is used in good faith and with reasonable care, the professional is protected from liability by s.139(1) of the Mental Health Act (MHA). However, as Article 3 of the European Convention on Human Rights expressly prohibits 'torture, inhuman or degrading treatment or punishment' it is possible that restraint or other treatment could be held to fall within the prohibition. However, the European Court of Human Rights has made it clear that where treatment is considered a therapeutic neces-

sity according to recognized medical science, Article 3 will not be engaged (*Herczegfalvy* v. *Austria* [1933] 15 HHRR 437).

Seclusion is the supervised confinement of a person in a room which may be locked to protect others from significant harm. The room must be safe and secure, adequately heated, lit, ventilated, with seating, giving the patient privacy but at the same time ensuring that there is complete observation. The goal is to give the client the opportunity to regain physical and emotional self-control. If the patient has been sedated, a nurse must always be present. In any event, a documented report is required every 15 minutes and a review by two nurses after 2 hours and by a doctor after 4 hours. An independent review by those not

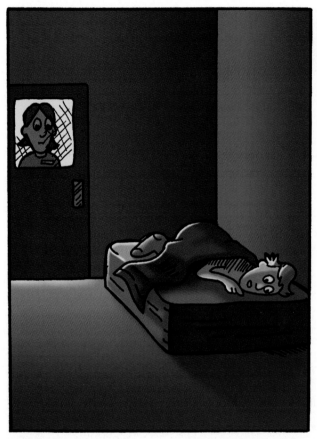

Seclusion

involved with the patient's care is required if seclusion lasts for more than 8 hours consecutively or 12 hours within a 48-hour period.

As soon as possible, staff members must explain to the patient what is needed for a decision to decrease or end the restraint or seclusion. Frequent contact by the nurse promotes ongoing assessment of the client's well-being and self-control, and encourages ongoing engagement. It also provides an opportunity for the nurse to reassure the client that restraint is intended to be a restorative, not a punitive, procedure.

The nurse should also be willing to offer support to the client's family – and to other patients – who may be angry or embarrassed when the client is restrained or secluded. A careful and thorough explanation about the client's behaviour and subsequent use of restraint or seclusion is important, while maintaining client confidentiality. If the client is an adult, however, such discussion requires a signed release of information. In the case of young children, signed consent is not required to inform parents or guardians about the use of restraint or seclusion. Providing the family with information may help prevent legal or ethical difficulties; it also keeps the family involved in the client's treatment.

PATIENTS LACKING MENTAL CAPACITY

In 2004 the European Court of Human Rights held that the lack of a process for independent review of the lawfulness of the detention of a person lacking capacity in a psychiatric hospital amounted to a breach of Article 5 of the European Convention on Human Rights. It didn't matter that the patient was 'compliant' in his deprivation of liberty (*HL* v, *United Kingdom* (Application no. 45508/00) 5 October 2004).

To deal with this problem, the Mental Health Act 2007 amends the Mental Capacity Act 2005. The new rules ensure that a person who lacks capacity, who is considered to be in need of psychiatric treatment but who does not meet the criteria for compulsory detention, can only be deprived of liberty after careful assessment by independent bodies. The assessments include:

- Mental health
- Mental capacity
- Best interests.

Authorization for detention will only be granted after the best interests assessor has recommended the period for which detention should be authorized. Additionally a person must be appointed to represent the detained person's interests (s.4(5) Mental Capacity Act 2005 and Schedule A1).

CLINICAL VIGNETTE: SECLUSION

The goal of seclusion is to give the client the opportunity to regain self-control, both emotionally and physically. Most clients who have been secluded, however, have very different feelings and thoughts about seclusion. Clients report feeling angry, agitated, bored, frustrated, helpless and afraid while in seclusion. They perceive seclusion as a punishment and receive the message that they were 'bad'. Many clients are not clear about the reasons for seclusion or the criteria for exiting seclusion, and they believe that seclusion lasted too long. In general, clients think that other interventions such as interaction with staff, a place to calm down or scream when needed or the presence of a family member could reduce or eliminate the need for seclusion. Clients who had not been secluded describe the seclusion of others in more positive terms such as *helpful, caring, fair* and *good*. However, these clients also express the wish that 'that never happens to me'.

RELEASE FROM HOSPITAL

Clients admitted to the hospital voluntarily have the right to leave the hospital against medical advice provided they have the capacity to make the decision. However, if the criteria for compulsory detention and treatment are met, the necessary steps for compulsory detention can be put in place.

While in the hospital, treatment being given may successfully alleviate/control symptoms so that the client can be discharged. Inevitably, some clients stop taking their medications after discharge – or disengage with services and support – and may once again become threatening, aggressive or dangerous to themselves and/or others. This situation contributed to the debate about how the public could be protected from patients who were free in the community but dangerous to others, and how the welfare of the patient could be best protected. An attempt was made to address these issues by the 2007 amendments.

COMMUNITY TREATMENT ORDERS

A **community treatment order** (CTO) is the mechanism for a detained client to be discharged subject to being recalled to hospital. The responsible clinician must order the discharge in writing, provided the criteria for compulsory detention are met and, additionally, the appropriate treatment can be provided without the client continuing to be detained in hospital. One condition which must be imposed is a requirement that the client makes himself or herself available for examination. Other conditions may include a requirement to live at a particular address and to attend for treatment.

A person who is subject to a CTO can be recalled to hospital if the responsible clinician is of the opinion that the person requires hospital treatment and there would be a risk of harm to the patient or others if they were not recalled to hospital. The patient may also be recalled if they do not comply with a condition imposed by the CTO.

GUARDIANSHIP

A patient may be received into guardianship if suffering from mental disorder which is of a nature or degree to warrant such a step and it is necessary in the interests of the patient's welfare or for the protection of others that this should happen (s.7(2) Mental Health Act 1983 (as amended)). A guardian has wide powers, for example, to specify where the patient is to live, to require the patient to attend for treatment, education or training, etc. The purpose of guardianship is intended to ensure that a patient accepts treatment so that compulsory detention is not necessary. There is one problem, however. It is a well-settled law that there is 'no power under the 1983 Act to give treatment to a mentally disordered person who withholds consent . . . unless he is detained in hospital' (per McCullough, J. in *R* v. *Hallstrom ex p W* (No 2) [1986] 2 All ER 306, 313; cited in Bartlett & Sandland, 2003, p. 558). Guardianship has not worked as originally envisaged because of this inability to impose treatment against the patient's wishes.

CONFIDENTIALITY

All health professionals must be aware that any information relating to the patient's health or other matters must be regarded as confidential. Information can be shared:

- With the patient's consent
- With others concerned with delivery of care to the patient – when it is necessary to do so
- When disclosure is required by law, e.g. child protection issues
- When disclosure is in the public interest, e.g. reporting a colleague who comes on duty under the influence of alcohol or drugs.

Breach of confidentiality is usually dealt with as a disciplinary matter by the relevant professional body (the Nursing and Midwifery Council for nurses) and/or by the employer.

The Data Protection Act 1998 sets out the legal principles which underpin the duty. The effect of the Act is to create a framework that determines the way in which information is collected and stored and the way in which it is protected. In relation to health records, 'Caldecott Guardians' are employed by NHS Trusts and primary care trusts (PCTs) to ensure that the rules are properly observed.

Privacy is further protected by Article 8 of the European Convention on Human Rights, which imposes a duty of respect for privacy and family life. The duty is not absolute, allowance being made for lawful disclosure to the extent that it can be justified. The duty of health professionals as outlined above is consistent with Article 8 requirements.

While in the US, there is a **duty to warn** identifiable third parties of threats made by clients, even if these threats were discussed during therapy sessions otherwise protected by privilege, there is no such provision under English law.

Some believe that these strict confidentiality policies may pose a barrier to collaboration among providers and families (Marshall & Solomon, 2003). In community mental health settings, compliance with the privacy rule has decreased communication and collaboration among providers, which may have a negative impact on patient care (Touchet *et al.*, 2004). Marshall and Solomon, as well as Touchet and colleagues, recommended a vigorous education programme for clients and families about confidentiality policies, as well as establishing open lines of communication between clients and families before a crisis occurs.

Insanity Defence

One legal issue that sparks controversy is the insanity defence, with *insanity* having a legal meaning but no medical definition. The defence is established if, at the time the act (crime) was committed, the person was labouring under such a defect of reason, from disease of the mind, as not to know the nature and quality of his act or, if he did know it, that he did not know that he was doing wrong. Once the defence is accepted, the accused will be held to be not guilty by reason of insanity (s.1 Criminal Procedure (Insanity) Act 1964). Until 1991 this meant that the person was immediately ordered to be detained indefinitely in a psychiatric hospital. The Criminal Procedure (Insanity and Unfitness to Plead) Act 1991 amended the 1964 Act to allow the judge to use discretion in sentencing (except in cases of murder) so that the accused may be made subject to an appropriate order, e.g. guardianship or, in trivial cases, be given an absolute discharge.

The defence remains controversial. Reforms have been proposed by the Law Commission's Criminal Code Bill in 1989 but to date no steps to effect reform have been taken.

Nursing Liability

Nurses are responsible for providing safe, competent, legal and ethical care to clients and families. Professional guidelines such as the Code of Practice published by the Nursing and Midwifery Council (2007) outline the nurse's responsibilities and provide guidance. Nurses are expected to meet **standards of care**, meaning the care they provide to clients meets set expectations and is what any nurse in a similar situation would do. Standards of care are enforced by the professional bodies, by employers and through civil and criminal law. Mental health law in the UK varies from country to country. The basic principles relating to Scotland are included to provide some guidance for Scottish practitioners (see Appendix B).

TORTS

A **tort** is 'a wrong which entitles the injured party to claim compensation from the wrongdoer' (Martin & Gibbins, 1999, p. 235). Torts may be either unintentional or intentional.

Unintentional Torts: Negligence. **Negligence** is an unintentional tort that involves causing harm by doing – or failing to do – what a reasonable and prudent person would do in similar circumstances. To succeed in an action the injured party must prove:

1. **Duty**: That the wrongdoer owed a legal duty of care to the victim; that the victim was someone whom it could be foreseen would be affected by the wrongdoer's act. In the health-care situation, a health-care professional owes a legal duty to anyone for whom responsibility has been taken, e.g. by accepting a patient onto a ward.
2. **Breach of duty**: The nurse (or doctor) failed to conform to standards of care, thereby breaching or failing the existing duty. The nurse did not act as a reasonable, prudent nurse would have acted in similar circumstances.
3. **Injury or damage**: As a result of the breach of duty, the patient suffered some type of loss, damage or injury. It is insufficient to say the breach might have caused the injury; it must be shown to have done so (*Wilsher* v. *Essex Area Health Authority* [1987] QB 730).

Not all injury or harm to a client can be prevented, nor do all client injuries result from negligence. The issues are whether or not the client's actions were predictable or foreseeable (and, therefore, preventable) and whether or not

the nurse carried out appropriate assessment, interventions and evaluation that met the standards of care. In the mental health setting, lawsuits most often are related to suicide and suicide attempts. Other areas of concern include clients harming others (staff, family, other clients), sexual assault and medication errors.

Intentional Torts. Psychiatric nurses also may be liable for intentional torts or voluntary acts that result in harm to the client. Examples include assault, battery and false imprisonment.

Assault involves any action that causes a person to fear being touched without either their consent or lawful authority. Examples include making threats to restrain the client to give him or her an injection following failure to co-operate. **Battery** involves actual contact with a client. Examples include touching a client without consent or unnecessarily restraining a client. **False imprisonment** is defined as the unjustifiable detention of a client, such as the inappropriate use of restraint or seclusion, again without the person's consent or lawful authority.

In the case of these torts, the injured party has, in fact, no need to prove that any fear, injury or damage happened. It is enough simply to establish that, for example, the touching happened. The amount of any compensation may, of course, be influenced by whether or not there was actual injury and the circumstances in which the tort occurred. A patient who is detained by virtue of the MHA cannot bring an action, provided the criteria for detention and treatment are properly observed.

PREVENTION OF LIABILITY

Nurses can minimize the risk for lawsuits through safe, competent nursing care and descriptive, accurate documentation. Box 9.3 highlights ways to minimize the risk for liability.

Box 9.3   STEPS TO AVOID LIABILITY

Practise within the scope of the law.

Be aware of developments in relation to practice and treatment.

Recognize the limits of one's own competence and act only with those limits.

Collaborate with colleagues to determine the best course of action.

Use established practice standards to guide decisions and actions.

Always put the client's rights and welfare first.

Develop effective interpersonal relationships with clients and families.

Accurately and thoroughly document all assessment data, treatments, interventions and evaluations of the client's response to care.

ETHICAL ISSUES

The nurse should respect the client's autonomy through ensuring that his or her rights are protected, through informed consent, and through encouraging the client to make choices about his or her health care. The nurse has a duty to take actions that promote the client's health (beneficence) and that do not harm the client (non-maleficence). The nurse must treat all clients fairly (justice), be truthful and honest (veracity), and honour all duties and commitments to clients and families (fidelity). These principles form the basis of an ethical approach to nursing.

Ethics is a branch of philosophy that deals with values of human conduct related to the rightness or wrongness of actions and to the goodness and badness of the motives and ends of such actions (King, 1984). Ethical theories are sets of principles used to decide what is right or wrong.

Two broad areas of ethical stance will be outlined here: utilitarianism and deontology. Mental health care offers a whole host of situations in which pragmatic utilitarian principles can come into conflict with the more individually focused, morality driven principles of a deontological approach (and the many years of debate over changes to the 1983 Mental Health Act offer an excellent example of these tensions).

Utilitarianism is a theory that bases decisions on 'the greatest good for the greatest number'. Decisions based on utilitarianism consider which action would produce the greatest benefit for the most people.

Deontology, meanwhile, is a theory that says decisions should be based on whether or not an action is morally right, with no regard for the result or consequences. Principles used as guides for decision making in deontology include autonomy, beneficence, non-maleficence, justice, veracity and fidelity.

Autonomy refers to the person's right to self-determination and independence. **Beneficence** refers to one's duty to benefit or to promote good for others. **Non-maleficence** is the requirement to do no harm to others either intentionally or unintentionally. **Justice** refers to fairness; that is, treating all people fairly and equally without regard for social or economic status, race, sex, marital status, religion, ethnicity or cultural beliefs. **Veracity** is the duty to be honest or truthful. **Fidelity** refers to the obligation to honour commitments and contracts.

Ethical Dilemmas in Mental Health

An **ethical dilemma** is a situation in which ethical principles conflict or when there is no one clear course of action in a given situation. For example, the client who refuses medication or treatment is allowed to do so based on the principle of autonomy. If the client presents an imminent threat of danger to self or others, however, the principle of non-maleficence (do no harm) is at risk. To protect the client or others from harm, the client may be compulsorily detained and treated in a hospital, even though some may argue that this action violates his or her right to autonomy. In this example, the utilitarian theory of doing the greatest good for the greatest number (involuntary commitment) overrides the individual client's autonomy (right to refuse treatment). Ethical dilemmas are often complicated and charged with emotion, making it difficult to arrive at fair or 'right' decisions.

Many dilemmas in mental health involve the client's right to self-determination and independence (autonomy) and concern for the 'public good' (utilitarianism). Examples include the following:

- Once a client is 'stabilized' on psychotropic medication, should he or she be forced to remain on medication through the use of enforced depot injections or the use of a CTO?
- Are clients who are psychotic necessarily incompetent, unable to give or decline consent, or do they still have the right to refuse hospitalization and medication?
- Can clients of mental health care ever truly be empowered if health-care professionals are able to 'step in' to make decisions for them 'for their own good'?
- Should nurses break confidentiality to report clients who drive cars at high speeds and recklessly?
- Should a client who is loud and intrusive to other clients on a hospital unit be secluded from the others?
- A CPN has an established relationship with a person who later becomes a client in the CMHT where the health-care worker practises. Can the CPN continue the relationship with the person who is now a client? If so should he or she make any changes?
- To protect the public, can clients with a history of violence toward others be detained after their symptoms are stable?
- When a therapeutic relationship has ended, can a health-care professional ever have a social or intimate relationship with someone he or she met as a client?
- Is it possible to maintain strict professional boundaries (i.e. no previous, current or future personal relationships with clients) in small communities and rural areas where all people in the community know one another?

The nurse will confront some of these dilemmas directly, and he or she will have to make decisions about a course of action. For example, the nurse may observe behaviour between another health-care worker and a client that seems flirtatious or inappropriate. Another dilemma might represent the policies or common practice of the agency where the nurse is employed. The nurse may have to decide whether to support current practice or to advocate for change on behalf of clients, such as laws permitting people to be detained after treatment is completed when there is a potential of future risk for violence.

Box 9.4   NMC STANDARDS OF CONDUCT, PERFORMANCE AND ETHICS FOR NURSES

The people in your care must be able to trust you with their health and well-being. To justify that trust, you must:

- Make the care of people your first concern, treating them as individuals and respecting their dignity
- Work with others to protect and promote the health and well-being of those in your care, their families and carers and the wider community

- Provide a high standard of practice and care at all times
- Be open and honest, act with integrity and uphold the reputation of your profession

As a professional, you are personally accountable for actions and omissions in your practice and must always be able to justify your decisions.

Nursing and Midwifery Council (2008). *The Code – Standards of conduct, performance and ethics for nurses and midwives.* London: NMC.
Available: http://www.nmc-uk.org/aArticle.aspx?ArticleID=3236

Ethical Decision-Making

Models for ethical decision making include gathering information, clarifying values, identifying options, identifying legal considerations and practical restraints, building consensus for the decision reached and reviewing and analysing the decision to determine what was learned (Abma & Widdershoven, 2006). The NMC issues a code setting out principles that assist the practitioner to reach an ethical decision (Box 9.4).

SELF-AWARENESS ISSUES

All nurses have beliefs about what is right or wrong and good or bad. That is, they have values just like all other people. Being a member of the nursing profession, however, presumes a duty to clients and families under the nurse's care: a duty to protect rights, to be an advocate and to act in the clients' best interests even if that duty is in conflict with the nurse's personal values and beliefs. The nurse is obligated to engage in self-awareness by identifying clearly and examining his or her own values and beliefs so they do not become confused with, or overshadow, a client's. For example, if a client is grieving over her decision to have an abortion, the nurse must be able to provide support to her even though the nurse may be opposed to abortion. If the nurse cannot do that, then he or she should talk to colleagues to find someone who can meet that client's needs.

Points to Consider When Confronting Ethical Dilemmas

- Talk to colleagues or seek professional supervision.
- Spend time thinking about ethical issues and determine what your values and beliefs are regarding situations before they occur.

- Be willing to discuss ethical concerns with colleagues or managers. Being silent is – potentially – condoning unprofessional behaviour.

Critical Thinking Questions

1. Some clients with mental disorders have made headlines when they've commited crimes against others that involve serious injury or death. With appropriate care and treatment, these clients may be rational and represent no threat to others, but often have a history of stopping their medications when discharged. Where and how should these clients be treated? What measures can protect their individual rights as well as the public right to safety?

2. Some critics of deinstitutionalization argue that taking people who are severely and persistently mentally disordered out of institutions and closing some or all those institutions have worsened the mental health crisis. The emphasis on community care has made it difficult for this minority of clients to receive necessary inpatient treatment. Opponents counter that institutions are harmful because they segregate 'the mentally ill' from the community, limit autonomy and contribute to the loss of social skills. With which viewpoint do you agree? Why? Is there a way of reconciling these two views?

KEY POINTS

- Clients can be involuntarily hospitalized if they are suffering mental disorder, present an imminent danger of harm to themselves or others to such an extent that appropriate treatment should be given in hospital.
- The interests of those lacking capacity who need to be deprived of their liberty are safeguarded by the requirement of assessment by an independent body.

- Patients' rights include the right to receive and refuse treatment, to be involved in the plan of care, to be treated in the least restrictive environment, to refuse to participate in research and to have unrestricted visitors, mail and phone calls.
- The use of seclusion (confinement in a locked room) and restraint (direct application of physical force) falls under the domain of the patient's right to the least restrictive environment. Short-term use is permitted only if the client is imminently aggressive and dangerous to himself or herself or to others.
- Nurses have the responsibility to provide safe, competent, legal and ethical care as outlined in the NMC Code (2008).
- A tort is a wrongful act that results in injury, loss or damage. Negligence is an unintentional tort causing harm through incompetent/inappropriate practice.
- Intentional torts include assault, battery and false imprisonment.
- Ethical theories are sets of principles used to decide what is morally right or wrong, such as utilitarianism (the greatest good for the greatest number) and deontology (using principles such as autonomy, beneficence, non-maleficence, justice, veracity and fidelity) to make ethical decisions.
- Ethical dilemmas are situations that arise when principles conflict or when there is no single clear course of action in a given situation.
- Many ethical dilemmas in mental health involve a conflict between the client's autonomy and concerns for the public good (utilitarianism).

REFERENCES

Abma, T. A. & Widdershoven, G. A. (2006). Moral deliberation in psychiatric nursing practice. *Nursing Ethics,*13(5), 546–557.

Bartlett, P. & Sandland, R. (2003). *Mental health law policy and practice* (2nd edn). Oxford: Oxford University Press.

Bowen, P. (2007). *Blackstone's guide to the Mental Health Act 2007.* Oxford: Oxford University Press.

Data Protection Act. (1998). London: OPSI. Available: http://www.opsi.gov.uk/Acts/Acts1998/ukpga_19980029_en_1

Department of Health. (2008). Code of Practice: Mental Health Act 1983. London: TSO. Availablet: http://www.dh.gov.uk/en/Publicationsandstatistics/Publications/PublicationsPolicyAndGuidance/DH_084597

King, E. C. (1984). *Affective education in nursing: A guide to teaching and assessment.* Rockville, MD: Aspen Systems.

Marshall, T. & Solomon, P. (2003). Professionals' responsibilities in releasing information to families of adults with mental illness. *Psychiatric Services, 54*(12), 1622–1628.

Martin, J. & Gibbins, M. (1999). *The complete A–Z law handbook.* London: Hodder & Stoughton,

Mental Capacity Act 2005 (as amended) (2007). London: OPSI.

Mental Health Act 1983 (as amended) (2007). London: OPSI. Available: http://www.dh.gov.uk/en/Healthcare/NationalServiceFrameworks/Mentalhealth/DH_089882

Nursing and Midwifery Council (2007). *The Code – Standards of conduct performance and ethics for nurses and midwives.* London: NMC.

Nursing and Midwifery Council. (2008). The Code: Standards of conduct, performance and ethics for nurses and midwives. Available: http://www.nmc-uk.org/aArticle.aspx?ArticleID=3056

Touchet, B. K., Drummond, S. R., & Yates, W. R. (2004). The impact of fear of HIPPA violation on patient care. *Psychiatric Services, 55*(5), 575–576.

ADDITIONAL READING

Bartlett, P. (2005). *Blackstone's guide to the Mental Capacity Act 2005.* Oxford: Oxford University Press.

Beauchamp,T. L. & Childress, J. F. (2001). *Principles of biomedical ethics* (5th edn). Oxford: Oxford University Press.

Dimond, B. (2008). *Legal aspects of nursing* (5th edn). Harlow, Essex: Pearson Education.

Herring, J. (2006). *Medical law and ethics.* Oxford: Oxford University Press.

Mason, J. K. & Laurie, G. T. (2006). *Mason & McCall Smith's law and medical ethics* (7th edn). Oxford: Oxford University Press.

Turner, C. & Hodge, S. (2007). *Unlocking torts* (2nd edn). London: Hodder Arnold.

INTERNET RESOURCES

RESOURCES	INTERNET ADDRESS
Department of Health	www.dh.gov.uk
MENCAP	www.mencap.org.uk
Mental Health (Care and Treatment) (Scotland) Act, 2003	http://www.opsi.gov.uk/legislation/scotland/acts2003/asp_20030013_en_1
Mental Health Tribunal Scotland	www.mhtscotland.gov.uk
Mental Welfare Commission for Scotland	www.mwcscot.org.uk
MIND	www.mind.org.uk
Nursing and Midwifery Council	www.nmc-uk.or/
Office of Public Sector Information	www.opsi.gov.uk
Royal College of Nursing	www.rcn.org.uk
Royal College of Psychiatrists	www.rcpsch.ac.uk
SANE	www.sane.org.uk
Scottish Development Centre for Mental Health	www.sdcmh.org.uk
Scottish Executive	www.scotland.gov.uk

Chapter Study Guide

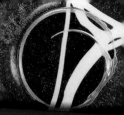

MULTIPLE-CHOICE QUESTIONS

Select the best answer for each of the following questions.

1. The client who is involuntarily committed to an inpatient psychiatric unit loses which of the following rights?
   a. Right to freedom
   b. Right to refuse treatment
   c. Right to sign legal documents
   d. The client loses no rights

2. A client in an inpatient unit is yelling again and again, 'The world's coming to an end. We must all run to safety!' When other clients complain that this client is loud and annoying, the nurse decides to put the client in seclusion. The client has made no threatening gestures or statements to anyone. The nurse's action is an example of
   a. Assault
   b. False imprisonment
   c. Negligence

3. The nurse gives the client quetiapine (Seroquel) in error when olanzapine (Zyprexa) was ordered. The client has no ill effects from the quetiapine. In addition to making a medication error, the nurse has committed which of the following?
   a. Fraud
   b. Negligence
   c. Tort (unintentional)
   d. None of the above

FILL-IN-THE-BLANK QUESTIONS

Identify the deontological principle being described.

_____ Telling the truth

_____ Doing no harm

_____ Keeping commitments

_____ Promoting good

_____ Being fair

_____ Exhibiting self-determination

GROUP DISCUSSION TOPICS

1. Describe the concept of the least restrictive environment.

2. Identify the steps involved in the ethical decision-making process.

3. Discuss minimum standards of care for nursing.

4. Discuss the elements necessary to prove liability in negligence lawsuits.

Anger, Hostility and Aggression

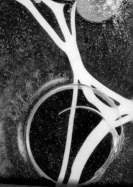

Key Terms

- acting out
- anger
- catharsis
- hostility
- impulse control
- physical aggression
- risk

Learning Objectives

After reading this chapter, you should be able to

1. Discuss anger, hostility and aggression.

2. Describe mental health problems that may be associated with an increased risk of hostility and physical aggression in people.

3. Describe the signs, symptoms and behaviours associated with the five phases of aggression.

4. Discuss appropriate nursing interventions for the client during the five phases of aggression.

5. Describe important issues for nurses to be aware of when working with angry, hostile or aggressive clients.

Anger, a normal human emotion, is a strong, uncomfortable, emotional response to a real or perceived provocation. Anger results when a person is frustrated, hurt or afraid. Handled appropriately and expressed assertively, anger can be a positive force that helps a person to resolve conflicts, solve problems and make decisions (Dunbar, 2004). Anger energizes the body physically for self-defence, when needed, by activating the 'fight-or-flight' response mechanisms of the sympathetic nervous system (the way in which the brain prepares the body to face threat). When expressed inappropriately or suppressed, however, anger can lead to physical or emotional problems or interfere with relationships.

Hostility, or *verbal aggression,* is an expression of anger or fear through verbal abuse, lack of co-operation, violation of rules or norms or threatening behaviour (Schultz & Videbeck, 2005). A person may express hostility when he or she feels threatened or powerless, or when his or her beliefs – about the way he or she should be, the way the world should be, the way other people should be – are challenged . Hostile behaviour is intended to intimidate or cause emotional harm to another, to attempt to change 'the way things are' and it can lead to physical aggression. **Physical aggression** is, obviously, behaviour in which a person attacks or injures another person or that involves destruction of property. Both verbal and physical aggression are meant to harm or punish another person, to force someone into compliance or – on occasion – to protect against possible attack.

A minority of people with mental health problems display hostile or physically aggressive behaviour that represents a challenge to nurses and other staff members. Violence and abuse are discussed in Chapter 11, and self-directed aggression such as suicidal behaviour is presented in Chapter 15. The focus of this chapter is the nurse's role in recognizing and managing hostile and aggressive behaviour that people direct toward others within psychiatric settings.

It is important to emphasize that the management of violence and aggression is exceptionally complex: it is hard to convey all the subtleties and nuances of aggression, anger, hostility and violence in words. Experience, reflection, feedback and supervision are essential in helping people develop in this area.

ONSET AND CLINICAL COURSE

Anger

Anger is, in essence, a complex series of interactions:

- Between the individual – and his or her environment
- Between the individual's beliefs about self, the world and others – and those of other people
- Between the individual's own feelings, thoughts and behaviour.

A cognitive-behavioural model of anger sees 'automatic' thoughts (themselves built on the core beliefs someone has) appearing in response to perceived external or internal

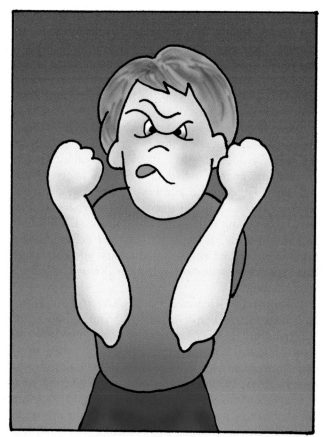
Hostility

threats and this leading, in turn, to uncomfortable feelings (although there is some evidence that feelings actually come *before* thoughts (Blackmore, 2003)): the individual then has a choice to behave in a number of ways, one of which is aggression or violence. Intervention at any or all of these stages can prove helpful.

Although the experience of anger is normal, its expression – particularly in sections of northern European and North American society, and particularly by women – is often perceived as being inherently negative. Many people are not comfortable expressing anger directly. Nevertheless, the expression of anger can be a normal and healthy reaction when situations or circumstances are unfair or unjust, personal rights are not respected, or realistic expectations are not met. If the person can express his or her anger assertively and respectfully, problem-solving or conflict resolution is possible.

Anger can become negative if the person denies it, suppresses it or expresses it inappropriately. A person may deny or suppress (i.e. hold in) angry feelings if he or she is uncomfortable expressing anger: possible consequences are physical problems such as migraine headaches, ulcers or coronary artery disease, and psychological problems such as depression and low self-esteem.

Anger that is expressed inappropriately can lead to hostility and aggression. One way in which the nurse can help people express anger appropriately is by acting as a role-model and by role-playing assertive communication techniques. Assertive communication uses 'I' statements that express feelings and are specific to the situation, for example, 'I feel angry when you interrupt me', or 'I am angry that you changed the work schedule without talking to me'. Statements such as these allow the appropriate expression of anger and can lead to productive problem-solving discussions – and reduced anger.

Some people try to express their angry feelings by engaging in aggressive but safe activities, such as hitting a punching bag or yelling. However, this kind of '**catharsis**' can, on occasion, increase rather than alleviate angry feelings and, therefore, cathartic activities may be contraindicated for angry clients. Activities that are not aggressive, such as walking or talking with another person, are more likely to be effective in decreasing anger (Jacob & Pelham, 2005). Meditation and mindfulness techniques are also excellent approaches to dealing with anger (Kabat-Zinn, 2005; Linehan, 2007).

Shapiro (2005) reported that high hostility is associated with increased risk of coronary artery disease and hypertension. Hostility can lead to angry outbursts that are not effective for anger expression. Effective methods of anger expression, such as using assertive communication to express anger, should replace angry, aggressive outbursts of temper such as yelling or throwing things. Controlling one's temper or managing anger effectively should not be confused with suppressing angry feelings, which can lead to the problems described earlier.

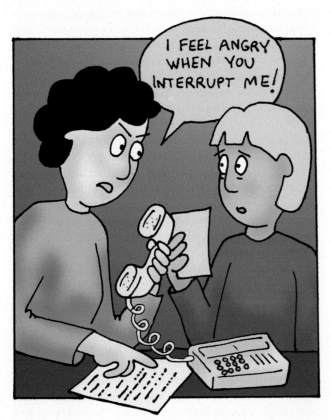

Assertive communication

Anger suppression is especially common in women, who have often been socialized to maintain and enhance relationships with others and to avoid the expression of so-called negative or unfeminine emotions such as anger. Women's anger often results when people deny them power or resources, treat them unjustly or behave irresponsibly toward them (Thomas, 2005); the 'offenders' are – frequently – not strangers, but people close to them. Manifestations of anger-suppression through somatic complaints and psychological problems may be more common among women than men.

Hostility and Aggression

Hostile and aggressive behaviour can be sudden and unexpected. Often, however, stages or phases can be identified in aggressive incidents: one model is to divide hostility and aggression into a triggering phase, an escalation phase, a crisis phase, a recovery phase and a postcrisis phase.

As a client's behaviour escalates toward the crisis phase, he or she loses the ability to perceive events accurately, solve problems, express feelings appropriately or control his or her behaviour; behavioural escalation may lead to physical aggression. Therefore, interventions during the triggering and escalation phases are key to preventing physically aggressive behaviour. The phases and their signs, symptoms and behaviours are discussed later in the chapter.

RELATED DISORDERS

The media gives a great deal of attention to people with 'mental illness' who commit aggressive acts. This helps give the general public (and, sadly, some professionals) the mistaken idea that most people with mental health problems are aggressive and to be feared. In reality, people with mental health problems are much more likely to hurt themselves than other people. According to the Mental Health Alliance:

> More than half a million people in England and Wales have a severe mental illness. The vast majority do not harm anyone and manage their illness without recourse to compulsory treatment . . . Homicides by people with mental health problems are rare: of 873 homicides in 2002, less than 5% were attributable to mental illness.
>
> (Mental Health Alliance, 2008)

Although most people with mental health disorders are not aggressive, individuals with a variety of diagnoses can, rarely, exhibit angry, hostile and aggressive behaviour. People experiencing paranoid delusions may believe others are out to get them; believing they are protecting themselves, they may retaliate with hostility or aggression. Some clients have auditory hallucinations that command them to hurt others. Aggressive behaviour is also seen in people diagnosed with dementia, delirium, head injuries, intoxication with alcohol or other drugs and antisocial and borderline personality disorders

Some people with depression have intense angry outbursts. These sudden spells of anger typically occur in situations in which the depressed person feels emotionally trapped. Anger attacks involve verbal expressions of anger or rage but no physical aggression. Clients described these anger attacks as uncharacteristic behaviour that was inappropriate for the situation and was followed by remorse. The anger attacks seen in some depressed clients may be related to irritable mood, overreaction to minor annoyances and decreased coping abilities (Akiskal, 2005).

'Intermittent explosive disorder' is a rare psychiatric diagnosis characterized by discrete episodes of aggressive impulses that result in serious assaults or destruction of property. The aggressive behaviour the person displays is grossly disproportionate to any provocation or precipitating factor. This diagnosis is made only if the client has no other co-morbid mental health disorders. The person describes a period of tension or arousal that the aggressive outburst seems to relieve. Afterwards, however, the person is remorseful and embarrassed, and there are no signs of aggressiveness between episodes (Greenberg, 2005). Intermittent explosive disorder develops between late adolescence and the third decade of life (American Psychiatric Association, 2000). Typically, clients with intermittent explosive disorder are men with dependent personality features who respond to feelings of uselessness or ineffectiveness with violent outbursts.

'**Acting out**' is an immature defence mechanism by which the person deals with emotional conflicts or stressors through actions rather than through reflection or feelings. The person engages in acting-out behaviour, such as verbal or physical aggression, to feel temporarily less helpless or powerless. Children and adolescents often 'act out' when they cannot handle intense feelings or deal with emotional conflict verbally. To understand acting-out behaviours, it is important to consider the situation and the person's ability to deal with feelings and emotions: and to beware of using the term to invalidate someone's sense of frustration or loss of control.

AETIOLOGY

Neurobiological Theories

Researchers have examined the role of neurotransmitters in aggression in animals and humans, but they have been unable to identify a single cause. Findings reveal that serotonin plays a major inhibitory role in aggressive behaviour; therefore, low serotonin levels may lead to increased aggressive behaviour (Johnson, 2004). This finding may be related to the anger attacks seen in some clients with depression. In addition, increased activity of dopamine and noradrenaline in the brain is associated with increased impulsively violent behaviour. Further, structural damage to the limbic system and the frontal and temporal lobes of the brain may alter the person's ability to modulate aggression; this can lead to aggressive behaviour.

Psychosocial Theories

Infants and toddlers express themselves loudly and intensely, which is normal for these stages of growth and development. Temper tantrums are a common response from toddlers whose wishes are not granted. As a child matures, he or she is expected to develop **impulse control** (the ability to delay gratification) and socially appropriate behaviour. Positive relationships with parents, teachers and peers, success in school and the ability to be responsible for oneself all foster development of these qualities. Children in dysfunctional families with poor parenting, children who receive inconsistent responses to their behaviour and children whose families are of lower socioeconomic status are at increased **risk** for failing to develop socially appropriate behaviour; this lack of development can result in a person who is impulsive, easily frustrated and prone to aggressive behaviour.

Leary and colleagues (2006) found a relationship between interpersonal rejection and aggression. Rejection can lead to anger and aggression when that rejection causes the individual emotional pain or frustration, or is a threat to self-esteem. Aggressive behaviour was often seen as a means of re-establishing control, improving mood or achieving retribution. It is important to note that nurses are often seen as rejecting clients; for example, when they hide behind a professional façade, when they objectify or belittle a client, when they treat the client as a 'person' but fail to allow the client to see *them* as a person or when they fail to carry out a promised action or dismiss someone's self-harming or angry behaviour as 'attention seeking' (Hem & Heggen, 2004).

CULTURAL CONSIDERATIONS

What a culture considers to be acceptable strongly influences the expression of anger. The nurse must be aware of cultural norms in order to provide culturally competent care. In the UK, women traditionally were not permitted to express anger openly and directly because doing so would not be 'feminine' and would challenge male authority. That cultural norm has changed slowly during the past 30 years. People from some cultures, such as some Asian people, see expressing anger as rude or disrespectful and try to avoid it at all costs. In these cultures, trying to help a client express anger verbally to an authority figure could prove unacceptable.

Spector (2001) conducted a literature review to study whether or not racial bias influences clinicians' perceptions of patient dangerousness in Britain and the US. She found that clinicians generally perceived patients with black skin (regardless of ethnicity or place of birth) as being more dangerous; this bias influenced treatment decisions (e.g. more compulsory hospitalizations, increased use of restraint and seclusion).

Two culture-bound syndromes involve aggressive behaviour. *Bouffée delirante*, a condition observed in West Africa and Haiti, is characterized by a sudden outburst of agitated and aggressive behaviour, marked confusion and psycho-motor excitement. These episodes may include visual and auditory hallucinations and paranoid ideation that resemble brief psychotic episodes. *Amok* is a dissociative episode characterized by a period of brooding followed by an outburst of violent, aggressive or homicidal behaviour directed at other people and objects. This behaviour is precipitated by a perceived slight or insult and is seen only in men. Originally reported from Malaysia, similar behaviour patterns are seen in Laos, the Philippines, Papua New Guinea, Polynesia (*cafard*), Puerto Rico (*mal de pelea*) and among the Navajo (*iich'aa*) (Moitabai, 2005).

CARE AND TREATMENT

The care and treatment of 'aggressive' clients often focuses on treating the underlying or co-morbid mental health problem, such as schizophrenia or bipolar disorder. Successful treatment of co-morbid disorders frequently results in successful treatment of aggressive behaviour. Lithium has been effective in treating 'aggressive' clients with bipolar disorder, conduct disorders (in children) and for people with learning disabilities. Carbamazepine (Tegretol) and valproic acid (Depakote) are sometimes used to treat aggression associated with dementia, psychosis and personality disorders. Atypical antipsychotic agents such as clozapine (Clozaril), risperidone (Risperdal) and olanzapine (Zyprexa) have been effective in treating aggressive clients with dementia, brain injury, learning disability and personality disorders. Benzodiazepines can reduce irritability and agitation in older adults with dementia, but they can result in the loss of social inhibition for other aggressive clients, thereby increasing rather than reducing their aggression.

This said, the relationship between mental disorder and anger is a complex one: it is far too easy for professionals to dismiss feelings of – and the expression of – anger as 'symptomatic', as part of a 'disease' process. The truth is often far more complex and – as with all of us – lies in the complex interaction between the neurological, the psychological and the social, between thoughts, feelings and behaviours, between people and their environment: anger and aggression are interpersonal and have a social dimension as well as an internal one. Nurses themselves can be a prime cause of aggression and violence in mental health services if they fail to act respectfully, if they fail to consider the impact of the environment and other people on individuals they're caring for, and if they fail to explore and develop their understanding of anger and aggression, including their own.

APPLICATION OF THE NURSING PROCESS

Effective assessment and sensitive engagement and intervention with angry or hostile clients can often prevent aggressive episodes. Early assessment, judicious use of medications, and skilled, respectful verbal interaction with an angry client can often prevent anger from escalating into physical aggression.

The nurse needs to assess individual clients carefully. A history of violent or aggressive behaviour is one of the best predictors of future aggression. Determining how the client with a history of aggression handles anger and what the client believes is helpful is important in assisting him or her to control or non-aggressively manage angry feelings. Clients who are angry and frustrated and believe that no one is listening to them are more prone to behave in a hostile or aggressive manner. In addition to a past history of violence, a history of being personally victimized and one of substance abuse increase a client's likelihood of aggressive behaviour. Individual cues can help the nurse recognize when aggressive behaviour is imminent (Pryor, 2005). These cues include: what the client is saying; changes in the client's voice – volume, pitch, speed; changes in the client's facial expression; and changes in the client's behaviour.

The nurse should assess the client's behaviour to determine which phase of the aggression cycle he or she is in, so that appropriate interventions can be implemented. The five phases of aggression and their signs, symptoms and behaviours are presented in Table 10.1. Assessment of clients must take place at a safe distance. The nurse can approach the client while maintaining an adequate distance so that the client does not feel trapped or threatened. To ensure staff safety and exhibit teamwork, and if it is possible, it may be prudent for two staff members to be with the client.

Data Analysis

Nursing formulations commonly used when working with aggressive clients include the following:

- Risk of violence towards others
- Ineffective coping.

If the client is intoxicated, depressed or psychotic, additional nursing formulations may be indicated.

Outcome Identification

Expected outcomes for aggressive clients may include the following:

1. The client will not harm or threaten others.
2. The client will refrain from behaviours that are intimidating or frightening to others.
3. The client will describe his or her feelings and concerns without aggression.
4. The client will attempt to work collaboratively with care and treatment.

Care of People in Inpatient Settings

The nurse should be aware of factors that influence aggression in an inpatient milieu. Predicting who might

Table 10.1   FIVE-PHASE AGGRESSION CYCLE

Phase	Definition	Signs, symptoms and behaviours
Triggering	An event or circumstances in the environment initiates the client's response, which is often one of anger or hostility	Restlessness, anxiety, irritability, pacing, muscle tension, rapid breathing, perspiration, loud voice, anger
Escalation	Client's responses represent escalating behaviours that indicate movement toward a loss of control	Pale or flushed face, yelling, swearing, agitated, threatening, demanding, clenched fists, threatening gestures, hostility, loss of ability to solve the problem or think clearly
Crisis	During a period of emotional and physical crisis, the client loses control	Loss of emotional and physical control, throwing objects, kicking, hitting, spitting, biting, scratching, shrieking, screaming, inability to communicate clearly
Recovery	Client regains physical and emotional control	Lowering of voice; decreased muscle tension; clearer, more rational communication; physical relaxation
Postcrisis	Client attempts reconciliation with others and returns to the level of functioning before the aggressive incident and its antecedents	Remorse; apologies; crying; quiet, withdrawn behaviour

Adapted from Keltner, N. L., Schwecke, L. H., & Bostrom, C. E. (2007). *Psychiatric nursing* (5th edn). St. Louis: Mosby.

become aggressive, when, and in what circumstances on an inpatient ward remains problematic. The research around the influence of historical factors, diagnosis and clinical factors, context factors and 'dispositional' factors, such as personality and demographics, has proved inconclusive (Anderson *et al.*, 2004; Woods & Ashley, 2007). However, high levels of planned engagement, a pleasant physical environment, well-supported, supervised and trained staff, purposeful activity, good leadership and good teamwork seem essential in reducing incidents (Huckshorn, 2004; Bowers *et al.*, 2006; Brennan *et al.*, 2006). Conversely, when predictability of meetings or groups and staff–client interactions are lacking, clients often felt frustrated and bored, and aggression is more common and intense. A lack of 'psychological space' – having no privacy, being unable to get sufficient rest – may be more important in triggering aggression than a lack of physical space.

Inevitably, some people will become angry, and care is most effective when that anger can be identified and defused at an early stage. The goal is to work with angry, hostile and potentially aggressive clients in learning to notice, understand and express their feelings verbally and safely, without threats or harm to others or destruction of property: 'de-escalation' is infinitely preferable to physical intervention.

Hostility or verbally aggressive behaviour can be intimidating or frightening even for experienced nurses. People exhibiting these behaviours can also be threatening to other clients, staff and visitors. In community settings, the most frequent response to hostile people is to get as far away from them as possible; in an inpatient setting, however, engaging the hostile person in dialogue may be most effective to prevent the behaviour from escalating to physical aggression.

It is NOT 'OK' or 'just part of the job' for nurses to be victims of violence; the Department of Health's zero tolerance campaign (Department of Health, 2000) and local policy initiatives have been part of an effort to counter this attitude. Violence does, nevertheless, happen, and it appears to be increasing: nurses need to work hard to find ways to collaborate with people, to be realistic about issues of risk and safety and to reduce the impact of violence on service users, on carers, on professionals and on society as a whole.

Intervention

As mentioned, interventions are most effective and least restrictive when implemented early in the cycle of aggression. This section presents interventions for the management of the milieu (which benefit all clients regardless of setting) and specific interventions for each phase of the aggression cycle.

MANAGING THE ENVIRONMENT: INPATIENT SETTINGS

It is important to consider the environment for all clients when trying to reduce or eliminate aggressive behaviour. Group and planned activities, such as playing card games, watching and discussing films or participating in informal discussions give clients the opportunity to talk about events or issues when they are calm. Activities also engage clients in the therapeutic process and minimize boredom. Scheduling one-to-one interactions with clients indicates the nurse's genuine interest in the client and a willingness to listen to the client's concerns, thoughts and feelings. Knowing what to expect enhances the client's feelings of security. The Star Wards project (2008) outlines hundreds of examples of good practice relating to ward milieu.

If clients have a conflict or dispute with one another, the nurse should offer the opportunity for problem-solving or conflict resolution. Expressing angry feelings appropriately, using assertive communication statements, and negotiating a solution are important skills that clients can practise. These skills will be useful for the client when he or she returns to the community.

If a client appears psychotic, hyperactive or intoxicated, the nurse must consider the safety and security of other clients, who may need protection from the intrusive or threatening demeanour of that client. Talking with other clients about their feelings is helpful, and close supervision of the client who is potentially aggressive is essential.

MANAGING AGGRESSIVE BEHAVIOUR IN INPATIENT UNITS

The management of aggressive behaviours starts with good collaborative engagement and trust. Where this has not been established, or has broken-down, 'de-escalation' (Box 10.1) may be necessary to help someone regain control of a situation and their response to it.

In the *triggering phase*, the nurse should approach the client in a non-threatening, calm manner in order to begin working with the person to de-escalate his or her thoughts, feelings and behaviour. Conveying empathy for the client's anger or frustration is important. The nurse can encourage the client to express his or her angry feelings verbally, suggesting that the client is still in control and can maintain that control. Use of clear, simple, short statements is helpful. The nurse should allow the client time to express himself or herself. The nurse can suggest that the client go to a quiet area or may get assistance to move other clients to decrease stimulation. When required, medications might be offered (if prescribed). As

the client's anger subsides, the nurse can help the client to use relaxation techniques and to look at ways to solve any problem or conflict that may exist (Marder, 2006). Physical activity, such as walking, may also help the client relax and become calmer.

If these techniques are unsuccessful and the client progresses to the *escalation phase*, the nurse must take control of the situation. The nurse should provide directions to the client in a calm, firm voice. The client should be directed to take time-out for cooling off in a quiet area or his or her room. The nurse should tell the client that aggressive behaviour is not acceptable here, and frightening for other people, and that the nurse is there to help the client regain control. If the client refused medications during the triggering phase, the nurse could offer them again.

If the client's behaviour continues to escalate and he or she is unwilling to accept direction to a quiet area, the nurse should obtain assistance from other staff members. Initially, four to six staff members should remain ready within sight of the client but not as close as the primary nurse talking with the client. This technique, sometimes called a 'show of force', indicates to the client that the staff will control the situation if the client cannot do so. Sometimes the presence of additional staff convinces the client to accept medication and take the time-out necessary to regain control. It may, however, also be counter-productive and feel threatening to the patient, thus potentially escalating the situation; knowledge of the patient and sensitivity to verbal and non-verbal cues is crucial here.

The short-term use of seclusion or restraint may be required during the *crisis phase* of the 'aggression cycle' (see Table 10.1) to protect the client and others from injury. Many legal and ethical safeguards govern the use of seclusion and restraint (see Chapter 9).

Box 10.1   DE-ESCALATION: NON-VERBAL AND VERBAL SKILLS AND TECHNIQUES

Skills, qualities and techniques:

- Beginning with compassion
- Ensuring space: physical and psychological
- Establishing rapport: attentiveness, concern and empathy
- Reflecting and active listening
- Displaying genuine curiosity: non-intrusive and gentle
- Using open questions
- Using non-alienating language
- Displaying confidence but being honest about impact of the person's behaviour

- Negotiating and co-operating: 'we' rather than 'you' and 'I'
- Modelling calmness: posture, voice, breathing, appropriate level of eye-contact
- Avoiding sudden movements
- Keeping hands visible
- Identifying source of person's anger
- Mutually understanding reasons for anger
- Drawing on previous coping techniques
- Exploring/suggesting alternatives
- Limit setting and maintaining clarity of goals

Adapted from Whittington, R. (2006). Preventing violence. In P. Callaghan & H. Waldock (Eds.), *Oxford handbook of mental health*. Oxford: Oxford University Press.

Seclusion and Restraint. If the client becomes physically aggressive (*crisis phase*), the staff must take charge of the situation for the safety of the client, staff and other clients. Mental health facilities offer training and practice in safe techniques for managing behavioural emergencies, and only staff with such training should participate in the restraint of a physically aggressive client. The nurse's decision to use seclusion or restraint should be based on the facility's protocols and standards for restraint and seclusion.

Restraint and its dangers (along with the prevalence of 'institutional racism' within the mental health services) were brought to the fore after the tragic death of David 'Rocky' Bennett in 1998 and the subsequent inquiry report, published in 2004 (Norfolk, Suffolk and Cambridgeshire Strategic Health Authority, 2004). As a result of lessons learned from this event, NICE guidelines were issued in 2005 (Box 10.2).

For aggressive clients with psychoses, rapid tranquillization can be used to decrease agitation and aggression, and provide sedation. An 'algorithm' for the safe and appropriate use of rapid tranquillization can be obtained from the following website: http://www.southstaffshealthcare.nhs.uk/corporate/policies/clinical/C.YEL.mm.C.pdfStaffs-.

As the client regains control (*recovery phase*), he or she is encouraged to talk about the situation or triggers that led to the aggressive behaviour. The nurse should help the client relax, perhaps sleep, and return to a calmer state.

It is important to help the client explore alternatives to aggressive behaviour by asking what the client or staff can do next time to avoid an aggressive episode. The nurse should also assess staff members for any injuries and complete the required documentation, such as incident reports and flow sheets. The staff should have a debriefing session to discuss the aggressive episode, how it was handled, what worked well or needed improvement and how the situation could have been defused more effectively. It also is important to encourage other clients to talk about their feelings regarding the incident. However, the aggressive client should not be discussed in detail with other clients.

In the *post-crisis phase*, the client is removed from restraint or seclusion as soon as he or she meets the behavioural criteria. The nurse should not lecture or chastise the client for the aggressive behaviour, but should discuss the behaviour in a calm, rational, adult-to-adult manner. The client should be reintegrated into the milieu and its activities as soon as he or she can participate.

A number of programmes are used in the UK to guide the management of aggression. Over the past decade these have become progressively more focused on de-escalation and prevention than on physical intervention. They include Management of Actual and Potential Aggression (MAPA) programmes and many others offered by the NHS and by private organizations.

Box 10.2   GUIDELINES FOR THE SHORT-TERM MANAGEMENT OF DISTURBED AND VIOLENT BEHAVIOUR

- Measures to reduce disturbed/violent behaviour need to be based on comprehensive risk assessment and risk management, and mental health service providers should ensure that there is a full risk-management strategy for all their services
- All staff whose need is determined by risk assessment should receive ongoing competency training to recognize anger, potential aggression, antecedents and risk factors of disturbed/violent behaviour and to monitor their own verbal and non-verbal behaviour. Training should include methods of anticipating, de-escalating or coping with disturbed/violent behaviour
- Rapid tranquillization, physical restraint and seclusion should only be considered once de-escalation and other strategies have failed to calm the service user. The intervention selected must be a reasonable and proportionate response to the risk posed by the service user

- Staff who may need to employ physical intervention (such as restraint) or seclusion and those involved in administering rapid tranquillization must be trained to an appropriate level in life support techniques (such as the use of defibrillators)
- During physical restraint one team member should be responsible for protecting and supporting the head and neck, where required. The team member who is responsible for supporting the head and neck should take responsibility for leading the team through the physical intervention process, and for ensuring that the airway and breathing are not compromised and that vital signs are monitored
- Service users identified to be at risk of disturbed/violent behaviour should be given the opportunity to have their needs and wishes recorded in the form of an advance directive

Adapted from http://www.nice.org.uk/nicemedia/pdf/cg025quickrefguide.pdf

CARE OF PEOPLE IN COMMUNITY SETTINGS

Engagement with people who may present with an increased level of risk in the community raises many issues. All Care Programme Approach care plans should consider issues of potential aggression and violence, and formal risk assessments and risk management plans are now common, if not yet universal. In addition to the risks involved in inpatient settings, nurses need to consider the dangers posed to people by their own family, 'friends' or neighbours *and* the dangers posed to the nurse by seeing people in their own homes. Community staff need to be aware of – and adhere strictly to – local 'lone worker' policies.

Assaults by clients in the community seem to be made more likely by stressful living situations, financial problems, alcohol and drugs and a reluctance to engage with services. Episodes of assault are often precipitated by denial of services, acute psychosis and/or excessive stimulation (Flannery *et al.*, 2006). Community mental health nurses and other professionals need to intervene to help alleviate social factors that may be leading to aggression and the risk of violence, and to ensure that engagement with services is beneficial, respectful and focused.

For many people who display aggressive behaviour, effective management of any co-morbid mental health problem can be the key to controlling aggression. Regular contact with care co-ordinators and other professionals; active, willing, informed participation in care and treatment (including medication if necessary); and participation in community support programmes can help the client to achieve stability. Cognitive-behavioural anger management groups and individual work – including dialectical behaviour therapy approaches – should be available to help clients recognize, acknowledge, notice and express their feelings, and to learn problem-solving, distress-tolerance and conflict-resolution techniques.

Post-Incident Support

Anger, aggression and violence can all be distressing to staff, other clients and, of course, the client themselves. There is a need for structured support – in teams and for individuals – to be in place for staff and clients, to deal with the emotional and practical aftermath of traumatic incidents. The effects of trauma on team and individual functioning can be severe and can radically affect the standard of care offered.

Some work has been carried out in the UK and other countries in offering support or 'debriefing' following incidents, although formal post-incident support remains the exception rather than the rule. It is vital that individuals involved in potentially traumatic incidents ensure that they seek out and obtain the support they feel they need, ideally from both within the service for which they work, and externally.

SELF-AWARENESS ISSUES

The nurse must be aware of how he or she deals with his or her own anger before helping clients do so. The nurse who is afraid of angry feelings may avoid a client's anger, which may allow the client's behaviour to escalate. If the nurse's response is angry, the situation can escalate into a power struggle, and the nurse may lose the opportunity to 'talk down' the client's anger.

It is important to practise and gain experience in using techniques for restraint and seclusion before attempting them with clients in crisis. There is a risk of staff injury whenever a client is aggressive. As outlined in the NICE guidelines (2003), ongoing education and practice of safe techniques are essential to minimize or avoid injury to both staff and clients. The nurse must be calm, non-judgemental and non-punitive when using techniques to control a client's aggressive behaviour. Inexperienced nurses can learn from watching and working alongside experienced nurses as they deal with clients who are hostile or aggressive.

When verbal techniques fail to defuse a client's anger and the client becomes aggressive, the nurse may feel frustrated or angry, as if he or she failed. The client's aggressive behaviour, however, does not necessarily reflect the nurse's skills and abilities. Some clients have a limited capacity to control their aggressive behaviours, and the nurse can help them to learn alternative ways to handle angry or aggressive impulses.

CLINICAL VIGNETTE: ESCALATION PHASE

John, 35 years of age, was admitted to the hospital on Section 2 after being assessed by the crisis resolution team. John has a history of aggressive behaviour, usually precipitated by voices telling him he will be harmed by staff and must kill them to protect himself. John had not been taking his prescribed medication for 2 weeks before hospitalization. The nurse observes John pacing in the hall, muttering to himself, and avoiding close contact with anyone else.

Suddenly, John begins to yell, 'I can't take it. I can't stay here!' His fists are clenched, and he is very agitated. The nurse approaches John, remaining 6 feet away from him, and says, 'John, tell me what's happening'. John runs to the end of the hall and won't talk to the nurse. The nurse asks John if he'd take some medication and go to his room, as she thinks it might help him. He refuses both. As he begins to pick up objects from a nearby table, the nurse summons other staff to assist

Points to Consider When Working With Clients Who Are Angry, Hostile or Aggressive

- Identify how *you* handle angry feelings; assess your use of assertive communication and conflict resolution.
- Increasing your skills in dealing with your angry feelings will help you to work more effectively with clients.
- Discuss situations or the care of potentially aggressive clients with experienced nurses.
- Do not take the client's anger or aggressive behaviour personally or as a measure of your effectiveness as a nurse.

Critical Thinking Questions

1. Many community-based residential services will not admit a client with a recent history of aggression. Is this fair to the client? What factors should influence such decisions?
2. If an aggressive client injures another client or a staff person, should criminal charges be filed against the client? Why/why not?

KEY POINTS

- Anger, expressed appropriately, can be a positive force that helps the person solve problems and make decisions.
- Hostility, also called verbal aggression, is behaviour meant to intimidate or cause emotional harm to another and can lead to physical aggression.
- Physical aggression is behaviour meant to harm, punish or force into compliance another person.
- Most people with mental health problems are not aggressive. Clients diagnosed with schizophrenia, bipolar disorder, dementia, head injury, antisocial or bor-

derline personality disorders or conduct disorder, and those intoxicated with alcohol or other drugs, may be aggressive. Anger and aggression may or may not be a direct result of 'symptoms': they are likely to be the result of a combination of factors – intrapersonal and interpersonal.
- Care and treatment of aggressive clients necessitates high-quality therapeutic engagement and sometimes involves treating the 'co-morbid' mental health disorder with mood stabilizers or antipsychotic medications.
- Collaborative assessment, psycho-education and effective intervention with angry or hostile clients can often prevent aggressive episodes.
- Aggressive behaviour is less common and less intense on units with strong leadership, clear staff roles and planned and adequate events, such as staff–client interaction, group interaction and activities.
- The nurse must be familiar with the signs, symptoms and behaviours associated with the triggering, escalation, crisis, recovery and post-crisis phases of the aggression cycle.
- In the triggering phase, nursing interventions include speaking calmly and non-threateningly, conveying empathy, listening, offering medication when required and suggesting retreat to a quiet area.
- In the escalation phase, interventions include using a directive approach, taking control of the situation, using a calm, firm voice for giving directions, directing the client to take a time-out in a quiet place, offering medication when required and, on occasion, making a 'show of force'.
- In the crisis phase, experienced, trained staff can use the techniques of seclusion or restraint to deal quickly with the client's aggression.
- During the recovery phase, interventions include helping clients to relax, assisting them to regain self-control and discussing the aggressive event rationally.
- In the post-crisis phase, the client is re-integrated into the milieu.
- Important self-awareness issues include examining how one handles angry feelings and deals with one's own reactions to angry clients.

INTERNET RESOURCES

RESOURCES	INTERNET ADDRESS
British Association of Anger Management	http://www.angermanage.co.uk/
Everyman Project	http://www.everymanproject.co.uk

Nursing Care Plan *Aggressive Behaviour*

Nursing Formulation

Risk of Violence Towards Others: *The person is at risk of behaviours in which he/she could be physically, emotionally and/or sexually harmful to others.*

RISK FACTORS

- Actual physical violence
- Destruction of/damage to property
- Homicidal or suicidal ideation
- Physical danger to self or others
- History of assaultive behaviour or other forensic history
- Neurological illness
- Disordered thoughts
- Agitation or restlessness
- Lack of impulse control
- Delusions, hallucinations or other psychotic experiences
- Diagnosis of personality disorder or other mental health disorders
- Manic/labile behaviour
- Conduct disorder
- Posttraumatic stress disorder (PTSD)
- Substance use

EXPECTED OUTCOMES

Immediate
The person will
- Not harm others or destroy property
- Be free of self-harming behaviours
- Decrease 'acting-out' behaviour
- Experience decreased restlessness or agitation
- Experience decreased fear, anxiety or hostility

Medium-term
The person will
- Demonstrate the ability to be mindful of, and exercise internal control over, his or her thoughts, feelings and behaviour
- Be free of psychotic or disturbed thoughts, feelings and behaviour
- Identify ways to deal with tension and aggressive feelings in a non-destructive manner
- Express feelings of anxiety, fear, anger or hostility verbally or in a non-destructive manner
- Verbalize an understanding of aggressive behaviour, associated disorder(s) and medications, if any

Longer-term
The person will
- Participate in therapy for underlying or associated mental health problems
- Demonstrate internal awareness and control of behaviour when confronted with stress

IMPLEMENTATION

Nursing Interventions *denotes collaborative interventions

Build a trusting relationship with this client as soon as possible, ideally well in advance of aggressive episodes.

Be aware of factors that increase the likelihood of violent behaviour or that signify a build-up of agitation. Use verbal communication or medication as required to intervene before the client's behaviour reaches a destructive or violent point and physical restraint becomes necessary.

Rationale

Familiarity with and trust in the staff members can decrease the client's fears and facilitate communication.

A period of building tension often precedes acting out or violent behaviour; however, a client who is intoxicated or psychotic may become violent without warning. Signs of increasing agitation include increased restlessness, verbal cues, motor activity (e.g. pacing), voice volume, verbal cues ('I'm afraid of losing control'), threats, decreased frustration tolerance and frowning or clenching fists.

continued ⋯⟩

Nursing Care Plan: Aggressive Behaviour, cont.

IMPLEMENTATION

Nursing Interventions *denotes collaborative interventions	**Rationale**
Decrease environmental stimulation by turning stereo or television off or lowering the volume; lowering the lights; if in inpatient unit, ask other clients, visitors or others to leave the area (or you can go with the client to another room).	If the client is feeling threatened, he or she can perceive any stimulus as a threat. The client is unable to deal with excess stimuli when agitated.
If the client tells you (verbally or non-verbally) that he or she feels hostile or destructive, try to help the client express these feelings in non-destructive ways (e.g. use communication techniques, or take the client to the gym for physical exercise).	The client may need to learn non-destructive ways to express feelings. The client can try out new behaviours with you in a non-threatening environment and learn to focus on expressing emotions rather than acting out.
Calmly and respectfully assure the client that you (the staff) will provide control if he or she can not control himself or herself, but do not threaten the client.	The client may fear loss of control and may be afraid of what he or she may do if he or she begins to express anger. Showing that you are in control without competing with the client can reassure the client without lowering his or her self-esteem.
Be aware of medication requirements and procedures for seclusion or restraint.	In an aggressive situation you will need to make decisions and act quickly. If the client is severely agitated, medication may be necessary to decrease the agitation. You must be prepared to act and direct other staff in the safe management of the client. You are legally accountable for your decisions and actions.
Always maintain control of yourself and the situation; remain calm. If you do not feel competent in dealing with a situation, obtain assistance as soon as possible.	Your behaviour provides a role model for the client and communicates that you can and will provide control.
If you are not properly trained or skilled in dealing safely with a client who has a weapon, do not attempt to remove the weapon. Keep something (like a pillow, mattress or a blanket wrapped around your arm) between you and the weapon.	Avoiding personal injury, summoning help, leaving the area or protecting other clients may be the only things you can realistically do. You may risk further danger by attempting to remove a weapon or subdue an armed client.
If it is necessary to remove the weapon, try to kick it out of the client's hand. (Never reach for a knife or other weapon with your hand.)	Reaching for a weapon increases your physical vulnerability.
Distract the client momentarily to remove the weapon (throw water in the client's face, or yell suddenly).	Distracting the client's attention may give you an opportunity to remove the weapon or subdue the client.
*You may need to summon outside assistance (especially if the client has a weapon). When this is done, total responsibility is delegated to the outside authorities.	Exceeding your abilities may place you in grave danger. It is not necessary to try to deal with a situation beyond your control or to assume personal risk.
*Notify the person in charge as soon as possible in a (potentially) aggressive situation; tell them your assessment of the situation and the need for help, the client's name, care plan and orders for medication, seclusion or restraint.	You may need assistance from staff members who are unfamiliar with this client. They will be able to help more effectively and safely if they are aware of this information.

continued ⋯⇢

Nursing Care Plan: Aggressive Behaviour, cont.

IMPLEMENTATION

Nursing Interventions *denotes collaborative interventions

Rationale

*Follow local emergency response procedures, then, if possible, have one staff member meet the additional staff at the unit door to give them the client's name, situation, goal, plan and so forth.

The need for help may be immediate in an emergency situation. Any information that can be given to arriving staff will be helpful in ensuring safety and effectiveness in dealing with this client.

Do not use physical restraints or techniques without sufficient reason (refer to local and national guidelines).

The client has a right to the fewest restrictions possible within the limits of safety and prevention of destructive behaviour.

Remain aware of the client's body space or territory; do not trap the client.

Potentially violent people have a body space zone up to four times larger than that of other people. That is, you need to stay farther away from them for them to not feel trapped or threatened.

Allow the client freedom to move around (within safe limits) unless you are trying to restrain him or her.

Interfering with the client's mobility without the intent of restraint may increase the client's frustration, fears or perception of threat.

Talk with the client in a low, calm voice. Call the client by name, tell the client your name, where you are, and so forth.

Using a low voice may help prevent increasing agitation. The client may be disoriented or unaware of what is happening.

Tell the client what you are going to do and what you are doing. Use simple, clear, direct speech; repeat if necessary. Do not threaten the client, but state limits and expectations.

The client's ability to understand the situation and to process information is impaired. Clear limits let the client know what is expected of him or her.

*When a decision has been made to subdue or restrain the client, act quickly and co-operatively with other staff members. Tell the client in a matter-of-fact manner that he or she will be restrained, subdued or secluded; allow no bargaining after the decision has been made. Reassure the client that he or she will not be hurt and that restraint or seclusion is to ensure safety.

Firm limits must be set and maintained. Bargaining interjects doubt and will undermine the limit.

*While subduing or restraining the client, talk with other staff members to ensure co-ordination of effort (e.g. do not attempt to carry the client until you are sure that everyone is ready).

Direct verbal communication will promote co-operation and safety.

Do not strike the client.

Physical safety of the client is a priority.

Do not help to restrain or subdue the client if you are angry (if enough other staff members are present). Do not restrain or subdue the client as a punishment.

Staff members must maintain self-control at all times and act in the client's best interest. There is no justification for being punitive to a client.

Do not recruit or allow other clients to help in restraining or subduing a client.

Physical safety of all clients is a priority. Other clients are not responsible for controlling the behaviour of a client and should not assume a staff role.

If possible, do not allow other clients to watch staff subduing the client. Take them to a different area, and involve them in activities or discussion.

Other clients may be frightened, agitated or endangered by an aggressive client. They need safety and reassurance at this time.

continued ⋯⟶

Nursing Care Plan: Aggressive Behaviour, cont.

IMPLEMENTATION

Nursing Interventions *denotes collaborative interventions	**Rationale**
*Develop and practise consistent techniques of restraint as part of nursing orientation and continuing education.	Consistent techniques let each staff person know what is expected and will increase safety and effectiveness.
*Develop instructions in safe techniques for carrying clients. Obtain additional staff assistance when needed. Have someone clear furniture and so forth from the area through which you will be carrying the client.	Consistent techniques increase safety and effectiveness. Transporting a client who is agitated can be dangerous if attempted without sufficient help and sufficient space.
When placing the client in restraints or seclusion, tell the client what you are doing and the reason (e.g. to regain control or protect the client from injuring himself, herself or others). Use simple, concise language in a non-judgemental, matter-of-fact manner.	The client's ability to understand what is happening to him or her may be impaired.
Tell the client where he or she is, that he or she will be safe and that staff members will check on him or her. Tell the client how to summon the staff. Reorient the client or remind him or her of the reason for restraint as necessary.	Being placed in seclusion or restraints can be terrifying to a client. Your assurances may help alleviate the client's fears.
Reassess the client's need for continued seclusion or restraint and release the client or decrease restraint as soon as it is safe and therapeutic. Base your decisions on the client's, not the staff's, needs.	The client has a right to the least restrictions possible within the limits of safety and prevention of destructive behaviour.
Remain aware of the client's feelings (including fear), dignity and rights.	The client is a worthwhile person regardless of his or her unacceptable behaviour.
Carefully observe the client, and promptly complete documentation in keeping with hospital policy. Bear in mind possible legal implications.	Accurate, complete documentation is essential, as restraint, seclusion, assault and so forth are situations that may result in legal action.
Administer medications safely; take care to prepare correct dosage, identify correct sites for administration, withdraw plunger to aspirate for blood, and so forth.	When you are in a stressful situation and under pressure to move quickly, the possibility of errors in dosage or administration of medication is increased.
Take care to avoid needlestick injury and other injuries that may involve exposure to the client's blood or body fluids.	Hepatitis C, HIV and other diseases are transmitted by exposure to blood or body fluids.
Monitor the client for effects of medications and intervene as appropriate.	Psychoactive drugs can have adverse effects such as allergic reactions, hypotension, and pseudoparkinsonian symptoms.
Talk with other clients after the situation is resolved; allow them to express feelings about the situation.	The other clients have their own needs and problems. Be careful not to give attention only to the client who is acting out.

Adapted from Schultz, M., & Videbeck, S. L. (2005). *Lippincott's manual of psychiatric nursing care plans* (7th edn). Philadelphia: Lippincott Williams & Wilkins.

REFERENCES

Akiskal, H. S. (2005). Mood disorders: Historical introduction and conceptual overview. In B. J. Sadock & V. A. Sadock (Eds.), *Comprehensive textbook of psychiatry, Vol. 1* (8th edn, pp. 1559–1575). Philadelphia: Lippincott Williams & Wilkins.

American Psychiatric Association. (2000). *Diagnostic and statistical manual of mental disorders* (4th edn, text revision). Washington, DC: American Psychiatric Association.

Anderson, T. R., Bell, C. C., Powell, T. E., et al. (2004). Assessing psychiatric patients for violence. *Community Mental Health Journal, 40*, 379–399.

Blackmore, S. (2003). *Consciousness: An introduction.* Oxford: Oxford University Press.

Bowers, L., Flood, C., Brennan, G., LiPang, M., & Oladapo, P. (2006). A trial to reduce conflict and containment on acute psychiatric wards: City Nurses. *Journal of Psychiatric and Mental Health Nursing, 13*, 165–172.

Brennan, G., Flood, C., & Bowers, L. (2006). Constraints and blocks to change and improvement on acute psychiatric wards – lessons from the City Nurses project. *Journal of Psychiatric and Mental Health Nursing, 13*, 475–482.

Bright. (2008). Star Wards. Available: http://starwards.org.uk/

Department of Health. (2000). *NHS zero tolerance zone campaign: Tackling violence in primary care, ambulance, mental health, and community settings. Available:* http://www.dh.gov.uk/en/Publicationsandstatistics/Lettersandcirculars/Dearcolleagueletters/DH_4002920

Dunbar, B. (2004). Anger management: a holistic approach. *Journal of the American Psychiatric Nurses Association, 10*(1), 16–23.

Flannery, R. J. Jr, Laudani, L., Levitre, V., & Walker, A. P. (2006). Precipitants of psychiatric patient assaults on staff: three-year empirical inquiry of the Assaulted Staff Action Program (ASAP). *International Journal of Emergency Mental Health, 8*(1), 15–22.

Greenberg, H. A. (2005). Impulse-control disorders not elsewhere specified. In B. J. Sadock & V. A. Sadock (Eds.), *Comprehensive textbook of psychiatry, Vol.1* (8th edn, pp. 2035–2054). Philadelphia: Lippincott Williams & Wilkins.

Hem, M. & Heggen, K. (2004). Rejection – a neglected phenomenon in psychiatric nursing. *Journal of Psychiatric and Mental Health Nursing, 11*, 55–59.

Huckshorn, K. A. (2004). Reducing seclusion and restraint use in mental health settings: core strategies for prevention. *Journal of Psychosocial Nursing, 42*(9), 22–33.

Jacob, R. G. & Pelham, W. E. (2005). Behaviour therapy. In B. J. Sadock & V. A. Sadock (Eds.), *Comprehensive textbook of psychiatry, Vol. 2* (8th edn, pp. 2498–2548). Philadelphia: Lippincott Williams & Wilkins.

Johnson, M. E. (2004). Violence on inpatient psychiatric units: State of the science. *Journal of the American Psychiatric Nurses Association, 10*(3), 113–121.

Kabat-Zinn, J. (2005). Coming to our senses: Healing ourselves and the world through mindfulness. London: Piatkus

Leary, M. R., Twenge, J. M., & Quinlivan, E. (2006). Interpersonal rejection as a determinant of anger and aggression. *Personality and Social Psychology Review, 10*(2), 1111–1132.

Linehan, M. (2007). *Dialectical behaviour therapy in clinical practice: Applications across disorders and settings.* New York: Guilford.

Marder, S. R. (2006). A review of agitation in mental illness: treatment guidelines and current therapies. *Journal of Clinical Psychiatry, 67* (Suppl. 10), 13–21.

Mental Health Alliance (2008) *Factbase: mental health and public safety.* Available: http://www.mentalhealthalliance.org.uk/policy/factbase.html

Moitabai, R. (2005). Culture-bound syndromes with psychotic features. In B. J. Sadock & V. A. Sadock (Eds.), *Comprehensive textbook of psychiatry, Vol. 1* (8th edn, pp. 1538–1542). Philadelphia: Lippincott Williams & Wilkins.

NICE. (2003). *Schizophrenia: Full national clinical guideline on core interventions in primary and secondary care.* Available: http://nccmh.claromentis.com/intranet/documents/1545/11999/cg001fullguideline.pdf

NICE. (2005). Violence: The short-term management of disturbed/violent behaviour in inpatient psychiatric settings and emergency departments. London: Royal College of Nursing.

Norfolk, Suffolk and Cambridgeshire Strategic Health Authority. (2004). *Independent inquiry into the death of David 'Rocky' Bennett chaired by Sir John Blofeld.* Available: http://image.guardian.co.uk/sys-files/Society/documents/2004/02/12/Bennett.pdf

Pryor, J. (2005). What cues do nurses use to predict aggression in people with acquired brain injury? *Journal of Neuroscience Nursing, 37*(2), 117–121.

Schultz, J. M. & Videbeck, S. L. (2005). *Lippincott's manual of psychiatric nursing care plans* (7th edn). Philadelphia: Lippincott Williams & Wilkins.

Shapiro, P. A. (2005). Cardiovascular disorders. In B. J. Sadock & V. A. Sadock (Eds.), *Comprehensive textbook of psychiatry, Vol. 2* (8th edn, pp. 2136–2148). Philadelphia: Lippincott Williams & Wilkins.

Spector, R. (2001). Is there racial bias in clinicians' perceptions of the dangerousness of psychiatric patients? A review of the literature. *Journal of Mental Health, 10*(1), 5–15.

Thomas, S. P. (2005). Women's anger, aggression, and violence. *Health Care for Women International, 26*(6), 504–522.

Woods, P. & Ashley, C. (2007). Violence and aggression: a literature review. *Journal of Psychiatric and Mental Health Nursing, 14*(7), 652–660.

ADDITIONAL READING

Bowers, L., Allan, T., Simpson, A., Nijman, H., & Warren, J. (2007). Adverse incidents, patient flow and nursing workforce variables on acute psychiatric wards: the Tompkins Acute Ward Study. *International Journal of Social Psychiatry, 53*(1),75–84.

Champagne, T. & Stromberg, N. (2004). Sensory approaches in inpatient psychiatric settings: innovative alternatives to seclusion and restraint. *Journal of Psychosocial Nursing, 42*(9), 35–44.

Dryden, W. (1996). *Overcoming anger: when anger helps and when it hurts.* London: Sheldon.

Foster, C., Bowers, L., & Nijman, H. (2007). Aggressive behaviour on acute psychiatric wards: prevalence, severity and management. *Journal of Advanced Nursing, 58*(2),140–149

Ilkiw-Lavalle, O. & Grenyer, B. F. S. (2003). Differences between patient and staff perceptions of aggression in mental health units. *Psychiatric Services, 54*(3), 389–393.

Needham, I., Abderhalden, C., Halfens, R. J., et al. (2005). Non-somatic effects of patient aggression on nurses: a systematic review. *Journal of Advanced Nursing, 49*(3), 283–296.

Nhat Hanh, T. (2001). *Anger: Buddhist wisdom for cooling the flames.* London: Rider.

Veltkamp, E., Nijman, H., Stolker, J., Frigge, K., Dries, P., & Bowers, L. (2008). Seclusion or forced medication, patient's preferences. *Psychiatric Services, 59*, 209–211.

Chapter Study Guide

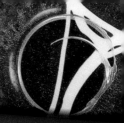

MULTIPLE CHOICE QUESTIONS

Select the best answer for each of the following questions.

1. Which of the following is an example of assertive communication?
   a. 'I wish you would stop making me angry.'
   b. 'I feel angry when you walk away when I'm talking.'
   c. 'You never listen to me when I'm talking.'
   d. 'You make me angry when you interrupt me.'

2. Which of the following statements about anger is true?
   a. Expressing anger openly and directly usually leads to arguments.
   b. Anger results from being frustrated, hurt or afraid.
   c. Suppressing anger is a sign of maturity.
   d. Angry feelings are a negative response to a situation.

3. Which of the following types of drugs requires cautious use with potentially aggressive clients?
   a. Antipsychotic medications
   b. Benzodiazepines
   c. Mood stabilizers
   d. Lithium

4. A client is pacing in the hallway with clenched fists and a flushed face. He is yelling and swearing. Which phase of the aggression cycle is he probably in?
   a. Anger
   b. Triggering
   c. Escalation
   d. Crisis

5. The nurse observes a client muttering to himself and pounding his fist in his other hand while pacing in the hallway. Which of the following principles should guide the nurse's action?
   a. Only one nurse should approach an upset client to avoid threatening the client.
   b. Clients who can verbalize angry feelings are less likely to become physically aggressive.
   c. Talking to a client with delusions is not helpful, because the client has no ability to reason.
   d. Verbally aggressive clients often calm down on their own if staff members don't bother them.

GROUP DISCUSSION

1. What makes you angry?

2. Explore together each of the phases of the aggression cycle.

3. Describe aspects of a nurse's behaviour that might contribute to a client feeling angry.

4. Describe aspects of the environment in an acute mental health unit that might contribute to someone feeling angry.

5. Discuss interventions the nurse might use for a client who becomes aggressive without warning.

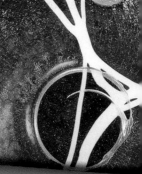

Chapter

11

Abuse and Violence

Key Terms

- abuse
- acute stress disorder
- child abuse
- cycle of violence
- date rape (acquaintance rape)
- dissociation
- elder abuse
- family violence
- grounding techniques
- intergenerational transmission process
- neglect
- physical abuse
- posttraumatic stress disorder
- psychological abuse (emotional abuse)
- rape
- repressed memories
- sexual abuse
- spouse or partner abuse
- stalking
- survivor

Learning Objectives

After reading this chapter, you should be able to:

1. Discuss the characteristics, risk factors and family dynamics of abusive and violent behaviour.

2. Examine the incidences of and trends in domestic violence, child and elder abuse and rape.

3. Describe responses to abuse, specifically posttraumatic stress disorder and dissociative identity disorder.

4. Apply the nursing process to the care of clients who have survived abuse and violence.

5. Provide education to clients, families and communities to promote prevention and early intervention of abuse and violence.

6. Evaluate your own experiences, feelings, attitudes and beliefs about abusive and violent behaviour.

According to the Office of National Statistics:

Men outnumber women across all major crime categories. Between 83 and 94 per cent of offenders found guilty of burglary, robbery, drug offences, criminal damage or violence against the person were male. Although the number of offenders was relatively small, 98 per cent of those found guilty of or cautioned for sexual offences were male … The 2005/06 British Crime Survey showed that the risk of being a victim of domestic violence was three times higher for women than for men – 0.6 per cent of women had been a victim of domestic violence, compared with 0.2 per cent of men. The risk of being involved in a violent incident caused by a stranger remains substantially greater for men than for women, with men being three times more likely than women to suffer this form of attack.

(Source: Office of National Statistics. (2008). *Focus on gender*.
Available: http://www.statistics.gov.uk/focuson/gender/)

See also Box 11.1.

Box 11.1   VIOLENT CRIME IN BRITAIN

According to the Home Office (2008a):

- In 2007–2008 there were 2,164,000 violent offences – 1,292,000 against men and 875,000 against women.
- There were:
  around 17,000 incidents of serious wounding
  228,000 incidents of harassment
  nearly 22,000 assaults on policemen
  around 2700 sexual assaults on male children
  nearly 17,000 assaults on females over 13
  over 4000 on female children
  53,540 sexual offences in total were recorded.

In addition (Home Office, 2008b):

- Domestic violence accounts for 15% of all violent incidents.
- One in four women and one in six men will be a victim of domestic violence in their lifetime, with women at greater risk of repeat victimization and serious injury.
- 89% of those suffering four or more incidents are women.
- One incident of domestic violence is reported to the police every minute.
- On average, two women a week are killed by a current or former male partner.

and

- It is estimated that 750,000 women in Britain have been the victims of rape (Home Office, 2002).

Violent behaviour is a major national concern: the media is crowded with stories and comment. The most alarming statistics relate to violence in the home; most abuse is perpetrated by someone the victim knows. Victims of abuse are found across the life span, and they can be spouses or partners, children or elderly parents. Mental health nurses are in a key position to help detect abuse, protect people and help prevent it happening.

This chapter discusses domestic abuse (spouse abuse, child abuse/neglect, elder abuse) and rape. Because many survivors of abuse suffer long-term emotional trauma, it also discusses disorders associated with abuse and violence: PTSD and dissociative disorders. Other major problems associated with abuse and trauma include psychosis (see Chapter 14), personality disorders (see Chapter 16), substance abuse (see Chapter 17) and depression (see Chapter 15).

CLINICAL PICTURE OF ABUSE AND VIOLENCE

Victims of abuse or violence will often, of course, have physical injuries, but they also experience short-term and longer-term psychological injuries. In the short term, some people are agitated and visibly upset; others are withdrawn and aloof, appearing numb or oblivious to their surroundings; others still may be avoidant of places and people that remind them of their experiences. In the longer term, substance misuse problems, anxiety and depression and PTSD may result.

Domestic violence often remains undisclosed for months, or even years, because victims fear their abusers or have been manipulated into protecting them. Victims thus frequently suppress their anger and resentment and tell no-one: this is particularly true in cases of childhood sexual abuse. Survivors of abuse often suffer in silence and continue to feel guilt and shame. Children, particularly, come to believe that somehow they are at fault and did something to deserve or provoke the abuse. They are more likely to miss school, are less likely to attend further education and continue to have problems through adolescence into adulthood. As adults, they often feel guilt or shame for not trying to stop the abuse. They may feel degraded, humiliated and dehumanized. Their self-esteem may be extremely low, and they may view themselves as unlovable. They may believe they are unacceptable to others, contaminated or ruined. Depression and other mental health problems, suicidal behaviour, marital and sexual difficulties are common.

Victims and survivors of abuse may have problems relating to others. They can find it difficult to trust others, especially authority figures. In relationships, their emotional reactions may well be erratic, intense and perceived as unpredictable. Intimate relationships may trigger extreme emotional responses such as panic, anxiety, fear and terror. Even when survivors of abuse desire closeness with another person, they may perceive that closeness as intrusive and threatening.

Nurses should be particularly sensitive to the abused client's need to feel safe, secure and in control of his or her body. They should take care to maintain the client's personal space, assess the client's anxiety level and ask permission before touching him or her for any reason. Because the nurse may not always be aware of a history of abuse when initially working with a client, he or she should apply these cautions to all clients in the mental health setting.

Asking about abuse – sensitively and respectfully – should be incorporated into the assessment process in all settings:

> If clinicians conducting an initial assessment decide to delay the inquiry they should record clearly that a trauma history has not been taken (and why) and take responsibility for following up when the client is less distressed. Clinicians who are tempted to wait for some magic moment when rapport is just right should remember that, for many abused clients, asking may be a crucial act that encourages rapport rather than creates a barrier to it. For some clients, it might even be a prerequisite.
>
> (Read *et al.*, 2007, p. 105)

CHARACTERISTICS OF VIOLENT FAMILIES

Family violence encompasses violence towards a partner; neglect and physical, emotional or sexual abuse of children; elder abuse; and marital rape. In many cases, family members tolerate abusive and violent behaviour from relatives that they would never accept from strangers. In violent families, the home, which is normally a safe haven of love and protection, may be the most dangerous place for victims.

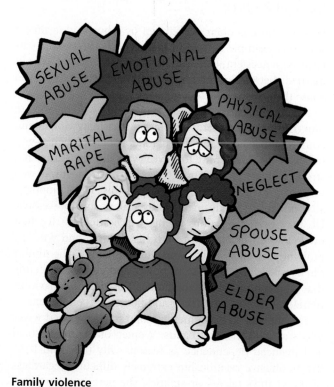

Family violence

<table>
<tr><td>Box 11.2</td><td>CHARACTERISTICS OF VIOLENT FAMILIES</td></tr>
</table>

Social isolation
Abuse of power and control
Alcohol and other drug abuse
Intergenerational transmission process

Research studies have identified some common characteristics of violent families regardless of the type of abuse that exists. They are discussed next and in Box 11.2.

Social Isolation

One characteristic of violent families is social isolation. Members of these families keep to themselves and do not usually invite others into the home or tell them what is happening. Often, abusers threaten victims with even greater harm if they reveal the secret. They may tell children that a parent, sibling or pet will die if anyone outside the family learns of the abuse. As a result, children keep the secret out of fear, which prevents others from 'interfering with private family business'.

Abuse of Power and Control

The abusive family member almost always holds a position of power and control over the victim (child, spouse or elderly parent). The abuser not only exerts physical power but also economic and social control. The abuser is often the only family member who makes decisions, spends money or spends time outside the home with other people. The abuser belittles and blames the victim, often by using threats and emotional manipulation. If the abuser perceives any indication, real or imagined, of victim independence or disobedience, violence usually escalates.

Alcohol and Other Drug Abuse

Substance abuse, especially alcoholism, has been associated with family violence. This finding does not imply a direct cause and effect relationship. Alcohol does not necessarily cause the person to be abusive; rather, an abusive person is also likely to use alcohol or other drugs. Although alcohol may not cause the abuse, many researchers believe that alcohol may diminish inhibitions and make violent behaviour more intense or frequent.

Alcohol is also a major factor in **acquaintance** or **date rape**. According to the US Marin Institute (2006), 40% of convicted rape and sexual assault offenders reported drinking alcohol at the time of their crime. Horvath & Brown (2006) found that alcohol played a role in three out of every four date rapes or sexual assaults. They concluded that alcohol was used by those intent on sexual assault, with attackers more likely to take advantage of victims who had been drinking. The use of the drugs Rohypnol and gamma hydroxybutyrate (GHB) to subdue potential victims of date rape, while clearly common, seemed to have far less influence.

Intergenerational Transmission Process

The concept of the **intergenerational transmission process** suggests that patterns of violence are perpetuated from one generation to the next through role-modelling and social learning (van der Kolk, 2005). Intergenerational transmission indicates that family violence is a learned pattern of behaviour. For example, children who witness violence between their parents learn that violence is a way to resolve conflict and is an integral part of a close relationship. Statistics show that one-third of abusive men are likely to have come from violent homes where they witnessed wife-beating or were abused themselves. Women who grew up in violent homes are 50% more likely to expect or accept violence in their own relationships. Not all persons exposed to family violence, however, become abusive or violent as adults. Therefore, this single factor does not explain the perpetuation of violent behaviour.

CULTURAL CONSIDERATIONS

Although domestic violence affects families of all ethnicities, races, ages, national origins, sexual orientations, religions and socioeconomic backgrounds, a specific population is particularly at risk: immigrant women. Abused immigrant women face legal, social and economic problems different from UK citizens who are assaulted, and from people of other cultural, racial and ethnic origins who are not assaulted:

- The abused woman may come from a culture that more easily condones violence against women.
- She may have – or believe she has – less access to legal and social services than do British citizens.
- If she is not a citizen, she may be forced to leave the UK if she seeks legal sanctions against her husband or attempts to leave him.
- She is isolated by cultural dynamics that may not permit her to leave her husband; economically, she may be unable to gather the resources to leave, work or go to school.
- Language barriers may interfere with her ability to call 999, learn about her rights or legal options and obtain shelter, financial assistance or food.

It may be necessary for the nurse to obtain the assistance of an interpreter whom the woman trusts, make referrals to legal services and assist the woman to contact local support organizations to help deal with these additional concerns.

SPOUSE OR PARTNER ABUSE

Spouse or partner abuse is the mistreatment or misuse of one person by another in the context of an intimate relationship. The abuse can be emotional or psychological, physical, sexual or a combination (which is common). **Psychological abuse (emotional abuse)** includes name-calling, belittling, screaming, yelling, destroying property and making threats, as well as subtler forms such as refusing to speak to, or ignoring, the victim. **Physical abuse** ranges from shoving and pushing to severe battering and choking, and may involve broken limbs and ribs, internal bleeding, brain damage and even murder. Sexual abuse includes assaults during sexual relations such as biting nipples, pulling hair, slapping and hitting and rape (discussed later).

Somewhere between 2.5 and 3.4% of women experience violence while pregnant. Violence during pregnancy leads to adverse outcomes, such as miscarriage and stillbirth, as well as to further physical and psychological problems for the woman. The increase in violence may often be due to the partner's jealousy, possessiveness, insecurity and lessened physical and emotional availability of the pregnant woman (Bacchus et al., 2006).

Domestic violence seems to occur in same-sex relationships with the same statistical frequency as in heterosexual relationships. Although same-sex violence mirrors heterosexual violence in prevalence, its victims receive less protection. The same-sex abuser has an additional possible weapon to use against the victim: the threat of revealing the partner's homosexuality to friends, family, employers or the community.

Clinical Picture

Because abuse is often perpetrated by a husband against a wife, that example is used in this section. These same patterns are consistent, however, between partners who are not married, between same-sex partners and with wives who abuse their husbands.

An abusive husband often believes his wife belongs to him (is his property) and becomes increasingly violent and abusive if she shows any sign of independence, such as getting a job or threatening to leave. Typically, the abuser has strong feelings of inadequacy and low self-esteem as well as poor problem-solving and social skills. He is emotionally immature, needy, irrationally jealous and possessive. He may even be jealous of his wife's attention to their own children or may beat both his children and wife. By bullying and physically punishing the family, the abuser often experiences a sense of power and control, a feeling that eludes him outside the home. The violent behaviour, therefore, is often rewarding and boosts his self-esteem.

Dependence is a commonly found trait in abused wives who stay with their husbands. Women often cite personal and financial dependence as reasons why they find leaving an abusive relationship extremely difficult. Regardless of the victim's talents or abilities, she perceives herself as unable to function without her husband. She, too, often suffers from low self-esteem and defines her success as a person by her ability to remain loyal to her marriage and 'make it work'. Some women internalize the criticism they receive and mistakenly believe they are to blame. Women also fear that their abuser will kill them if they try to leave. This fear is realistic, given that US statistics show 65% of women murdered by spouses or boyfriends were attempting to leave or had left the relationships (Bureau of Justice Statistics, 2006).

Cycle of Abuse and Violence

The **cycle of violence** or abuse is another reason often cited for why women have difficulty leaving abusive relationships. A typical pattern exists: usually, the initial episode of battering or violence is followed by a period of the abuser expressing regret, apologizing and promising it will never happen again. He professes his love for his wife and may even engage in romantic behaviour (e.g. buying gifts and flowers). This period of contrition or remorse sometimes is called the *honeymoon period*. The woman naturally wants to believe her husband and hopes the violence was an isolated incident. After this honeymoon period, the tension-building phase begins; there may be arguments, stony silence or complaints from the husband. The tension ends in another violent episode after which the abuser once again feels regret and remorse and promises to change. This cycle continually repeats itself. Each time, the victim keeps hoping the violence will stop.

Initially, the honeymoon period may last weeks or even months, causing the woman to believe that the relationship has improved and her husband's behaviour has changed. Over time, however, the violent episodes are more frequent, the period of remorse disappears altogether, and the level of violence and severity of injuries worsen. Eventually, the violence is routine – several times a week or even daily.

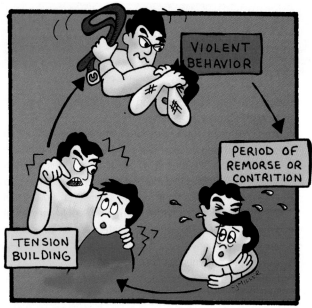

Cycle of violence

Assessment

Because most abused people do not seek direct help for the problem, nurses have an obligation to help identify them in all settings. Nurses may encounter abused people in inpatient units, CMHT appointments, or their own home. Some victims may be seeking treatment for problems not clearly related to the abuse. Identifying, protecting and helping abused women who need assistance should be a key nursing priority.

Table 11.1 summarizes techniques for working with victims of partner violence.

Many hospitals, clinics and CMHTs ask women about safety issues as part of all health histories or intake interviews. Because this issue is delicate and sensitive, and many abused women are afraid or embarrassed to admit the problem, nurses must be skilled in asking appropriate questions about abuse. Box 11.3 gives an example of questions to

Table 11.1 DO'S AND DON'TS OF WORKING WITH VICTIMS OF PARTNER ABUSE	
Don'ts	**Do's**
Don't disclose client communications without the client's consent	Do ensure and maintain the client's confidentiality
Don't preach, moralize or imply that you doubt the client	Do listen, affirm, and say, 'I am sorry you have been hurt'
Don't minimize the impact of violence	Do express, 'I'm concerned for your safety'
Don't express outrage with the perpetrator	Do tell the victim, 'You have a right to be safe and respected'
Don't imply that the client is responsible for the abuse	Do say, 'The abuse is not your fault'
Don't recommend couples' counselling	Do recommend a support group or individual counselling
Don't direct the client to leave the relationship	Do identify community resources and encourage the client to develop a safety plan
Don't take charge and do everything for the client	Do offer to help the client contact a shelter, the police or other resources

Box 11.3   SAFE QUESTIONS

- **S**tress/**S**afety: What stress do you experience in your relationships? Do you feel safe in your relationships? Should I be worried about your safety?
- **A**fraid/**A**bused: Have there been situations in your relationships where you've felt afraid? Has your partner ever threatened or abused you or your children? Have you ever been physically hurt or threatened by your partner? Are you in a relationship like that now? Has your partner ever forced you to engage in sexual intercourse that you didn't want? People in relationships/ marriages often fight; what happens when you and your partner disagree?
- **F**riends/**F**amily: Are your friends aware that you've been hurt? Do your parents or siblings know about this abuse? Do you think you could tell them, and would they be able to give you support?
- **E**mergency plan: Do you have a safe place to go and the resources you (and your children) need in an emergency? If you are in danger now, would you like help in locating a shelter? Would you like to talk to a social worker/your GP/me to develop an emergency plan?

Adapted from Ashur, M. L. C. (1993). Asking about domestic violence: SAFE questions. *Journal of the American Medical Association, 269*(18), 2367. © American Medical Association.

ask using the acronym SAFE (Stress/Safety, Afraid/Abused, Friends/Family and Emergency plan). The first two categories are designed to detect abuse. The nurse should ask questions in the other two categories if abuse is present. He or she should ask these questions when the woman is alone. The questions can be paraphrased or edited as needed for any given situation.

Nurses have a moral and statutory obligation to help protect victims of violence, and one of the key aspects of that obligation is an awareness of legal and civil rights and available resources: the police, colleagues in social services, Refuge and Women's Aid and other support groups can all help.

Even after a victim of violence has 'ended' the relationship, problems may continue. **Stalking**, or repeated and persistent

CLINICAL VIGNETTE: SPOUSE ABUSE

Diana sat in the bathroom trying to regain her balance and holding a cold flannel to her face. She looked in the mirror and saw a large, red, swollen area around her eye and cheek where her husband, Steve, had hit her. They had been married for only 6 months, and this was the second time that he had become angry and struck her in the face before storming out of the house. Last time, he was so sorry the day after it happened that he brought her flowers and took her out to dinner to apologize. He said he loved her more than ever and felt terrible about what had happened. He said it was because he had had an argument with his boss about not getting a pay rise and went out drinking after work before coming home. He had promised not to go out drinking any more and that it would never happen again. For several weeks after he stopped drinking, he was wonderful, and it felt like it was before they got married. She remembered thinking that she must try harder to keep him happy because she knew he really did love her.

But during the past 2 weeks, Steve had been increasingly silent and sullen, complaining about everything. He didn't like the dinners she cooked and said he wanted to go out to eat

even though money was tight and their credit cards were up to the limit. He began drinking again. After a few hours of drinking tonight, he yelled at her and said she was the cause of all his money problems. She tried to reason with him, but he hit her and this time he knocked her to the floor and her head hit the table. She was really frightened now, but what should she do? She couldn't move out; she had no money of her own and her job just didn't pay enough to support her. Should she go to her parents? She couldn't tell them about what happened because they never wanted her to marry Steve in the first place. They would probably say, 'We told you so and you didn't listen. Now you've married him and you'll have to deal with his problems'. She was too embarrassed to tell her friends, most of whom were 'their' friends and had never seen this violent side of Steve. They probably wouldn't believe her. What should she do? Her face and head were really beginning to hurt now. 'I'll talk to him tomorrow when he is sober and tell him he must get some help for the drinking problem. When he's sober, he is reasonable and he'll see that this drinking is causing a big problem for our marriage', she thought.

attempts to impose unwanted communication or contact on another person, is a problem. Stalkers are usually people pursuing relationships that have ended – or never even existed. One in 10 British women reported being stalked in the previous 12 months, according to Finney's (2006) online report on the previous year's British Crime Survey.

Safe houses run by organizations such as Refuge can provide temporary housing and food for abused women and their children when they decide to leave the abusive relationship. The woman leaving an abusive relationship may have no financial support and limited job skills or experience. Often she has dependent children. These barriers are difficult to overcome, and public or private assistance is limited.

In addition to the many physical injuries that abused women may experience, there are emotional and psychological consequences. Individual psychotherapy or counselling, group therapy or support and self-help groups can help abused people deal with their trauma and begin to build new, healthier relationships. Violence may also result in PTSD, which is discussed later in this chapter.

CHILD ABUSE

Child abuse is generally defined as the intentional injury of a child. It can include physical abuse or injuries, neglect or failure to prevent harm, failure to provide adequate physical or emotional care or supervision, abandonment, sexual assault or intrusion, and overt torture or maiming (Bernet, 2005).

In 2000, an eight-year-old girl called Victoria Climbie died in London, killed by her guardians. The post-mortem examination found 128 separate injuries on her body. She had been emotionally and physically abused over months following 'a gross failure of the system …' that was, according to the inquiry into her murder 'inexcusable' (Laming, 2003). Social workers, policemen, nurses, doctors and church pastors all failed Victoria.

Despite the outcry and subsequent policy, organizational and procedural changes (see Her Majesty's Government, 2006), children continued to be killed at the rate of 1–2 a week by those looking after them, some of them while clients of Health and Social Services. In 2007, 'Baby P', a 17-month-old boy living in North London, died as a result of over 50 injuries sustained while in the care of his mother, her boyfriend and their lodger. Social workers, doctors, lawyers, health visitors and nurses had all been involved in the case: they failed, ultimately, to protect the little boy.

It is absolutely vital that all nurses are aware of the facts of Baby P and Victoria's lives and awful deaths, that they remain vigilant for signs of abuse of children and are fully aware of local procedures for raising concerns effectively and quickly. They must be prepared to promote the rights of children assertively, even in the face of unresponsive or hostile senior managers.

The Royal College of Nursing (2005) shows that reviews and inquiries over the past 30 years have shared three key concerns:

- Poor communication and information-sharing between agencies
- Inadequate training and support
- A failure to listen to children.

The safety and well-being of children is one area in which routine standards of professional confidentiality may not be appropriate.

According to the National Society for the Prevention of Cruelty to Children (2008), drawing on Cawson et al. (2000) and Cawson (2002):

- 7% of children experienced serious physical abuse at the hands of their parents or carers.
- 1% of children aged under 16 experienced sexual abuse by a parent or carer, and a further 3% by another relative.
- 11% of children experienced sexual abuse by people known but unrelated to them.
- 5% of children experienced sexual abuse by an adult stranger or someone they had just met.
- 6% of children experienced serious absence of care at home.
- 5% of children experienced serious absence of supervision.
- 6% of children experienced frequent and severe emotional maltreatment.

Estimates are that 15 million women in the US were sexually abused as children, and one-third of all sexually abused victims were abused when they were younger than 9 years of age. Accurate UK statistics on sexual abuse are difficult to obtain because many incidences are unreported as a result of threats, shame and embarrassment but Cawson's figures of up to 11% may well be a significant underestimate. In many cases, women do not acknowledge sexual abuse until they are adults, if then. Significantly for mental health professionals, risks of depression, suicide attempts, marital problems and marriage to an alcoholic are increased among adults with a history of childhood sexual abuse (Dube et al., 2005).

Types of Child Abuse

Physical abuse of children often results from unreasonably severe corporal punishment or unjustifiable punishment, such as hitting an infant for crying or soiling his or her nappies. Intentional, deliberate assaults on children include burning, biting, cutting, poking, twisting limbs or scalding with hot water. The victim often has evidence of old injuries (e.g. scars, untreated fractures, multiple bruises of various ages) that the history given by parents or caregivers does not explain adequately.

Sexual abuse involves sexual acts performed by an adult on a child younger than 18 years. Examples include incest, rape and sodomy performed directly by the person or with an object, oral–genital contact and acts of molestation such as rubbing, fondling or exposing the adult's genitals. Sexual abuse may consist of a single incident or multiple episodes over a protracted period. A second type of sexual abuse – one that frequently involves the first – involves exploitation, such as making, promoting or selling pornography involving minors and the coercion of minors to participate in obscene acts. A third type of sexual abuse, again overlapping with the first, involves the 'new' offence of 'grooming', brought into law in part as a result of the multiplicity of emerging internet-related sexual offences. In England and Wales, it is an offence to arrange a meeting with a child, for oneself or someone else, with the intent of sexually abusing the child. The meeting itself is also now a criminal activity.

Neglect is malicious or ignorant withholding of physical, emotional or educational necessities for the child's well-being. Child abuse by neglect is the most prevalent type of maltreatment and includes refusal to seek health care or delay in doing so; abandonment; inadequate supervision; reckless disregard for the child's safety; punitive, exploitive or abusive emotional treatment; spousal abuse in the child's presence; giving the child permission to be truant; or failing to enrol the child in school.

Psychological abuse (emotional abuse) includes verbal assaults, such as blaming, screaming, name-calling and using sarcasm; constant family discord characterized by fighting, yelling and chaos; and emotional deprivation or withholding of affection, nurturing and normal experiences that engender acceptance, love, security and self-worth. Emotional abuse often accompanies other types of abuse (e.g. physical or sexual abuse). Exposure to parental alcoholism, drug use or prostitution – and the neglect that results – also falls within this category.

Clinical Picture

Parents who abuse their children often have limited parenting knowledge and skills. They may not understand or know what their children need, or they may be angry or frustrated because they are emotionally or financially unequipped to meet those needs. Although a lack of education and poverty contribute to child abuse and neglect, they by no means explain the entire phenomenon. Many incidences of abuse and violence occur in families who seem to have everything – the parents are well educated with successful careers, and the family is financially stable.

Parents who abuse their children are often emotionally immature, needy and incapable of meeting their own needs, let alone those of a child. As in spousal abuse, the abuser frequently views his or her children as property belonging to the abusing parent. The abuser does not value the children as human beings with rights and feelings. In some instances, the parent feels the need to have children to replace his or her own faulty and disappointing childhood; the parent wants to feel the love between child and parent that he or she missed as a child. The reality of the tremendous emotional, physical and financial demands that comes with raising children usually shatters these unrealistic expectations. When the parent's unrealistic expectations are not met, he or she often reverts to using the same methods that his or her parents used.

This tendency for adults to raise their children in the same way they were raised perpetuates the cycle of family violence. Adults who were victims of abuse as children frequently abuse their own children (Bernet, 2005).

Assessment

As with all types of family violence, detection and accurate identification are the first steps. Box 11.4 lists signs that might lead the nurse to suspect neglect or abuse. Burns or scalds may have an identifiable shape, such as cigarette marks, or may have a 'stocking and glove' distribution, indicating scalding. The parent of an infant with a severe skull fracture may report that he or she 'rolled off the couch', even though the child is too young to do so or the injury is much too severe for a fall of 20 inches. Bruises may have familiar, recognizable shapes, such as belt buckles or teeth marks (Ryan, 2003).

The nurse does not have to decide with certainty that abuse has occurred. Nurses are responsible for reporting suspected child abuse with accurate and thorough documentation of assessment data (http://www.rcn.org.uk/__data/assets/pdf_file/0004/78583/002045.pdf).

Children who have been sexually abused may have urinary tract infections; bruised, red or swollen genitalia; tears of the rectum or vagina; and bruising. The emotional response of these children varies widely. Often, these children talk or behave in ways that indicate more advanced knowledge of sexual issues than would be expected for their ages. Other times, they are frightened and anxious, and may either cling to an adult or reject adult attention entirely. The key is to recognize when the child's behaviour is different from that normally expected for his or her age and developmental stage. Seemingly unexplained behaviour, from refusal to eat to aggressive behaviour with peers, may indicate abuse.

Box 11.4 **WARNING SIGNS OF ABUSED/ NEGLECTED CHILDREN**

- Serious injuries such as fractures, burns or lacerations with no reported history of trauma
- Delay in seeking treatment for a significant injury
- Child or parent gives a history inconsistent with severity of injury, such as a baby with *contrecoup* injuries to the brain (shaken baby syndrome) that the parents claim happened when the infant rolled off the sofa
- Inconsistencies or changes in the child's history during the evaluation by either the child or the adult
- Unusual injuries for the child's age and level of development, such as a fractured femur on a 2-month-old or a dislocated shoulder in a 2-year-old
- High incidence of urinary tract infections; bruised, red or swollen genitalia; tears or bruising of rectum or vagina
- Evidence of old injuries not reported, such as scars, fractures not treated, multiple bruises that parent/carer cannot explain adequately

CLINICAL VIGNETTE: CHILD ABUSE

Michael, 7 years old, is the son of a client of the community mental health team. Today, when the CPN visits, he's home from school after being sent to the school nurse because of a large bruise on his face.

Michael's mother describes him as clumsy, always tripping and falling down. She says he's a 'daredevil', always trying stunts with his bike or rollerblades or climbing trees and falling

or jumping to the ground. She says she has tried everything but can't slow him down.

When the nurse talks to Michael, he is reluctant to discuss the bruise on his face. He does not make eye contact with the nurse and gives a vague explanation for his bruise: 'I guess I ran into something'. The nurse suspects that someone – perhaps even her own client – is abusing Michael.

Treatment and Intervention

The first intervention for child abuse or neglect is to ensure the child's safety and well-being (Bernet, 2005). This may involve removing the child from the home, which can be traumatic in itself. Given the high risk of psychological problems, a thorough mental health evaluation may also be indicated. A relationship of trust between any therapist and child is crucial to help the child deal with the trauma of abuse. Depending on the severity and duration of abuse and the child's response, therapy may be indicated over a significant period.

Long-term treatment for the child usually involves professionals from several disciplines, such as nursing, psychiatry, social work and psychology, many working within child and adolescent mental health services (CAMHS). The very young child may communicate best through play therapy, where he or she draws or acts out situations with puppets or dolls, rather than talking about what has happened or his or her feelings. Multi-agency child protection teams are involved in determining whether returning the child to the parental home is possible, based on whether parents can show benefit from treatment. Family therapy may be indicated if reuniting the family is feasible. Parents may require mental health or substance abuse treatment. If the child is unlikely to return home, short-term or long-term foster care services may be indicated.

The media has focused much attention on the theory of **repressed memories** in victims of abuse. Many professionals believe that memories of childhood abuse can be buried deeply in the subconscious mind or repressed, because they are too painful for the victims to acknowledge, and that victims can be helped to recover or remember such painful memories. If a person comes to a mental health professional experiencing serious problems in relationships, symptoms of PTSD, or flashbacks involving abuse, the mental health professional may help the person remember or recover those memories of abuse. Some believe that mental health professionals may be overzealous in helping clients 'remember' abuse that really did not happen, or encouraging clients to see themselves as having many parts or as having inner children (Piper & Merskey, 2004). This so-called *false memory syndrome* has created

problems in families when clients made groundless accusations of abuse. Fears exist, however, that people abused in childhood will be more reluctant to talk about their abuse history because, once again, no one will believe them. Still other therapists argue that people thought to have dissociative identity disorder are suffering anxiety, terror and intrusive ideas and emotions and therefore need help, and the therapist should remain open-minded about the diagnosis (Middleton *et al.*, 2005).

ELDER ABUSE

Elder abuse is the mistreatment of older adults by family members or others (including nurses) providing care. It may include physical and sexual abuse, psychological abuse, neglect, self-neglect, financial exploitation and denial of adequate medical treatment (Box 11.5). Abuse is more likely when the older person has multiple chronic mental and physical health problems and when he or she is dependent on others for food, medical care and various activities of daily living. It can occur in the person's own home (accounting for 64% of cases identified by the Action on Elder Abuse helpline), in residential care (23%) or in hospitals (5%).

Box 11.5 THE FACTS ABOUT ELDER ABUSE

- 500,000 older people are believed to be abused at any one time in the UK.
- Two-thirds of abuse is committed at home by someone in a position of trust.
- Those aged between 80 and 89 are the most vulnerable to abuse.

From Help The Aged. (2008). *Enough is Enough: the Issues*. http://www.helptheaged.org.uk/en-gb/Campaigns/ElderAbuse/EnoughIsEnough/default.htm

WARNING ● Signs of Elder Abuse

There are five types of elder abuse: psychological, physical, financial, sexual and neglect. There are a number of signs that someone might be experiencing abuse or neglect. These include:

- Withdrawing from usual activities
- Talking and interacting less than before
- Becoming angry or aggressive for little reason
- Seeming depressed or very lethargic, tearful or sad
- Being reluctant to be left on their own or with certain individuals
- Seeming uncharacteristically jolly and inappropriately lighthearted.

From Help the Aged. (2008). *Frequent questions about elder abuse.* http://www.helptheaged.org.uk/en-gb/Campaigns/ElderAbuse/EnoughIsEnough/default.htm

People who abuse older people are almost always in a caregiver position, or the elders depend on them in some way. Many cases of elder abuse occur when one older spouse is taking care of another. This type of spousal abuse usually happens over many years after a disability renders the abused spouse unable to care for himself or herself. When the abuser is an adult child, it is twice as likely to be a son as a daughter. A psychiatric disorder or a problem with substance abuse also may aggravate abuse of elders (Goldstein, 2005).

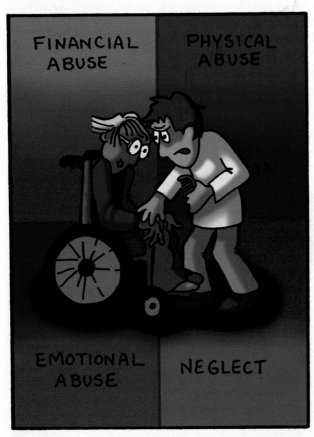

Elder abuse

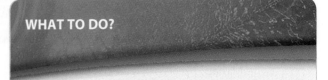

WHAT TO DO?

If you have been affected by elder abuse – whether you are personally coping with abuse or whether you are concerned about the abuse of another – you are not alone. You can speak to someone in confidence, please call the freephone Action on Elder Abuse helpline on **0808 808 8141**.

Older people are often reluctant to report abuse, even when they can, especially when the abuse involves family members whom the older person wishes to protect. Victims may often fear losing their support and being moved to an institution, if in their own home, or risking further abuse or homelessness if in a care home.

Clinical Picture

The victim may have bruises or fractures; may lack needed eyeglasses or hearing aids; may be denied food, fluids or medications; or may be restrained in a bed or chair. The abuser may misuse the victim's financial resources while the older person cannot afford food or medications. Abusers may withhold medical care itself from an elder with acute or chronic illness. Self-neglect involves the elder's failure to provide for himself or herself.

Assessment

Careful assessment of older people and their caregiving relationships is essential in detecting elder abuse. Often, determining whether the older person's condition results from deterioration associated with a chronic illness or from abuse is difficult. Several potential indicators of abuse require further assessment and careful evaluation (Box 11.6). These indicators by themselves, however, do not necessarily signify abuse or neglect.

The nurse should suspect abuse if injuries have been hidden or untreated, or are incompatible with the explanation provided. Such injuries can include cuts, lacerations, puncture wounds, bruises, welts or burns. Burns can be cigarette burns, scaldings, acid or caustic burns or friction burns of the wrists or ankles caused from being restrained by ropes, clothing or chains. Signs of physical neglect include a pervasive smell of urine or faeces, dirt, rashes, sores, lice or inadequate clothing. Dehydration or malnourishment not linked with a specific illness also strongly indicates abuse.

Possible indicators of emotional or psychological abuse include an older person who is hesitant to talk openly to the nurse or who is fearful, withdrawn, depressed and helpless.

Box 11.6   POSSIBLE INDICATORS OF ELDER ABUSE

PHYSICAL ABUSE INDICATORS

- Frequent, unexplained injuries accompanied by a habit of seeking medical assistance from various locations
- Reluctance to seek medical treatment for injuries or denial of their existence
- Disorientation or grogginess indicating misuse of medications
- Fear or edginess in the presence of a family member or carer

PSYCHOLOGICAL OR EMOTIONAL ABUSE INDICATORS

- Helplessness
- Reluctance to talk openly
- Anger or agitation
- Withdrawal or depression

FINANCIAL ABUSE INDICATORS

- Unusual or inappropriate activity in bank accounts
- Signatures on cheques that differ from the older person's
- Recent changes in will or power of attorney when the older person is not capable of making those decisions
- Missing valuable belongings that are not just misplaced
- Lack of television, clothes or personal items that are easily affordable
- Unusual concern by the carer over the expense of the older person's treatment when it is not the carer's money being spent

NEGLECT INDICATORS

- Dirt, faecal or urine smell or other health hazards in the older person's living environment

- Rashes, sores or lice on the person
- The person has an untreated medical condition or is malnourished or dehydrated not related to a known illness
- Inadequate clothing

INDICATORS OF SELF-NEGLECT

- Inability to manage personal finances, such as hoarding, squandering or giving away money while not paying bills
- Inability to manage activities of daily living, such as personal care, shopping or housework
- Wandering, refusing needed medical attention, isolation, substance use
- Failure to keep needed medical appointments
- Confusion, memory loss, unresponsiveness
- Lack of toilet facilities, living quarters infested with animals or vermin

WARNING INDICATORS FROM CARER

- The older person is not given the opportunity to speak for himself or herself, to have visitors or to see anyone without the presence of the carer
- Attitudes of indifference or anger toward the older person
- Insincere statements of caring about and interest in the older person
- Blaming the older person for his or her illness or limitations
- Defensiveness
- Conflicting accounts of the older person's abilities, problems and so forth
- Previous history of abuse or problems with alcohol or drugs

The older person may also exhibit anger or agitation for no apparent reason. He or she may deny any problems, even when the facts indicate otherwise.

Possible indicators of self-neglect include inability to manage money (hoarding or squandering while failing to pay bills), inability to perform activities of daily living (personal care, shopping, food preparation and cleaning), and changes in intellectual function (confusion, disorientation, inappropriate responses and memory loss and isolation). Other indicators of self-neglect include signs of malnutrition or dehydration, rashes or sores on the body, an odour of urine or faeces or failure to keep needed medical appointments.

For self-neglect to be diagnosed, the elder must be evaluated as unable to manage day-to-day life and take care of him or herself. Self-neglect cannot be established based solely on family members' beliefs that the elder cannot manage his or her finances. For example, an older adult cannot be considered to have self-neglect just because he or she gives away large sums of money to a group or charity or invests in some venture of which family members disapprove.

Warnings of financial exploitation or abuse may include numerous unpaid bills (when the client has enough money to pay them), unusual activity in bank accounts, cheques signed by someone other than the older person or recent

CLINICAL VIGNETTE: ELDER ABUSE

Josephine is an elderly woman who has moved in with her son, daughter-in-law, and two grandchildren after the death of her husband. She lives in a 'granny annex' with her own bath. Friction with her daughter-in-law begins to develop when Josephine tries to help out around the house. She comments on the poor manners and outlandish clothes of her teenage grandchildren. She adds garlic and pepper to food her daughter-in-law is cooking on the stove. She comments on how late the children stay out, their friends and how hard her son works. All this is annoying but harmless.

Josephine's daughter-in-law gets very impatient, telling her husband, 'I'm the one who has to deal with your mother all day long'. One day, after more criticism from Josephine, the daughter-in-law slaps her. She then tells Josephine to go downstairs to her room and stay out of sight if she wants to have a place to live. A friend of Josephine's calls on the phone and the daughter-in-law lies and tells her Josephine is sleeping.

Josephine spends more time alone in her room, becomes more isolated and depressed, and is eating and sleeping poorly. She is afraid she will be placed in a nursing home if she doesn't get along with her daughter-in-law. Her son seems too busy to notice what is happening, and Josephine is afraid to tell him for fear he won't believe her or will take his wife's side. Her friends don't seem to call much any more, and she has no one to talk to about how miserable she is. She just keeps herself to herself most of the day.

changes in a will or power of attorney when the older person cannot make such decisions. The older person may lack amenities that he or she can afford, such as clothing, personal products or a television. He or she may report losing valuable possessions and report that he or she has no contact with friends or relatives.

The nurse may also detect possible indicators of abuse from the caregiver. The caregiver may complain about how difficult caring for the elder is, about incontinence, difficulties in feeding or excessive costs of medication. He or she may display anger or indifference toward the elder and try to keep the nurse from talking with the elder alone. Elder abuse is more likely when the caregiver has a history of family violence or alcohol or drug problems.

As well as an ethical and moral obligation, nurses have an obligation under the NMC's Code of Professional Conduct to raise any concerns about the abuse of an older person immediately. The Department of Health document *No secrets* (Department of Health and Home Office, 2000) outlined clearly for the first time that the prevention, identification and treatment of elder abuse was a multi-agency task in which individuals, teams and organizations all had responsibility. The guidance defined 'vulnerable adults', outlined an inter-agency framework for tackling the issue strategically and practically (including mandatory training) and set out the correct procedures for dealing with individual cases in which vulnerable adults – including older people – were being abused or neglected or were at risk of being abused or neglected.

Treatment and Intervention

Elder abuse may develop gradually as the burden of care exceeds the caregiver's physical or emotional resources. Relieving the caregiver's stress and providing additional resources may help to correct an abusive situation and leave the caregiving relationship intact. In other cases, the neglect or abuse is intentional and designed to provide personal gain to the caregiver, such as access to the victim's financial resources. In these situations, removal of the elder or caregiver is necessary.

RAPE AND SEXUAL ASSAULT

Rape is a crime of violence, power and humiliation of the victim expressed through sexual means, and the person who is raped may or may not also be physically beaten and injured.

Definitions of rape vary in different countries. Under the Sexual Offences Act, 2003, in England and Wales 'rape' as an offence involves non-consensual penile penetration of the vagina, anus or mouth and can, thus, be carried out by a man against a women or against another man. The 2003 Act introduces a new sexual offence in England and Wales of 'assault by penetration'. It is committed when someone penetrates the vagina or anus of someone without that person's consent.

Under Scottish law, at present, an assault is only defined as rape if a man penetrates a non-consenting *woman*'s vagina. There is no separate offence at present of 'assault by penetration'.

Rape and sexual assault can occur between strangers, acquaintances, married persons and people of the same sex. People known to the victims commit the majority of rapes and sexual assaults. A phenomenon called **date rape (acquaintance rape)**, mentioned earlier in this chapter, may occur on a first date, on a ride home from a party, or when the two people have known each other for some time. It is more prevalent near college and university campuses. See Table 11.2 for UK data on rape and sexual assault.

Rape is a highly under-reported crime: estimates in the US are that only 1 rape is reported for every 4 to 10 rapes that occur.

Table 11.2	UK DATA ON RAPE AND SEXUAL ASSAULT	
Finding	**Source**	**Method**
1 in 4 women have experienced rape or attempted rape	Painter, 1991	Survey of 1007 women in 11 cities, northern England
1 in 7 women have been coerced into sex, rising to 1 in 3 among divorced and separated women	Painter, 1991	Survey of 1007 women in 11 cities, northern England
The most common perpetrators of rape are husbands and partners	Painter, 1991	Survey of 1007 women in 11 cities, northern England
97% of callers to rape crisis lines knew their assailant prior to the assault	Rape Crisis Federation of England and Wales	Analysis of RCF members' records, England and Wales
The majority of perpetrators are known to the victim	Kelly *et al.*, 2005	
During 2001 it is estimated that there were 190,000 incidents of serious sexual assault and 47,000 female victims of rape/attempted rape	Walby & Allen, 2004	British Crime Survey 2002

From Rape Crisis England and Wales. (2008). *Statistics.* http://www.cer.truthaboutrape.co.uk/3.html

The under-reporting is attributed to the victim's feelings of shame and guilt, the fear of further injury and the belief that she has no recourse in the legal system. Victims of rape can be any age: reported cases have victims ranging in age from 15 months to 82 years. The highest incidence is in girls and women 16 to 24 years of age. Girls younger than 18 years were the victims in 61% of rapes reported (van der Kolk, 2005). Rape against women most commonly occurs in a woman's local area, often inside or near her home. Rape results in pregnancy about 10% of the time (van der Kolk, 2005).

Male rape is a significantly under-reported crime. It can occur between gay partners or strangers but seems to be most prevalent in institutions such as prisons or maximum-security hospitals. Estimates are that 2 to 5% of male inmates are sexually assaulted, but the figure may be much higher. This type of rape is particularly violent, and the dynamics of power and control are similar to those for heterosexual rape.

Dynamics of Rape

In the US, most men who commit rape are 25 to 44 years of age. In terms of race, 51% are white and tend to rape white victims, and 47% are African–American and tend to rape African–American victims; the remaining 2% come from all other races. Alcohol is involved in 34% of cases. Rape often accompanies another crime. Almost 75% of arrested rapists have prior criminal histories, including other rapes, assaults, robberies and homicides (van der Kolk, 2005). Barring those for specific ethnicity, findings for the UK are likely to be similar.

Recent research (van der Kolk, 2005) has categorized male rapists into four categories:

- Sexual sadists who are aroused by the pain of their victims
- Exploitive predators who impulsively use their victims as objects for gratification
- Inadequate men who believe that no woman would voluntarily have sexual relations with them and who are obsessed with fantasies about sex
- Men for whom rape is a displaced expression of anger and rage.

Feminist ideologies propose that women have historically served as objects for aggression, dating back to when women (and children) were legally the property of men. Armies have historically – and continue to – use rape as a weapon to terrify and subdue civilian populations; men use rape to enforce particular – usually religiously driven – standards of behaviour. Although already recognized as rape in Scotland, it was only in 1991 in England and Wales, for the first time, that a married man could be convicted of raping his wife, signalling a legal end to the notion that the act of marriage offered a husband lifelong consent.

Women who are raped are frequently in life-threatening situations, so their primary motivation is to stay alive. At times, attempts to resist or fight the attacker succeed; in other situations, fighting and yelling result in more severe physical injuries or even death. Degree of submission is higher when the attacker has a weapon such as a gun or knife. In addition to forcible penetration, the more violent rapist may urinate or defecate on the woman or insert foreign objects into her vagina and rectum.

The physical and psychological trauma that rape victims suffer is severe. Related medical problems can include acute physical injury, sexually transmitted diseases, pregnancy and lingering medical complaints. A cross-sectional study of medical patients found that women who had been raped rated themselves as significantly less healthy, visited a doctor twice as often and incurred medical costs more than twice as high as women who had not experienced any criminal victimization (American Medical Association, 2004). The level of violence experienced during the assault was found to be a powerful predictor of future use of medical services. Many victims of rape experience fear, helplessness, shock and disbelief, guilt, humiliation and embarrassment. They also may avoid the place or circumstances of the rape; give up previously pleasurable activities; and experience depression, sexual dysfunction, insomnia and impaired memory (American Medical Association, 2004).

Until recently, the rights of rape victims were often ignored. For example, when rape victims reported a rape to the police, they often faced doubt and embarrassing questions from male officers. The courts, equally, did not protect the rights of victims; for example, a woman's past sexual behaviour was admissible in court – although the past criminal record of her accused attacker was not. Action has slowly been taken to address these issues, but society still has a long way to go to properly tackle the pain and distress of rape and sexual assault

Although the treatment of rape victims and the prosecution of rapists have improved in the past two decades, many people still believe that somehow a woman provokes rape by her behaviour and that the woman is partially responsible for this crime. Box 11.7 summarizes common myths and misunderstandings about rape.

Treatment and Intervention

Victims of rape fare best when they receive immediate support and can express fear and rage to family members, nurses, doctors and policemen who *believe* them. Education about rape and the needs of victims is an ongoing requirement for health-care professionals, the police and the general public.

Box 11.7   COMMON MYTHS ABOUT RAPE

- When a woman submits to rape, she really wants it to happen.
- Women who dress provocatively are asking for trouble.
- Some women like rough sex but later call it rape.
- Once a man is aroused by a woman, he cannot stop his actions.
- Walking alone at night is an invitation for rape.
- Rape cannot happen between persons who are married.
- Rape is exciting for some women.
- Rape only occurs between heterosexual couples.
- If a woman has an orgasm, it can't be rape.

Box 11.8   WARNING SIGNS OF RELATIONSHIP VIOLENCE

- Emotionally abuses you (insults, makes belittling comments, acts sulky or angry when you initiate an idea or activity)
- Tells you with whom you may be friends or how you should dress, or tries to control other elements of your life
- Talks negatively about women in general
- Gets jealous for no reason
- Drinks heavily, uses drugs or tries to get you drunk
- Acts in an intimidating way by invading your personal space, such as standing too close or touching you when you don't want him to
- Cannot handle sexual or emotional frustration without becoming angry
- Does not view you as an equal: sees himself as smarter or socially superior
- Guards his masculinity by acting tough
- Is angry or threatening to the point that you have changed your life or yourself so you won't anger him
- Goes through extreme highs and lows; is kind one minute, cruel the next
- Berates you for not getting drunk or high, or not wanting to have sex with him
- Is physically aggressive, grabbing and holding you or pushing and shoving

Adapted from the State University of New York at Buffalo Counseling Center. (2006). Relationship violence warning signs. Available: http://ub-counseling.buffalo.edu/warnings.shtml

---

Box 11.8 lists warning signs of relationship violence. These signs, used at the State University of New York at Buffalo (2006) to educate students about date rape, can alert women to the characteristics of men who are likely to commit dating violence. Examples include expressing negativity about women, acting tough, engaging in heavy drinking, exhibiting jealousy, making belittling comments, expressing anger and using intimidation.

Giving as much control back to the victim as possible is important. Ways to do so include allowing her to make decisions when possible, about who to call, what to do next, what she would like done, and so on. It is the woman's decision about whether or not to press charges and give evidence against her attacker.

Prophylactic treatment for sexually transmitted diseases such as chlamydia or gonorrhoea may be offered. Doing so is cost effective: many victims of rape will not return to get definitive test results for these diseases. HIV testing is strongly encouraged at specified intervals because seroconversion to positive status does not occur immediately.

CLINICAL VIGNETTE: RAPE

Cynthia is a 22-year-old university student who spent Saturday afternoon with a group of friends at a football match. That evening, they decided to go to a party at the college. Cynthia quickly became separated from her friends but started talking to Ron, whom she recognized from her course. They spent the rest of the evening together, talking, dancing and drinking. She had had more drinks then she was used to, as Ron kept bringing her more every time her glass was empty. At the end of the night, Ron asked if she wanted him to drive her home. Her friends had decided to stay a bit longer at the party.

When Ron and Cynthia arrived at her flat, she asked Ron to come in. She was feeling a bit drunk, and they began kissing. She could feel Ron getting really excited. He began to try to remove her skirt, but she said, 'No' and tried to move away from him. She remembered him saying, 'What's the matter with you? Are you a virgin or what?' She told him she had had a good time but didn't want to go further. He responded, 'Come on, you've been trying to turn me on all night. You want this as much as I do.' He forced himself on top of her and held his arm over her neck and raped her.

When her roommates return about an hour later, Cynthia is huddled in the corner of her room, seems stunned, and is crying uncontrollably. She feels sick and confused. Did she do something to cause this whole thing? She keeps asking herself whether she might not have got into that situation had she not had so much to drink. She is so confused.

Women are also encouraged to engage in safe-sex practices until the results of HIV testing are available. Prophylaxis with ethinylestradiol and norgestrel (Ovral) can be offered to prevent pregnancy. Some women may elect to wait to initiate intervention until they have a positive pregnancy test result or miss a menstrual period.

Rape crisis centres, women's advocacy groups and other local resources often provide a counsellor or volunteer to be with the victim from A&E or the police station through longer-term follow-up. This person provides emotional support, serves as an advocate for the woman throughout the process, and can be totally available to the victim. This type of complete and unconditional support is often crucial to recovery.

Therapy is usually supportive in approach and focuses on restoring the victim's sense of control; relieving feelings of helplessness, dependency and obsession with the assault that frequently follow rape; regaining trust; improving daily functioning; finding adequate social support; and dealing with feelings of guilt, shame and anger. Group therapy with other women who have been raped is a particularly effective treatment. Some women attend both individual and group therapies.

It often takes a year or more for survivors of rape to regain previous levels of functioning. In some cases, survivors of rape have long-term consequences, such as PTSD, which is discussed later in this chapter.

BULLYING

Violence – physical and verbal – in UK schools appears to be increasing. Figures from Keele University suggested that, in 2007, 40% of children reported being bullied in the previous year, with 4% being bullied every single day. Recent shifts in patterns of bullying have included the development of bullying by text and over the internet.

Children who were bullied reported more loneliness and difficulty making friends, and those who bullied were more likely to have poor grades and to use alcohol and tobacco. Children with special physical health-care needs are bullied more often, and children with a chronic emotional, behavioural or developmental problem are more likely to be both a bully and a victim of bullying (Van Cleave & Davis, 2006).

Exposure to community violence – on TV, on the street, on the internet – tremendously affects children and young adults. When children witness violence they experience stress-related symptoms that seem to increase with the amount of violence they see. In addition, witnessing violence can lead to future problems with aggression, depression, relationships, achievement and abuse of drugs and alcohol (Skybo, 2005). Addressing the problem of violence exposure may help to alleviate the cycle of dysfunction and further violence.

COMMUNITY VIOLENCE

On a larger scale, violence such as the terrorist attacks in New York, Washington and Pennsylvania in 2001 or those on the London Underground in 2005 also have far-reaching effects on people. In the immediate aftermath, many children were afraid to go to school or have their parents leave them for any reason. Adults had difficulty going to work, leaving their homes, using public transportation, and flying. Research is now showing that 1 in 10 New York area residents were still experiencing lingering stress and depression as a result of September 11 some 4 years on, and an additional 532,240 cases of PTSD have been reported in the New York City metropolitan area alone (Schlenger et al., 2002). In addition, people are reporting higher relapse rates of depression and anxiety disorders. However, the study showed no increase of PTSD nationwide as a result of individuals watching the attacks and associated coverage on television, which had been an initial concern.

According to the NHS Trauma Response (London bombings) Screening Team, around a quarter of adults (1000 out of 4000 people) directly affected by the 7 July attacks may have PTSD; a large proportion of the children of these people may also have psychological problems as a result

Early intervention and treatment are key to dealing with victims of violence. Over the past few years, immediate responses to the psychological impact of violence on individuals, services and communities have become better co-ordinated and focused. Nevertheless, despite such efforts, many people will continue to experience long-term difficulties, as described in the next section.

MENTAL DISORDERS RELATED TO ABUSE AND VIOLENCE

Posttraumatic Stress Disorder

Posttraumatic stress disorder is a disturbing pattern of behaviour demonstrated by someone who has experienced a traumatic event such as a natural disaster, combat or an assault. The person with PTSD was exposed to an event that posed a threat of death or serious injury and he or she responded with intense fear, helplessness or terror. Three clusters of symptoms are present: reliving the event, avoiding reminders of the event and being on guard or experiencing *hyperarousal*. The person persistently re-experiences the trauma through memories, dreams, flashbacks or reactions to external cues about the event, and therefore avoids stimuli associated with the trauma. The victim feels a numbing of general responsiveness and shows persistent signs of increased arousal, such as insomnia, hyperarousal or hypervigilance, irritability or angry outbursts. He or she reports losing a sense of connection and control over his or her life. In PTSD, the symptoms occur 3 months or more after the trauma, which distinguishes PTSD from **acute stress disorder**. The latter diagnosis from the *DSM-IV-TR* (American Psychiatric Association, 2000) is appropriate when symptoms appear within the first month after the trauma and do not persist longer than 4 weeks.

PTSD can occur at any age, including during childhood. Estimates are that up to 60% of people at risk, such as combat veterans and victims of violence and natural disasters, develop PTSD. Complete recovery occurs within 3 months for about 50% of people. The severity and duration of the trauma and the proximity of the person to the event are the most important factors affecting the likelihood of developing PTSD (American Psychiatric Association, 2000). One-quarter of all victims of physical assault develop PTSD. Victims of rape have one of the highest rates of PTSD – approximately 70% (van der Kolk, 2005).

Dissociative Disorders

Dissociation is a subconscious defence mechanism that helps a person protect his or her emotional self from recognizing the full effects of some horrific or traumatic event, by

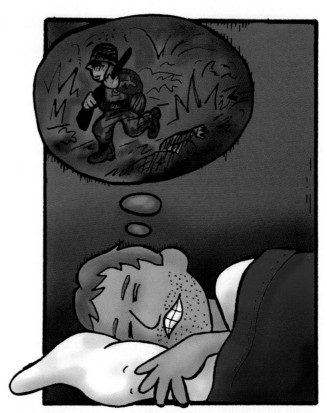

Posttraumatic stress disorder

DSM-IV-TR DIAGNOSTIC CRITERIA: MAJOR SYMPTOMS OF POSTTRAUMATIC STRESS DISORDER

- Recurrent, intrusive, distressing memories of the event
- Nightmares
- Flashbacks
- Avoidance of thoughts, feelings or conversations associated with the trauma
- Avoidance of activities, places or people that arouse memories of the trauma
- Inability to recall important aspect of the trauma
- Marked decrease in interest or participation in significant events
- Feeling detached or estranged from others
- Restricted range of affect
- Sense of foreshortened future
- Difficulty falling or staying asleep
- Irritability or anger outbursts
- Difficulty concentrating
- Hypervigilance
- Exaggerated startle response

Adapted from *DSM-IV-TR*, American Psychiatric Association 2000.

CLINICAL VIGNETTE: POSTTRAUMATIC STRESS DISORDER

Julie sat up in bed. She felt her heart pounding, she was perspiring, and she felt like she couldn't breathe. She was gasping for breath and felt the pressure on her throat . . . The picture of that dark figure knocking her to the ground and his hands around her throat was vivid in her mind. Her heart was pounding and she was reliving it all over again, the pain and the terror of that night. It had been 2 years since she was attacked and raped in the park while jogging, but sometimes it felt like just yesterday. She had nightmares of panic almost every night. She would never be rid of that night. Never.

Lately, the dread of reliving the nightmare made Julie afraid to fall asleep, and she wasn't getting much sleep. She felt exhausted. She didn't feel much like eating and was losing weight. This ordeal had ruined her life. She was missing work more and more. Even while at work, she often felt an overwhelming sense of dread. Sometimes even in the daytime, the memories of that night and flashbacks would come.

Her friends didn't seem to want to be around her any more because she was often moody and couldn't seem to enjoy herself. Sure, they were supportive and listened to her for the first 6 months, but now it was 2 years since the rape. Before the rape, she was always ready to go to a party or out to dinner and a film with friends. Now she just felt like staying home. She was tired of her mother and friends telling her she needed to go out and have some fun. Nobody could understand what she had gone through and how she felt. Julie had had several boyfriends since then, but the relationships just never seemed to work out. She was moody and would often become anxious and depressed for no reason and cancel dates at the last minute. Everyone was getting tired of her moods, but she felt she had no control over them.

allowing the mind to forget or remove itself from the painful situation or memory. Dissociation can occur both during and after the event. As with any other protective coping mechanism, dissociating becomes easier with repeated use.

Treatment and Interventions

Survivors of trauma and abuse who have PTSD or dissociative disorders are often involved in group or individual therapy in the community to address the short- and longer-term effects of their experiences. Cognitive-behavioural therapy seems to be effective in helping trauma and abuse survivors cope with their thoughts and subsequent feelings and behaviour. Both paroxetine (Seroxat) and sertraline (Lustral) have been used to help treat PTSD successfully. Clients with dissociative disorders may be treated symptomatically, that is, with medications for anxiety or depression (or both), if these symptoms are predominant.

Clients with PTSD are found in all areas of health care, from clinics to CMHTs to inpatient units. The nurse is most likely to encounter these clients in acute care settings, when there are concerns for their safety or the safety of others, or when acute symptoms have become intense and require stabilization. Treatment in acute care is usually short term, with the client returning to community-based treatment as quickly as possible.

Crucially, there seems to be a significant relationship between a number of mental health problems and trauma: not only anxiety and depressive disorders but also psychosis seem to be correlated significantly with trauma.

Cognitive-behavioural approaches and (more controversially) other treatment options, such as eye movement desensitization and re-processing, seem to be developing a good body of evidence.

APPLICATION OF THE NURSING PROCESS

Assessment

BACKGROUND

An assessment interview will often reveal that the client has a history of trauma or abuse. This may be abuse as a child or in a current or recent relationship. It is generally not necessary or desirable for the client to detail specific events of the abuse or trauma; rather, in-depth discussion of the actual abuse is usually undertaken during any subsequent individual psychotherapy or counselling sessions.

GENERAL APPEARANCE AND MOTOR BEHAVIOUR

The nurse assesses the client's overall appearance and motor behaviour. The client often appears hyperalert and reacts to even small environmental noises with a startle response. He or she may be very uncomfortable if the nurse is too close physically and may require greater distance or personal space than most people. The client may appear anxious or agitated and may have difficulty sitting still, often needing to pace or move around the room. Sometimes the client may sit very still, seeming to curl up with arms around knees.

MOOD AND AFFECT

In assessing mood and affect, the nurse must remember that a wide range of emotions is possible, from passivity to anger. The client may look frightened or scared, or agitated and hostile, depending on his or her experience. When the client experiences a flashback, he or she appears terrified and may cry, scream or attempt to hide or run away. When the client is dissociating, he or she may speak in a different tone of voice or appear numb with a vacant stare. The client may report intense rage or anger, or feeling dead inside and unable to identify any feelings or emotions.

THOUGHT PROCESS AND CONTENT

The nurse asks questions about thought process and content. Clients who have been abused or traumatized report reliving the trauma, often through nightmares or flashbacks. Intrusive, persistent thoughts about the trauma interfere with the client's ability to think about other things or to focus on daily living. Some clients report hallucinations or buzzing voices in their heads. Self-destructive thoughts and impulses, as well as intermittent suicidal ideation, are also common. Some clients report fantasies in which they take revenge on their abusers.

SENSORY AND INTELLECTUAL PROCESSES

During assessment of sensory and intellectual processes, the nurse usually finds that the client is oriented to reality except if the client is experiencing a flashback or dissociative episode. During those experiences, the client may not respond to the nurse or may be unable to communicate at all. The nurse also may find that clients who have been abused or traumatized have *memory gaps*, which are periods for which they have no clear memories. These periods may be short or extensive and are usually related to the time of the abuse or trauma. Intrusive thoughts or ideas of self-harm often impair the client's ability to concentrate or pay attention.

JUDGEMENT AND INSIGHT

The client's insight is often related to the duration of his or her problems with dissociation or PTSD. Early in treatment, the client may report little idea about the relationship of past trauma to his or her current symptoms and problems. Other clients may be quite knowledgeable if they have progressed further in treatment. The client's ability to make decisions or solve problems may be impaired.

SELF-CONCEPT

The nurse is likely to find that these clients have low self-esteem. They may believe they are bad people who somehow deserve or provoke the abuse. Many clients believe they are unworthy or damaged by their abusive experiences, to the point that they will never be worthwhile or valued. Clients may believe they are going crazy and are out of control, with no hope of regaining control. Clients may see themselves as helpless, hopeless and worthless.

ROLES AND RELATIONSHIPS

People may report a great deal of difficulty with all types of relationships. Problems with authority figures often lead to difficulties at work, such as being unable to take directions from another or have another person monitor his or her performance. Close relationships are difficult or impossible because the person's ability to trust others is severely compromised. Often the person has given up work or has been fired, and he or she may be estranged from family members. Intrusive thoughts, flashbacks or dissociative episodes may interfere with the client's ability to socialize with family or friends, and the client's avoidant behaviour may keep him or her from participating in social or family events.

PHYSIOLOGICAL CONSIDERATIONS

Most clients report difficulty sleeping because of nightmares or anxiety over anticipating nightmares. Overeating or lack of appetite is also common. Frequently, these clients use alcohol or other drugs to attempt to sleep or to blot out intrusive thoughts or memories.

Data Analysis

Nursing formulations commonly used in the acute care setting when working with clients who dissociate or have PTSD related to trauma or abuse include consideration of the following:

- Risk of Self-harm
- Ineffective Coping Strategies
- Distressing Posttrauma Responses
- Chronic Low Self-esteem
- Powerlessness.

In addition, the following nursing formulations may be pertinent for clients over longer periods, although not all formulations apply to each client:

- Disturbed Sleep Pattern
- Sexual Dysfunction
- Spiritual Distress
- Social Isolation.

Outcome Identification

Care and treatment outcomes for clients who have survived trauma or abuse may include the following:

1. The client will be physically safe.
2. The client will distinguish between ideas of self-harm and taking action on those ideas.
3. The client will demonstrate healthy, effective ways of dealing with stress.
4. The client will express emotions non-destructively.
5. The client will establish (or re-establish) a social support system in the community.

Intervention

PROMOTING THE CLIENT'S SAFETY

The client's safety is a priority. The nurse must assess continually the client's potential for self-harm or suicide, and take action accordingly. The nurse and treatment team must provide safety measures when the client cannot do so (see Chapters 10 and 15). To increase the client's sense of personal control, he or she must begin to manage safety needs as soon as possible. The nurse can talk with the client about the difference between having self-harm thoughts and taking action on those thoughts: having the thoughts does not mean the client must act on those thoughts. Training in essential DBT skills may be helpful: gradually, the nurse can help the client to find ways to tolerate the thoughts until they diminish in intensity.

The nurse can help the client learn to go to a safe place during destructive thoughts and impulses, so that he or she can calm down and wait until they pass. Initially, this may mean just sitting with the nurse or around others. Later, the client can find a safe place at home, often a closet or small room, where he or she feels safe. The client may want to keep a blanket or pillows there for comfort, and pictures or a tape recording to serve as reminders of the present.

HELPING THE CLIENT COPE WITH STRESS AND EMOTIONS

Grounding techniques are helpful to use with the client who is dissociating or experiencing a flashback. Grounding techniques remind the client that he or she is in the present, is an adult and is safe. Validating what the client is feeling during these experiences is important: 'I know this is frightening, but you're safe now.' In addition, the nurse can increase contact with reality and diminish the dissociative experience by helping the client focus on what he or she is currently experiencing through the senses:

- 'What are you feeling?'
- 'Are you hearing something?'
- 'What are you touching?'
- 'Can you see me and the room we're in?'
- 'Do you feel your feet on the floor?'
- 'Do you feel your arm on the chair?'
- 'Do you feel the watch on your wrist?'

For the client experiencing dissociative symptoms, the nurse can use grounding techniques to focus the client on the present. For example, the nurse approaches the client and speaks in a calm, reassuring tone. First, the nurse calls the client by name and then introduces himself or herself by name and role. If the area is dark, the nurse turns on the lights. He or she can reorient the client by saying – carefully, slowly, warmly and conversationally – the following:

'Janet, I'm here with you. My name's Sheila. I'm the nurse working with you today. Today is Thursday, 8 February 2007. You're here in the hospital. This is your room at the hospital. Can you open your eyes and look at me? Janet, my name's Sheila.'

The nurse repeats this re-orienting information as needed. Asking the client to look around the room encourages the client to move his or her eyes and avoid being locked in a daze or flashback.

As soon as possible, the nurse may encourage the client to change positions. Often, during a flashback, the client might curl up in a defensive posture. Getting the client to stand and walk around helps to dispel the dissociative or flashback experience. At this time, the client can focus on his or her feet moving on the floor or the swinging movements of his or her arms. The nurse must not grab the client or attempt to force him or her to stand up or move. The client experiencing a flashback may respond to such attempts aggressively or defensively, even striking out at the nurse. Ideally, the nurse asks the client how he or she responds to touch when dissociating or experiencing a flashback before one occurs; then the nurse knows if using touch is beneficial for that client. The nurse may also ask the client to touch the nurse's arm. If the client does so, then supportive touch may well be beneficial for this client.

Many clients have difficulty identifying or gauging the intensity of their emotions. They also may report that extreme emotions appear out of nowhere with no warning. The nurse can help clients to get in touch with their feelings by using a log or journal. Initially, clients may use a 'feelings list' so they can select the feeling that most closely matches their experience. The nurse encourages the client to write down feelings throughout the day at specified intervals, for example, every 30 minutes. Once clients have identified their feelings, they can gauge the intensity of those feelings, for example, rating each feeling on a scale of 0 to 10. Using this process, clients have a greater awareness of their feelings and the different intensities; this step is important in managing and expressing those feelings.

After identifying feelings and their intensities, clients can begin to find triggers, or feelings that precede the flashbacks or dissociative episodes. Clients can then begin to use grounding techniques to diminish or avoid these episodes. They can use deep breathing and relaxation, focus on sensory information or stimuli in the environment, or engage in positive distractions until the feelings subside. Such distractions may include physical exercise, listening to music, talking to others or engaging in a hobby or activity. Clients must find which distractions work for them; they should then write them down and keep the list and the necessary materials for the activities close at hand. When clients begin to experience intense feelings, they can look at the list and pick up a book, listen to a tape or draw a picture, for instance.

HELPING TO PROMOTE THE CLIENT'S SELF-ESTEEM

Often it is useful to view the client as a **survivor** of trauma or abuse rather than as a victim. For those clients who believe they are worthless and have no power over the situation, it may help re-focus their view of themselves from being *victims* to being *survivors*. Defining themselves as survivors allows them to see themselves as strong enough to survive their ordeal: it is a more empowering image than seeing oneself as a victim.

NURSING INTERVENTIONS

Promote Client's Safety

- Discuss self-harm thoughts.
- Help the client develop a plan for going to safe place when having destructive thoughts or impulses.

Help Client Cope with Stress and Emotions

- Use grounding techniques to help the client who is dissociating or experiencing flashbacks.
- Validate the client's feelings of fear, but try to increase contact with reality.
- During dissociative experiences or flashbacks, help the client change body position, but do not grab or force the client to stand up or move.
- Use a supportive touch if client responds well to it.

- Teach deep-breathing and relaxation techniques.
- Use distraction techniques, such as participating in physical exercise, listening to music, talking with others or engaging in a hobby or other enjoyable activity.
- Help to make a list of activities and keep materials on hand to engage the client when his or her feelings are intense.

Help Promote Client's Self-esteem

- Refer to the client as a 'survivor' rather than a 'victim' (if he or she is comfortable with this).
- Ensure connections with social support systems.
- Make a list of people and activities for the client to contact when he or she needs help.

ESTABLISHING SOCIAL SUPPORT

The client needs to find support people or activities in the community. The nurse can help the client to prepare a list of support people. Problem-solving skills are difficult for these clients when under stress, so having a prepared list eliminates confusion or stress. This list should include a local crisis hotline to call when the client experiences self-harm thoughts or urges, and friends or family to call when the client is feeling lonely, anxious or depressed. The client can also identify local activities or groups that provide a diversion and a chance to get out of the house.

Evaluation

Long-term treatment outcomes for clients who have survived trauma or abuse may take years to achieve. These clients usually make gradual progress in protecting themselves, learning to manage stress and emotions and functioning in their daily lives. Although clients learn to manage their feelings and responses, the effects of trauma and abuse can be far reaching and last a lifetime. This said, people can grow and develop as a result of trauma: their beliefs about themselves, the world and other people can become more realistic, more integrated, more positive and more valued than before.

Nursing Care Plan *for a Client with PTSD*

Nursing Formulation

PTSD: *Sustained maladaptive response to a traumatic, overwhelming event.*

ASSESSMENT DATA

- Flashbacks or re-experiencing the traumatic event(s)
- Nightmares or recurrent dreams of the event or other trauma
- Sleep disturbances (e.g. insomnia, early awakening, crying out in sleep)
- Depression
- Denial of feelings or emotional numbness
- Projection of feelings
- Difficulty in expressing feelings
- Anger (may not be overt)

EXPECTED OUTCOMES

Immediate
The client will

- Identify the traumatic event
- Demonstrate decreased physical symptoms
- Verbalize need to grieve loss(es)
- Establish an adequate balance of rest, sleep and activity
- Demonstrate decreased anxiety, fear, guilt and so forth
- Participate in care and treatment programme

continued ⋯⊹

Nursing Care Plan: for a Client with PTSD, cont.

ASSESSMENT DATA

- Guilt or remorse
- Low self-esteem
- Frustration and irritability
- Anxiety, panic or separation anxiety
- Fears – may be displaced or generalized (as in fear of men in rape victims)
- Decreased concentration
- Difficulty expressing love or empathy
- Difficulty experiencing pleasure
- Difficulty with interpersonal relationships, marital problems, divorce
- Abuse in relationships
- Sexual problems
- Substance use
- Employment problems
- Physical symptoms

EXPECTED OUTCOMES

Medium-term
The client will

- Begin a grieving process
- Express feelings directly and openly in non-destructive ways
- Identify strengths and weaknesses realistically
- Demonstrate an increased ability to cope with stress
- Eliminate substance use
- Verbalize knowledge of illness, treatment plan or safe use of medications, if any

Longer-term
The client will

- Demonstrate initial integration of the traumatic experience into his or her life
- Identify and use support systems in the community
- Implement plans for follow-up or ongoing therapy, if indicated

IMPLEMENTATION

Nursing Interventions *denotes collaborative interventions	Rationale
When you approach the client, be non-threatening and professional.	The client's fears may be triggered by perceived authority figures, by someone of a particular gender or from a particular ethnic background.
Initially, on a ward, assign the same staff members to the client if possible; try to respect the client's fears and feelings. Gradually increase the number and variety of staff members interacting with the client.	Limiting the number of staff members who interact with the client at first will facilitate familiarity and trust. The client may have strong feelings of fear or mistrust about working with staff members with certain characteristics. These feelings may have been reinforced in previous encounters with professionals and may interfere with the therapeutic relationship.
*Educate yourself and other staff members about the client's experience and about posttraumatic behaviour.	Learning about the client's experience will help prepare you for the client's feelings and the details of his or her experience.
Examine and remain aware of your own feelings regarding both the client's traumatic experience and his or her feelings and behaviour. Talk with other staff members to air and work through your feelings.	Traumatic events engender strong feelings in others and may be quite threatening. You may be reminded of a related experience or of your own vulnerability, or issues related to sexuality, morality, safety or well-being. It is essential that you remain aware of your feelings so that you do not unconsciously project feelings, avoid issues or be otherwise non-therapeutic with the client.
Remain non-judgemental in your interactions with the client.	It is important not to reinforce blame that the client may have internalized related to the experience.
Be consistent with the client; convey acceptance of him or her as a person while setting and maintaining limits regarding behaviours.	The client may test limits or the therapeutic relationship. Problems with acceptance, trust or authority often occur with posttraumatic behaviour.

continued ⋯⟩

Nursing Care Plan: for a Client with PTSD, cont.

IMPLEMENTATION

Nursing Interventions *denotes collaborative interventions	Rationale
*Assess the client's history of substance use (information from significant others might be helpful).	Clients often use substances to help repress (or release) emotions.
Be aware of the client's use or abuse of substances. Set limits and consequences for this behaviour; it may be helpful to allow the client or group to have input into these decisions.	Substance use undermines therapy and may endanger the client's health. Allowing input from the client or group may minimize power struggles.
*If substance use is a major problem, refer the client to a substance dependence treatment programme.	Substance use must be dealt with because it may affect all other areas of the client's life.
Encourage the client to talk about his or her experience(s); be accepting and non-judgemental of the client's accounts and perceptions.	Re-telling the experience can help the client to identify the reality of what has happened and help to identify and work through related feelings.
Encourage the client to express his or her feelings through talking, writing, crying or other ways in which the client is comfortable.	Identification and expression of feelings are central to the grieving process.
Especially encourage the expression of anger, guilt and rage.	These feelings often occur in clients who have experienced trauma. The client may feel survivor's guilt that he or she survived when others did not, or guilt about the behaviour he or she undertook to survive (killing others in combat, enduring a rape, not saving others).
*Teach the client and the family or significant others about posttraumatic behaviour and treatment.	Knowledge about posttraumatic behaviour may help alleviate anxiety or guilt and may increase hope for recovery.
*As tolerated, encourage the client to share his or her feelings and experiences in group therapy, in a support group related to posttrauma recovery, or with other clients informally.	The client needs to know that his or her feelings are acceptable to others and can be shared. Peer or support groups can offer understanding, support and the opportunity for sharing experiences.
Give the client positive feedback for expressing feelings and sharing experiences. Remain non-judgemental toward the client.	The client may feel that he or she is burdening others with his or her problems. It is important not to reinforce the client's internalized blame.
*If the client has a religious or spiritual orientation, referral to an appropriate member of the clergy or a chaplain may be appropriate.	Guilt and forgiveness are often religious or spiritual issues for the client.
Encourage the client to make realistic plans for the future, integrating his or her traumatic experience.	Integrating traumatic experiences and making future plans are important resolution steps in the grief process.
Help the client learn and practise stress-management and relaxation techniques, assertiveness or self-defence training or other skills as appropriate.	The client's traumatic experience may have resulted in a loss or decrease in self-confidence, sense of safety or ability to deal with stress.
*Provide social skills and leisure time counselling, or refer the client to an occupational therapist or a STAR worker, as appropriate.	Social isolation and lack of interest in recreational activities are common problems following trauma.
*Talk with the client about employment, job-related stress and so forth. Refer the client to vocational services as needed.	Problems with employment frequently occur in clients with posttraumatic behaviour.
*Help the client arrange for follow-up therapy as needed.	Recovering from trauma may be a long-term process. Follow-up therapy can offer continuing support in the client's recovery.

Adapted from Schultz, J. M. & Videbeck, S. L. (2005). *Lippincott's manual of psychiatric nursing care plans* (7th edn.). Philadelphia: Lippincott Williams & Wilkins.

SELF-AWARENESS ISSUES

Nurses are sometimes reluctant to ask people about abuse, partly because they may believe some common myths about abuse. They may believe that questions about abuse will offend the client, or fear that incorrect interventions will worsen the situation. Nurses may even believe, say, that a woman who stays in an abusive relationship might deserve or enjoy the abuse, or that abuse between husband and wife is private. Some nurses may believe abuse to be a societal or legal, not a health, problem and therefore one that doesn't fall within the nursing remit.

Listening to stories of family violence or rape is difficult; the nurse may feel horror or revulsion. Because clients often watch for the nurse's reaction, containing these feelings and focusing on the client's needs are important. The nurse must be prepared to listen to the client's story, no matter how disturbing, and support and validate the client's feelings with comments such as 'That must have been terrifying' or 'Sounds like you were afraid for your life'. The nurse must convey acceptance and regard for the client as a person with worth and dignity, regardless of the circumstances. These clients often have low self-esteem and guilt. They must learn to accept and face what has occurred. If the client believes that the nurse can accept him or her after hearing what has happened, he or she then may gain self-acceptance. Although this acceptance is often painful, it is essential to healing. The nurse must remember that he or she cannot fix or change things; the nurse's role is to listen and convey acceptance and support for the client.

Nurses with a personal history of abuse or trauma themselves must seek professional assistance to deal with these issues before working with survivors of trauma or abuse. Such nurses can be very effective and supportive of other survivors, but usually only after engaging in therapeutic work and accepting and understanding their own trauma.

Points to Consider When Working With Abused or Traumatized Clients

- These clients have many strengths that they – and others – may not realize. The nurse can help them move from being *victims* to being *survivors*.
- Nurses should be aware of a need sometimes to ask clients about abuse, and always to consider its possible relevance to someone's current difficulties. Sometimes a client may be offended and angry, but it is important not to miss the opportunity of helping the woman who replies, 'Yes. Can you help me?'
- The nurse should help the client focus on the present and – if appropriate – on experiences in the past.
- Sometimes, a nurse may work best with either the survivors of abuse or the abusers themselves. Many can find it too difficult emotionally to work with both groups. Nevertheless, all clients – including 'abusers' and 'survivors' – deserve respect and sensitive, focused and compassionate care.

Critical Thinking Questions

1. Is smacking a child an acceptable form of discipline, or is it abusive? What determines the appropriateness of discipline? Who should make these decisions, and why?
2. How can the nurse continue to have a positive relationship with the client who returns again and again to an abusive relationship? What should the nurse say to the client who has decided to return to an abusive relationship?
3. A client has just told the nurse that in the past he has lost his temper and has beaten his child. How should the nurse respond? What factors would affect the nurse's response?

KEY POINTS

- Violence and abusive behaviour are major national health and social concerns.
- There is a clear link between the experience of trauma and a variety of mental health problems.
- Women and children are the most likely victims of abuse and violence.
- Characteristics of violent families include an intergenerational transmission process, social isolation, power and control and the use of alcohol and other drugs.
- Spousal abuse can be emotional, physical, sexual or all three.
- Women may have difficulty leaving abusive relationships because of financial and emotional dependence on the abusers and the risk for suffering increased violence or death.
- Nurses in various settings can uncover abuse by asking people about their sense of safety in relationships.
- Many services routinely ask women about safety issues as an integral part of the assessment interview or health history.
- Rape is a crime of violence and humiliation through sexual means. Most reported cases are perpetrated by someone the victim knows.
- Child abuse includes neglect and physical, emotional and sexual abuse.
- Elder abuse may include physical and sexual abuse, psychological abuse, neglect, exploitation and medical abuse.
- Survivors of abuse and trauma often experience guilt and shame, low self-esteem, substance abuse, depression, PTSD and dissociative disorders.
- PTSD is a response to a traumatic event. It can include flashbacks, nightmares, insomnia, mistrust, avoidance behaviours and intense psychological distress.

INTERNET RESOURCES

RESOURCES*	INTERNET ADDRESS
• Action on Elder Abuse	http://www.elderabuse.org.uk/
• Anti-Bullying Alliance	http://www.anti-bullyingalliance.org.uk/Page.asp
• End Violence Against Women	http://www.endviolenceagainstwomen.org.uk/
• National Association for People Abused in Childhood	http://www.napac.org.uk/
• Parentlineplus	http://www.parentlineplus.org.uk/index.php?id=11
• Rape Crisis and Sexual Abuse Centre, Northern Ireland	http://www.rapecrisisni.com/whatwedo.php
• Rape Crisis England and Wales	http://www.rapecrisis.org.uk/stats.html
• Rape Crisis Scotland	http://www.rapecrisisscotland.org.uk
• Refuge	http://www.refuge.org.uk/homepage.html
• Women's Aid	http://www.womensaid.org.uk/

*All of these websites have multiple links to other sites on the topic.

- Dissociation is a defence mechanism that protects the emotional self from the full reality of abusive or traumatic events during and after those events.
- Survivors of trauma and abuse may be admitted to the hospital for safety concerns or stabilization of intense symptoms such as flashbacks or dissociative episodes.
- The nurse can help the client to minimize dissociative episodes or flashbacks through grounding techniques and reality orientation.
- Important nursing interventions for survivors of abuse and trauma include protecting the client's safety, helping the client learn to manage stress and emotions and working with the client to build a network of community support.
- Important self-awareness issues for the nurse include managing his or her own feelings and reactions about abuse, being willing to ask about abuse and recognizing and dealing with any abuse issues he or she may have experienced personally.

REFERENCES

American Medical Association. (2004). Available: http://www.ama-assn.org/.

American Psychiatric Association. (2000). *Diagnostic and statistical manual of mental disorders* (4th edn, text revision). Washington, DC: American Psychiatric Association.

Bacchus, L., Mezey, G., & Bewley, S. (2006). A qualitative exploration of the nature of domestic violence in pregnancy. *Violence Against Women, 12*(6), 558–604.

Bernet, W. (2005). Child maltreatment. In B. J. Sadock & V. A. Sadock (Eds.), *Comprehensive textbook of psychiatry, Vol. 2* (8th edn, pp. 3412–3424). Philadelphia: Lippincott Williams & Wilkins.

Bureau of Justice Statistics. (2006). Available: http://www.ojp.usdoj.gov/bjs

Cawson, P. (2002). *Child maltreatment in the family: The experience of a national sample of young people.* NSPCC.

Cawson, P., Wattam, C., Brooker, S., & Kelly, G. (2000). *Child maltreatment in the UK: A study of the prevalence of child abuse and neglect.* NSPCC.

Department of Health and Home Office. (2000). *No secrets: guidance on developing and implementing multi-agency policies and procedures to protect vulnerable adults from abuse.* Available: http://www.dh.gov.uk/en/Publicationsandstatistics/Publications/PublicationsPolicyAndGuidance/DH_4008486

Dube, S. R., Anda, R. F., Whitfield, C. L., et al. (2005). Long-term consequences of childhood sexual abuse by gender of victim. *American Journal of Preventative Medicine, 28*(5), 430–438.

Finney, A. (2006). *Domestic violence, sexual assault and stalking: findings from the 2004/05British Crime Survey.* Home Office Online Report 12/06. London: Home Office. Available: http://www.homeoffice.gov.uk/rds/pdfs06/rdsolr1206.pdf

Goldstein, M. Z. (2005). Elder abuse, neglect, and exploitation. In B. J. Sadock & V. A. Sadock (Eds.), *Comprehensive textbook of psychiatry, Vol. 2* (8th edn, pp. 3828–3834). Philadelphia: Lippincott Williams & Wilkins.

Her Majesty's Government. (2006). *Working together to safeguard children: A guide to inter-agency working to safeguard and promote the welfare of children.* Available: http://www.everychildmatters.gov.uk/_files/AE53C8F9D7AEB1B23E403514A6C1B17D.pdf

Home Office. (2002). *Rape and sexual assault of women: findings from the British Crime Survey.* Available: http://www.homeoffice.gov.uk/rds/pdfs2/r159.pdf

Home Office. (2008a). *Crime in England and Wales 2007/08. Findings from the British Crime Survey and police recorded crime.* Available: http://www.homeoffice.gov.uk/rds/pdfs07/hosb1107.pdf

Home Office. (2008b). *Crime reduction: domestic violence minisite.* Available: http://www.crimereduction.homeoffice.gov.uk/dv/dv01.htm

Horvath, M. A. H. & Brown, J. (2006). The role of alcohol and drugs in rape. Medicine, Science and the Law, 46(3), 219–228.

Laming, Lord (2003). *The Victoria Climbié Inquiry.* Available: http://www.victoria-climbie-inquiry.org.uk/finreport/finreport.htm

Marin Institute. (2006). *Alcohol and violence.* Available: http://www.marininstitue.org/print/alcohol_policy/violence.htm (accessed 31 December 2006).

Middleton, W., Cromer, L. M., & Freyd, J. (2005). Remembering the past, anticipating a future. *Australasian Psychiatry, 13*(3), 223–233.

National Society for the Prevention of Cruelty to Children. (2008). *Professional practice.* Available: http://www.nspcc.org.uk/Inform/resourcesforprofessionals/resources_wda49819.html

Office of National Statistics. (2008). *Crime.* Available: http://www.statistics.gov.uk/cci/nugget.asp?id=1661

Piper, A. & Merskey, H. (2004). The persistence of folly: Critical examination of dissociative identity disorder. II. The defence and decline of multiple personality or dissociative identity disorder. *Canadian Journal of Psychiatry, 49*(10), 678–683.

Rape Crisis England and Wales. (2008). *Statistics*. Available: http://www.rapecrisis.org.uk/stats.html

Read, J., Hammersley, P., & Rudegeir, T. (2007). Why, when and how to ask about childhood abuse *Advances in Psychiatric Treatment, 13*, 101–110.

Royal College of Nursing. (2005). *Child protection – every nurse's responsibility*. Available: http://www.rcn.org.uk/__data/assets/pdf_file/0004/78583/002045.pdf

Ryan, B. A. (2003). Do you suspect child abuse? *RN, 66*(9), 73–74, 76–79.

Schlenger, W. E., Caddell, J. M., Ebert, L., *et al.* (2002). Psychological reactions to terrorist attacks: Findings from the national study of Americans' reactions. *Journal of the American Medical Association, 288*(5), 581–588.

Sexual Offences Act. (2003). London: OPSI. Available: http://www.opsi.gov.uk/Acts/acts2003/ukpga_20030042_en_1

Skybo, T. (2005). Witnessing violence: Biopsychosocial impact on children. *Pediatric Nursing, 31*(4), 263–270.

State University of New York at Buffalo Counseling Center. (2006). Relationship violence warning signs. Available: http://ub-counseling.buffalo.edu/warnings.shtml

Van Cleave, J. & Davis M. M. (2006). Bullying and peer victimization among children with special health care needs. *Pediatrics, 118*(4), e1212–1219.

Van der Kolk, B. A. (2005). Physical and sexual abuse of adults. In B. J. Sadock & V. A. Sadock (Eds.), *Comprehensive textbook of psychiatry Vol. 2* (8th edn, pp. 2393–2398). Philadelphia: Lippincott Williams & Wilkins.

ADDITIONAL READING

Action on Elder Abuse. (2004). *Hidden voices: Older people's experience of abuse*. Help the Aged. Available: http://www.elderabuse.org.uk/

Basile, K. C., Swahn, M. H., Chen, J., & Saltzman, L. E. (2006). Stalking in the United States: recent national prevalence rates. *American Journal of Preventative Medicine, 31*(2), 172–175.

Johnson, D. M. & Zlotnick, C. (2006). A cognitive-behavioural treatment for battered women with PTSD in shelters: Findings from a pilot study. *Journal of Traumatic Stress, 19*(4), 559–564.

McCabe, M. P. & Wauchope, M. (2005). Behavioural characteristics of men accused of rape: Evidence for different types of rapists. *Archives of Sexual Behaviour, 34*(2), 241–253.

Sheehan, K., Kim, L. E., & Galvin, J. P. Jr. (2004). Urban children's perceptions of violence. *Archives of Pediatric and Adolescent Medicine, 158*(1), 74–77.

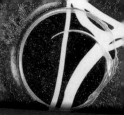

MULTIPLE-CHOICE QUESTIONS

Select the best answer for each of the following questions.

1. Which of the following is the best action for the nurse to take when assessing a child who might be abused?
   a. Confront the parents with the facts and ask them what happened.
   b. Consult with a professional member of the health team about contacting the Child Protection Team.
   c. Ask the child which of his parents caused this injury.
   d. Say or do nothing; the nurse has only suspicions, not evidence.

2. Which of the following interventions would be most helpful for a client with dissociative disorder having difficulty expressing feelings?
   a. Distraction
   b. Reality orientation
   c. Journaling
   d. Grounding techniques

3. Which of the following is true about touching a client who is experiencing a flashback?
   a. The nurse should stand in front of the client before touching.
   b. The nurse should never touch a client who is having a flashback.
   c. The nurse should touch the client only after receiving permission to do so.
   d. The nurse should touch the client to increase feelings of security.

4. Which of the following is true about domestic violence between same-sex partners?
   a. Such violence is less common than that between heterosexual partners.
   b. The frequency and intensity of violence are greater than between heterosexual partners.
   c. Rates of violence are about the same as between heterosexual partners.
   d. None of the above.

5. The nurse working with a client during a flashback says, 'I know you're scared, but you're in a safe place. Do you see the bed in your room? Do you feel the chair you're sitting on?' The nurse is using which of the following techniques?
   a. Distraction
   b. Reality orientation
   c. Relaxation
   d. Grounding

6. Which of the following assessment findings might indicate self-neglect in an older person?
   a. Hesitancy to talk openly with nurse
   b. Inability to manage personal finances
   c. Missing valuables that are not misplaced
   d. Unusual explanations for injuries

7. Women in violent and abusive relationships often remain in those relationships as a result of faulty or incorrect beliefs. Which of the following beliefs is valid?
   a. If she tried to leave, she would be at increased risk for violence.
   b. If she would do a better job of meeting his needs, the violence would stop.
   c. No one else would put up with her dependent, clinging behaviour.
   d. She often does things that provoke the violent episodes.

FILL-IN-THE-BLANK QUESTIONS

Identify the type of abuse described in the following situations.

_____ A parent does not see a doctor or give medicine to a 3-month-old with a fever of 103°F (39°C).

_____ An elderly woman's utilities are cut off for non-payment of bills, yet she has three uncashed Giros in her possession.

_____ An adult daughter tells her elderly mother, 'I'll send you to a nursing home if you don't give me your benefit money!'

_____ A parent repeatedly tells a child, 'You're stupid. You'll never amount to anything!'

GROUP DISCUSSION TOPICS

Discuss and give examples to illustrate each of the following concepts:

• Cycle of violence or abuse

• Blaming the victim of abuse or rape

• Survivor's guilt

• Intergenerational transmission process in violent families

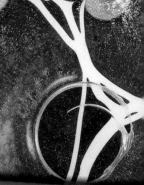

Chapter

12

Grief and Loss

Key Terms

- acculturation
- adaptive denial
- anticipatory grieving
- attachment behaviours
- attentive presence
- bereavement
- complicated grieving
- disenfranchised grief
- dysfunctional grieving
- grief
- grieving
- homeostasis
- mourning
- phase of disorganization and despair
- phase of numbing
- phase of reorganization
- phase of yearning and searching
- spirituality

Learning Objectives

After reading this chapter, you should be able to:

1. Identify the types of loss we might all encounter in our lives.

2. Discuss various theories related to understanding the grief process.

3. Describe the five dimensions of grieving.

4. Discuss universal and culturally specific mourning rituals.

5. Discuss disenfranchised grief and the vulnerability of people who experience it.

6. Identify factors that increase a person's susceptibility to complications related to grieving.

7. Discuss factors that are critical to integrating loss into life.

8. Apply the nursing process to facilitate productive grieving for clients and families.

Experiences of loss are normal and essential in human life. Letting go, relinquishing and moving on are unavoidable passages as a person moves through the stages of growth and development. People frequently say goodbye to places, people, dreams and familiar objects. Examples of necessary losses accompanying growth include abandoning a favourite blanket or toy, leaving a primary school teacher and (particularly traumatic for many people involved in nurse education) giving up the adolescent hope of becoming a famous rock star. Loss allows a person to change, develop and fulfil innate human potential. It may be planned, expected or sudden. Although it can be difficult, loss is inevitable and, frequently, a beneficial part of development and personal growth. Sometimes, though, loss can be devastating and debilitating.

Grief refers to the subjective cognitions, emotions and affect that are a normal response to the experience of loss. **Grieving**, also known as **bereavement**, refers to the process by which a person experiences the grief. It involves not only the content (*what* a person thinks, says and feels) but also the process (*how* a person thinks, says and feels). All people grieve when they experience life's changes and losses. Often, grieving is one of the most difficult and challenging processes of human existence; rarely is it comfortable or pleasant. **Anticipatory grieving** occurs when people facing an imminent loss begin to grapple with the very real possibility of the loss or death in the near future (Ziemba & Lynch-Sauer, 2005). **Mourning** is the outward expression of grief. Rituals of mourning include having a wake, sitting Shiva, holding religious ceremonies and arranging funerals.

This chapter examines the human experience of loss and the process by which a person moves through bereavement and integrates loss into his or her life. To support and care for the grieving person, the nurse must understand these phases as well as cultural responses to loss. At times, grief may be the focus of care and treatment. The nursing process section outlines the nurse's role in grieving, and gives guidelines for offering support and for teaching coping skills to clients. The chapter also outlines the importance of the nurse's self-awareness and interpersonal competence in helping clients and families during bereavement.

TYPES OF LOSSES

A helpful way to examine different types of losses is to use Abraham Maslow's hierarchy of human needs. According to Maslow (1954), a hierarchy of needs motivates human actions. The hierarchy begins with physiological needs (food, air, water, sleep), safety needs (a safe place to live and work), and security and belonging needs (satisfying relationships). The next set of needs includes self-esteem needs, which lead to feelings of adequacy and confidence. The last and final need is self-actualization, the ability to realize one's full innate potential. When these human needs are taken away or not met for some reason, a person experiences loss. Examples of losses related to specific human needs in Maslow's hierarchy are as follows:

- *Physiological loss*: Examples include amputation of a limb, loss of adequate air exchange or decrease in pancreatic functioning.
- *Safety loss*: Loss of a safe environment is evident in domestic or public violence. A person may perceive a breach of confidentiality in a professional relationship as a loss of psychological safety secondary to broken trust of self and the care provider.
- *Loss of security and a sense of belonging*: The loss of a loved one affects the need to love and be loved. Loss accompanies changes in relationships, such as birth, marriage, divorce, illness and death; as the meaning of a relationship changes, a person may lose roles within a family or group.
- *Loss of self-esteem*: Any change in how a person is valued at work or in relationships can threaten his or her self-esteem needs. A change in self-perception can challenge one's sense of self-worth. A loss of role function and the self-perception and worth tied to that role may accompany the death of a loved one.
- *Loss related to self-actualization*: An external or internal crisis that blocks or inhibits strivings toward fulfilment may threaten personal goals and individual potential. A change in goals or direction will precipitate an inevitable period of grief as the person gives up a creative thought to make room for new ideas and directions. Examples include having to give up plans to attend university or losing the hope of marriage and family.

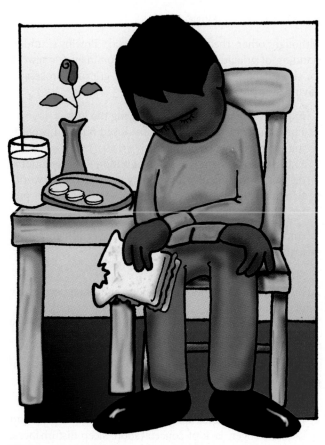

Grief

The fulfilment of human needs requires dynamic movement throughout the various levels in the hierarchy. The simultaneous maintenance of needs in the areas of physiological integrity, safety, security and sense of belonging, self-esteem and self-actualization is challenging and demands flexibility and focus. At times, a focus on protection may take priority over professional or self-actualization goals. Likewise, human losses demand a grieving process that simultaneously challenges each level of need. Specific examples include the loss of a pregnancy or loss of sight or hearing.

THE GRIEVING PROCESS

Nurses interact with people responding to a myriad of losses along the continuum of health and illness. Regardless of the type of loss, nurses must have a basic understanding of what is involved to meet the challenges that grief brings to people. By understanding the phenomena that we all experience as we deal with the discomfort of loss, nurses can promote the expression and release of emotional as well as physical pain during grieving. Supporting this process means ministering to psychological – and physical – needs.

Establishing an effective therapeutic relationship based on core skills such as active listening is vital when assisting people who are grieving (see Chapters 5 and 6). Recognizing the verbal and non-verbal communication content of the various stages of grieving can help nurses to select interventions that meet the client's psychological and physical needs. Above all, compassion is paramount.

Theories of the Grieving Process

KUBLER-ROSS'S STAGES OF GRIEVING

Elisabeth Kubler-Ross (1969) established a basis for understanding how loss affects human life. As she attended to clients with terminal illnesses, a *process* of dying became apparent to her. Through her observations and work with dying people and their families, Kubler-Ross developed a model of five stages to explain what people experience as they grieve and mourn:

1. *Denial* is shock and disbelief regarding the loss.
2. *Anger* may be expressed toward God, relatives, friends or health professionals.
3. *Bargaining* occurs when the person asks God or fate for more time to delay the inevitable loss.
4. *Depression* results when awareness of the loss becomes acute.
5. *Acceptance* occurs when the person shows evidence of coming to terms with death.

This model became a prototype for clinicians as they looked for ways to understand and assist their clients in the grieving process.

BOWLBY'S THEORY OF ATTACHMENT BEHAVIOURS

John Bowlby, a British psychoanalyst, proposed a theory that humans instinctively attain and retain affectional bonds with significant others through **attachment behaviours**. These attachment behaviours are crucial to the development of a sense of security and survival. Examples of attachment behaviours include following, clinging, calling out and crying. Bowlby saw that human beings modified these attachment behaviours as they matured from childhood into adulthood, but he also noticed that patterns of attachment behaviour formed early in life endure throughout the life cycle. People experience the most intense emotions when *forming* a bond such as falling in love, *maintaining* a bond such as loving someone, *disrupting* a bond such as in a divorce and *renewing* an attachment, such as resolving a conflict or renewing a relationship (Bowlby, 1980).

An attachment that is maintained is a source of security; an attachment that is renewed is a source of joy. When a bond is threatened or broken, however, the person responds with anxiety, protest and anger. Actual loss leads to sorrow. According to Bowlby, these emotions reflect affectional bonds. Loss strongly activates or arouses attachment behaviours. Thus, the clinical picture of increased anxiety, sorrow, anger, looking for the lost person or object, calling out, crying and protesting is an attempt to restore the lost affectional bond.

PHASES OF THE GRIEVING PROCESS

Although other theories are described, Bowlby's understanding of grieving serves as the predominant framework for this chapter. Bowlby described the grieving process as having four phases:

1. Experiencing numbness and denying the loss
2. Emotionally yearning for the lost loved one and protesting the permanence of the loss
3. Experiencing cognitive disorganization and emotional despair, with difficulty functioning in the everyday world
4. Reorganizing and reintegrating the sense of self to pull life back together.

Another theorist, John Harvey (Harvey & Miller, 1998), described similar phases of grieving:

1. Shock, outcry and denial
2. Intrusion of thoughts, distractions and obsessive review of the loss
3. Confiding in others as a way to emote and to cognitively restructure an account of the loss.

Rodebaugh and colleagues (1999) viewed the process of grief as a journey through four stages:

1. *Reeling*: The person feels shock, disbelief or denial.
2. *Feeling*: The person experiences anguish, guilt, profound sadness, anger, lack of concentration, sleep disturbances, appetite changes, fatigue and general physical discomfort.

3. *Dealing*: The person begins to adapt to the loss by engaging in support groups, grief therapy, reading and spiritual guidance.
4. *Healing*: The person integrates the loss as part of life. Acute anguish lessens. Healing does not imply, however, that the person has forgotten or accepted the loss.

Table 12.1 compares these theories of grieving.

Nurses should not expect everyone to follow predictable steps in the grieving process. Indeed, such an expectation may put added pressure or stress on someone when he or she most needs acceptance, reflection and support from others. Interventions that nurses can use to facilitate the grieving process are discussed later in this chapter.

Tasks of the Grieving Process

Rando (1984) described tasks inherent to grieving:

- Undoing psychosocial bonds to the loved one and, eventually, creating new ties
- Adding new roles, skills and behaviours and revising old ones into a 'new identity and sense of self
- Pursuing a healthy lifestyle that includes people and activities
- Integrating the loss into life, which does not mean ending the grieving but accommodating the reality of the loss.

The accompanying *Clinical Vignette*: *Grief* gives an example of integrating loss into life. Margaret has come to view James's death and the painful period of grief as a profound and poignant 'search for meaning in life'. The sense of his presence remains with her as she pursues her life without him, and she often pictures him before he became ill. Viewing the grieving process more positively, she believes

that his death in some way has encouraged her to become more independent and to participate in new opportunities.

DIMENSIONS OF GRIEVING

People have many and varied responses to loss. They express their bereavement in their thoughts, words, feelings and actions, as well as through their physiological responses. Nurses, must, therefore, use a holistic model of grieving that encompasses cognitive, emotional, spiritual, behavioural and physiological dimensions (Lobb *et al.*, 2006).

Cognitive Responses to Grief

In some respects, the pain that accompanies grieving results from a disturbance in the person's beliefs. The loss disrupts, if not shatters, basic assumptions about life's meaning and purpose. Grieving often causes a person to change beliefs about self, other people and the world, such as perceptions of the world's benevolence, the meaning of life and its relationship to justice and a sense of destiny or life-path. Other changes in thinking and attitude include reviewing and ranking values, becoming wiser, shedding illusions about immortality and permanence, viewing the world more realistically and re-evaluating religious or spiritual beliefs (Zisook & Zisook, 2005).

QUESTIONING AND TRYING TO MAKE SENSE OF THE LOSS

The grieving person needs to make sense of the loss. He or she undergoes self-examination and questions accepted ways of thinking. The loss challenges old assumptions about life. For example, when a loved one dies prematurely, the grieving person often questions the belief that 'life is fair' or

Table 12.1	THEORETICAL UNDERSTANDING OF THE GRIEVING PROCESS			
Theorist/Clinician	**Phase I**	**Phase II**	**Phase III**	**Phase IV**
Kubler-Ross (1969)	Stage I: denial	Stage II: anger Stage III: depression	Stage IV: bargaining	Stage V: acceptance
Bowlby (1980)	Numbness, denial	Emotional yearning for the loved one, protesting permanence of the loss	Cognitive disorganization, emotional despair, difficulty functioning	Cognitive reorganization, reintegrating sense of self
Harvey & Miller (1998)	Shock, outcry, denial	Intrusion of thoughts, distractions; obsessive reviewing of the loss	Confiding in others to emote and to cognitively restructure account of loss	
Rodebaugh *et al.* (1999)	Reeling: shock, disbelief or denial	Feeling: anguish, guilt, sadness, anger, lack of concentration, sleep disturbances, appetite changes, fatigue, general discomfort	Dealing: adapting to the loss	Healing: integration of loss, acute anguish dissipated, loss may or may not be forgotten or accepted

CLINICAL VIGNETTE: GRIEF

'If I had known what the grief process was like, I would never have married, or I would have prayed every day of my married life that I would be the first to die', reflects Margaret, 9 years after the death of her husband.

She recalls her initial thought, denying and acknowledging reality simultaneously, when James was diagnosed with multiple myeloma in October 1988: 'It's a mistake . . . but I know it isn't'.

For 2½ years, Margaret and James diligently followed his regime of treatment while taking time for work and play, making the most of their life together in the moment. 'We were not melodramatic people. We told ourselves, "This is what's happening; we'll deal with it".'

For Margaret, it was a shock to realize that some friends who had been so readily present for social gatherings were no longer available. She waited alone in the dark and stillness of early morning when James had emergency surgery. She was shocked when she told a priest who came into the room, 'My husband is having surgery', and his reply was 'Oh, sorry to bother you; I'm looking for the paper.'

Margaret began to undergo a shift in her thinking: 'You begin to evaluate your perceptions of others. I asked myself, "Who is there for me?" Friends, *are* they *really*? It can be painful to find out they really aren't. It frees you later, though. You can let them go.'

When James died, Margaret remained 'level-headed and composed' until one day shortly after the funeral when she suddenly became aware of her exhaustion. While shopping, she found herself protesting at the emotional pain and wanting to shout, 'Doesn't anybody know that I have just lost my husband?'

Surprised with how overwhelmed she felt, one of her hardest moments was putting her sister on the plane and going home to 'an empty house'. It was at this time that she began to feel the initial shock of her loss. Her body felt like it was 'wired with electricity'. She felt as though she was 'just going through the motions', doing routine chores like grocery shopping and putting petrol in the car, all the while feeling numb.

Crying spells lasted 6 months. She became 'tired of mourning' and would ask herself, 'When is this going to get easier?' She also felt anger. 'I was upset with James, wondering why he didn't go for his complete physical. Maybe James's death might not have happened so soon.'

After a few months and well into the grief process, Margaret knew she needed to 'do something constructive'. She did. She attended support groups, travelled and became involved with church activities.

Her faith in God was a plus. Exercising this faith, she trusted that eventually her emotions would catch up with the intellectual understanding of all that had transpired in James's dying. She developed an 'inner knowing that God is all-seeing, all-knowing'. This belief gave her spiritual strength and empowered her as she grieved.

Nearly a decade after James's death, Margaret viewed the grief process as a profound and poignant 'search for meaning in life. If he had not gone, I would not have come to where I am in life. I am content, confident and happy with how authentic life is.'

Even so, a sense of James's presence remains with her as she pictures the way he was before he became ill. She states, 'This is good for me.'

---

that 'one has control over life or destiny'. He or she searches for answers to why the trauma occurred. The goal of the search is to give meaning and purpose to the loss. The nurse might hear the following questions:

- 'Why did this have to happen? He took such good care of himself!'
- 'Why did such a young person have to die?'
- 'He was such a good person! Why did this happen to him?'

Questioning may help the person accept the reality of why someone died. For example, perhaps the death is related to the person's health practices – maybe he did not take good care of himself and have regular check-ups. Questioning may result in realizing that loss and death are realities that everyone must face one day. Others may discover explanations and meaning and even gain comfort from a religious or spiritual perspective, such as believing that the dead person is with God and at peace (Neimeyer *et al.*, 2006).

ATTEMPTING TO KEEP THE LOST ONE PRESENT

Belief in an afterlife and the idea that the lost one has become a personal guide are cognitive responses that serve to keep the lost one present. Carrying on an internal dialogue with the loved one while doing an activity is an example: 'John, I wonder what you would do in this situation. I wish you were here to show me. Let's see, I think you would probably . . . .' This method of keeping the lost one present may help soften the effects of the loss while assimilating its reality.

Humanists and others may take solace in the knowledge that people live on in their work, their impact on others during their life, their children and in others' memories of them.

Emotional Responses to Grief

Anger, sadness and anxiety are the predominant emotional responses to loss. The grieving person may direct anger and resentment toward the dead person and his or her health practices, family members or health-care providers or institutions. Common reactions the nurse might hear are as follows:

- 'He should have stopped smoking years ago.'
- 'If I had taken her to the doctor earlier, this might not have happened.'
- 'It took you too long to diagnose his illness.'

Guilt over things not done or said in the lost relationship is another painful emotion. Feelings of hatred and revenge are common when death has resulted from extreme circumstances such as suicide, murder or war (Zisook & Zisook, 2005). In addition to despair and anger, some people may also experience feelings of loss of control in their lives, uncharacteristic feelings of dependency on others and even anxiety about their own death.

Emotional responses are evident in all phases of Bowlby's grief process. During the **phase of numbing**, the common first response to the news of a loss is to be stunned, as though not perceiving reality. Emotions vacillate in frequency and intensity. Contrasting emotions are common, such as experiencing an impulsive outburst of anger toward the deceased, oneself or others at one moment, and then feeling unexpected elation at a sense of union with the deceased the next (Bowlby, 1980). The person may function automatically in a state of calm and then suddenly become overwhelmed with panic. In the clinical vignette, Margaret discusses having felt 'numbness' while going through routine functions immediately after her husband's death and then one day finding herself in a department store overwhelmed with frustration and wanting to shout, 'Doesn't anyone realize I've just lost my husband?'

In the second **phase of yearning and searching**, reality begins to set in. The grieving person exhibits anger, profound sorrow and crying. He or she often reverts to the attachment behaviours of childhood by acting similar to a child who loses his or her mother in a shop or at the park. The grieving person may express irritability, bitterness and hostility toward clergy, medical providers, relatives, comforters and even the dead person. The hopeless, yet intense, desire to restore the bond with the lost person compels the bereaved to search for and recover him or her. The grieving person interprets sounds, sights and smells associated with the lost one as signs of the deceased's presence, which may intermittently provide comfort and ignite hope for a reunion. For example, the ring of the telephone at a time in the day when the deceased friend regularly called will trigger the excitement of hearing his or her voice. Or the scent of his wife's perfume will spur her late husband to scan the room for her smiling face. As hopes for the lost one's return diminish, sadness and loneliness become constant.

In the vignette, Margaret became angry with her husband for not having his physical examination sooner and upset with friends who seemed to disappear after James became critically ill. Such emotional tumult may last several months and seems necessary for the person to begin to acknowledge the true permanence of the loss.

During the **phase of disorganization and despair**, the bereaved person begins to understand the loss's permanence. He or she recognizes that the patterns of thinking, feeling and acting attached to life with the deceased must change. As the person relinquishes all hope of recovering the lost one, he or she inevitably experiences moments of depression, apathy or despair. Night can be a time of acute loneliness during this phase.

In the final phase, the **phase of reorganization**, the bereaved person begins to re-establish a sense of personal identity, direction and purpose for living. He or she gains independence and confidence (Bowlby, 1980). By experimenting with and accomplishing newly defined roles and functions, the bereaved becomes personally empowered. This emotional and affective experience is associated closely with the inherent cognitive recognition that life without the loved one is a reality and therefore must be different. In this phase, the person still misses the deceased, but thinking of him or her no longer evokes painful feelings. In the vignette, hearing Spanish music, which Margaret associated with James's love and her sense of being loved, was unbearable for many months. Spanish music now inspires warm memories of their love for each other and comforts Margaret.

Spiritual Responses to Grief

Closely associated with the cognitive and emotional dimensions of grief are the deeply embedded personal values that give meaning and purpose to life. These values and the belief systems that sustain them are central components of **spirituality** and the spiritual response to grief. During loss, it is within the spiritual dimension of human experience that a person may be most comforted, challenged or devastated. The grieving person may become disillusioned and angry with God or other religious figures, such as the priest who, in Margaret's situation, seemed more concerned about getting a paper than being aware of her loneliness in the waiting room. The anguish of abandonment, loss of hope or loss of meaning can cause deep spiritual suffering.

Ministering to the spiritual needs of those grieving is an essential aspect of nursing care. The client's emotional and spiritual responses become intertwined as he or she grapples with pain. With an astute awareness of such suffering, nurses can promote a sense of well-being. Providing opportunities for clients to share their suffering assists in the psychological and spiritual transformation that can evolve through grieving. Finding explanations and meaning through religious, humanist or other spiritual beliefs, the client may begin to identify positive aspects of grieving. The grieving person can also experience loss as significant to his or her own growth and development. In the vignette, although Margaret was 'disillusioned' with aspects of her religious support system, she eventually finds much comfort, hope and strength in her spiritual beliefs. She begins to see that her husband's death gave her life new direction and empowered her to act in new ways. She states, 'If he hadn't gone, I wouldn't be the person I am today. I'm very content and peaceful about who I am and what I am doing.' Through her voluntary work, she comforts others who have terminal illness.

Behavioural Responses to Grief

Behavioural responses to grief are often the easiest to observe. By recognizing behaviours common to grieving, the nurse can provide supportive guidance for the client's journey over emotionally and cognitively rocky terrain. To promote the process, the nurse must provide a context of acceptance in which the client can explore his or her behaviour. For example, noticing that the grieving person seems to be functioning 'automatically' or routinely, without much thought, can indicate that the person is in the phase of numbness – the reality of the loss has not set in. Tearfully sobbing, crying uncontrollably, showing great restlessness and searching are evidence of yearning and seeking. The person may actually call out for the deceased or visually scan the room for him or her. Irritability and hostility toward others reveal anger and frustration in the process. Seeking out as well as avoiding places or activities once shared with the deceased, and keeping or wanting to discard valuables and belongings of the deceased, illustrate fluctuating emotions and perceptions of hope for a reconnection.

During the phase of disorganization, the cognitive act of redefining self-identity is essential, but difficult. Although superficial at first, efforts made in social or work activities are behavioural means to support the person's cognitive and emotional shifts. Drug or alcohol abuse indicates a maladaptive behavioural response to the emotional and spiritual despair. Suicide and homicide attempts may be extreme responses if the bereaved person cannot move through the grieving process.

In the phase of reorganization, the bereaved person participates in activities and reflection that are personally meaningful and satisfying. After finding creative outlets and building her personal growth, Margaret states, 'I'm happy with who I am and what I do. My life is more *authentic*, somehow.'

Physiological Responses to Grief

Physiological symptoms and problems associated with grief responses are often a source of anxiety and concern for the grieving person, as well as for friends or carers. Those grieving may complain of insomnia, headaches, impaired appetite, weight loss, lack of energy, palpitations, indigestion and changes in the immune and endocrine systems. Sleep disturbances are among the most frequent and persistent bereavement-associated symptoms (Zisook & Zisook, 2005).

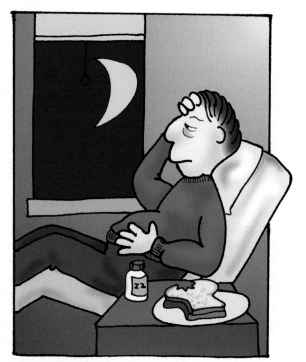

Physiological symptoms

CULTURAL CONSIDERATIONS

Working Compassionately and Effectively when a Patient Dies

In many settings, mental health nurses may be required to work with people who are dying or who die within the care of the services. Compassionate and effective care alongside families and friends is essential.

The Department of Health (2005) outlines the following set of principles that should guide all health-care professionals:

- *Respect for the individual* – when a patient dies a bereavement service should be available that respects confidentiality and individual preferences, values, culture and beliefs at all times in respect of both the person who has died and the bereaved family, partners or others.
- *Equality of provision* – all bereaved people are entitled to a service that responds to and respects their basic needs. Trusts may wish to consider policies that describe a core service which is inclusive and can accommodate the range and variety of users' needs equally.
- *Communication* – communication with people around the time of a death and afterwards should be clear, sensitive and honest. This is particularly important when addressing issues such as postmortem or donation of organs.
- *Information* – people who are dying, and those who are bereaved, need accurate information, appropriate to their needs, communicated clearly, sensitively and at the appropriate time (the role of the voluntary sector can be of particular importance here).

- *Partnership* – when a patient dies, services should be responsive to the experiences of the patient and people who are bereaved; these experiences should inform both service development and provision. In one-to-one contact, patients and families should be enabled to express their needs and preferences, through sharing expertise and responsibility and facilitating informed choice. There should be sufficient information, time and support available to enable this to happen.
- *Recognizing and acknowledging loss* – people who are bereaved need others to recognize and acknowledge their loss. Recognition by professionals, appropriately expressed, may be especially valued. Professionals should be aware of the importance of time and timing, and should try to work at the pace dictated by people's feelings and needs.
- *Environment and facilities* – every effort should be made to conduct discussions and/or counselling in a private, sympathetic environment away from interruptions.
- *Staff training and development* – it is essential that staff involved in caring for people who are dying and for people who are bereaved are well informed so they feel confident about the care and support they give. They should have adequate opportunities to develop their knowledge, understanding, self-awareness and skills.
- *Staff support* – staff need to be supported by the knowledge that they are working within a carefully designed, well-managed, high-quality service. In addition, it is essential that all those who care for and support dying and bereaved people, regardless of their role, should be provided with support for themselves.
- *Health and safety* – consideration should be given to the health and safety both of the bereaved and of staff working with the bereaved, to ensure that the health and safety of an individual is not compromised by issues relating to the cause of death (e.g. infectious disease or similar) or by the reaction of the bereaved to the death.
- *Review and audit* – systems need to be in place to enable appropriate reviews and audits of bereavement services to be carried out, and the results of these evaluations to be disseminated and acted upon.

Universal Reactions to Loss

Although people across all cultures grieve for lost loved ones, rituals and habits surrounding death vary. Each culture defines the context in which grieving, mourning and integrating loss into life are given meaningful expression. The context for expression is consistent with beliefs about life, death and an afterlife. Certain aspects of the experience are more important than other aspects for each culture (Kemp, 2005; Ng, 2005).

Universal reactions include the initial response of shock and social disorientation, attempts to continue a relationship with the deceased, anger with those perceived as responsible for the death and a time for mourning. Each culture, however, defines specific acceptable ways to exhibit shock and sadness, display anger and mourn (Bowlby, 1980). Cultural awareness of rituals for mourning can help nurses understand an individual's or a family's behaviour.

Culture-Specific Rituals

As people immigrate to the UK, they may lose rich ethnic and cultural roots during the adjustment of **acculturation** (altering cultural values or behaviours as a way to adapt to another culture). For example, health-care professionals, friends or funeral directors may discourage specific rites of passage that celebrate or mourn the loss of loved ones, or they may be reluctant to allow behavioural expressions they perceive as disruptive or inappropriate. Many such expressions are culturally related, and health-care providers must be aware of such instances. For example, the Hmong (people of a mountainous region of South-East Asia) believe that the deceased person enters the next world appearing as she or he did at the time of death. This may lead to a request for removal of needles, tubes or other 'foreign objects' before death (Johnson & Hang, 2005).

Because most cultural bereavement rituals have roots in several of the world's major religions (i.e. Buddhism, Christianity, Hinduism, Islam, Judaism), religious or spiritual beliefs and practices regarding death frequently guide the client's mourning. In the UK, a huge variety of mourning rituals and practices exist. Three of the major, non-Christian ones are summarized next for illustrative purposes, although it is important to bear in mind that group, family and individual differences may be significant even within a particular culture: once again, it is vital the nurse works with people to find out what they, their family and their friends want.

PEOPLE FROM A MUSLIM BACKGROUND

Islam does not permit cremation. It is important to follow the five steps of the burial procedure, which specify washing, dressing and positioning of the body. The first step is traditional washing of the body by a Muslim of the same gender (Yasien-Esmael & Rubin, 2005). There may be – as with other groups – significant differences to the specifics of mourning, dependent on level of devotion, gender, culture, class and nationality.

PEOPLE FROM A HINDU BACKGROUND

Hindu approaches to death and mourning tend to follow a process drawn from the Vedas, though there are variations according to sect, region, caste and family tradition. All members of the family – including children – are likely to be fully involved throughout the process. The dead are cremated. Organ donation is not acceptable

PEOPLE FROM AN ORTHODOX JEWISH BACKGROUND

An Orthodox Jewish custom is for a relative to stay with a dying person so that the soul does not leave the body while the person is alone. To leave the body alone after death is disrespectful. The family of the deceased may request to cover the body with a sheet. The eyes of the deceased should be closed, and the body should remain covered and untouched until family, a rabbi, or a Jewish undertaker can begin rites. Although organ donation is permitted, autopsy is not; burial must occur within 24 hours unless delayed by the Sabbath (Weinstein, 2003).

Nurse's Role

The diverse cultural environment of the UK offers the sensitive nurse many opportunities to individualize care when working with grieving clients. In extended families, varying expressions and responses to loss can exist, depending on the degree of acculturation to the dominant culture of society. Rather than assuming that he or she understands a particular culture's grieving behaviours, the nurse must encourage clients to discover and use what is effective and meaningful for them. For example, the nurse could ask a Polish client who also is a practising Catholic if he or she would like to pray for the deceased. If an Orthodox Jewish person has just died, the nurse could offer to stay with the body while the client notifies relatives.

The loosening grip of religion in the UK on indigenous people and the pressures of acculturation for others have caused many people to lose, minimize or modify specific culture-related rituals. Many Europeans and Americans, however, seem, in the past decade or so, to have experienced a renewed and deepened awareness of – and need for – meaningful mourning through ritual, in the UK sparked (or first identified) after the death of Princess Diana. The planting of a flag in the debris at Ground Zero during the immediate aftermath of the terrorist attack on the World Trade Center in September 2001 signalled the beginnings of such a ritual. As bodies were recovered and removed, the caring diligence and attentive presence of those facilitating their transport continued this meaningful rite of passage. For a while, through television and the internet, the US and much of the world became 'companions in grief'. Ceremonies held for those struck down in the 7 July 2005 London bombings seemed, similarly, to reflect a desire for a cross-cultural, public and ritual sharing of grief.

DISENFRANCHISED GRIEF

Disenfranchised grief is grief over a loss that is not, or cannot, be acknowledged openly, mourned publicly or supported socially. Three categories of circumstances can result in disenfranchised grief:

- A relationship has no legitimacy
- The loss itself is not recognized
- The griever is not recognized.

In each situation, there was an attachment followed by a loss that leads to grief. The grief process is more complex because the usual supports that facilitate grieving and healing are absent (Schultz & Videbeck, 2005).

In our culture, kin-based relationships receive the most attention in cases of death. Relationships between lovers, friends, neighbours, foster parents, colleagues and carers may be long-lasting and intense, but people suffering loss in these relationships may not be able to mourn publicly with the social support and recognition given to family members. In addition, some relationships are not always recognized publicly or sanctioned socially. Possible examples include same-sex relationships (Smolinski & Colon, 2006), cohabitation without marriage and extramarital affairs.

Other losses are not recognized or seen as socially significant; thus, the accompanying grief is not legitimized, expected or supported. Examples in this category include prenatal death, abortion, relinquishing a child for adoption, death of a pet (Kaufman & Kaufman, 2006) or other losses not involving death, such as job loss, separation, divorce and children leaving home. Though these losses can lead to intense grief for the bereaved, other people may perceive them as minor (Schultz & Videbeck, 2005).

Some people who experience a loss may not be recognized or fully supported as people who are grieving. For example, older adults and children experience limited social recognition for their losses and the need to mourn. As people grow older, they 'should expect' others their age to die. Adults sometimes view children as 'not understanding or comprehending' the loss, and may assume wrongly that their children's grief is minimal. Children may experience the loss of a 'nurturing parental figure' from death, divorce or family dysfunction such as alcoholism or abuse. These losses are very significant, yet they may not be recognized.

Another largely unrecognized sphere of loss directly involves mental health and mental disorder: the impact of first contact with mental health services, of admission to an acute unit, of a psychotic episode, of a diagnosis of schizophrenia or of Alzheimer's disease, may all lead to a distressing sense of loss, change and threat, and necessitate sensitive transitional support from professionals and others.

Nurses themselves may experience disenfranchised grief when their own need to grieve is not recognized. For example, nurses who work in elderly care may be involved intimately with the death of clients. The daily intensity of relationships between nurses and clients/families in all settings creates strong bonds among them. The emotional effects of loss are significant for these nurses; however, there is seldom a socially ordained place or time to grieve. The solitude in which the grieving occurs usually provides little or no comfort (Doka, 2006).

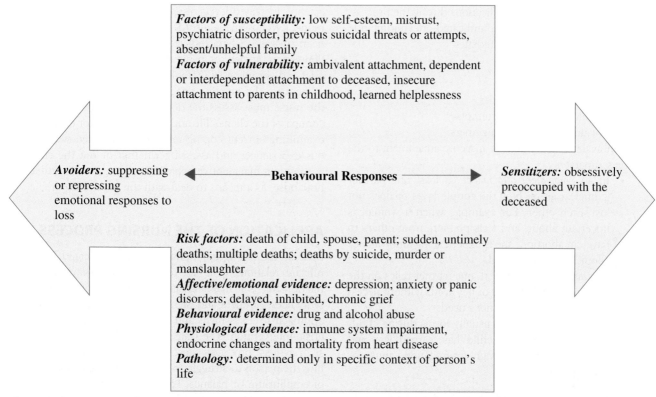

Factors of susceptibility: low self-esteem, mistrust, psychiatric disorder, previous suicidal threats or attempts, absent/unhelpful family
Factors of vulnerability: ambivalent attachment, dependent or interdependent attachment to deceased, insecure attachment to parents in childhood, learned helplessness

Avoiders: suppressing or repressing emotional responses to loss ← **Behavioural Responses** → *Sensitizers:* obsessively preoccupied with the deceased

Risk factors: death of child, spouse, parent; sudden, untimely deaths; multiple deaths; deaths by suicide, murder or manslaughter
Affective/emotional evidence: depression; anxiety or panic disorders; delayed, inhibited, chronic grief
Behavioural evidence: drug and alcohol abuse
Physiological evidence: immune system impairment, endocrine changes and mortality from heart disease
Pathology: determined only in specific context of person's life

Figure 12.1. Overview of complicated grief. (Adapted from Groot *et al.*, 2006; Zhang *et al., 2006*; Zisook & Zisook, 2005.)

COMPLICATED GRIEVING

Some consider **complicated grieving** to be a response outside 'the norm', occurring when a person is void of emotion, grieves for prolonged periods or has expressions of grief that seem disproportionate to the event. People may suppress emotional responses to the loss or become obsessively preoccupied with the deceased person or lost object. Others may actually move into an experience of clinical depression when they cannot make progress in the grief process (Zhang *et al.*, 2006). Figure 12.1 depicts an overview of complicated grieving.

Previously existing mental disorders also may complicate the grief process, so nurses must be particularly alert to clients with mental disorders who also are grieving. Grief can precipitate major depression in a person with a history of the disorder. These clients can also experience grief and a sense of loss when they encounter changes in treatment settings, routine, environment or even staff.

Although nurses must recognize that complications may arise in the grief process, the process remains unique and dynamic for each person. Immense variety exists in terms of the cultural determinants in communicating the experience and the individual differences in emotional reactions, depth of pain and time needed to acknowledge and grasp the personal meaning or assimilate the loss. Box 12.1 discusses styles of grieving.

Characteristics of Susceptibility

For some, the effects of grief are particularly devastating because their personalities, emotional states or situations

---

Box 12.1 STYLES OF GRIEVING

When determining whether a person may be experiencing a complicated grieving process, the nurse should consider viewing the person's behaviour as a unique style of grieving. Silver & Wortman (1980) suggested three styles of grieving:

- The bereaved vacillates from high to low distress over time.
- The bereaved shows no distress, either as an immediate response to loss or subsequently.
- The bereaved remains in a high state of distress for a period beyond that which others would consider appropriate.

Silver, R. L. & Wortman, C. B. (1980). Coping with undesirable life events. In J. Garber & M. E. P. Seligman (Eds.), *Human helplessness: Theory and applications* (pp. 279–340). New York: Academic Press.

make them susceptible to complications during the process. People who are vulnerable to complicated grieving include those with the following characteristics:

- Low self-esteem
- Low trust in others
- A previous psychiatric disorder
- Previous suicide threats or attempts
- Absent or unhelpful family members
- An ambivalent, dependent or insecure attachment to the deceased person
  - In an *ambivalent attachment*, at least one partner is unclear about how the couple loves or does not love each other. For example, when a woman is uncertain about, and feels pressure from others to have, an abortion, she is experiencing ambivalence about her unborn child.
  - In a *dependent attachment*, one partner relies on the other to provide for his or her needs without necessarily meeting the partner's needs.
  - An *insecure attachment* usually forms during childhood, especially if a child has learned fear and helplessness (i.e. through intimidation, abuse or control by parents).

A person's perception is another factor contributing to vulnerability: perception, or how a person thinks or feels about a situation, is not always reality. After the death of a loved one, a person may believe that he or she really cannot continue and is at a great disadvantage. He or she may become increasingly sad and depressed, not eat or sleep and perhaps experience suicidal thoughts.

Risk Factors Leading to Vulnerability

Zhang *et al.* (2006) and Zisook and Zisook (2005) identified experiences that increase the risk for complicated grieving for the vulnerable parties previously mentioned. These experiences are related to trauma or individual perceptions of vulnerability, and include the following:

- Death of a spouse or child
- Death of a parent (particularly in early childhood or adolescence)
- Sudden, unexpected and untimely death
- Multiple deaths
- Death by suicide or murder.

Based on the experiences previously identified, those most intimately affected by the terrorist attacks on 7 July 2005 could be considered at increased risk for complicated grieving.

Complicated Grieving as a Unique and Varied Experience

The person with complicated grieving can also experience physiological and emotional reactions. Physical reactions can include an impaired immune system, increased adrenocortical activity, increased levels of serum prolactin and growth hormone, psychosomatic disorders and increased mortality from heart disease. Characteristic emotional responses include depression, anxiety or panic disorders, delayed or inhibited grief and chronic grief (Zisook & Zisook, 2005).

Because the grieving process is unique to each person, the nurse must assess the degree of impairment within the context of the client's life and experiences – for example, by examining current coping responses compared with previous experiences and assessing whether or not the client is engaging in maladaptive behaviours, such as drug and alcohol abuse, as a means to deal with the painful experience.

APPLICATION OF THE NURSING PROCESS

Because the strong emotional attachment created in a significant relationship is not released easily, the loss of that relationship is a major crisis, often with momentous consequences. Aquilera and Messick (1982) developed a broad approach to assessment and intervention in their work on crisis intervention. The state of disequilibrium that a crisis, such as loss, produces causes great consternation, compelling the person to struggle to return to **homeostasis**, a state of equilibrium or balance. Factors that influence the grieving person's return to homeostasis are adequate perception of the situation, adequate situational support and adequate coping. These factors help the person to regain balance and return to previous functioning, or even to use the crisis as an opportunity to grow. Because any loss may be perceived as a personal crisis, it seems appropriate for the nurse to link understanding of crisis theory with the nursing process.

> Perhaps the most important principle is allowing the bereaved person to take control, letting them set the tone, pace and content of any discussion or interaction. Nurses need to display active listening skills, that is, listening with all the senses. Nurses must hear what is being said, accept it and adopt a non-judgemental attitude.
>
> (Walsh, 2008)

For the nurse to support and facilitate the grief process for clients, he or she must observe and listen for cognitive, emotional, spiritual, behavioural and physiological cues. Although the nurse must be familiar with the phases, tasks and dimensions of human response to loss, he or she must realize that each client's experience is unique. Skilful communication is the key to performing collaborative assessment, exchanging information and offering effective interventions.

To meet clients' needs effectively, the nurse must examine his or her own personal attitudes, maintain an attentive presence and provide a psychologically safe environment for deeply intimate sharing. Awareness of one's own beliefs and attitudes is essential so that the nurse can avoid imposing them on the client. **Attentive presence** is being with the client and focusing intently on communicating with and understanding him or her. The nurse can maintain attentive presence by using open body language, such as standing or sitting with arms down, facing the client and maintaining moderate eye contact, especially as the client speaks. Creating a psychologically safe environment includes ensuring the client of confidentiality, refraining from judging or giving specific advice and allowing the client to share thoughts and feelings freely (Larson, 2005).

HOPE

Research seems to suggest that a maintenance of hope throughout a therapeutic relationship (while never invalidating the client's sense of hopelessness and negativity) is crucial to that relationship being effective. Cutcliffe (2006a,b) identifies the following five 'categories' that help forge an effective connection with someone who is bereaved:

- Experiencing a caring, human–human connection
- Countering the projection of hopelessness
- Unwavering commitment
- Rediscovering trust
- Permeating hope throughout the counselling encounter.

Assessment

Effective assessment involves observing all dimensions of human response: what the person is thinking (cognitive), how the person is feeling (emotional), what the person's values and beliefs are (spiritual), how the person is acting (behavioural), and what is happening in the person's body (physiological) (Box 12.2). Effective communication skills during assessment

Box 12.2 DIMENSIONS (RESPONSES) AND SYMPTOMS OF THE GRIEVING CLIENT

Cognitive responses
- Disruption of assumptions and beliefs
- Questioning and trying to make sense of the loss
- Attempting to keep the lost one present
- Believing in an afterlife and as though the lost one is a guide

Emotional responses
- Anger, sadness, anxiety
- Resentment
- Guilt
- Feeling numb
- Vacillating emotions
- Profound sorrow, loneliness
- Intense desire to restore bond with lost one or object
- Depression, apathy, despair during phase of disorganization
- Sense of independence and confidence as phase of reorganization evolves

Spiritual responses
- Disillusioned and angry with God
- Anguish of abandonment or perceived abandonment
- Hopelessness; meaninglessness

Behavioural responses
- Functioning 'automatically'
- Tearful sobbing; uncontrollable crying
- Great restlessness; searching behaviours
- Irritability and hostility
- Seeking and avoiding places and activities shared with lost one
- Keeping valuables of lost one while wanting to discard them
- Possibly abusing drugs or alcohol
- Possible suicidal or homicidal gestures or attempts
- Seeking activity and personal reflection during phase of reorganization

Physiological responses
- Headaches, insomnia
- Impaired appetite, weight loss
- Lack of energy
- Palpitations, indigestion
- Changes in immune and endocrine systems

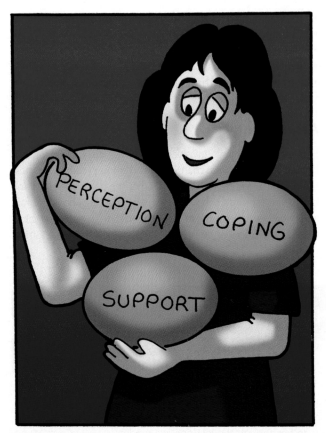

Three major areas to explore to facilitate a grieving client

can lead the client toward understanding his or her experience. Thus, assessment facilitates the client's grief process.

While observing for client responses in the dimensions of grieving, the nurse explores three critical components in assessment:

- Adequate perception regarding the loss
- Adequate support while grieving for the loss
- Adequate coping behaviours during the process.

PERCEPTION OF THE LOSS

Assessment begins with exploration of the client's perception of the loss. What does the loss mean to the client? For the woman who has spontaneously lost her first unborn child and the woman who has elected to abort a pregnancy, this question could have similar or different answers. Nevertheless, the question is valuable for beginning to facilitate the grief process.

Other questions that assess perception and encourage the client's movement through the grief process include the following:

- What does the client think and feel about the loss?
- How is the loss going to affect the client's life?
- What information does the nurse need to clarify or share with the client?

Assessing the client's 'need to know' in plain and simple language invites the client to verbalize perceptions that may need clarification. This is especially true for the person who is anticipating a loss, such as one facing a life-ending illness

or the loss of a body part. The nurse uses open-ended questions and helps to clarify any misperceptions.

Consider the following. The doctor has just informed Ms Morrison, a CPN's client, that the lump on her breast is cancerous and that she is scheduled for a mastectomy in 2 days. The CPN visits the client on her ward and finds her quietly watching television.

Nurse: *'Hi. How are you?' (offering presence; giving a broad opening)*
    Client: *'Oh, I'm fine. Really, I am.'*
    Nurse: *'I gather the doctor was just here? Tell me, what do you understand about what he said?'*
(using open-ended questions for description of perception)
    Client: *'Well, I think he said I'll have to have surgery on my breast.'*
    Nurse: *'How do you feel about that?' (using open-ended question for what it means to the client)*

Exploring what the person believes about the grieving process is another important assessment. Does the client have preconceived ideas about when or how grieving should happen? The nurse can help the client realize that grieving is very personal and unique: each person grieves in his or her own way.

The next day, the CPN visits and finds Ms Morrison hitting her pillow and crying. She's apparently eaten very little food and has been refusing visitors.

    Nurse: *'Ms Morrison, I can see you're upset. Tell me, what's happening right now?' (sharing observation; encouraging description)*
    Client: *'Oh, I'm disgusted with myself. I'm sorry you had to see me act this way. I should be able to handle this. Other people have lost their breasts to cancer, and they're doing OK.'*
    Nurse: *'You're pretty upset with yourself, thinking you should feel differently?' (using reflection)*
    Client: *'Yes, exactly. Don't you think so?'*
    Nurse: *'You've had to deal with quite a shock today. Sounds to me like you're expecting quite a bit of yourself. What do you think?' (using reflection; sharing perceptions; seeking validation)*
    Client: *'I don't know, maybe. How long is this going to go on? I'm a wreck emotionally.'*
    Nurse: *'You're starting to go through a sort of grieving process, and there's no fixed timetable for what you're dealing with. Everyone has a unique time and way of coping with something as major as this.' (informing; validating experience)*

SUPPORT

Purposeful assessment of support systems provides the grieving client with an awareness of those who can meet his or her emotional and spiritual needs for security and love. The nurse can help the client to identify his or her support systems and reach out and accept what they can offer.

    Nurse: *'Who in your life should or would really want to know what you've just heard from the doctor?' (seeking information about situational support)*

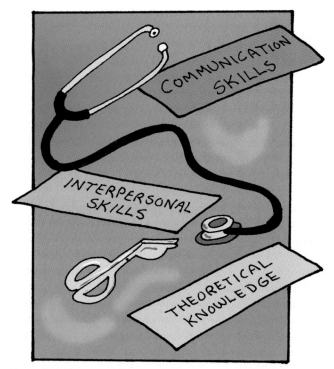

Nurses' tools

Client: *'Oh, I'm really alone. I'm not married and don't have any relatives in town.'*

Nurse: *'There's no one who would care about this news?'* (voicing doubt)

Client: *'Oh, maybe a friend I talk with on the phone now and then.'*

COPING BEHAVIOURS

The client's behaviour is likely to give the nurse the easiest and most concrete information about coping skills. The nurse must be careful to observe the client's behaviour throughout the grief process and never assume that a client is at a particular phase. The nurse must use effective communication skills to assess how the client's behaviour reflects coping, as well as emotions and thoughts.

The following day, the CPN has heard that Ms Morrison had a restless night. She enters Ms Morrison's room and sees her crying with a full tray of food untouched. After a few pleasantries:

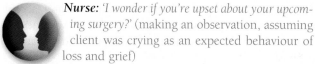

Nurse: *'I wonder if you're upset about your upcoming surgery?'* (making an observation, assuming client was crying as an expected behaviour of loss and grief)

Client: *'I'm not having surgery. No way. I don't need it.'* (using denial to cope)

The nurse must also consider several other questions when assessing the client's coping. How has the person dealt with loss previously? How is the person currently impaired? How does the current experience compare with previous experiences? What does the client perceive as a problem? Is

it related to unrealistic ideas about what he or she should feel or do? (McBride, 2001). The interaction of the dimensions of human response is fluid and dynamic. What a person thinks about during grieving affects his or her feelings, and those feelings influence his or her behaviour. The critical factors of perception, support and coping are interrelated as well, and provide a framework for assessing and assisting the client.

Analysis and Planning

The nurse must base nursing formulations for the person experiencing loss on subjective and objective assessment data. Nursing formulations used for clients experiencing grief include the following:

- **Grieving**, related to actual or perceived loss such as a physiological loss (e.g. loss of a limb). Loss of security and sense of belonging (e.g. loss of a loved one) is defined as a normal process in the human experience of loss.
- **Anticipatory grieving**, related to the intellectual and emotional responses and behaviours by which individuals, families and communities work through the process of modifying self-concept based on the perception of potential loss.
- **Dysfunctional grieving**, related to the extended unsuccessful use of intellectual and emotional responses by which individuals, families and communities attempt to work through the process of modifying self-concept based on the perception of loss.

Outcome Identif ication

Examples of outcomes for the three nursing formulations are as follows:

- Grieving: The client will
  - Identify the effects of his or her loss
  - Seek and receive adequate support
  - Apply effective coping strategies while expressing and assimilating all dimensions of human response to loss in his or her life.
- Anticipatory Grieving: The client will
  - Identify the meaning of the expected loss in his or her life
  - Seek and receive adequate support while expressing grief
  - Develop a plan for coping with the loss as it becomes a reality.
- Dysfunctional Grieving: The client will
  - Identify the meaning of his or her loss
  - Recognize the negative effects of the loss on his or her life
  - Seek or accept professional assistance to promote the grieving process.

Interventions

The nurse's guidance helps the client examine and make changes. Changes imply movement as the client progresses through the grief process. Sometimes the client takes one painful step at a time. Sometimes he or she may seem to go over the same ground repeatedly.

INTERVENTIONS REGARDING THE PERCEPTION OF LOSS

Cognitive responses are connected significantly with the intense emotional turmoil that accompanies grieving. For example, in the vignette, Margaret's disillusionment with those friends unavailable after her husband's death added great pain to her loss. She had counted on them to be there as she dealt with James's death. A cognitive shift occurred when she realized they would not be there, meaning she was alone and they no longer cared. She felt abandoned. She then had two immediate losses: James's death and realizing that people she had counted on were unavailable.

Exploring the client's perception and meaning of the loss is a first step that can help alleviate the pain of what some would call the initial emotional overload in grieving. Using the example of Margaret, the nurse could ask what being alone means to her and explore the possibility of others being supportive. Further exploration could focus on her perception that those who had abandoned her no longer cared. Perhaps Margaret would then discover that others could meet her need to be cared for. She may begin to believe that it was fear or discomfort about death that kept former friends away. In fact, it was in just this way that she could accept the caring of some friends and release the importance of those who would not, or could not, be there for her. In this situation, exploring perceptions and the meaning of the loss helped the bereaved to make cognitive shifts that valuably influenced her emotional experience.

When loss occurs, especially if it is sudden and without warning, the cognitive defence mechanism of denial acts as a cushion to soften the effects. Typical verbal responses are, 'I can't believe this has happened,' 'It can't be true,' and 'There's been a mistake.'

Adaptive denial, in which the client gradually adjusts to the reality of the loss, can help the client let go of previous (before the loss) perceptions while creating new ways of thinking about himself or herself, others and the world. For example, Margaret had to face the reality that although she believed that a priest (because he was a priest) would care about her being alone in the surgery waiting room, he actually was only concerned about getting a paper. Gradually, she was able to relinquish this assumption.

Effective communication skills can be useful in helping the client in adaptive denial move toward acceptance. Note the intervention the nurse makes in the scenario with Ms Morrison. The nurse enters Ms Morrison's room and sees her crying with a full tray of food untouched.

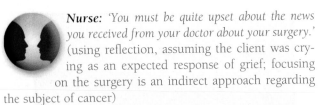

Nurse: 'You must be quite upset about the news you received from your doctor about your surgery.' (using reflection, assuming the client was crying as an expected response of grief; focusing on the surgery is an indirect approach regarding the subject of cancer)

Client: 'I'm not having surgery. No way. I don't need it.' (denial)

Nurse: 'I saw you crying and was wondering what was upsetting you. I'm interested in how you're feeling.' (focusing on behaviour and sharing observation while indicating concern and accepting the client's denial)

Client: 'I'm just not hungry. I don't have an appetite and . . . I'm not clear about what the doctor said.' (focusing on physiological response; non-responsive to nurse's encouragement to talk about feelings; acknowledging doctor's visit but unsure of what he said – beginning to adjust cognitively to reality of condition)

Nurse: 'I wonder if not wanting to eat may be related to what you are feeling. Are there times when you don't have an appetite and you feel upset about something?' (suggesting a connection between physiological response and feelings; promoting adaptive denial)

Client: 'Well, as a matter of fact, yes. But I can't think what I would be upset about.' (acknowledging a connection between behaviour and feeling; continuing to deny reality)

Nurse: 'You said you were unclear about what the doctor said. I wonder if things didn't seem clear because it may have upset you to hear what he had to say. And now, tonight, you don't have an appetite.' (using client's experience to make connection between doctor's news and client's physiological response and behaviour)

Client: 'What did he say, do you know?' (requesting information; demonstrating a readiness to hear it again while continuing to adjust to reality)

Nurse: Begins to outline her knowledge of what's going on, checking understanding frequently with her client and, where necessary, enlisting the help of ward staff, leaflets and other sources of information.

In this example, the nurse gently but persistently guides the client toward acknowledging the reality of her impending loss.

INTERVENTIONS REGARDING SUPPORT

The nurse can help the client to reach out and accept what others want to give in support of his or her grieving process. Note the assessment is developed into a plan for support.

Nurse: 'Who in your life would really want to know what you've just heard from the doctor?' (seeking information about situational support for the client)

Client: 'Oh, I'm really alone. I'm not married.'

Nurse: 'There's no one who would care about this news?' (voicing doubt)

Client: 'Oh, maybe a friend I talk with on the phone now and then.'

Nurse: 'Why don't I get the phone book for you and you can call her?' (continuing to offer presence; suggesting an immediate source of support; developing a plan of action providing further support)

There are many groups available who can provide access to information about death and dying to professionals and clients (see references below)

INTERVENTIONS REGARDING COPING BEHAVIOURS

When attempting to focus Ms Morrison on the reality of her surgery, the nurse was helping her shift from an unconscious mechanism of denial to conscious coping with reality. The nurse used communication skills to encourage Ms Morrison to examine her experience and behaviour as possible ways in which she might be coping with the news of loss. Margaret and James's logical approach to life allowed them to cope by continuing to have fun together while attending to medical necessities as they faced the reality of his impending death.

Intervention involves giving the client the opportunity to compare and contrast ways in which he or she has coped with significant loss in the past, and helping him or her to review strengths and renew a sense of personal power. Remembering and practising old behaviours in a new situation may lead to experimentation with new methods and self-discovery. Having a historical perspective helps the person's grief work by allowing shifts in thinking about himself or herself, the loss, and perhaps the meaning of the loss. Margaret's religious practices of prayer and spiritual reading helped her to discover new depths of meaning and purpose in her life.

Encouraging the client to care for himself or herself is another intervention that helps the client cope. The nurse can offer food without pressuring the client to eat. Being careful to eat, sleep well, exercise and take time for comforting activities are ways that the client can nourish himself or herself. Just as the tired hiker needs to stop, rest and replenish himself or herself, so must the bereaved person take a break from the exhausting process of grieving. Going back to a routine of work or focusing on other members of the family may provide that respite. Volunteer activities – volunteering at a hospice or botanical garden, taking part in church activities or speaking to bereavement education groups, for example – can affirm the client's talents and abilities and can renew feelings of self-worth.

Communication and interpersonal skills are the key tools of the effective nurse. In helping people cope with loss (as in other areas of mental health nursing) compassion – a genuine human-to-human connection and a desire to relieve suffering – is essential. The client trusts that the nurse will have what it takes to assist him or her in grieving. In addition to previously mentioned skills, these tools include the following:

- Using simple non-judgemental statements to acknowledge loss: 'I want you to know I'm thinking of you.'
- Referring to a loved one or object of loss by name (if acceptable in the client's culture)
- Remembering words are not always necessary; a light touch on the elbow, shoulder or hand, or just being there, indicates caring
- Respecting the client's unique process of grieving
- Respecting the client's personal beliefs
- Being honest, dependable, consistent and worthy of the client's trust.

A welcoming smile and eye contact from the client during intimate conversations can help indicate the nurse's humanity and care.

Evaluation

Evaluation of progress depends on the goals established for the client. A review of the tasks and phases of grieving (discussed earlier in the chapter) can be useful in making a statement about the client's status at any given moment. We could say that although Margaret, in the vignette, still misses James, she is in the reorganization phase of grieving. She has a sense of independence and confidence and has accomplished several tasks of grieving: creating new ties, developing a new sense of self, pursuing new activities and integrating the loss into her life.

SELF-AWARENESS ISSUES

Clients who are grieving need more than someone who is equipped with skills and basic knowledge; they need the compassion and support of someone they can trust with their emotions and thoughts. For clients to see nurses as trustworthy, nurses must be willing to examine their personal attitudes about loss and the grieving process.

Points to Consider When Working With Clients With Grief and Loss

Taking a self-awareness inventory means periodic reflection on questions, such as the following:

- What have been the major losses in my life, and how have they affected me?
- Am I currently grieving for a significant loss? How does my loss affect my ability to be present for my client?
- Who is there for me as I grieve?
- How am I coping with my loss?
- Is the pain of my personal grief spilling over as I listen and watch for cues of the client's grieving?
- Am I making assumptions about the client's experience based on my own process?
- Can I keep appropriate nurse–client boundaries as I attend to the client's needs?

NURSING INTERVENTIONS FOR GRIEF

Explore client's perception and meaning of his or her loss.

Allow adaptive denial.

Encourage or assist client to reach out for and accept support.

Encourage client to examine patterns of coping in past and present situation of loss.

Encourage client to review personal strengths and personal power.

Encourage client to care for himself or herself.

Offer client food without pressure to eat.

Use effective communication:
• Offer presence and give broad openings.
• Use open-ended questions
• Encourage description
• Share observations
• Use reflection
• Seek validation of perceptions
• Provide information
• Voice doubt
• Use focusing
• Attempt to translate into feelings or verbalize the implied.

Establish rapport and maintain interpersonal skills, such as:
• Attentive presence
• Respect for client's unique grieving process
• Respect for client's personal beliefs
• Being trustworthy: honest, dependable, consistent
• Periodic self-inventory of attitudes and issues related to loss.

• Do I have the strength to be present and to facilitate the client's grief?
• What might my supervisor or a trusted colleague think about my current ability to support a client in the grief process?

Ongoing self-examination is an effective method of keeping the therapeutic relationship goal-directed and acutely attentive to the client's needs.

KEY POINTS

• Grief refers to the subjective emotions and affect that are normal responses to the experience of loss.
• Grieving is the process through which a person travels as he or she experiences grief.

• Types of losses can be identified as unfulfilled or unmet human needs. Maslow's hierarchy of human needs is a useful model by which to understand loss as it relates to unfulfilled human needs.
• Grief work is one of life's most difficult challenges. The challenge of integrating a loss requires all that the person can give of mind, body and spirit.
• Because the nurse constantly interacts with clients at various points on the health–illness continuum, he or she must understand loss and the process of grieving.
• Loss of a 'significant other' activates attachment behaviours that range from quiet glances toward that person, to following, clinging to, searching for and calling out for the other person, to wails of protest when the significant other or object is gone.
• The process of grieving has been described in terms of dynamically interrelated phases: numbness and denial, yearning and protesting, cognitive disorganization and emotional despair and reorganization and reintegration.
• Dimensions of human response include cognitive, emotional, spiritual, behavioural and physiological. People may be experiencing more than one phase of the grieving process.
• Culturally bound reactions to loss are often lost in the acculturation to dominant societal norms. Both universal and culture-specific rituals can facilitate grieving.
• Nurses and other clinicians who are constantly interacting with dying clients are vulnerable to disenfranchised grief.
• Complicated grieving is a response that lies outside the norm. The person may be void of emotion, grieve for a

Critical Thinking Questions

1. Although grieving is explained in terms of a process of stages, the client experiences a myriad of emotions and thoughts. What phenomena of the grieving process might give the nurse concrete information about the client's progress? Of these phenomena, which is easiest to observe? How should the nurse investigate the meaning of this phenomenon?

2. What issues of loss does the nurse deal with every day? What are the nurse's most valuable tools for dealing with these losses? How might the nurse use these tools across health-care settings?

3. A client in a mental health setting has recently lost his mother. How must the nurse differentiate between the client's mental health problems and a 'normal' response to grief? How will the nurse determine the risk for complicated grief for this client?

4. How might the nurse maintain his or her professional responsibility toward the therapeutic relationship with those who are grieving for a loss? What components of trustworthiness must the nurse cultivate in relation to the client who is grieving?

prolonged period or express feelings that seem out of proportion. With so many variables in the grieving process, what may appear to be complicated grieving may be only the person's unique style of grieving.

- Low self-esteem, distrust of others, a psychiatric disorder, previous suicide threats or attempts and absent or unhelpful family members increase the risk for complicated grieving.
- Situations considered risk factors for complicated grief in those already vulnerable include death of a spouse or child, a sudden unexpected death and murder.
- During assessment, the nurse observes and listens for cues in what the person thinks and feels, and how he or she behaves, and then uses these relevant data to guide the client in the grieving process.

- Crisis theory can be used to help the nurse working with a grieving client. Adequate perception, adequate support and adequate coping are critical factors.
- Compassion and effective communication skills are the key to successful assessment and interventions.
- Interventions focused on the perception of loss include exploring the meaning of the loss and allowing adaptive denial, which is the process of gradually adjusting to the reality of a loss.
- Being there to help the client, while assisting him or her to seek other sources of support, is an essential intervention.
- Encouraging the client to care for himself or herself promotes adequate coping.
- To earn the client's trust, the nurse must examine his or her own attitudes about loss and periodically undertake a self-awareness inventory.

Nursing Care Plan   *Grief*

Nursing Formulation

Grieving: *A normal response to the human experience of loss.*

ASSESSMENT DATA

Cognitive Responses
- Questioning and trying to make sense of the loss
- Experiencing disillusionment
- Attempting to make sense of the loss

Emotional Responses
- Feeling numb
- Experiencing sorrow, loneliness
- Crying, sobbing
- Having vacillating emotions, including anger
- Experiencing hopelessness
- Feeling helpless, powerless

Behavioural Responses
- Experiencing great restlessness; searching for the deceased
- Seeking and avoiding places and activities once shared with the lost one
- Functioning 'automatically'

Physiological Responses
- Headaches
- Insomnia
- Lack of energy

Critical Component of Perception – questions to explore and listen for while talking with the client:
- What is the meaning of the loss for the client?

EXPECTED OUTCOMES

The client will
- Identify the loss and its meaning for self (adequate perception)
- Express feelings, verbally and non-verbally
- Establish and maintain adequate nutrition, hydration and elimination (adequate coping)
- Establish and maintain an adequate balance of rest, sleep and activity (adequate coping)
- Establish and maintain an adequate support system
- Verbalize knowledge of the grief process
- Demonstrate initial integration of loss into his or her life (adequate coping)
- Verbalize realistic future plans integrating loss (adequate perception)

continued ⋯⊹

Nursing Care Plan: Grief, cont.

ASSESSMENT DATA

- What is the client's understanding of his or her current experience in grieving?
- Are the client's perceptions adequate? (Do the client's perceptions reflect the process of grieving?)

Critical Component of Support – questions to explore with the client:
- Who in the client's life needs to be present to offer adequate support for the client?
- How can resources be established to offer optimum support for the client?

Critical Component of Coping – questions to keep in mind during planning and implementation of care:
- How has the client handled past crises?
- How can the client use skills that have helped in the past for this current situation?
- Considering the phase of his or her grieving process, how is the client's current experience a reflection of adequate coping?

IMPLEMENTATION

Nursing Interventions *denotes collaborative interventions	**Rationale**
After establishing rapport with the client, bring up the loss in a supportive manner; if the client refuses to discuss it, withdraw and state your intention to return. ('I can understand you don't want to talk to me about this now. I'll come to talk to you again at 11:00. Maybe we can talk about it then.') Return at the stated time, then continue to be as supportive as possible rather than confronting the client.	Your presence demonstrates interest and caring. Telling the client you will return conveys your support. The client may need emotional support to face and express uncomfortable or painful feelings. Confronting the client or pushing him or her to express feelings may increase anxiety and lead to further denial or avoidance.
Talk with the client realistically about his or her loss; discuss concrete changes that the client must now begin to make as a result of the loss.	Discussing the loss on this level may help to make it more real for the client.
Encourage the expression of feelings in ways the client is comfortable – for example, talking, writing, drawing, crying, wailing or yelling. Convey your acceptance of these feelings and means of expression. Offer the client verbal support for attempts to express feelings.	Expression of feelings can help the client to identify, accept and work through his or her feelings, even if these are painful or otherwise uncomfortable for the client.
Encourage the client to recall experiences, talk about what was involved in his or her relationship with the lost person or object and so forth. Discuss with the client the changes in his or her feelings toward self, others and the lost person or object as a result of the loss and grief process.	Discussing the lost object or person can help the client to identify and express the loss, what the loss means to him or her, and his or her emotional response.

continued ⋯⟶

Nursing Care Plan: Grief, cont.

IMPLEMENTATION

Nursing Interventions *denotes collaborative interventions	**Rationale**
Encourage appropriate (that is, safe) expression of all feelings that the client has toward the lost person or object and convey acceptance. Assure the client that even 'negative' feelings, such as anger and resentment, are normal and healthy in grieving.	Feelings are not inherently bad or good. Giving the client support for expressing feelings may help the client to accept uncomfortable feelings.
Convey to the client that, although feelings may be uncomfortable, they are natural and necessary to this process, that he or she can withstand having these feelings, and that the feelings will not harm him or her.	The client may fear the intensity of his or her feelings.
Discourage rumination if the client is dwelling on his or her guilt or worthlessness. After listening to the client's feelings, tell the client you will talk about other aspects of grief and feelings.	The client needs to identify and express the feelings that underlie the rumination and to proceed through the grief process.
Referral to a hospital chaplain, clergy or other spiritual resource person may be indicated. Encourage a connection with those in his or her life who may be a source of support.	The client may be more comfortable discussing spiritual issues with an advisor who shares his or her belief system.
Provide opportunities for the release of tension, anger, guilt and so forth through physical activities. Promote regular exercise as a healthy means of dealing with stress and tension.	Physical activity provides a way to relieve tension in a healthy, non-destructive manner.
Limit times and frequency of therapeutic interactions with the client. Encourage independent, spontaneous expression of feelings (writing, initiating interactions with other clients or with other staff members, getting involved in a physical activity). Plan staff-initiated interactions at times that allow the client to fulfil responsibilities (activities, unit duties) and maintain personal care (sleeping, eating, hygiene).	The client needs to develop independent skills of communicating feelings and to integrate the loss into his or her daily life, while meeting his or her own basic needs.
Encourage the client to talk with others, individually and in small groups (larger as tolerated), about the loss in terms of his or her own and others' feelings, and about experiences and changes resulting from the loss.	The client needs to develop independent skills of communicating feelings and expressing grief to others.
Promote sharing, communicating, expressing feelings and support among clients. Use larger groups (such as open report) for a general discussion of loss and grief (with or without focusing on this client's loss). Also help the client to realize that there are limits to sharing grief in a social context.	Sharing grief and experiences with others can help the client to identify and express feelings and to feel normal in grieving. Dwelling on grief in social interactions, however, can result in other people's discomfort with their own feelings, and may lead to friends and significant others avoiding the client.
Point out to the client that a major aspect of loss is a real physical stress. Encourage good nutrition, hydration and elimination, as well as adequate rest and daily physical exercise (such as walking, running, swimming or cycling) in the hospital and after discharge.	The client may be unaware of the physical stress of the loss or may lack interest in activities of daily living. Physical exercise can relieve tension or pent-up feelings in a healthy, non-destructive manner.

continued ···⟩

Nursing Care Plan: Grief, cont.

IMPLEMENTATION

Nursing Interventions *denotes collaborative interventions	Rationale
Teach the client (and his or her family or significant others) about the grief process.	These people may have little or no knowledge of grief or the process involved in recovery.
Point out to the client that time spent grieving can be nurturing, that it is a time of learning and growth from which to gather the strength to go forward.	The grief process allows the client to adjust to a change in his or her life and to begin to move toward future opportunities.

Adapted from Schultz, J. M. & Videbeck, S. L. (2005). *Lippincott's manual of psychiatric nursing care plans* (7th edn). Philadelphia: Lippincott Williams & Wilkins.

INTERNET RESOURCES

RESOURCES	INTERNET ADDRESS
• Association for Death Education and Counselling	http://www.adec.org/
• Cruse Bereavement Care	http://www.crusebereavementcare.org.uk/
• Cruse Scotland	http://www.crusescotland.org.uk/
• The Compassionate Friends	http://www.tcf.org.uk/

REFERENCES

Aquilera, D. C. & Messick, J. M. (1982). *Crisis intervention: Theory and methodology.* St. Louis: C. V. Mosby.

Bowlby, J. (1980). *Attachment and loss, Vol. 3: Loss, sadness, and depression.* New York: Basic Books.

Cutcliffe, J. (2006a). The principles and processes of inspiring hope in bereavement counselling: a modified grounded theory study – part one. *Journal of Psychiatric and Mental Health Nursing, 13*(5), 598–603.

Cutcliffe, J. (2006b). The principles and processes of inspiring hope in bereavement counselling: a modified grounded theory study – part two. *Journal of Psychiatric and Mental Health Nursing, 13*(5), 604–610.

Department of Health. (2005). *When a patient dies: Advice on developing bereavement services in the NHS.* Available: http://www.dh.gov.uk/en/Publicationsandstatistics/Publications/PublicationsPolicyAndGuidance/DH_4122191

Doka, K. J. (2006). Grief: The constant companion of illness. *Anesthesiology Clinics, 24*(1), 205–212.

Groot, M. H., Keijser, J., & Neeleman, J. (2006). Grief shortly after suicide and natural death: A comparative study among spouses and first-degree relatives. *Suicide & Life-threatening Behaviour, 36*(4), 418–431.

Harvey, J. H. & Miller, E. D. (1998). Toward a psychology of loss. *Psychological Science, 9*(6), 429.

Johnson, S. K., & Hang, A. L. (2005). Hmong. In J. G. Lipson & Dibble, S. L. (Eds.), *Culture & clinical care* (pp. 250–263). San Francisco: University of California San Francisco Press.

Kaufman, K. R. & Kaufman, N. D. (2006). And then the dog died. *Death Studies, 30*(1), 61–76.

Kemp, C. (2005). Cultural issues in palliative care. *Seminars in Oncology Nursing, 21*(1), 44–52.

Kubler-Ross, E. (1969). *On death and dying.* New York: Macmillan.

Larson, D. G. (2005). Becky's legacy: More lessons. *Death Studies, 29*(8), 745–757.

Lobb, E. A., Clayton, J. M., & Price, M. A. (2006). Suffering, loss and grief in palliative care. *Australian Family Physician, 35*(10), 772–775.

Maslow, A. H. (1954). *Motivation and personality.* New York: Harper.

McBride, J. (2001). Death in the family: adapting a family systems framework to the grief process. *American Journal of Family Therapy, 29*(1), 59–73.

Neimeyer, R. A., Baldwin, S. A., & Gillies, J. (2006). Continuing bonds and reconstructing meaning: Mitigating complications in bereavement. *Death Studies, 30*(8), 715–738.

Ng, B. Y. (2005). Grief revisited. *Annals of the Academy of Medicine, Singapore, 34*(5), 352–355.

Rando, T. A. (1984). *Grief, dying, and death: Clinical interventions for caregivers.* Champaign, IL: Research Press.

Rodebaugh, L. S., Schwindt, R. G., & Valentine, F. M. (1999). How to handle grief with wisdom. *Nursing, 29,* 52.

Schultz, J. M. & Videbeck, S. L. (2005). *Lippincott's manual of psychiatric nursing care plans* (7th edn). Philadelphia: Lippincott Williams & Wilkins.

Silver, R. L. & Wortman, C. B. (1980). Coping with undesirable life events. In J. Garber & M. E. P. Seligman (Eds.), *Human helplessness: Theory and applications* (pp. 279–340). New York: Academic Press.

Smolinski, K. M. & Colon, Y. (2006). Silent voices and invisible walls: exploring end of life care with lesbians and gay men. *Journal of Psychosocial Oncology, 24*(1), 51–64.

Walsh, H. (2008). Caring for bereaved people, part 2: models of bereavement. *Nursing Times*, 104(1), 32–37.

Weinstein, L. B. (2003). Bereaved orthodox Jewish families and their community: a cross-cultural perspective. *Journal of Community Health Nursing*, 20(4), 233–243.

Yasien-Esmael, H. & Rubin, S. S. (2005). The meaning structures of Muslim bereavements in Israel: religious traditions, mourning practices, and human experience. *Death Studies*, 29(6), 495–518.

Zhang, B., El-Jawahri, A., & Prigerson, H. G. (2006). Update on bereavement research: evidence-based guidelines for the diagnosis and treatment of complicated bereavement. *Journal of Palliative Medicine*, 9(5), 1188–1203.

Ziemba, R. A. & Lynch-Sauer, J. M. (2005). Preparedness for taking care of elderly parents: 'First, you get ready to cry'. *Journal of Women & Aging*, 17(1–2), 99–113.

Zisook, S. & Zisook, S. A. (2005). Death, dying, and bereavement. In B. J. Sadock & V. A. Sadock (Eds.), *Comprehensive textbook of psychiatry*, Vol. 2. (8th edn, pp. 2367–2393). Philadelphia: Lippincott, Williams, & Wilkins.

ADDITIONAL READING

Beliefnet: Transition Rituals. Available: http://www.beliefnet.com/story/78/story_7894.html

Fahey-McCarthy, E. (2003). Exploring theories of grief: personal reflection. *British Journal of Midwifery, 11*(10), 595–612.

MIND. (2008). *Understanding bereavement*. Available: http://www.mind.org.uk/Information/Booklets/Understanding/Understanding+bereavement.htm

Stroebe, M. S., Folkman, S., Hansson, R. O., & Schut, H. (2006). The prediction of bereavement outcome: development of an integrative risk factor framework. *Social Science & Medicine*, 63(9), 2440–2451.

Walsh, H. (2007). Caring for bereaved people, part 1: models of bereavement. *Nursing Times*, 103(51), 26–27.

Wimpenny, P., Unwin, R., & Dempster, P. (2007). A literature review on bereavement and bereavement care: developing evidence-based practice in Scotland. Bereavement Care, 26(1), 7–10.

Chapter Study Guide

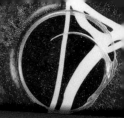

MULTIPLE-CHOICE QUESTIONS

Select the best answer for each of the following questions.

1. Which of the following accurately lists Bowlby's phases of the grieving process?
   a. Denial, anger, depression, bargaining, acceptance
   b. Shock, outcry and denial; intrusion of thought, distractions and obsessive reviewing of the loss; confiding in others to emote and cognitively restructure an account of the loss
   c. Numbness and denial of the loss, emotional yearning for the loved one and protesting permanence of the loss, cognitive disorganization and emotional despair, reorganizing and reintegrating a sense of self
   d. Reeling, feeling, dealing, healing

2. Which of the following give cues to the nurse that a client may be grieving for a loss?
   a. Sad affect, anger, anxiety and sudden changes in mood
   b. A range of thoughts, feelings, behaviour and physiological complaints
   c. Hallucinations, panic level of anxiety and sense of impending doom
   d. Complaints of abdominal pain, diarrhoea and loss of appetite

3. Situations that are considered risk factors for complicated grief are
   a. Inadequate support and old age
   b. Childbirth, marriage and divorce
   c. Death of a spouse or child, death by suicide and sudden and unexpected death
   d. Inadequate perception of the grieving crisis

4. Physiological responses of complicated grieving include
   a. Tearfulness when recalling significant memories of the person who has died.
   b. Impaired appetite, weight loss, lack of energy, palpitations
   c. Depression, panic disorders, chronic grief
   d. Impaired immune system, increased serum prolactin level, increased mortality rate from heart disease

5. Critical factors for successful integration of loss during the grieving process are
   a. The client's adequate perception, adequate support and adequate coping
   b. The nurse's trustworthiness and healthy attitudes about grief
   c. Accurate assessment and intervention by the nurse or helping person
   d. The client's predictable and steady movement from one stage of the process to the next

FILL-IN-THE-BLANK QUESTIONS

Identify the dimension of grieving for each of the following client expressions or behaviours.

_____   'I have this insatiable yearning to be with him.'

_____   Irritability and hostility toward others

_____   'I thought a priest would definitely understand my need for support at this time. Why didn't he ask how I was feeling when I told him my husband was having surgery?'

_____   'Why has God done this to me?'

_____   'I've lost my appetite, and I just can't seem to get to sleep at night when I go to bed.'

GROUP DISCUSSION TOPICS

Discuss examples of each of the following:

Styles of grieving

Critical factor of adequate support

Emotional response during phase of numbing in the grieving process

SHORT ANSWER QUESTIONS

For each of the following client statements, identify responses that the nurse might make and the rationale for the nurse's response:

'This is unbearable. I can't believe she's gone.'

'No one will want to hire me at this age.'

'There's nowhere for me to turn.'

'Get out of here! Leave me alone! I don't need your help.'

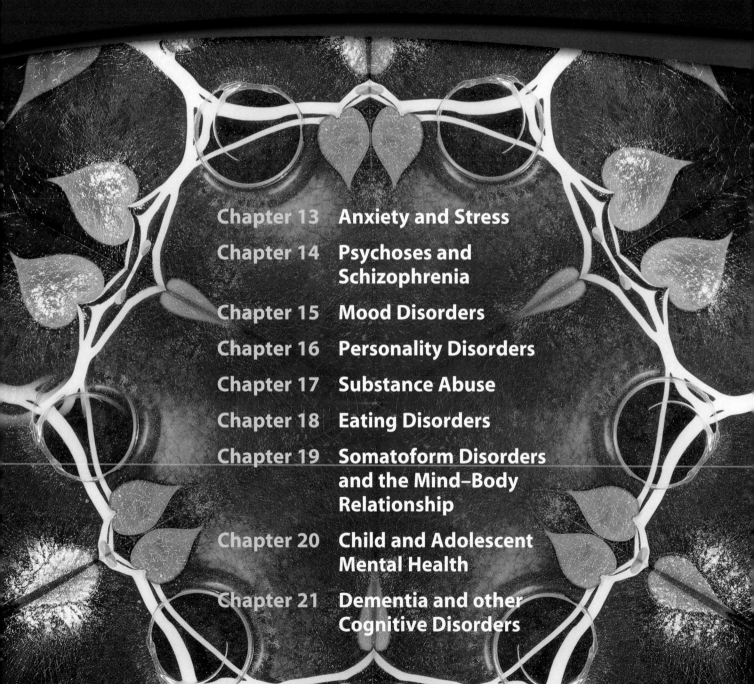

Unit 4

Nursing Practice for Specific Mental Health Problems

Unit

4

Nursing Practice for Specific Mental Health Problems

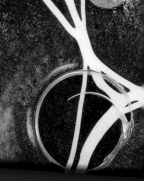

Chapter

13

Anxiety and Stress

Key Terms

- agoraphobia
- anxiety
- anxiety disorders
- assertiveness training
- automatisms
- avoidance behaviour
- compulsions
- decatastrophizing
- defence mechanisms
- depersonalization
- derealization
- exposure
- fear
- flooding
- mild anxiety
- moderate anxiety
- obsessions
- panic anxiety
- panic attack
- panic disorder
- phobia
- primary gain
- reframing
- response prevention
- secondary gain
- severe anxiety
- stress
- systematic desensitization

Learning Objectives

After reading this chapter, you should be able to:

1. Describe cognitive, affective and behavioural dimensions of anxiety as a response to stress.

2. Describe the 'levels' of anxiety and the behavioural changes related to each level.

3. Discuss the use of defence mechanisms by people with anxiety disorders.

4. Describe the current theories regarding the aetiologies of major anxiety disorders.

5. Evaluate the effectiveness of care and treatment – including medication – for clients with anxiety disorders.

6. Apply the nursing process to the care of clients coping with anxiety and anxiety disorders.

7. Provide teaching to clients, families, other carers and communities to increase understanding of anxiety and stress.

8. Examine your feelings, beliefs and attitudes regarding clients with anxiety disorders.

Anxiety is a feeling of dread or apprehension, accompanied by specific thoughts and actions; it is a response to external or internal stimuli that has behavioural, emotional, cognitive and physical aspects. Anxiety can be distinguished from **fear**, which is a feeling of being afraid of, or threatened by, a clearly identifiable external stimulus that represents danger to the person. Anxiety is unavoidable in life and can serve many positive functions, such as motivating the person to take action to solve a problem or to resolve a crisis. It can be considered 'normal' when it is appropriate to the situation and dissipates when the situation has been resolved.

Anxiety disorders comprise a group of conditions that share a key feature of 'excessive' anxiety with ensuing behavioural, emotional, cognitive and physiological responses. People suffering from anxiety disorders can demonstrate 'unusual' behaviours such as panic without apparent reason, unwarranted fear of objects or life conditions, uncontrollable repetitive actions, re-experiencing of traumatic events or unexplainable or overwhelming worry. They experience significant distress over time, and the disorder significantly impairs their daily routines, social lives and occupational functioning.

Anxiety – and its management – play a key role in many other mental health disorders; there is a close relationship between anxiety and depression, between anxiety and psychoses, between anxiety and personality disorders, between anxiety and substance misuse.

ANXIETY AS A RESPONSE TO STRESS

Stress is a much-used (and abused) term within both professional and public domains, and runs the risk of being so vague as to be meaningless. According to Hans Selye (1956), stress consists of the wear and tear that life causes *on the body*; this 'wear and tear' can be short term or longer term and is the result of the complex interactions between a person's physiological and neurological status, their cognitive make-up (in particular, their core beliefs about themselves, the world and others), external events and the social context in which challenges or demands occur. The wear and tear occurs when someone perceives the resources they have to be actually or potentially overwhelmed by the challenges they face.

Stress occurs when a person has difficulty dealing with life situations, challenges, problems and goals. Each person, of course, handles stress differently: one person can thrive in a situation that creates great distress for another; many people view public speaking as scary, but for many teachers and actors, it is an everyday, enjoyable experience. Marriage, having children, airplanes, snakes, a new job, a new school and leaving home are examples of stress-causing events (or 'stressors').

Selye (1956, 1974), an endocrinologist, identified the physiological aspects of stress, which he labelled the *general adaptation syndrome*. He used laboratory animals to assess biological system changes; the stages of the body's physical responses to pain, heat, toxins and restraint; and, later, the mind's emotional responses to real or perceived stressors. He determined three stages of reaction to stress:

- In the *alarm reaction stage,* stress stimulates the body to send messages from the hypothalamus to the glands (such as the adrenal gland, to send out adrenaline and noradrenaline for fuel) and organs (such as the liver, to reconvert glycogen stores to glucose for food) to prepare for potential defence needs.
- In the *resistance stage,* the digestive system reduces function to shunt blood to areas needed for defence. The lungs take in more air, and the heart beats faster and harder so it can circulate this highly oxygenated and highly nourished blood to the muscles to defend the body by fight, flight or freeze behaviours. If the person adapts to the stress, the body responses relax, and the gland, organ and systemic responses abate.
- The *exhaustion stage* occurs when the person has responded negatively to anxiety and stress: body stores are depleted or the emotional components are not resolved, resulting in continual arousal of the physiological responses and little reserve capacity.

Autonomic nervous system responses to fear and anxiety generate the involuntary activities of the body that are involved in self-preservation. Sympathetic nerve fibres 'charge up' the vital signs at any hint of danger, to prepare the body's defences. The adrenal glands release adrenaline, which causes the body to take in more oxygen, dilate the pupils and increase arterial pressure and heart rate, while

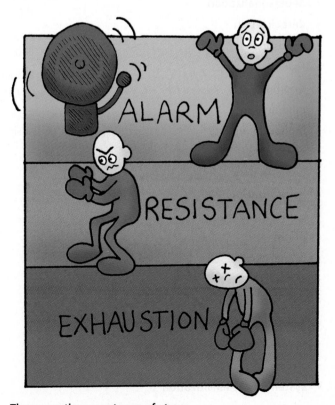

Three reactions or stages of stress

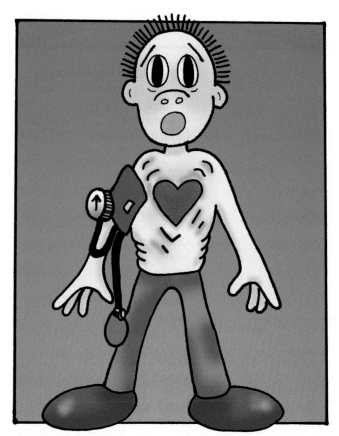

Physiological response

constricting the peripheral vessels and shunting blood from the gastrointestinal and reproductive systems and increasing glycogenolysis to free glucose for fuel for the heart, muscles and central nervous system. When the danger has passed, parasympathetic nerve fibres reverse this process and return the body to normal operating conditions until the next sign of threat reactivates the sympathetic responses.

Anxiety causes uncomfortable cognitive, psychomotor and physiological responses, such as difficulty with logical thought, increasingly agitated motor activity and elevated heart rate. To reduce these uncomfortable feelings, the person tries to reduce the level of discomfort by implementing new adaptive behaviours or defence mechanisms. Adaptive behaviours can be positive and help the person to learn; for example, meditation and mindfulness techniques, using imagery techniques to refocus attention on a pleasant scene, practising sequential relaxation of the body from head to toe, and breathing slowly and steadily to reduce muscle tension and vital signs. Negative responses to anxiety can result in maladaptive behaviours such as tension headaches, pain syndromes and stress-related responses that reduce the efficiency of the immune system.

People can communicate anxiety to others both verbally and non-verbally. If someone yells 'fire', others around them can become anxious as they picture a fire and the possible threat that represents. Viewing a distraught mother searching for her lost child in a shopping mall can cause anxiety in others as they imagine the panic she is experiencing. People can convey anxiety non-verbally through empathy, which might – in this case – be defined as the sense of walking in another person's shoes for a moment in time (Sullivan, 1952). Examples of non-verbal empathetic communication are when the family of a client undergoing surgery can tell from the surgeon's body language that their loved one has died, when the nurse reads a plea for help in a client's eyes, or when a person 'feels the tension' in a room where two people have been arguing and are now not speaking to each other.

Levels of Anxiety

Anxiety has both healthy and harmful aspects depending on its degree and duration, as well as on how well the person copes with it. Anxiety can be seen as having four levels: mild, moderate, severe and panic (Table 13.1). Each level causes both physiological and emotional changes in the person.

Mild anxiety is a sensation that something is different and warrants special attention. Sensory stimulation increases and helps the person focus attention to learn, solve problems, think, act, feel and protect himself or herself. Mild anxiety often motivates people to make changes or to engage in goal-directed activity. For example, it helps students to focus on studying for an examination.

Moderate anxiety is the disturbing feeling that something is definitely wrong; the person becomes nervous or agitated. In moderate anxiety, the person can still process information, solve problems and learn new things with assistance from others. He or she has difficulty concentrating independently but can be redirected to the topic. For example, a nurse might be explaining ECT to a client who is anxious about the procedure. As the nurse is talking, the client's attention wanders but he or she can regain the client's attention and help gently direct him or her back to the task at hand.

As the person progresses to **severe anxiety** and **panic**, more primitive survival skills take over, defensive responses ensue and cognitive skills decrease significantly. A person with severe anxiety has trouble thinking and reasoning. Muscles tighten and vital signs increase. The person paces; is restless, irritable and angry; or uses other similar emotional–psychomotor means to release tension. In panic, the emotional–psychomotor realm predominates with accompanying fight, flight or freeze responses. Adrenaline surge greatly increases vital signs. Pupils enlarge to let in more light, and the only cognitive process focuses on the person's defence.

Working with Anxious Clients

Mental health nurses encounter anxious clients and families in a wide variety of situations in inpatient and community settings. First and foremost, the nurse must engage with and then assess with the person his or her anxiety level (and any

Table 13.1	LEVELS OF ANXIETY	
Anxiety Level	**Psychological Responses**	**Physiological Responses**
Mild	Wide perceptual field Sharpened senses Increased motivation Effective problem solving Increased learning ability Irritability	Restlessness Fidgeting GI 'butterflies' Difficulty sleeping Hypersensitivity to noise
Moderate	Perceptual field narrowed to immediate task Selectively attentive Cannot connect thoughts or events independently Increased use of automatisms	Muscle tension Diaphoresis Pounding pulse Headache Dry mouth High voice pitch Faster rate of speech GI upset Frequent urination
Severe	Perceptual field reduced to one detail or scattered details Cannot complete tasks Cannot solve problems or learn effectively Behaviour geared toward anxiety relief and is usually ineffective Doesn't respond to redirection Feels awe, dread or horror Cries Ritualistic behaviour	Severe headache Nausea, vomiting and diarrhoea Trembling Rigid stance Vertigo Pale Tachycardia Chest pain
Panic	Perceptual field reduced to focus on self Cannot process any environmental stimuli Distorted perceptions Loss of rational thought Doesn't recognize potential danger Can't communicate verbally Possible delusions and hallucination May be suicidal	May bolt and run OR Totally immobile and mute Dilated pupils Increased blood pressure and pulse Flight, fight or freeze

GI, gastrointestinal.

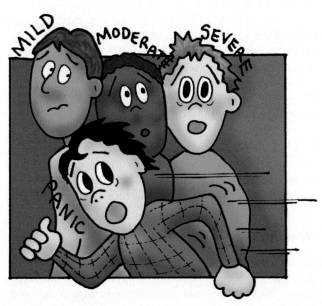

Levels of anxiety

previously employed anxiety-reduction strategies), because these can determine the interventions that are likely to be effective.

Mild anxiety is almost invariably an asset to the client and requires no direct intervention. People with mild anxiety can learn and solve problems and are even eager for information. Teaching can be very effective when a client is mildly anxious.

In moderate anxiety, the nurse must be certain that the client is following what he or she is saying. The client's attention can wander, and he or she may have some difficulty concentrating over time. Speaking in short, simple and easy-to-understand sentences is effective; the nurse must stop to ensure that the client is still taking in information correctly. The nurse may need to redirect the client back to the topic if the client goes off on an unrelated tangent.

When anxiety becomes severe, the client can no longer pay attention or take in information. The nurse's goal must be to work collaboratively to lower the person's anxiety level to moderate or mild before proceeding with anything else. It is also essential to remain with the person because

Table 13.2   ANXIOLYTIC DRUGS

Non-propietary Name	Side-effects	Nursing Implications
Diazepam Alprazolam Chlordiazepoxide Lorazepam (shorter-acting Oxazepam (shorter-acting)	Dizziness, clumsiness, sedation, headache, fatigue, sexual dysfunction, blurred vision, dry throat and mouth, constipation, high potential for abuse and dependence, ataxia, confusion, muscle weakness	Long-term use must be avoided Avoid other CNS depressants such as antihistamines and alcohol Avoid caffeine Take care with potentially hazardous activities such as driving Rise slowly from lying or sitting position Use sugar-free beverages or hard sweets Drink adequate fluids
Buspirone (Buspar)	Dizziness, restlessness, agitation, drowsiness, headache, weakness, nausea, vomiting, paradoxical excitement or euphoria	Take only as prescribed Do not stop taking the drug abruptly Rise slowly from sitting position Take care with potentially hazardous activities such as driving Take with food Report persistent restlessness, agitation, excitement, or euphoria immediately

anxiety may well worsen if he or she is left alone. Talking to the client in a low, calm and soothing voice can help. If the person cannot sit still, walking with him or her while talking can be effective. What the nurse talks about matters less than how he or she says the words. Helping the person to take deep, even breaths can help lower anxiety.

During panic-level anxiety, the person's safety is the primary concern. He or she cannot perceive potential harm and may have no capacity for rational thought. The nurse must keep talking to the person in a comforting manner, even though the client cannot process what the nurse is saying. Going to a small, quiet and non-stimulating environment may help to reduce anxiety. The nurse can reassure the person that this is anxiety, that it will pass, and that he or she is in a safe place. The nurse should remain with the client until the panic recedes. Panic-level anxiety is not sustained indefinitely but can last for up to 30 minutes.

When working with an anxious person, the nurse must be aware of his or her own anxiety level. It is easy for the nurse to become increasingly anxious. Remaining calm and in control is essential if the nurse is going to work effectively with the client.

Short-term anxiety can be treated with anxiolytic medications (Table 13.2). Many of these drugs are benzodiazepines, which are still commonly prescribed for anxiety. Benzodiazepines have a high potential for abuse and dependence, however, so their use should be short term, ideally no longer than 4 to 6 weeks. These drugs are designed to relieve anxiety so that the person can deal more effectively with whatever crisis or situation is causing stress. Unfortunately, many people see these drugs as a 'cure' for anxiety and continue to use them instead of learning more effective coping skills or making needed changes.

Overview of Anxiety Disorders

Anxiety disorders are diagnosed when anxiety no longer functions as a signal of danger or a motivation for needed change but becomes chronic and permeates major portions of the person's life, resulting in maladaptive behaviours and emotional disability. Anxiety disorders have many manifestations, but anxiety is the key feature of each (American Psychiatric Association, 2000). Types of anxiety disorders include the following:

- Agoraphobia with or without panic disorder
- Panic disorder
- Specific phobia
- Social phobia
- OCD
- Generalized anxiety disorder (GAD)
- Acute stress disorder
- PTSD.

For the purposes of this chapter, these *DSM-IV* classifications will be used. Panic disorder and OCD seem to be the most common anxiety disorders and are the focus of this chapter. PTSD was addressed in Chapter 11.

INCIDENCE

In the UK (according to NICE, 2004), around 1 in 20 people has generalized anxiety disorder and 1 in 100 have panic disorder. Many more have high levels of anxiety in particular situations or aspects of life, or as a concomitant part of another mental health problem. Anxiety disorders seem to be more prevalent in women, people younger than 45, people who are divorced or separated and people of lower

DSM-IV-TR DIAGNOSTIC CRITERIA: SYMPTOMS OF ANXIETY DISORDERS

Disorder

Agoraphobia is anxiety about, or avoidance of, places or situations from which escape might be difficult or help might be unavailable.

Panic disorder is characterized by recurrent, unexpected panic attacks that cause constant concern. **Panic attack** is the sudden onset of intense apprehension, fearfulness or terror associated with feelings of impending doom.

Specific phobia is characterized by significant anxiety provoked by a specific feared object or situation, which often leads to avoidance behaviour.

Social phobia is characterized by anxiety provoked by certain types of social or performance situations, which often leads to avoidance behaviour.

OCD involves obsessions (thoughts, impulses or images) that cause marked anxiety and/or compulsions (repetitive behaviours or mental acts) that attempt to neutralize anxiety.

GAD is characterized by at least 6 months of persistent and excessive worry and anxiety.

Acute stress disorder is the development of anxiety, dissociation and other symptoms within 1 month of exposure to an extremely traumatic stressor; it lasts 2 days to 4 weeks.

PTSD is characterized by the re-experiencing of an extremely traumatic event, avoidance of stimuli associated with the event, numbing of responsiveness and persistent increased arousal; it begins within 3 months to years after the event and may last a few months or years.

Symptoms

Avoids being outside alone or at home alone; avoids travelling in vehicles; impaired ability to work; difficulty meeting daily responsibilities (e.g. grocery shopping, going to appointments); knows response is extreme.

A discrete episode of panic lasting 15 to 30 minutes with four or more of the following: palpitations, sweating, trembling or shaking, shortness of breath, choking or smothering sensation, chest pain or discomfort, nausea, derealization or depersonalization, fear of dying or going crazy, paraesthesias, chills or hot flushes.

Marked anxiety response to the object or situation; avoidance or suffered endurance of object or situation; significant distress or impairment of daily routine, occupation or social functioning; adolescents and adults recognize their fear as excessive or unreasonable.

Fear of embarrassment or inability to perform; avoidance or dreaded endurance of behaviour or situation; recognition that response is irrational or excessive; belief that others are judging him or her negatively; significant distress or impairment in relationships, work or social life; anxiety can be severe or panic level.

Recurrent, persistent, unwanted, intrusive thoughts, impulses or images beyond worrying about realistic life problems; attempts to ignore, suppress or neutralize obsessions with compulsions that are mostly ineffective; adults and adolescents recognize that obsessions and compulsions are excessive and unreasonable.

Apprehensive expectations more days than not for 6 months or more about several events or activities; uncontrollable worrying; significant distress or impaired social or occupational functioning; three of the following symptoms: restlessness, easily fatigued, difficulty concentrating or mind going blank, irritability, muscle tension, sleep disturbance.

Exposure to traumatic event causing intense fear, helplessness or horror; marked anxiety symptoms or increased arousal; significant distress or impaired functioning; persistent re-experiencing of the event; three of the following symptoms: sense of emotional numbing or detachment, feeling dazed, derealization, depersonalization, dissociative amnesia (inability to recall important aspect of the event).

Exposure to traumatic event involving intense fear, helplessness or horror; re-experiencing (intrusive recollections or dreams, flashbacks, physical and psychological distress over reminders of the event); avoidance of memory-provoking stimuli and numbing of general responsiveness (avoidance of thoughts, feelings, conversations, people, places, amnesia, diminished interest or participation in life events, feeling detached or estranged from others, restricted affect, sense of foreboding); increased arousal (sleep disturbance, irritability or angry outbursts, difficulty concentrating, hypervigilance, exaggerated startle response); significant distress or impairment.

Adapted from American Psychiatric Association. (2000). *DSM-IV-TR: Diagnostic and statistical manual of mental disorders* (4th edn, text revision). Washington DC: American Psychiatric Association.

socioeconomic status. The exception is OCD, which is equally prevalent in men and women but is more common among boys than girls.

ONSET AND CLINICAL COURSE

The onset and clinical course of anxiety disorders are extremely variable, depending on the specific disorder. These aspects are discussed later in this chapter within the context of each disorder.

RELATED DISORDERS

Anxiety disorder due to a general medical condition is diagnosed when the prominent symptoms of anxiety are judged to result directly from a physiological condition. The person may have panic attacks, generalized anxiety or obsessions or compulsions. Medical conditions causing this disorder can include endocrine dysfunction, chronic obstructive pulmonary disease, congestive heart failure and neurological conditions.

Substance-induced anxiety disorder is anxiety directly caused by drug abuse, a medication or exposure to a toxin. Symptoms include prominent anxiety, panic attacks, phobias, obsessions or compulsions.

Separation anxiety disorder is excessive anxiety concerning separation from home or from persons, parents or carers to whom the client is attached. It occurs when it is no longer developmentally appropriate and before 18 years of age.

Adjustment disorder is an emotional response to a stressful event, such as one involving financial issues, medical illness or a relationship problem, that results in clinically significant symptoms such as marked distress or impaired functioning.

AETIOLOGY

Biological Theories

GENETIC THEORIES

Anxiety may have an inherited component because first-degree relatives of clients with increased anxiety have higher rates of developing anxiety. *Heritability* refers to the proportion of a disorder that can be attributed to genetic factors:

- High heritabilities are greater than 0.6 and indicate that genetic influences dominate.
- Moderate heritabilities are 0.3 to 0.5 and suggest the influence of genetic and non-genetic factors.
- Heritabilities less than 0.3 mean that genetics are negligible as a primary cause of the disorder.

Panic disorder and social and specific phobias, including agoraphobia, have moderate heritability. GAD and OCD tend to be more common in families, indicating a strong genetic component, but still require further in-depth study (McMahon & Kassem, 2005). At this point, current research indicates a clear genetic susceptibility to, or vulnerability for, anxiety disorders; however, additional factors are necessary for these disorders to actually develop.

NEUROCHEMICAL THEORIES

GABA is the amino acid neurotransmitter believed to be dysfunctional in anxiety disorders. GABA, an inhibitory neurotransmitter, functions as the body's natural anti-anxiety agent by reducing cell excitability, thus decreasing the rate of neuronal firing. It is available in one-third of the nerve synapses, especially those in the limbic system and in the locus coeruleus, the area where the neurotransmitter noradrenaline, which excites cellular function, is produced. Because GABA reduces anxiety and noradrenaline increases it, researchers believe that a problem with the regulation of these neurotransmitters occurs in anxiety disorders.

Serotonin, the indolamine neurotransmitter usually implicated in psychosis and mood disorders, has many subtypes. 5-Hydroxytryptamine type 1a plays a role in anxiety, and it also affects aggression and mood. Serotonin is believed to play a distinct role in OCD, panic disorder and GAD. An excess of noradrenaline is suspected in panic disorder, GAD and posttraumatic stress disorder (Neumeister *et al.*, 2005).

Psychodynamic Theories

INTRAPSYCHIC/PSYCHOANALYTIC THEORIES

Freud (1936) saw a person's innate anxiety as the stimulus for behaviour. He described defence mechanisms as the human being's attempt to control awareness of and to reduce anxiety (see Chapter 2). **Defence mechanisms** are cognitive distortions that a person uses unconsciously to maintain a sense of being in control of a situation, to lessen discomfort and to deal with stress. Because defence mechanisms arise from the unconscious, the person is unaware of using them. Some people overuse defence mechanisms, which stops them from learning a variety of appropriate methods to resolve anxiety-producing situations. The dependence on one or two defence mechanisms can also inhibit emotional growth, lead to poor problem-solving skills, and create difficulty with relationships.

INTERPERSONAL THEORY

Harry Stack Sullivan (1952) viewed anxiety as being generated from problems in interpersonal relationships. Carers can communicate anxiety to infants or children through inadequate nurturing, agitation when holding or handling the child and distorted messages. Such communicated anxiety can result in dysfunction, such as failure to achieve age-appropriate developmental tasks. In adults, anxiety often arises from the person's need to conform to the norms and values of his or her cultural group. The higher the level of anxiety, the lower the ability to communicate and to solve problems and the greater chance for anxiety disorders to develop.

Hildegard Peplau (1952) understood that humans exist in interpersonal and physiological realms; thus the nurse can better help the client to achieve health by attending to both areas. She identified the four levels of anxiety and developed nursing interventions and interpersonal communication techniques based on Sullivan's interpersonal view of anxiety; she described an understanding of the 'relief behaviours' of 'acting out,' 'somatizing' and 'withdrawal' as key to helping people cope with anxiety.

BEHAVIOURAL THEORY

Behavioural theorists view anxiety as being learned through experiences. Conversely, people can change or 'unlearn' behaviours through new experiences. Behaviourists believe that people can modify maladaptive behaviours without gaining insight into the causes for them. They contend that disturbing behaviours that develop and interfere with a person's life can be extinguished or unlearned by repeated experiences guided by a trained therapist.

COGNITIVE-BEHAVIOURAL THEORIES

Cognitive-behavioural theorists see anxiety as emerging from the interplay between the environment and someone's thoughts, feelings and behaviour. Core beliefs – about the self, the world and other people – interact with

environmental and developmental stressors and produce a way of approaching the world that is manifested in 'automatic thoughts' in stressful situations. These produce further anxious feelings and physiological discomfort and then lead, often, to the avoidance of difficult situations; anxiety thus becomes 'connected' to those situations.

CULTURAL CONSIDERATIONS

Each culture has rules governing the appropriate ways to express and deal with anxiety. Culturally competent nurses should be aware of them, while being careful not to stereotype clients. People from some Asian and African cultures may more readily express anxiety through somatic symptoms such as headaches, backaches, fatigue, dizziness and stomach problems.

CARE AND TREATMENT

Treatment for anxiety disorders usually involves medication (Table 13.3) and/or psychotherapeutic help (usually, though not exclusively, CBT. Formal treatment for people in community settings may take place in health centres, in CMHTs and in the person's own house or workplace. Because the person with an anxiety disorder often believes that any sporadic symptoms are related to medical problems, the GP or practice nurse can often be the first healthcare professional to evaluate him or her. Other community resources, such as anxiety management groups or self-help

Table 13.3	DRUGS USED TO TREAT ANXIETY DISORDERS	
Drug Name Generic (Trade)	**Classification**	**Used to Treat**
Alprazolam (Xanax)	Benzodiazepine	Anxiety, panic disorder, OCD, social phobia, agoraphobia
Buspirone (Buspar)	Non-benzodiazepine anxiolytic	Anxiety, OCD, social anxiety disorder, GAD
Chlordiazepoxide (Librium)	Benzodiazepine	Anxiety
Citalopram (Cipramil)	SSRI antidepressant	Panic disorder
Clomipramine (Anafranil)	Tricyclic antidepressant	OCD, phobias
Clonazepam	Benzodiazepine	Anxiety, panic disorder, OCD
Diazepam	Benzodiazepine	Anxiety
Escitalopram (Cipralex)	SSRI antidepressant	GAD, OCD, panic disorder, social anxiety disorder
Fluoxetine (Prozac)	SSRI antidepressant	Panic disorder, OCD, GAD
Fluvoxamine (Faverin)	SSRI antidepressant	OCD
Hydroxyzine (Atarax)	Antihistamine	Anxiety
Lorazepam (Ativan)	Benzodiazepine	Anxiety
Oxprenolol (Trasicor)	Beta-blocker	Anxiety
Oxazepam	Benzodiazepine	Anxiety
Paroxetine (Seroxat)	SSRI antidepressant	Social phobia, GAD
Propranolol (Inderal)	Beta-blocker	Anxiety, panic disorder, GAD
Sertraline (Lustral)	SSRI antidepressant	Panic disorder, PTSD, OCD, social phobia, GAD

GAD, generalized anxiety disorder; OCD, obsessive-compulsive disorder; PTSD, posttraumatic stress disorder; SSRI, selective serotonin reuptake inhibitor. Adapted using British National Formulary Online (2008) http://www.bnf.org/bnf/bnf/55/

Nursing Care Plan

Anxious Behaviour

Nursing Formulation

Anxiety: *Vague, uneasy feeling of discomfort or dread accompanied by an autonomic response (the source often non-specific or unknown to the individual); a feeling of apprehension caused by anticipation of danger. It is an alerting signal that warns of impending danger and enables the individual to take measures to deal with the threat.*

ASSESSMENT DATA

- Decreased attention span
- Restlessness, irritability
- Poor impulse control
- Feelings of discomfort, apprehension or helplessness
- Hyperactivity, pacing
- Wringing hands
- Perceptual field deficits
- Decreased ability to communicate verbally

In addition, in panic anxiety
- Inability to discriminate harmful stimuli or situations
- Disorganized thought processes
- Delusions

EXPECTED OUTCOMES

Immediate
The client will
- Be safe and free from injury
- Discuss feelings of dread and anxiety and collaboratively work towards solutions
- Respond to relaxation techniques with a decreased anxiety level

Stabilization
The client will
- Demonstrate the ability to perform relaxation techniques
- Reduce own anxiety level

Community
The client will
- Be free from anxiety attacks
- Manage the anxiety response to stress effectively

ASSESSMENT DATA

Nursing Interventions *denotes collaborative interventions

Remain with the client at all times when levels of anxiety are high (severe or panic).

Move the client to a quiet area with minimal or decreased stimuli, such as a small room or seclusion area.

Remain calm in your approach to the client.

Use short, simple and clear statements.

Avoid asking or forcing the client to make choices.

Medications may be indicated for high levels of anxiety, delusions, disorganized thoughts and so forth.

Be aware of your own feelings and level of discomfort.

Encourage the client's participation in relaxation exercises, such as deep breathing, progressive muscle relaxation, meditation and imagining being in a quiet, peaceful place.

Teach the client to use relaxation techniques independently.

Help the client see that mild anxiety can be a positive catalyst for change and does not need to be avoided.

Rationale

The client's safety is a priority. A highly anxious client should not be left alone – his or her anxiety may well escalate.

Anxious behaviour can be escalated by external stimuli. In a large area, the client can feel lost and panicked, but a smaller room can enhance a sense of security.

The client will feel more secure if you are calm and if the client feels you are in control of the situation.

The client's ability to deal with abstractions or complexity is impaired.

The client may not make sound decisions or may be unable to make decisions or solve problems.

Medication may be necessary to decrease anxiety to a level at which the client can feel safe.

Anxiety is communicated interpersonally. Being with an anxious client can raise your own anxiety level.

Relaxation exercises are effective, non-chemical ways to reduce anxiety.

Using relaxation techniques can give the client confidence in having control over anxiety.

The client may feel that all anxiety is bad and not useful.

Adapted from Schultz, J. M. & Videbeck, S. L. (2005). *Lippincott's manual of psychiatric care plans* (7th edn). Philadelphia: Lippincott Williams & Wilkins.

groups, can provide support and help the client feel less isolated and lonely.

Cognitive-Behavioural Approaches

CBT approaches to anxiety include thorough assessment of triggers and of the cognitive, affective and behavioural responses to those triggers. It involves helping people towards behavioural change through working with the automatic thoughts that may arise in anxiety-provoking situations. CBT adopts very pragmatic approaches to anxiety, encouraging – through the medium of a formal collaborative and educational relationship – regular sessions, goal-setting and the use of diaries, self-screening tools and journals to record and monitor changes. Interventions may be at the level of physical symptoms: learning relaxation techniques; behaviour: finding ways to confront avoidance; affect: noticing and being non-judgemental towards feelings of dread; and cognition: both challenging automatic thoughts in the here-and-now and validating, understanding and beginning to change core beliefs about the self, others and the world.

Reframing – turning negative messages into realistic messages – involves the therapist coaching the person to create more positive messages for use during panic episodes. For example, instead of thinking, 'My heart is pounding. I'm going to die!' the client thinks, 'I can stand this. This is just anxiety. It will go away.' The client can write down these messages and keep them readily accessible such as in an address book, calendar or wallet.

Decatastrophizing involves the therapist's use of questions to more realistically appraise the situation. The therapist may ask, 'What's the worst thing that could happen? Is that likely? Could you survive that? Is that as bad as you imagine?' The client may be helped to use thought-stopping and distraction techniques to jolt him or herself from focusing on negative thoughts. Splashing the face with cold water, snapping a rubber band worn on the wrist or shouting are all techniques that can break the cycle of negative thoughts.

Assertiveness training helps the person take more control over life situations. Techniques help the person negotiate interpersonal situations and foster self-assurance. They involve using 'I' statements to identify feelings and to communicate concerns or needs to others. Examples include 'I feel angry when you turn your back while I'm talking,' 'I want to have 5 minutes of your time for an uninterrupted conversation about something important,' and 'I would like to have about 30 minutes in the evening to relax without interruption.'

CONSIDERATIONS WHEN WORKING WITH THE OLDER PERSON WHO IS ANXIOUS

Anxiety that starts for the first time in late life is frequently associated with another condition such as depression, dementia, physical illness or medication toxicity or withdrawal. Phobias, particularly agoraphobia, and GAD are the most common late-life anxiety disorders. Most people with late-onset agoraphobia attribute the start of the disorder to the abrupt onset of a physical illness or as a response to a traumatic event such as a fall, a burglary or mugging. Late-onset GAD is usually associated with depression. Though less common, panic attacks can occur in later life and are often related to depression or a physical illness, such as cardiovascular, gastrointestinal or chronic pulmonary diseases. Ruminative thoughts are common in late-life depression and can take the form of obsessions, such as contamination fears, pathological doubt or fear of harming others. The pharmacological treatment of choice for anxiety disorders in the elderly is selective SSRI antidepressants. Initial treatment involves doses lower than the usual starting doses for adults, to ensure that the elderly client can tolerate the medication: if started on too high a dose, SSRIs can exacerbate anxiety symptoms in elderly clients (Flint, 2004).

MENTAL HEALTH PROMOTION

Too often, 'stress' or anxiety are viewed negatively as things to avoid at all costs; life, though, is inevitably anxiety-provoking and to grow and develop, every one of us needs to encounter challenges and fears and difficulties. Peplau's 'relief behaviours' may, in the end, be destructive for us. For many people, though, anxiety can be a warning they are not dealing with stress effectively. Learning to heed this warning and to make needed changes is a healthy way to deal with the stress of daily events.

Stress and resulting anxiety are not associated exclusively with life 'problems'. Events that are 'positive' or desired, such as going away to university, getting a first job, getting married and having children, are stressful and cause anxiety. Managing the effects of stress and anxiety in one's life is important to being healthy. Tips for managing stress include the following:

- Keep a realistically positive attitude and believe in yourself
- Accept there are events you cannot control
- Communicate assertively with others
- Talk about your feelings to others
- Express your feelings through laughing, crying and so forth
- Learn to relax
- Exercise regularly
- Eat well-balanced meals
- Limit intake of caffeine and alcohol
- Get enough rest and sleep
- Set realistic goals and expectations
- Find an activity that is personally meaningful
- Learn stress management techniques such as relaxation, yoga, guided imagery, mindfulness and meditation; practise them as part of your daily routine.

For people with anxiety disorders, it is important to emphasize that the goal is effective management of stress and anxiety, their integration into one's life: it is not the total elimination of anxiety. Although medication can be important to relieve excessive anxiety, it does not solve or eliminate the problem entirely. Learning anxiety management techniques and effective methods for coping with life and its stresses is essential for overall improvement in life quality.

GENERALIZED ANXIETY DISORDER

A person with GAD worries excessively and feels highly anxious at least 50% of the time for 6 months or more. Unable to control this focus on worry, the person has three or more of the following symptoms: uneasiness, irritability, muscle tension, fatigue, difficulty thinking and sleep alterations. GAD seems to affect 50% more women than men; far more people experiencing it are seen in primary care than by specialist mental health services. The majority of people with GAD suffer with other mood and anxiety disorders as well; GAD seems to make the likelihood of full recovery from other conditions – both physical and psychological – much more difficult.

CBT and SSRI antidepressants seem to be effective treatments, although anxiety management therapy (incorporating key elements of CBT – education, relaxation training and **exposure** – but without cognitive restructuring) may well be as effective as CBT (NICE, 2004; Starcevic, 2006; Gale & Davidson, 2007).

If the anxiety becomes acutely distressing, bezodiazepines (for a maximum of 2–4 weeks) and rapid supportive and educational psychological interventions may be indicated.

PANIC DISORDER

Panic disorder is composed of discrete episodes of **panic attacks**, that is, perhaps, 15 to 30 minutes of rapid, intense, escalating anxiety in which the person experiences great emotional fear as well as physiological discomfort. During a panic attack, the person has overwhelmingly intense feelings of, and thoughts about, anxiety and displays four or more of the following symptoms: palpitations, sweating, tremors, shortness of breath, sense of suffocation, chest pain, nausea, abdominal distress, dizziness, paraesthesias, chills or hot flushes.

Panic disorder is diagnosed when the person has recurrent, unexpected panic attacks followed by at least 1 month of persistent concern or worry about future attacks or their meaning, or a significant behavioural change related to them. Slightly more than 75% of people with panic disorder have spontaneous initial attacks with no environmental trigger. Half of those with panic disorder have accompanying agoraphobia. Panic disorder is more common in people with less educational attainment and who are not married. The risk increases by 18% in people with depression (Merikangas, 2005).

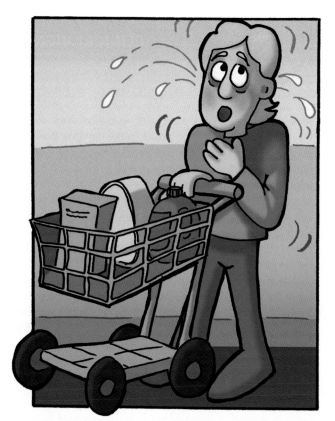

Panic attack

Clinical Course

The onset of panic disorder peaks in late adolescence and the mid-30s. Although **panic anxiety** might be normal in someone experiencing a life-threatening situation, a person with panic disorder experiences these emotional and physiological responses without this stimulus. The memory of the panic attack coupled with the fear of having more can lead to **avoidance behaviour**. In some cases, the person becomes housebound or stays in a very limited area around their home. This behaviour is known as **agoraphobia** (literally, 'fear of the marketplace', but used to mean a fear of being outside). Some people with agoraphobia fear stepping outside the front door because a panic attack may occur as soon as they leave the house. Others can leave the house but feel safe from the anticipatory fear of having a panic attack only within a limited area. Agoraphobia can also occur alone, without panic attacks.

The behaviour patterns of people with agoraphobia clearly demonstrate the concepts of primary and secondary gain associated with many anxiety disorders. **Primary gain** is the relief of anxiety achieved by performing the specific anxiety-driven behaviour, such as staying in the house to avoid the anxiety of leaving a safe place. **Secondary gain** is the attention received from others as a result of these behaviours. For instance, the person with agoraphobia may receive attention and caring concern from family members, who also assume all the responsibilities of family life outside the home (e.g.

CLINICAL VIGNETTE: PANIC DISORDER

Nancy spent as much time at her friend Jen's flat as she did in her own home. It was at Jen's place that Nancy had her first panic attack. For no reason at all, she felt the walls closing in on her, no air to breathe and her heart pounding out of her chest. She needed to get out – Hurry! Run! – so she could live. While a small, still-rational part of her mind assured her there was no reason to run, the need to flee was overwhelming. She ran out of the flat and down the hall, repeatedly smashing the lift button with the heel of her hand in hope of an instant response. 'What if the lift doesn't come?' Where were the stairs she so desperately wanted but couldn't find?

The lift door slid open. Scurrying into the lift and not realizing she had been holding her breath, Nancy exhaled with momentary relief. She had the faint perception of someone following her ask, 'What's wrong?' She couldn't answer! She still couldn't breathe. She held on to the rail on the wall of the lift because it was the only way to keep herself from falling.

'Breathe,' she told herself as she forced herself to inhale. She searched for the right button to push, the one for the ground floor. She couldn't make a mistake, couldn't push the wrong button, couldn't have the lift take more time, because she might not make it. Heart pounding, no air, run, run!!! When the lift doors opened, she ran outside and then bent forward, her hands on her knees. It took 5 minutes for her to realize she was safe and would be all right. Sliding on to a bench, breathing more easily, she sat there long enough for her heart rate to decrease. Exhausted and scared, she wondered, 'Am I having a heart attack? Am I going crazy? What's happening to me?'

Instead of returning to Jen's, Nancy walked across the street to her own flat. She couldn't face going into Jen's place until she recovered. She really hoped she would never have this happen to her again; in fact, it might not be a good idea to go to Jen's for a few days. As she sat in her apartment, she thought about what had happened to her that afternoon and how to prevent it from ever happening again.

---

work, shopping). Essentially, these compassionate 'helpers' can become enablers of the self-imprisonment of the person with agoraphobia.

Treatment

Panic disorder can be treated with CBT, information/self-help approaches, computerized CBT and medications, such as benzodiazepines, beta-blockers such as propranolol and antidepressants. Formalized psychological treatments seem to have the most sustained effect (NICE, 2004). There is some evidence that a guided self-help approach may be beneficial (Ricketts *et al.*, 2008).

APPLICATION OF THE NURSING PROCESS: PANIC DISORDER

Assessment

Box 13.1 presents the Hamilton Rating Scale for Anxiety. The nurse can use this tool along with the following detailed discussion to guide his or her assessment of the client with panic disorder.

HISTORY

The client usually seeks treatment for panic disorder after he or she has experienced several panic attacks. The client may report, 'I feel like I'm going mad. I thought I was having a heart attack, but the doctor says it's anxiety.' Usually, the client cannot identify any trigger for these events.

GENERAL APPEARANCE AND MOTOR BEHAVIOUR

The nurse assesses the client's general appearance and motor behaviour. The client may appear entirely 'normal' or may have signs of anxiety if he or she is apprehensive about having a panic attack in the next few moments. If the client is anxious, speech may increase in rate, pitch and volume, and he or she may have difficulty sitting in a chair. **Automatisms**, which are automatic, unconscious mannerisms, may be apparent. Examples include tapping fingers, jingling keys or twisting hair. Automatisms are geared toward anxiety relief and increase in frequency and intensity with the client's anxiety level.

MOOD AND AFFECT

Assessment of mood and affect may reveal that the person is anxious, worried, tense, depressed, serious or sad. When discussing the panic attacks, he or she may be tearful. He or she may express anger at himself or herself for being 'unable to control myself.' Most people are distressed about the intrusion of anxiety attacks in their lives. During a panic attack, the person may describe feelings of being disconnected from himself or herself (**depersonalization**) or sensing that things are not real (**derealization**).

THOUGHT PROCESSES AND CONTENT

During a panic attack, the person feels overwhelmed, believing that he or she is dying, losing control or 'going insane'. The person may even consider suicide. Thoughts are disorganized, and the person loses the ability to think rationally. At other times, he or she may be consumed with worry about when the next panic attack will occur or how to deal with it.

Box 13.1 HAMILTON RATING SCALE FOR ANXIETY

Instructions: This checklist is to assist the professional in evaluating each patient as to his or her degree of anxiety and pathological condition. Please fill in the appropriate rating:

NONE = 0,　　MILD = 1,　　MODERATE = 2,　　SEVERE = 3,　　SEVERE,　　GROSSLY DISABLING = 4

Item		Rating	Item		Rating
Anxious mood	Worries, anticipation of the worst, anticipation, irritability	_____	Cardiovascular symptoms	Tachycardia, palpitations, pain in chest, throbbing of vessels, fainting feelings, missing beat	_____
Tension	Feelings of tension, fatigability, startle response, moved to tears easily, trembling, feelings of restlessness, inability to relax	_____	Respiratory symptoms	Pressure or constriction in chest, choking feelings, sighing, dyspnoea	_____
Fears	Of dark, of strangers, of being left alone, of animals, of traffic, of crowds	_____	Gastrointestinal symptoms	Difficulty in swallowing, wind, abdominal pain, burning sensations, abdominal fullness, nausea, vomiting, borborygmi, looseness of bowels, loss of weight, constipation	_____
Insomnia	Difficulty in falling asleep, broken sleep, unsatisfying sleep and fatigue on waking, dreams, nightmares, night terrors	_____	Genitourinary symptoms	Frequency of micturition, urgency of micturition, amenorrhoea, menorrhagia, development of frigidity, premature ejaculation, loss of libido, impotence	_____
Intellectual (cognitive)	Difficulty in concentration, poor memory	_____	Autonomic symptoms	Dry mouth, flushing, pallor, tendency to sweat, giddiness, tension headache, raising of hair	_____
Depressed mood	Loss of interest, lack of pleasure in hobbies, depression, early waking, diurnal swing	_____	Behaviour at interview	Fidgeting, restlessness or pacing, tremor of hands, furrowed brow, strained face, sighing or rapid respiration, facial pallor, swallowing, belching, brisk tendon jerks, dilated pupils, exophthalmos	_____
Somatic (muscular)	Pains and aches, twitching, stiffness, myoclonic jerks, grinding of teeth, unsteady voice, increased muscular tone	_____			
Somatic (sensory)	Tinnitus, blurring of vision, hot and cold flushes, feelings of weakness, pricking sensation	_____			

Additional Comments:

Investigator's Signature:

_____

Reprinted with permission from the *British Journal of Medical Psychology* (1959), 32, 50–55. © British Psychological Society.

SENSORY AND INTELLECTUAL PROCESSES

During a panic attack, the person may become confused and disoriented. He or she cannot take in environmental cues and respond appropriately. These functions are restored to normal after the panic attack subsides.

JUDGEMENT AND INSIGHT

Judgement is suspended during panic attacks; in an effort to escape, the person can run out of a building and into the street in front of a speeding car before the ability to assess safety has returned. Insight into panic disorder occurs only after the client has been involved in a collaborative process of information-giving about the disorder. Even then, people may still initially believe they are helpless and have no control over their anxiety attacks.

SELF-CONCEPT

It is important for the nurse to assess self-concept in clients with panic disorder. These clients often make self-blaming statements such as 'I can't believe I'm so weak and out of control' or 'I used to be a happy, well-adjusted person.' They may evaluate themselves negatively in all aspects of their lives. They may find themselves consumed with worry about impending attacks and unable to do many of the things they did before having panic attacks.

ROLES AND RELATIONSHIPS

Because of the intense anticipation of having another panic attack, the person may report alterations in his or her social, occupational or family life. The person typically avoids people, places and events associated with previous panic attacks. For example, the person may no longer travel by bus if he or she has had a panic attack on a bus. Although avoiding these objects does not stop the panic attacks, the person's sense of helplessness is so great that he or she may take even more restrictive measures to avoid them, such as stopping going to work and remaining at home.

PHYSIOLOGICAL AND SELF-CARE CONCERNS

The client often reports problems with sleeping and eating. The anxiety of apprehension between panic attacks may interfere with adequate, restful sleep even though the person may spend hours in bed. Clients may experience loss of appetite or eat constantly in an attempt to ease the anxiety.

Data Analysis

The following nursing formulations may apply to the client with panic disorder:

- Risk of Injury
- Anxiety
- Situational Low Self-Esteem (panic attacks)
- Ineffective Coping

- Powerlessness
- Ineffective Role Performance
- Disturbed Sleep Pattern.

Outcome Identification

Outcomes for clients with panic disorders include the following:

- The client will be free from injury.
- The client will verbalize thoughts and feelings.
- The client will demonstrate use of effective coping mechanisms.
- The client will demonstrate effective use of methods to manage anxiety response.
- The client will verbalize a sense of personal control.
- The client will re-establish adequate nutritional intake.
- The client will sleep at least 6 hours per night.

Intervention

PROMOTING SAFETY AND COMFORT

During a panic attack, the nurse's first concern is to provide a safe environment and to ensure the client's privacy. If the environment is overstimulating, the client should move to a less stimulating place. A quiet place reduces anxiety and provides privacy for the client.

The nurse remains with the client to help calm him or her down and to assess client behaviours and concerns. After getting the client's attention, the nurse uses a soothing, calm voice and gives brief directions to assure the client that he or she is safe:

'John, look around. It's safe, and I'm here with you. Nothing is going to happen. Take a deep breath.'

Reassurances and a calm demeanour can help to reduce anxiety. When the client feels out of control, the nurse can

NURSING INTERVENTIONS FOR PANIC DISORDER

- Provide a safe environment and ensure client's privacy during a panic attack.
- Remain with the client during a panic attack.
- Help client to focus on deep breathing.
- Talk to client in a calm, reassuring voice.
- Teach client to use relaxation techniques.
- Help client to use cognitive restructuring techniques.
- Engage client to explore how to decrease stressors and anxiety-provoking situations.

let the client know that the nurse is in control until the client regains self-control.

USING THERAPEUTIC COMMUNICATION

As with other mental health difficulties, the nurse should always actively collaborate with clients with anxiety disorders in the assessment, planning, intervention and evaluation of their care; rapport between nurse and client is vital. Communication should be simple and calm, because the client with severe anxiety cannot pay attention to lengthy messages and may pace to release energy. The nurse can walk with the client who feels unable to sit and talk. The nurse should evaluate carefully the use of touch because clients with high anxiety may interpret touch by a stranger as a threat and pull away abruptly.

As the client's anxiety diminishes, more rational cognition begins to return. When anxiety has subsided to a manageable level, the nurse uses open-ended communication techniques to discuss the experience:

> **Nurse:** *'It seems your anxiety is getting a bit better. Is that right?' or 'Can you tell me what it was like a few minutes ago?'*

At this point, the client can discuss his or her emotional responses to physiological processes and behaviours and can try to regain a sense of control.

MANAGING ANXIETY

Mindfulness and meditation techniques can be invaluable. The nurse can also teach the client relaxation techniques to use when he or she is experiencing stress or anxiety. Deep breathing is simple; anyone can do it. Guided imagery and progressive relaxation are methods to relax taut muscles. Guided imagery involves imagining a safe, enjoyable place to relax. In progressive relaxation, the person progressively tightens, holds and then relaxes muscle groups while letting tension flow from the body through rhythmic breathing. Cognitive restructuring techniques (discussed earlier) may also help the client to manage his or her anxiety response.

For any of these techniques, it is important for the client to learn and to practise them when he or she is relatively calm. When adept at these techniques, the client is more likely to use them successfully during panic attacks or periods of increased anxiety. Clients are likely to believe that self-control is returning when using these techniques helps them to manage anxiety. When clients believe they can manage the panic attack, they spend less time worrying about and anticipating the next one, which reduces their overall anxiety level.

PROVIDING CLIENT AND FAMILY EDUCATION

Collaborative client and family education is of primary importance when working with clients who have anxiety disorders. The client learns ways to manage stress and to

> ### CLIENT/FAMILY EDUCATION FOR PANIC DISORDER
>
> - Review breathing control and relaxation techniques.
> - Discuss positive coping strategies.
> - Encourage regular exercise.
> - Emphasize the importance of maintaining prescribed medication regimen and regular follow-up.
> - Describe time management techniques such as creating 'to do' lists with realistic estimated deadlines for each activity, crossing off completed items for a sense of accomplishment, and saying 'no'.
> - Stress the importance of maintaining contact with community and participating in supportive organizations.

cope with reactions to stress and stress-provoking situations. With education about the efficacy of psychotherapeutic approaches and/or medication, and the effects of any prescribed medication, the client needs to become the chief treatment manager of the anxiety disorder. It is important for the nurse to educate the client and family members about the physiology of anxiety and the merits of using combined psychotherapeutic interventions and drug management. Such a combined treatment approach, along with cognitive-behavioural stress-reduction techniques, can help the client to manage these drastic reactions and allow him or her to gain a sense of self-control. The nurse should help the client to understand that these therapies and drugs do not 'cure' the disorder but are methods to help him or her to control and manage it. Client and family education regarding medications should include the recommended dosage and dosage regime, expected effects, side-effects and how to handle them and substances that have a synergistic or antagonistic effect with the drug.

The nurse encourages the client to exercise regularly. Routine exercise helps to metabolize adrenaline, reduces panic reactions and increases production of endorphins; all these activities increase feelings of well-being.

Evaluation

Evaluation of the plan of care must, of course, be individualized. Ongoing assessment provides data to nurse and client, and can determine whether the client's outcomes have been achieved. The client's perception of the success of treatment also plays a part in evaluation. Even if all outcomes are achieved, the nurse must ensure with the client that he or she is comfortable or satisfied with the quality of life.

Evaluation of the treatment of panic disorder is based on the following:

- Does the client understand any prescribed medication regime, and is he or she committed to adhering to it?

- Have the client's episodes of anxiety decreased in frequency or intensity?
- Does the client understand various coping methods and when to use them?
- Does the client believe that his or her quality of life is satisfactory?

PHOBIAS

A **phobia** is an illogical, intense, persistent fear of a specific object or a social situation that causes extreme distress and interferes with normal functioning. Phobias do not always result from past negative experiences: in fact, the person may never have had contact with the object of the phobia. People with phobias understand that their fear is unusual and irrational and may even joke about how 'silly' it is. Nevertheless, they often feel powerless to stop it (Andreasen & Black, 2006).

People with phobias develop anticipatory anxiety even when thinking about possibly encountering the dreaded phobic object or situation. They engage in avoidance behaviour that often severely limits their lives. Such avoidance behaviour usually does not relieve the anticipatory anxiety for long.

There are three categories of phobia:

- Agoraphobia (discussed earlier)
- Specific phobia, which is an irrational fear of an object or situation
- Social phobia, which is anxiety provoked by certain social or performance situations.

Many people express 'phobias' about snakes, spiders, rats or similar objects. These fears are very specific, easy to avoid and cause no anxiety or worry. The diagnosis of a phobic disorder is made only when the phobic behaviour significantly interferes with the person's life by creating marked distress or difficulty in interpersonal or occupational functioning.

Specific phobias can be subdivided into the following categories:

- Natural environmental phobias: fear of storms, water, heights or other natural phenomena
- Blood-injection phobias: fear of seeing one's own or others' blood, traumatic injury or an invasive medical procedure such as an injection
- Situational phobias: fear of being in a specific situation such as on a bridge or in a tunnel, lift, small room, hospital or airplane
- Animal phobia: fear of animals or insects (usually a specific type). Often this fear develops in childhood and can continue through adulthood in both men and women. Cats and dogs are the most common phobic objects
- Other types of specific phobias: for example, fear of getting lost while driving if not able to make all right (and no left) turns to get to one's destination.

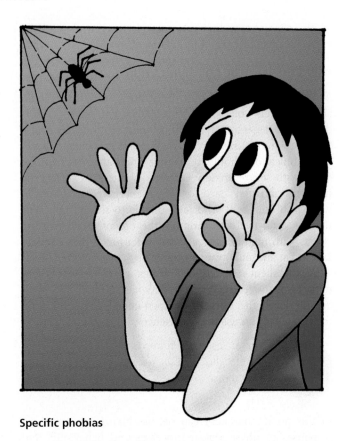

Specific phobias

In *social phobia*, also known as *social anxiety disorder*, the person becomes severely anxious to the point of panic or incapacitation when confronting situations involving people. Examples include making a speech, attending a social engagement alone, interacting with the opposite sex or with strangers and making complaints. The fear is rooted in low self-esteem and concern about others' judgements. The person fears looking socially inept, appearing anxious or doing something embarrassing such as burping or spilling food. Other social phobias include fear of eating in public, using public bathrooms, writing in public or becoming the centre of attention. A person may have one or several social phobias; the latter is known as generalized social phobia (Culpepper, 2006).

Onset and Clinical Course

Specific phobias usually occur in childhood or adolescence. In some cases, merely thinking about or handling a plastic model of the dreaded object can create fear. Specific phobias that persist into adulthood are lifelong 80% of the time.

The peak age of onset for social phobia is middle adolescence; it sometimes emerges in a person who was shy as a child. The course of social phobia is often continuous, although the disorder may become less severe during adulthood. Severity of impairment fluctuates with life stress and demands.

Treatment

Cognitive-behavioural therapy works well. Cognitive-behavioural therapists initially focus on teaching what anxiety is, helping the client to identify thoughts, feelings and behaviours involved in anxiety responses, teaching relaxation techniques, setting goals discussing methods to achieve those goals and helping the client to visualize phobic situations. Therapies that help the client to develop self-esteem and self-control are common and include positive reframing and assertiveness training (explained earlier).

One behavioural therapy often used to treat phobias is **systematic** (serial) **desensitization**, in which the therapist progressively exposes the client to the threatening object in a safe setting until the client's anxiety decreases. During each exposure, the complexity and intensity of exposure gradually increase, but the client's anxiety decreases. The reduced anxiety serves as a positive reinforcement until the anxiety is ultimately eliminated. For example, for the client who fears flying, the therapist would encourage the client to hold a small model airplane while talking about his or her experiences; later, the client would hold a larger model airplane and talk about flying. Even later exposures might include walking past an airport, sitting in a parked airplane and, finally, taking a short ride in a plane. Each session's challenge is based on the success achieved in previous sessions (Andreasen & Black, 2006).

Flooding is a form of rapid desensitization in which a therapist confronts the client with the phobic object (either a picture or the actual object) until it no longer produces anxiety. Because the client's worst fear has been realized and the client did not die, there is little reason to fear the situation any more. The goal is to rid the client of the phobia in one or two sessions. This method is highly anxiety producing and should be conducted only by a trained clinician under controlled circumstances and with the client's full consent.

OBSESSIVE-COMPULSIVE DISORDER

Obsessions are recurrent, persistent, intrusive and unwanted thoughts, images or impulses that cause marked anxiety and interfere with interpersonal, social or occupational function. The person knows these thoughts are excessive or unreasonable but believes he or she has no control over them. **Compulsions** are ritualistic or repetitive behaviours or mental acts that a person carries out continuously in an attempt to neutralize anxiety. Usually, the theme of the ritual is associated with that of the obsession, such as repetitive hand-washing when someone is obsessed with contamination, or repeated prayers or confession for someone obsessed with blasphemous thoughts. Common compulsions include the following:

- Checking rituals (repeatedly making sure the door is locked or the oven is turned off)
- Counting rituals (each step taken, ceiling tiles, concrete blocks, desks in a classroom)
- Washing and scrubbing until the skin is raw
- Praying or chanting

- Touching, rubbing or tapping (feeling the texture of each material in a clothing store; touching people, doors, walls or oneself)
- Hoarding items (for fear of throwing away something important)
- Ordering (arranging and rearranging furniture or items on a desk or shelf into perfect order; vacuuming the rug pile in one direction)
- Exhibiting rigid performance (getting dressed in an unvarying pattern)
- Having aggressive urges (for instance, to throw one's child against a wall).

OCD is diagnosed only when these thoughts, images and impulses consume the person, or he or she is compelled to act out the behaviours to a point at which they interfere with personal, social and occupational function. Examples include a man who can no longer work because he spends most of his day aligning and realigning all items in his home, or a woman who feels compelled to wash her hands after touching any object or person.

OCD can be manifested through many behaviours, all of which are repetitive, meaningless (to the onlooker) and difficult to conquer. The person understands that these rituals are unusual and unreasonable but feels forced to perform them to alleviate anxiety or to prevent terrible thoughts. Obsessions and compulsions are a source of distress and shame to the person, who may go to great lengths to keep them secret.

Onset and Clinical Course

OCD can start in childhood, especially in men. In women, it more commonly begins in the twenties. Overall, distribution between the sexes is equal. Onset is usually gradual, although there have been cases of acute onset with periods of waxing and waning symptoms. Exacerbation of symptoms may be related to stress. Eighty per cent of those treated with behaviour therapy and medication report success in managing obsessions and compulsions (American Psychiatric Association, 2000).

Treatment

Like other anxiety disorders, optimal treatment for OCD often combines medication and CBT. CBT may specifically include exposure and response prevention. **Exposure** involves assisting the client to deliberately confront the situations and stimuli that he or she usually avoids. **Response prevention** focuses on delaying or avoiding performance of rituals. The person learns to tolerate the anxiety and to recognize that it will recede without the disastrous imagined consequences. Other techniques discussed previously, such as deep breathing and relaxation, can also assist the person to tolerate and eventually manage the anxiety (Geffken *et al.*, 2004).

APPLICATION OF THE NURSING PROCESS: OBSESSIVE-COMPULSIVE DISORDER

Assessment

Box 13.2 presents the Yale–Brown Obsessive-Compulsive Scale. The nurse could use this tool along with the following detailed discussion to guide his or her assessment of the client with OCD.

HISTORY

The client usually seeks treatment only when obsessions become too overwhelming, when compulsions interfere with daily life (e.g. going to work, cooking meals, participating in leisure activities with family or friends), or both. Clients are hospitalized only when they have become completely unable to carry out their daily routines. Most care and treatment is carried out in the community. The client

---

Box 13.2   YALE–BROWN OBSESSIVE-COMPULSIVE SCALE

For each item, circle the number identifying the response which best characterizes the patient.

1. Time occupied by obsessive thoughts
   How much of your time is occupied by obsessive thoughts?
   How frequently do the obsessive thoughts occur?
   0 None
   1 Mild (less than 1 h/day) or occasional (intrusion occurring no more than 8 times a day)
   2 Moderate (1–3 h/day) or frequent (intrusion occurring more than 8 times a day, but most of the hours of the day are free of obsessions)
   3 Severe (greater than 3 and up to 8 h/day) or very frequent (intrusion occurring more than 8 times a day and occurring during most of the hours of the day)
   4 Extreme (greater than 8 h/day) or near consistent intrusion (too numerous to count and an hour rarely passes without several obsessions occurring)

2. Interference due to obsessive thoughts
   How much do your obsessive thoughts interfere with your social or work (or role) functioning?
   Is there anything that you don't do because of them?
   0 None
   1 Mild, slight interference with social or occupational activities, but overall performance not impaired
   2 Moderate, definite interference with social or occupational performance but still manageable
   3 Severe, causes substantial impairment in social or occupational performance
   4 Extreme, incapacitating

3. Distress associated with obsessive thoughts
   How much distress do your obsessive thoughts cause you?
   0 None
   1 Mild, infrequent and not too disturbing
   2 Moderate, frequent and disturbing but still manageable
   3 Severe, very frequent and very disturbing
   4 Extreme, nearly constant and disabling distress

4. Resistance against obsessions
   How much of an effort do you make to resist the obsessive thoughts?
   How often do you try to disregard or turn your attention away from these thoughts as they enter your mind?
   0 Makes an effort to always resist, or symptoms so minimal doesn't need to actively resist
   1 Tries to resist most of the time
   2 Makes some effort to resist
   3 Yields to all obsessions without attempting to control them, but does so with some reluctance
   4 Completely and willingly yields to all obsessions

5. Degree of control over obsessive thoughts
   How much control do you have over your obsessive thoughts?
   How successful are you in stopping or diverting your obsessive thinking?
   0 Complete control
   1 Much control, usually able to stop or divert obsessions with some effort and concentration
   2 Moderate control, sometimes able to stop or divert obsessions
   3 Little control, rarely successful in stopping obsessions
   4 No control, experienced as completely involuntary, rarely able to even momentarily divert thinking

6. Time spent performing compulsive behaviours
   How much time do you spend performing compulsive behaviours?
   How frequently do you perform compulsions?
   0 None
   1 Mild (less than 1 h/day performing compulsions) or occasional (performance of compulsions occurring no more than 8 times a day)
   2 Moderate (1–3 h/day performing compulsions) or frequent (performance of compulsions occurring more than 8 times a day, but most of the hours of the day are free of compulsive behaviours)

Box 13.2: Yale–Brown Obsessive-Compulsive Scale, cont.

3 Severe (greater than 3 and up to 8 h/day performing compulsions) or very frequent (performance of compulsions occurring more than 8 times a day and occurring during most of the hours of the day)

4 Extreme (greater than 8 h/day performing compulsions) or near consistent performance of compulsions (too numerous to count and an hour rarely passes without several compulsions being performed)

7. Interference due to compulsive behaviours

How much do your compulsive behaviours interfere with your social or work (or role) functioning?

Is there anything that you don't do because of the compulsions?

0 None

1 Mild, slight interference with social or occupational activities, but overall performance not impaired

2 Moderate, definite interference with social or occupational performance but still manageable

3 Severe, causes substantial impairment in social or occupational performance

4 Extreme, incapacitating

8. Distress associated with compulsive behaviour

How would you feel if prevented from performing your compulsions?

How anxious would you become?

How anxious do you get while performing compulsions until you are satisfied they are completed?

0 None

1 Mild, only slightly anxious if compulsions prevented, or only slightly anxious during performance of compulsions

2 Moderate, reports that anxiety would mount but remain manageable if compulsions prevented, or

that anxiety increases but remains manageable during performance of compulsions

3 Severe, prominent and very disturbing increase in anxiety if compulsions interrupted, or prominent and very disturbing increases in anxiety during performance of compulsions

4 Extreme, incapacitating anxiety from any intervention aimed at modifying activity, or incapacitating anxiety develops during performance of compulsions

9. Resistance against compulsions

How much of an effort do you make to resist the compulsions?

0 Makes an effort to always resist, or symptoms so minimal doesn't need to actively resist

1 Tries to resist most of the time

2 Makes some effort to resist

3 Yields to all compulsions without attempting to control them but does so with some reluctance

4 Completely and willingly yields to all compulsions

10. Degree of control over compulsive behaviour

0 Complete control

1 Much control, experiences pressure to perform the behaviour but usually able to exercise voluntary control over it

2 Moderate control, strong pressure to perform behaviour, can control it only with difficulty

3 Little control, very strong drive to perform behaviour, must be carried to completion, can only delay with difficulty

4 No control, drive to perform behaviour experienced as completely involuntary

Reprinted with permission from Goodman, W. K., Price, L. H., Rasmussen, S. A., *et al.* (1989). The Yale–Brown Obsessive-Compulsive Scale, I: Development, use, and reliability. *Archives of General Psychiatry*, 46, 1006.

often reports that rituals began many years before; some begin as early as childhood. The more responsibility the client has as he or she gets older, the more the rituals interfere with the ability to fulfil those responsibilities.

GENERAL APPEARANCE AND MOTOR BEHAVIOUR

The nurse assesses the person's appearance and behaviour. Clients with OCD often seem tense, anxious, worried and fretful. They may have difficulty relating symptoms because of embarrassment. Their overall appearance is unremarkable, that is, nothing observable seems to be 'out of the ordinary'. The exception is the client who is almost immobilized by her or his thoughts and the resulting anxiety.

MOOD AND AFFECT

During assessment of mood and affect, clients report ongoing, overwhelming feelings of anxiety in response to the obsessive thoughts, images or urges. They may look sad and anxious.

THOUGHT PROCESSES AND CONTENT

The nurse explores the client's thought processes and content with the person. Many clients describe the obsessions as 'arising from nowhere' during the middle of normal activities. The harder the client tries to stop the thought or image, the more intense it becomes. The client may describe how these obsessions are not what he or she wants to think about, and that he or she would never willingly have such ideas or images.

CLINICAL VIGNETTE: OCD

Sam had just returned home from work. He immediately got undressed and entered the shower. As he showered, he soaped and resoaped his flannel and rubbed it vigorously over every inch of his body. 'I can't miss anything! I must get all the germs off,' he kept repeating to himself. He spent 30 minutes scrubbing and scrubbing. As he stepped out of the shower, Sam was very careful to step on the clean, white bath towel on the floor. He dried himself thoroughly, making sure his towel didn't touch the floor or sink. He had intended to put on clean clothes after his shower and make something to eat. But now he wasn't sure he had actually got himself completely clean. He couldn't get dressed if he wasn't clean. Slowly, Sam turned around, got back in the shower, and started all over again.

Assessment usually reveals intact intellectual functioning. The client may describe difficulty concentrating or paying attention when obsessions are strong. There is no impairment of memory or sensory functioning.

JUDGEMENT AND INSIGHT

The nurse should examine the client's judgement and 'insight' with him or her. The client usually recognizes that the obsessions are irrational, but he or she cannot stop them. He or she can make sound judgements (e.g. 'I know the house is safe') but cannot act on them. The client still engages in ritualistic behaviour when the anxiety becomes overwhelming.

SELF-CONCEPT

During exploration of self-concept, the client may voice concern that he or she is 'going crazy'. Feelings of powerlessness to control the obsessions or compulsions contribute to low self-esteem. The client may believe that if he or she were 'stronger' or had more willpower, he or she could possibly control these thoughts and behaviours.

ROLES AND RELATIONSHIPS

It is important for the nurse to assess with the client the effects of OCD on the client's roles and relationships. As the time spent performing rituals increases, the client's ability to fulfil life roles successfully decreases. Relationships also suffer as family and friends tire of the repetitive behaviour, and the client is less available to them as he or she is more consumed with anxiety and ritualistic behaviour.

PHYSIOLOGICAL AND SELF-CARE CONSIDERATIONS

The nurse examines the effects of OCD on physiology and self-care. As with other anxiety disorders, clients with OCD may have trouble sleeping. Performing rituals may take time away from sleep, or anxiety may interfere with the ability to go to sleep and wake refreshed. Clients also may report a loss of appetite or unwanted weight loss. In severe cases, personal hygiene may suffer because the client cannot complete needed tasks.

Data Analysis

Depending on the particular obsession and its accompanying compulsions, clients have varying symptoms. Nursing formulations can include the following:

- Anxiety
- Ineffective Coping
- Fatigue
- Situational Low Self-Esteem
- Impaired Skin Integrity (if scrubbing or washing rituals).

Outcome Identification

Outcomes for clients with OCD include the following:

- The client will demonstrate effective use of relaxation techniques.
- The client will complete daily routine activities within a realistic time frame.
- The client will discuss feelings with another person.
- The client will demonstrate effective use of CBT techniques.
- The client will spend less time performing rituals.

Intervention

USING THERAPEUTIC COMMUNICATION

Offering support and encouragement to the client is important to help him or her manage anxiety responses. The nurse can validate the overwhelming feelings the client experiences, while indicating the belief that the client can make needed changes and regain a sense of control. The nurse should encourage the client to talk about the feelings and to describe them in as much detail as the client can tolerate. Because many clients try to hide their rituals and to keep obsessions secret, discussing these thoughts, behaviours and resulting feelings with the nurse is an important step. Doing so can begin to relieve some of the 'burden' the client has been keeping to himself or herself.

TEACHING RELAXATION AND BEHAVIOURAL TECHNIQUES

The nurse can teach the client about mindfulness and relaxation techniques such as deep breathing, progressive muscle relaxation and guided imagery. This intervention should take place when the client's anxiety is relatively low, so he or she can learn more effectively. Initially, the nurse can demonstrate and practise the techniques with the client. Then, the nurse encourages the client to practise these techniques until he or she is comfortable

NURSING INTERVENTIONS FOR OCD

- Offer encouragement, support and compassion.
- Be clear with the client that you believe he or she can change.
- Encourage the client to talk about feelings, obsessions and rituals in detail.
- Gradually decrease time for the client to carry out ritualistic behaviours.
- Assist client to use exposure and response prevention behavioural techniques.
- Encourage client to use techniques to manage and tolerate anxiety responses.
- Assist client to complete daily routine and activities within agreed-on time limits.
- Encourage the client to develop and follow a written schedule with specified times and activities.

CLIENT/FAMILY EDUCATION FOR OCD

- Teach about OCD.
- Review the importance of talking openly about obsessions, compulsions and anxiety.
- Emphasize medication compliance as an important part of treatment.
- Discuss necessary behavioural techniques for managing anxiety and decreasing prominence of obsessions.

doing them alone. When the client has mastered relaxation techniques, he or she can begin to use them when anxiety increases. In addition to decreasing anxiety, the client gains an increased sense of control that can lead to improved self-esteem.

To manage anxiety and ritualistic behaviours, a baseline of frequency and duration is necessary. The client can keep a diary to chronicle situations that trigger obsessions, the intensity of the anxiety, the time spent performing rituals and the avoidance behaviours. This record provides a clear picture for both client and nurse. The client then can begin to use exposure and response prevention behavioural techniques. Initially, the client can decrease the time he or she spends performing the ritual or delay performing the ritual while experiencing anxiety. Eventually, the client can eliminate the ritualistic response or decrease it significantly to the point that interference with daily life is minimal. Clients can use relaxation techniques to assist them in managing and tolerating the anxiety they are experiencing.

It is important to note that the client must be willing to engage in exposure and response prevention. These are not techniques that can ever be forced on the client.

COMPLETING A DAILY ROUTINE

To accomplish tasks efficiently, the client may initially need additional time to allow for rituals. For example, if breakfast is at 8:00 AM and the client has a 45-minute ritual before eating, the nurse must plan that time into the client's schedule. It is important for the nurse not to interrupt or to attempt to stop the ritual, because doing so may well escalate the client's anxiety dramatically. Again, the client must be willing to make changes in his or her behaviour. The nurse and client can agree on a plan to limit the time spent performing rituals. They may decide to limit the morning ritual to

40 minutes, then to 35 minutes and so forth, taking care to decrease this time gradually at a rate the client can tolerate. When the client has completed the ritual or the time allotted has passed, the client then must engage in the expected activity. This may cause anxiety and is a time when the client can use relaxation and stress-reduction techniques. At home, the client can continue to follow a daily routine or written schedule that helps him or her to stay on tasks and accomplish activities and responsibilities.

PROVIDING CLIENT AND FAMILY EDUCATION

It is important for both the client and family to learn about OCD. They often are relieved to find the client is not 'going mad' and that the obsessions are unwanted, rather than a reflection of any 'dark side' to the client's personality. Helping the client and family to talk openly about the obsessions, anxiety and rituals eliminates the client's need to keep these things secret and to carry the guilty burden alone. Family members are also better able to give the client needed emotional support when they are fully informed.

Teaching about the importance of medication compliance to combat OCD is essential. The client may need to try different medications until his or her response is satisfactory. The chances for improved OCD symptoms are enhanced when the client takes medication and uses behavioural techniques.

Evaluation

Treatment has been effective when OCD symptoms no longer interfere with the client's ability to carry out a 'normal' life. When obsessions occur, the client manages resulting anxiety without engaging in complicated or time-consuming rituals. He or she reports regained control over his or her life and the ability to tolerate and manage anxiety with minimal disruption.

POSTTRAUMATIC STRESS DISORDER

PTSD can occur in a person who has witnessed an extraordinarily terrifying and potentially deadly event. After the traumatic event, the person may re-experience all or some of it through dreams or waking recollections, and responds defensively to these flashbacks. New behaviours may develop related to the trauma, such as sleep difficulties, hypervigilance, thinking difficulties, severe startle response and agitation (American Psychiatric Association, 2000; see Chapter 11).

ACUTE STRESS DISORDER

Acute stress disorder is similar to posttraumatic stress disorder in that the person has experienced a traumatic situation, but the response is more dissociative. The person has a sense that the event was unreal, believes he or she is unreal and forgets some aspects of the event through amnesia, emotional detachment and muddled obliviousness to the environment (American Psychiatric Association, 2000).

SELF-AWARENESS ISSUES

Working with people who have anxiety disorders can offer a real challenge to the nurse. These clients *know* that their symptoms may seem unusual but feel unable to stop them. They can experience huge frustration and feelings of helplessness and failure. Their lives may seem out of their control, and they live in fear of the next episode. They go to extreme measures to try to prevent episodes by avoiding people and places where previous events occurred.

It may be difficult for nurses and others to understand why the person cannot simply stop performing the bizarre behaviours interfering with his or her life. Why does the hand-washer who has scrubbed himself raw keep washing his poor, sore hands every hour on the hour? Nurses must understand what and how anxiety behaviours work, not just for client care but to help understand the role anxiety plays in performing nursing responsibilities. Nurses are expected to function at a high level and to avoid allowing their own feelings and needs to hinder the care of their clients. But as emotional beings, nurses are just as vulnerable to stress and anxiety as others, and they have needs of their own.

Points to Consider When Working With Clients With Anxiety and Stress-Related Problems

- Remember that we all experience stress and anxiety that can interfere with daily life and work.
- Avoid falling into the pitfall of trying to 'fix' the client's problems.
- Discuss any uncomfortable feelings with a more experienced person for suggestions on how to deal with your feelings toward these clients.
- Remember to practise techniques to manage stress and anxiety in your own life.

Critical Thinking Questions

1. Because all people occasionally experience anxiety, it is important for nurses to be aware of their own coping mechanisms. Be honest and do a self-assessment: What causes you anxiety? What physical, emotional and cognitive responses occur when you are anxious? What coping mechanisms do you use? Are they healthy?

2. Some clients take benzodiazepine anxiolytics for months or even years even though these medications are designed for short-term use. Why does this happen? What, if anything, should be done for these clients? How would you approach the situation?

KEY POINTS

- Anxiety is a vague feeling of dread or apprehension. It is a response to external or internal stimuli that can have behavioural, emotional, cognitive and physical symptoms.
- Anxiety has positive and negative side-effects. The positive effects produce growth and adaptive change. The negative effects produce poor self-esteem, fear, inhibition and anxiety disorders (in addition to other disorders).
- The four levels of anxiety are mild anxiety (helps people learn, grow and change); moderate anxiety (increases focus on the alarm; learning is still possible); severe anxiety (greatly decreases cognitive function, increases preparation for physical responses, increases space needs); and panic (fight, flight or freeze response; no learning is possible; the person is attempting to free himself or herself from the discomfort of this high stage of anxiety).
- Defence mechanisms are intrapsychic distortions that a person uses to feel more in control. Some theorists believe that these defence mechanisms are overused when a person develops an anxiety disorder.
- Peplau outlined three 'relief behaviours' which can become destructive; these are 'acting out', 'somatizing' and 'withdrawal'.
- Current aetiological theories and studies of anxiety disorders have shown a familial incidence and have implicated the neurotransmitters GABA, noradrenaline and serotonin.
- Treatment for anxiety disorders involves medication (anxiolytics, SSRIs and tricyclic antidepressants and clonidine and propranolol) and psychotherapy – usually CBT.
- Cognitive-behavioural techniques include positive reframing, decatastrophizing, thought stopping and distraction. Behavioural techniques for OCD include exposure and response prevention.
- In a panic attack, the person often feels as if he or she is dying. Symptoms can include palpitations, sweating, tremors, shortness of breath, a sense of suffocation, chest

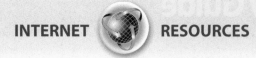

INTERNET RESOURCES

RESOURCES	INTERNET ADDRESS
• NATIONAL PHOBICS' SOCIETY	http://www.phobics-society.org.uk/
• NO MORE PANIC	http://www.nomorepanic.co.uk/
• OCD-UK	http://www.ocduk.org/
• SOCIAL ANXIETY UK	http://www.social-anxiety.org.uk/

pain, nausea, abdominal distress, dizziness, paraesthesias and vasomotor lability. The person has a fight, flight or freeze response.

- Phobias are excessive anxiety about being in public or open places (agoraphobia), a specific object or social situations.

- OCD involves recurrent, persistent, intrusive and unwanted thoughts, images or impulses (obsessions) and ritualistic or repetitive behaviours or mental acts (compulsions) carried out to eliminate the obsessions or to neutralize anxiety.

- Self-awareness about one's anxiety and responses to it greatly improves both personal and professional relationships.

REFERENCES

American Psychiatric Association. (2000). *DSM-IV-TR: Diagnostic and statistical manual of mental disorders* (4th edn, text revision). Washington, DC: American Psychiatric Association.

Andreasen, N. C. & Black, D. W. (2006). *Introductory textbook of psychiatry* (4th edn). Washington DC: American Psychiatric Publishing.

Culpepper, L. (2006). Social anxiety disorder in the primary care setting. *Journal of Clinical Psychiatry, 67*(Suppl 12), 31–37.

Flint, A. J. (2004). Anxiety disorders. In J. Sadavoy, L. F. Jarvik, G. T. Grossberg, *et al.* (Eds.), *Comprehensive textbook of geriatric psychiatry* (3rd edn, pp. 687–699). New York: W. W. Norton and Company.

Freud, S. (1936). *The problem of anxiety.* New York: W. W. Norton.

Gale, C. & Davidson, O. (2007). Clinical Review: generalised anxiety disorder. *British Medical Journal, 334*(7593), 579.

Geffken, G. R., Storch, E. A., Gelfand, K. M., Adkins, J. W., & Goodman, W. K. (2004). Cognitive-behavioural therapy for obsessive-compulsive disorder: review of treatment techniques. *Journal of Psychosocial Nursing, 42*(12), 44–51.

McMahon, F. J. & Kassem, L. (2005). Anxiety disorders: genetics. In B. J. Sadock & V. A. Sadock (Eds.), *Comprehensive textbook of psychiatry, Vol. 1* (8th edn, pp. 1759–1762). Philadelphia: Lippincott Williams & Wilkins.

Merikangas, K. R. (2005). Anxiety disorders: epidemiology. In B. J. Sadock & V. A. Sadock (Eds.), *Comprehensive textbook of psychiatry, Vol. 1* (8th edn, pp. 1720–1728). Philadelphia: Lippincott Williams & Wilkins.

Neumeister, A., Bonne, O., & Charney, D. S. (2005). Anxiety disorders: neurochemical aspects. In B. J. Sadock & V. A. Sadock (Eds.), *Comprehensive textbook of psychiatry, Vol. 1* (8th edn, pp. 1739–1748). Philadelphia: Lippincott Williams & Wilkins.

NICE. (2004). Anxiety: management of anxiety (panic disorder, with or without agoraphobia, and generalised anxiety disorder) in adults in primary, secondary and community care. Available: http://www.nice.org.uk/guidance/index.jsp?action=byID&o=10960

Peplau, H. (1952). *Interpersonal relations.* New York: Putnam.

Ricketts, T., Parry, G., Forrest, J., Mettam, L., Houghton, S., & Saxon, D. (2008). An uncontrolled evaluation of guided self-help for panic disorder. *Journal of Psychiatric and Mental Health Nursing, 15*(1), 72–74.

Selye, H. (1956). *The stress life.* St. Louis: McGraw-Hill.

Selye, H. (1974). *Stress without distress.* Philadelphia: J. B. Lippincott.

Starcevic, V. (2006). Anxiety states: A review of conceptual and treatment issues. *Current Opinion in Psychiatry, 19*(1), 79–83.

Sullivan, H. S. (1952). *Interpersonal theory of psychiatry.* New York: W. W. Norton.

ADDITIONAL READING

Cameron, C. (2007). Obsessive-compulsive disorder in children and adolescents. *Journal of Psychiatric and Mental Health Nursing, 14*(7), 696–704.

Mataix-Cois, D., do Rosario-Campos, M. C., & Leckman, J. F. (2005). A multidimensional model of obsessive-compulsive disorder. *American Journal of Psychiatry, 162*(2), 228–238.

Uhlenhuth, E. H., Leon, A. C., & Matuzas, W. (2006). Psychopathology of panic attacks in panic disorder. *Journal of Affective Disorders, 92*(1), 55–62.

Chapter Study Guide

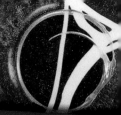

MULTIPLE-CHOICE QUESTIONS

Select the best answer for each of the following questions.

1. The nurse observes a client who is becoming increasingly upset. He is rapidly pacing, hyperventilating, clenching his jaw, wringing his hands and trembling. His speech is high-pitched and random; he seems preoccupied with his thoughts. He is pounding his fist into his other hand. The nurse identifies his anxiety level as
   a. Mild
   b. Moderate
   c. Severe
   d. Panic

2. When assessing a client with anxiety, the nurse's questions should be
   a. Avoided until the anxiety is gone
   b. Open ended
   c. Postponed until the client volunteers information
   d. Specific and direct

3. During the assessment, the client tells the nurse that she cannot stop worrying about her appearance and that she often removes 'old' make-up and applies fresh make-up every hour or two throughout the day. The nurse identifies this behaviour as possibly indicative of a(n)
   a. Acute stress disorder
   b. Generalized anxiety disorder
   c. Panic disorder
   d. Obsessive-compulsive disorder

4. The best goal for a client learning a relaxation technique is that the client will
   a. Confront the source of anxiety directly
   b. Experience anxiety without feeling overwhelmed
   c. Report no episodes of anxiety
   d. Suppress anxious feelings

5. Which of the four classes of medications used for panic disorder is considered the safest because of low incidence of side-effects and lack of physiological dependence?
   a. Benzodiazepines
   b. Tricyclics
   c. Monoamine oxidase inhibitors
   d. Selective serotonin reuptake inhibitors

6. Which of the following would be the best intervention for a client having a panic attack?
   a. Involve the client in a physical activity.
   b. Offer a distraction such as music.
   c. Remain with the client.
   d. Teach the client a relaxation technique.

7. A client with generalized anxiety disorder states, 'I have learned that the best thing I can do is to forget my worries.' How would the nurse evaluate this statement?
   a. The client is developing insight.
   b. The client's coping skills have improved.
   c. The client needs encouragement to verbalize feelings.
   d. The client's treatment has been successful.

8. A client with anxiety is beginning treatment with lorazepam (Ativan). It is most important for the nurse to assess the client's
   a. Motivation for treatment
   b. Family and social support
   c. Use of coping mechanisms
   d. Use of alcohol

FILL-IN-THE-BLANK QUESTIONS

Identify the level of anxiety represented by the following descriptions.

_____ 1. Severe muscle tension, limited perceptual field, frantic

_____ 2. Attentive, impatient, optimal learning level

_____ 3. Flight, fight or freeze; out of control; irrational

_____ 4. Selective inattention, voice changes, decreased perceptual field

GROUP DISCUSSION TOPIC

1. Discuss the role of anxiety in the assessment and management of risk.

2. Discuss ways in which anxiety has been beneficial or harmful to you in your career.

3. Explore the idea that anxiety is caused primarily by political, social and economic factors.

CLINICAL EXAMPLE

Mr Noe has discussed in detail with the CPN how his wife cannot be expected to walk 2 to 3 miles a day after her triple-bypass operation because she is afraid to leave the house. He has been taking care of her for the past 13 years, during which time she has rarely left the house and then only with great distress and only accompanied by him. His wife gets so anxious that if she tries to go outside, she just feels like screaming and running back in. She feels something terrible will happen to her because- all those years ago- she left the house to go to her GP and ended up having triple-bypass surgery the next day. Mr Noe takes care of necessary chores outside the house, attends parents' weekends at their children's colleges, does the grocery shopping and so forth.

Mrs Noe has asked the nurse to 'figure out how I can get outside and walk every day,' but for each suggestion the nurse makes, Mrs Noe finds some reason it will not work. The nurse is getting frustrated with Mrs Noe's constant rejection of her suggestions and sternly says, 'If you aren't going to try any of my suggestions, then I guess we're wasting our time.'

1. Rather than giving Mrs Noe suggestions to get her outside, what might be a better plan?

2. How is Mr Noe's behaviour affecting Mrs Noe's agoraphobia? What does the nurse need to explain and to recommend to Mr Noe about his response to her behaviour?

3. What other care and treatment is available for Mrs Noe?

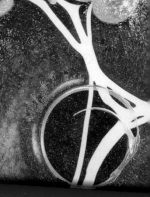

Chapter 14

Psychoses and Schizophrenia

Key Terms

- **Abnormal Involuntary Movement Scale (AIMS)**
- **akathisia**
- **alogia**
- **anhedonia**
- **blunted affect**
- **catatonia**
- **collaboration**
- **command hallucinations**
- **delusions**
- **depersonalization**
- **depression**
- **dystonic reactions**
- **echolalia**
- **echopraxia**
- **engagement**
- **extrapyramidal side-effects (EPS)**
- **flat affect**
- **hallucination**
- **ideas of reference**
- **latency of response**
- **meaning and purpose**
- **neuroleptic malignant syndrome (NMS)**
- **neuroleptics**
- **non-stigmatizing**
- **polydipsia**
- **pseudoparkinsonism**
- **psychomotor retardation**
- **psychosis**
- **recovery**
- **schizophrenia**
- **tardive dyskinesia**
- **thought blocking**
- **thought broadcasting**
- **thought insertion**
- **thought withdrawal**
- **trauma**
- **waxy flexibility**
- **word salad**

Learning Objectives

After reading this chapter, you should be able to:

1. Outline 'recovery' principles and their impact on the care and treatment of people with a diagnosis of schizophrenia.

2. Discuss the concept of psychosis.

3. Discuss various theories of the aetiology of 'schizophrenia'.

4. Describe the 'positive' and 'negative' symptoms of different types of schizophrenia.

5. Describe key aspects of assessment for someone diagnosed with schizophrenia.

6. Apply the nursing process to the care of a client diagnosed with schizophrenia.

7. Evaluate the effectiveness of antipsychotic medications for clients diagnosed with schizophrenia.

8. Provide teaching to clients, families, carers and community members to increase knowledge and understanding of schizophrenia.

9. Evaluate your own feelings, beliefs and attitudes regarding clients diagnosed with schizophrenia.

266

SCHIZOPHRENIA AND RECOVERY PRINCIPLES

Systematic evaluation and research, including an increasing focus on the voice of the person diagnosed with schizophrenia, has begun – falteringly – to transform services in the UK. Policy drivers such as SIGN's *Psychosocial interventions in the management of schizophrenia* (1998), the work of the Clinical Standards Board For Scotland (2001), the development of NICE guidelines (2002), the national review of mental health nursing in Scotland (*Scottish Government,* 2006), the Chief Nursing Officer's review of mental health nursing (Department of Health, 2006) and guidance from Care Services Improvement Partnership, Royal College of Psychiatrists and Social Care Institute For Excellence (CSIP/RCP and SCIE) (2007) have all focused on the crucial role mental health nurses have to play, and on the need to work within an holistic, collaborative framework: a framework that draws on the evidence, that puts relationships at the heart of care and that fully engages people in their own care and treatment, taking into account social, political and economic, as well as intrapersonal and interpersonal, factors.

It is hoped that the subsequent shift in policy and, in particular, attitude is reflected in this chapter. Ideas about schizophrenia and '**recovery**' have been moving from a focus on professionals' definitions of illness and wellness to people's own self-definitions. No longer is it enough for professionals to be content with merely 'relieving symptoms': they need to be working towards standing alongside people and supporting them as they take control of their lives and find **meaning and purpose**. No longer is it OK for professionals to see 'schizophrenia' as inevitably 'chronic', its sufferers as inevitably doomed to a disabled and bleak life. No longer can they look down with pity on people with the diagnosis as broken or partial in some way. And no longer can they avoid the voice of carers, of the general public or the complexities of the relationships we all have.

Nursing people with a diagnosis of schizophrenia is about working with equals, about identifying strengths and competencies and dreams, as much as it is about identifying deficits, 'symptoms' and fears. It is about validating the terrible distress schizophrenia can cause *and* helping people to build on what they have and to change. Nursing people with the diagnosis is about learning what schizophrenia is really like for them, and finding ways together to enhance the positive aspects and reduce the negative. It is about open, transparent assessments of risk and safety, using those assessments to deepen the therapeutic relationship and enhance the safety of clients and the people around them. It is about finding what works for each individual – whether that is CBT, medication or neither. If nurses can do all this, if they can be optimistic and realistic, be prepared to be student *and* teacher, then they can make a real difference to people's lives.

Psychosis

'**Psychosis**' is a term used widely in mental health care. A defining characteristic is that people who are psychotic fail to perceive the world, fail to perceive 'reality', in the way that most other people from the same culture and background experience it. Psychotic experiences can include hallucinations, delusional thoughts and beliefs, confused or restricted thinking and major interpersonal and social problems. People who are psychotic frequently fail to acknowledge the 'strangeness' or seeming unreality of their own thoughts (unlike, say, someone who is anxious).

Many see psychosis as being a symbolic expression of internal conflict, rather than a purely chemical or neurological phenomenon. 'Insight' – a term bandied about frequently within the mental health system – is a debatable concept: rarely do people – psychotic or not – either have full insight or completely lack insight: it can be argued that insight is a construction made between two or more people – it is interpersonal rather than intrapersonal – and it is often used, unfortunately, as a label to dismiss people's feelings, experiences or beliefs.

'Psychosis' can be short or long term. Some elements of it can be pervasive, others may come and go. Psychotic experiences are common to a number of mental health problems (indeed some, including hallucinations, can, on occasion, occur in the absence of any mental health problem): in particular, psychosis can be part of bipolar disorder, schizophrenia, major depression and can, in addition, be the result of alcohol or drug misuse or neurological or other physiological problems.

This chapter will primarily deal with the group of experiences – many of which can be labelled 'psychotic' – termed 'schizophrenia'.

'**Schizophrenia**' manifests itself in distorted and bizarre thoughts, perceptions, emotions, movements and behaviour. It should not be seen as a single illness; rather, schizophrenia can be more usefully thought of as a syndrome or group of disease processes or experiences with many different manifestations and symptoms. Louis Sass (1993, 1998) sees the two defining characteristics of schizophrenia as 'hyperreflexivity' and 'alienation': people with the disorder tend to think almost entirely with the left brain, which 'runs out of control' – they are constantly self-conscious, wary, scrutinizing, monitoring, trying unsuccessfully to make sense of things. The broader, more right-brain ways of thinking – creativity, imagination, intuition – are seen as too difficult to engage with or not to be trusted. The person thus sees himself or herself – and the world – less as a whole, more as lots of bits and pieces, incoherent and fragmented: as a result, he or she feels profoundly alienated and isolated from himself and the world.

For decades, the public has misunderstood schizophrenia, fearing it as dangerous and uncontrollable and causing wild disturbances and violent outbursts. Many people still believe that those diagnosed with schizophrenia need to be locked away from society. Only recently have mental health services come themselves to learn and to educate the community at large, that schizophrenia involves many different symptoms and presentations and is a syndrome that both medication and psychosocial approaches can help. Thanks to the increased effectiveness of newer atypical antipsychotic drugs and advances in psychotherapeutic and psychosocial community-based treatment, many clients diagnosed with schizophrenia live successfully in the community, working and enjoying an excellent quality of life. As mentioned at the start of the chapter, this quality of life has begun to improve further (it is hoped) with the recent service-wide adoption of 'recovery' approaches, in which clinical evidence and feedback from service users is beginning to be built on to develop a genuinely collaborative, hopeful, positive and **non-stigmatizing** approach to people diagnosed with schizophrenia: people who were previously discarded as helpless victims of a crippling chronic illness.

Yet, schizophrenia remains a controversial field in mental health care (Bentall (2004), Laing (1990), Szasz (1984)). As well as the stigma wrapped up in the term, its cause remains unclear, its diagnosis sometimes open to interpretation and the relationship between genetic, biochemical, psychological, social and environmental components much debated. Its presentation can vary hugely, and two people with the diagnosis may appear to have very little in common in terms of their cognitions, their affect and their behaviour. There is increasing evidence that psychological **trauma** may have a significant part

to play in the development of 'schizophrenia' and there is little doubt that the experience of psychosis (and its treatment) can produce posttraumatic stress symptoms for people.

What is vital to understand, regardless of all the controversies, is that 'schizophrenia' can be incredibly distressing – and ultimately potentially fatal – for the client, his family and friends and for carers, and that mental health nurses are a key professional group – perhaps *the* key professional group – in caring for people with the diagnosis.

Schizophrenia is usually diagnosed in late adolescence or early adulthood. Rarely does it seem to manifest in childhood. The peak incidence of onset is 15 to 25 years of age for men and 25 to 35 years of age for women . The prevalence of schizophrenia has been estimated at about 1% of the total population (NICE, 2002). The incidence and the lifetime prevalence seem to be roughly the same throughout the world (Buchanan & Carpenter, 2005). Around 20% of people are never ill again after an initial episode. At least 70% experience two or more acute episodes, with the second usually happening within 5–7 years of the first (NICE, 2002).

The 'symptoms' of schizophrenia can be divided into two major categories: *positive* or *hard symptoms/signs,* which include delusions, hallucinations and grossly disorganized thinking, speech and behaviour; and *negative* or *soft symptoms/signs,* which include flat affect, lack of volition and

---

DSM-IV-TR DIAGNOSTIC CRITERIA: POSITIVE AND NEGATIVE SYMPTOMS OF SCHIZOPHRENIA

Positive or Hard Symptoms

Ambivalence: Holding seemingly contradictory beliefs or feelings about the same person, event or situation
Associative looseness: Fragmented or poorly related thoughts and ideas
Delusions: Fixed false beliefs that have no basis in reality
Echopraxia: Imitation of the movements and gestures of another person whom the client is observing
Flight of ideas: Continuous flow of verbalization in which the person jumps rapidly from one topic to another
Hallucinations: False sensory perceptions or perceptual experiences that do not exist in reality
Ideas of reference: False impressions that external events have special meaning for the person
Perseveration: Persistent adherence to a single idea or topic; verbal repetition of a sentence, word, or phrase; resisting attempts to change the topic

Negative or Soft Symptoms

Alogia: Tendency to speak very little or to convey little substance of meaning (poverty of content)
Anhedonia: Feeling no joy or pleasure from life or any activities or relationships
Apathy: Feelings of indifference toward people, activities and events
Blunted affect: Restricted range of emotional feeling, tone or mood
Catatonia: Psychologically induced immobility occasionally marked by periods of agitation or excitement; the client seems motionless, as if in a trance
Flat affect: Absence of any facial expression that would indicate emotions or mood
Lack of volition: Absence of will, ambition or drive to take action or accomplish tasks

Adapted from American Psychiatric Association. (2000). *Diagnostic and Statistical Manual of Mental Disorders* (4th edn, text revision). Washington, DC: American Psychiatric Association.

social withdrawal or discomfort. For *DSM-IV-TR* diagnostic criteria for schizophrenia (American Psychiatric Association, 2000), please refer to the box below. Medication can control the positive symptoms, but frequently the negative symptoms persist after positive symptoms have abated.

The persistence of these negative symptoms over time presents a major barrier to recovery and improved functioning in the client's daily life. They can be intensified by 'cognitive deficits' – neurological changes associated with schizophrenia and identified by recent literature (including Gopal & Variand, 2005) as being significant in understanding negative symptomatology. Broadly, these deficits are:

- Memory: immediate and delayed recall, verbal and spatial memory
- Attention processes: slowed cognitive speed
- Executive functioning: sequencing, organization and flexibility.

Engagement with other (including professionals) is significantly hampered as a result. Cognitive remediation has been developed as a psychological approach to lessening these deficits and is showing promising results: Wykes *et al.* (2007) have demonstrated that, among other effects, cognitive remediation had a beneficial effect on memory, which in turn helped overall social functioning

The relationship between cognitive function, 'symptoms' and quality of life in schizophrenia is a complex one, but it seems certain that each impacts on the other and must be addressed in a separate, but linked way (Savilla *et al.*, 2008). There seems little doubt either that social factors, such as unemployment, stigma, social isolation and poverty, contribute significantly to quality of life and to someone's ability to cope with cognitive deficits and with both positive and negative symptoms.

The following are the types of schizophrenia according to the *DSM-IV-TR* (American Psychiatric Association, 2000). The diagnosis is made according to the client's predominant symptoms:

- *Schizophrenia, paranoid type*: characterized by persecutory (feeling victimized or spied on) or grandiose delusions, hallucinations and, occasionally, excessive religiosity (delusional religious focus) or hostile and aggressive behaviour.
- *Schizophrenia, disorganized type (equivalent to 'Hebephrenic' schizophrenia in ICD-10)*: characterized by grossly inappropriate or flat affect, incoherence, loose associations and extremely disorganized behaviour.
- *Schizophrenia, catatonic type*: characterized by marked psychomotor disturbance, either motionless or excessive motor activity. Motor immobility may be manifested by catalepsy (waxy flexibility) or stupor. Excessive motor activity is apparently purposeless and is not influenced by external stimuli. Other features include extreme negativism, mutism, peculiarities of voluntary movement, echolalia and echopraxia.

- *Schizophrenia, undifferentiated type*: characterized by mixed schizophrenic symptoms (of other types) along with disturbances of thought, affect and behaviour.
- *Schizophrenia, residual type*: characterized by at least one previous, though not a current, episode; social withdrawal; flat affect; and looseness of associations.

RELATED DISORDERS

Other disorders are related to but distinguished from schizophrenia in terms of presenting symptoms and the duration or magnitude of impairment. The *DSM-IV-TR* (American Psychiatric Association, 2000) categorizes these disorders as follows:

- *Schizophreniform disorder*: The client exhibits the symptoms of schizophrenia but for less than the 6 months necessary to meet the diagnostic criteria for schizophrenia. Social or occupational functioning may or may not be impaired.
- *Schizoaffective disorder*: The client exhibits the symptoms of psychosis and, at the same time, all the features of a mood disorder, either depression or mania.
- *Delusional disorder*: The client has one or more non-bizarre delusions – that is, the focus of the delusion is believable. Psychosocial functioning is not markedly impaired, and behaviour is not obviously odd or bizarre.
- *Brief psychotic disorder*: The client experiences the sudden onset of at least one psychotic symptom, such as delusions, hallucinations or disorganized speech or behaviour, which lasts from 1 day to 1 month. The episode may or may not have an identifiable stressor or may follow childbirth.
- *Shared psychotic disorder* (folie à deux): Two people share a similar delusion. The person with this diagnosis develops this delusion in the context of a close relationship with someone who has psychotic delusions.

Two other diagnoses, schizoid personality disorder and schizotypal personality disorder, are not psychotic disorders and should not be confused with schizophrenia even though the names sound similar and there is some clinical overlap. These two diagnoses are covered in Chapter 16.

CLINICAL COURSE

Although the 'symptoms' of schizophrenia are nearly always severe, the long-term course does *not* always involve progressive deterioration. The clinical course varies significantly between people.

Onset

Onset may be abrupt or insidious, but most clients slowly and gradually develop signs and symptoms such as social withdrawal, unusual behaviour, loss of interest in school or work and neglected hygiene. The diagnosis of schizophrenia is often made when the person begins to display more actively positive symptoms of delusions, hallucinations and disordered thinking (psychosis). Regardless of when and how 'the illness' begins and the type of schizophrenia, consequences for clients and their families can be substantial and enduring.

When and how schizophrenia develops seems to affect the outcome. Age at onset appears to be an important factor in how well the client fares: those who develop the illness earlier show worse outcomes than those who develop it later. Younger clients display a poorer premorbid adjustment, more prominent negative signs and greater cognitive impairment than do older clients. Those who experience a gradual onset of the disease (about 50%) tend to have both a poorer immediate and long-term course than those who experience an acute and sudden onset (Buchanan & Carpenter, 2005).

Immediate Course

In the years immediately after the onset of psychotic symptoms, three typical clinical patterns emerge. In one pattern, the client experiences ongoing psychosis and never fully recovers, although symptoms may shift in severity over time. In another pattern, the client experiences episodes of psychotic symptoms that alternate with episodes of relatively complete recovery from the psychosis. In a third, the person makes a full recovery.

Long-Term Course

The intensity of psychosis tends to diminish with age. Many clients with long-term impairment regain some degree of social and occupational functioning. Over time, symptoms become less disruptive to the person's life and easier to manage. In later life, these clients may live independently or in a structured family-type setting and may succeed at jobs with stable expectations and a supportive work environment. However, many clients with schizophrenia have difficulty functioning in the community, and few lead fully independent lives (Carter, 2006). This is primarily due to persistent negative symptoms, impaired cognition or treatment-refractory positive symptoms.

Antipsychotic medications often play a crucial role in the course of schizophrenia and individual outcomes. They do not 'cure' the disorder as such; they are, however, crucial to its successful management for many people. Frequently, the more effective the client's response and adherence to his or her medication regime, the better the outcome. Marshall and Rathbone (2006) found that early detection and aggressive treatment of the first psychotic episode were associated with improved outcomes.

The longer psychosis is untreated, the poorer the outcome (at least in the short term). The first 3 years of psychosis appear to be a period in which repeated breakdowns can occur, disabling symptoms become established and social, interpersonal and occupational disabilities rapidly develop. Two-thirds of suicides among this population occur within 5 years of the start of a psychotic illness. Early Intervention Teams have been developed to try to change the course of the process (Singh & Fisher, 2005).

Early intervention in schizophrenia is an emerging focus of research investigating the earliest signs of the illness that occur predominately in adolescence and young adulthood (Borgmann-Winter *et al.*, 2006). Accurate

---

CLINICAL VIGNETTE: PSYCHOSIS

Ricky was staying with his father for a few weeks on a visit. During the first week, things had gone pretty well, but Ricky forgot to take his medication for a few days. His father knew Ricky wasn't sleeping well at night, and he could hear Ricky talking to himself in the next room.

One day while his father was at work, Ricky began to hear some voices outside the flat. The voices grew louder, saying 'You're no good; you can't do anything right. You can't take care of yourself or protect your dad. We're going to get you both.' Ricky grew more frightened and went to the cupboard where his dad kept his tools. He grabbed a hammer and ran outside. When his father came home from work early, Ricky wasn't in the flat, though his coat and wallet were still there. Ricky's father called a neighbour, and they drove around the estate looking for Ricky. They finally found Ricky crouched behind some bushes. Although the temperature was only just above freezing, he was wearing only a T-shirt and shorts and no shoes. Ricky's neighbour called an ambulance. Meanwhile Ricky's father tried to coax Ricky into the car, but Ricky wouldn't come. The voices had grown louder, and Ricky was convinced that the devil had kidnapped his father and was coming for him too. He saw someone else in the car with his dad. The voices said they would crash the car if he got in. They were laughing at him! He couldn't get into the car; it was only a trap. His dad had tried his best, but he was trapped, too. The voices told Ricky to use the hammer and to destroy the car to kill the devil. He began to swing the hammer into the windscreen, but someone held him back.

The police and ambulancemen arrived and spoke quietly and firmly as they removed the hammer from Ricky's hands. They told Ricky they were taking him to the hospital where he and his father would be safe. They gently coaxed him into the back of the ambulance and took him to hospital.

identification of individuals at greatest risk is the key to early intervention. Many 'early intervention' initiatives – focused on early detection, intervention and prevention of psychosis – have now been established in the UK. These multidisciplinary, often nurse-led, teams work with CMHTs, AOTs, crisis teams, primary-care providers, and child and adolescent mental health service (CAMHS) teams to recognize prodromal signs that are predictive of later psychotic episodes, such as sleep difficulties, change in appetite, loss of energy and interest, odd speech, hearing voices, peculiar behaviour, inappropriate expression of feelings, paucity of speech, ideas of reference and feelings of unreality. After these high-risk individuals are identified, individualized intervention is implemented that may include CBT-based psychotherapeutic interventions, education, stress management or neuroleptic medication or a combination of these. Treatment also includes family involvement, individual and vocational counselling and coping strategies to enhance self-mastery. Interventions are intensive, using home visits and daily sessions if needed. Early intervention teams – at their best – focus on holistic approaches, way beyond traditional CMHT approaches to psychosis; even if someone becomes 'symptom-free', their social and interpersonal circumstances may still need active intervention and support and good teams will continue their involvement beyond apparent resolution, helping someone 'regain their life'.

Studies in Switzerland (Simon *et al.*, 2006) focused on identifying at-risk individuals demonstrating a core deficit of prodromal symptoms, including cognitive impairment, affective symptoms, social isolation and a decline in social functioning. In Germany, comprehensive CBT has been developed for patients in the early initial prodromal phase, whereas those in the late initial prodromal phase receive low-dose antipsychotic medication along with CBT (Bechdolf *et al.*, 2006b; Hafner & Maurer, 2006).

Early interventions implemented in Germany, Australia and the UK have resulted in the improvement of prodromal symptoms, prevention of social stagnation or decline and prevention or delay of progression to psychosis (Bechdolf *et al.*, 2006a).

Schizophrenia, Depression and Suicide

Depression is very common in people diagnosed with schizophrenia. Depression may occur in the 'prodromal' period before an acute breakdown, during acute episodes (when it is most common), after the resolution of psychosis or during the more chronic stages of the process (when rates are lower but still significant) (Mulholland & Cooper, 2000). It can be the result of attempting to cope with an acute psychotic episode and its consequences, as a result of the social and psychological meaning of the diagnosis for that individual, as a result of a loss of hope and sense of control and autonomy, as a result of feeling ground down by cognitive deficits and positive or negative symptoms. It may also be an integral part of the process of schizophrenia for some people. It is vital that clinicians

take the possibility of depression in someone diagnosed with schizophrenia seriously and act to help alleviate the distress it causes and its potentially fatal consequences: approximately 30–40% of people with the diagnosis attempt suicide; around 10% are successful (RETHINK, 2006).

Street Drugs and Alcohol

The use of street drugs – particularly ecstasy, speed, LSD and crack – seem to have the potential to 'spark' the onset of schizophrenia in those already vulnerable; at the same time, many people struggling with both positive and negative symptoms may use street drugs and alcohol to help them cope. Cannabis use can also lead to acute, transient psychotic episodes and appears to double the risk of developing schizophrenia, although cannabis seems to be 'a component cause, part of a complex constellation of factors leading to psychosis' rather than having a direct causal link (Arseneault *et al.*, 2004).

AETIOLOGY

Whether schizophrenia is an organic disease with underlying physical brain pathology has been an important question for researchers and clinicians for as long as they have studied it. In the first half of the 20th century, studies focused on trying to find a particular pathological structure associated with the disease, largely through autopsy: such a site was not discovered. In the 1950s and 1960s, the emphasis shifted to examination of psychological and social causes. Interpersonal theorists suggested that schizophrenia resulted from dysfunctional relationships in early life and adolescence. None of the interpersonal theories has been proved, despite strong coherent arguments, and, in the 1970s, studies began to focus on possible neurochemical causes, which remain the primary focus of research and theory today. These neurochemical/neurological theories are supported by the effects of antipsychotic medications, which help to control psychotic symptoms, and neuroimaging tools such as computed tomography, which have shown that the brains of people with schizophrenia differ in structure and function from those of control subjects.

Some therapists still believe that schizophrenia results from dysfunctional parenting or family dynamics. For parents or family members of persons diagnosed with schizophrenia, such beliefs run the risk of causing agony over what they did 'wrong' or what they could have done to help prevent it. There is no doubt, though, that psychosocial factors play a major part in the aetiology, development and prognosis. Cognitive therapy in psychosis has an ever-expanding evidence-base (Morrison *et al.*, 2008) and there appear to be clear links between psychosis and the experience of psychological trauma in childhood, and between the experience of psychosis and subsequent posttraumatic symptoms. An open, responsive, multifaceted approach, one that ensures people's active, autonomous involvement in their own care and treatment and the support of friends and family can play a vital part in people living a fulfilling life. The traditionally negative, pessimistic medical view that professionals have had of schizophrenia has contributed to thousands of lives being lived in a narrow, confined and depressing way; at the same time, we should bear in mind that careful, informed, collaborative use of medication can be liberating for many.

Biological Theories

The biological theories of schizophrenia focus on genetic factors, neuroanatomical and neurochemical factors (structure and function of the brain) and immunovirology (the body's response to exposure to a virus).

GENETIC FACTORS

Most genetic studies have focused on immediate families (i.e. parents, siblings, offspring) to examine whether schizophrenia is genetically transmitted or inherited. Few have focused on more distant relatives. The most important studies have centred on twins; these findings have demonstrated that identical twins have a 50% risk for schizophrenia; that is, if one twin has schizophrenia, the other has a 50% chance of developing it as well. Fraternal twins have only a 15% risk (Kirkpatrick & Tek, 2005). This finding indicates that schizophrenia is at least partially inherited.

Other important studies have shown that children with one biological parent with schizophrenia have a 15% risk; the

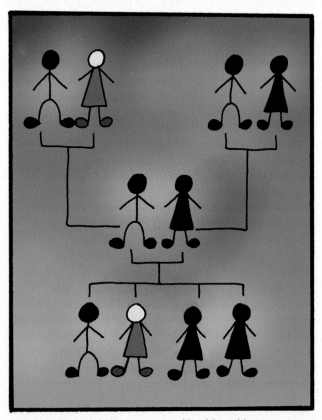

Genetics plays a role in many mental health problems

risk rises to 35% if both biological parents have schizophrenia. Children adopted at birth into a family with no history of schizophrenia but whose biological parents have a history of schizophrenia still reflect the genetic risk of their biological parents. All these studies have indicated a genetic risk or tendency for schizophrenia, but genetics cannot be the only factor: identical twins have only a 50% risk even though their genes are 100% identical (Riley & Kendler, 2005).

NEUROANATOMICAL AND NEUROCHEMICAL FACTORS

With the development of non-invasive imaging techniques such as computed tomography, magnetic resonance imaging and positron emission tomography in the past 25 years, scientists have been able to study the brain structure (neuroanatomy) and activity (neurochemistry) of people with schizophrenia. Findings have demonstrated that people with schizophrenia have relatively less brain tissue and cerebrospinal fluid than people who do not have schizophrenia (Schneider-Axmann et al., 2006); this could represent a failure in development or a subsequent loss of tissue. Computed tomography scans have shown enlarged ventricles in the brain and cortical atrophy. Positron emission tomography studies suggest that glucose metabolism and oxygen are diminished in the frontal cortical structures of the brain. The research consistently shows decreased brain volume and abnormal brain function in the frontal and temporal areas of persons with schizophrenia. This pathology correlates with the positive signs of schizophrenia (temporal lobe), such as psychosis, and the negative signs of schizophrenia (frontal lobe), such as lack of volition or motivation and anhedonia. It is unknown whether these changes in the frontal and temporal lobes are the result of a failure of these areas to develop properly or if a virus, trauma or immune response has damaged them. Intrauterine influences such as poor nutrition, tobacco, alcohol and other drugs and stress also are being studied as possible causes of the brain pathology found in people with schizophrenia (Buchanan & Carpenter, 2005).

Neurochemical studies have consistently demonstrated alterations in the neurotransmitter systems of the brain in people with schizophrenia. The neuronal networks that transmit information by electrical signals from a nerve cell through its axon and across synapses to postsynaptic receptors on other nerve cells seem to malfunction. The transmission of the signal across the synapse requires a complex series of biochemical events. Studies have implicated the actions of dopamine, serotonin, noradrenaline, acetylcholine, glutamate and several neuromodulatory peptides.

Currently, the most prominent neurochemical theories involve dopamine and serotonin. One theory suggests excess dopamine as a cause. This theory was developed based on two observations: first, drugs that increase activity in the dopaminergic system, such as amphetamine and levodopa, sometimes induce a paranoid psychotic reaction similar to schizophrenia. Second, drugs blocking postsynaptic dopamine receptors reduce psychotic symptoms; in fact, the greater the ability of the drug to block dopamine receptors, the more effective it is in decreasing symptoms of schizophrenia (Buchanan & Carpenter, 2005).

More recently, serotonin has been included among the leading neurochemical factors affecting schizophrenia. The theory regarding serotonin suggests that serotonin modulates and helps to control excess dopamine. Some believe that excess serotonin itself contributes to the development of schizophrenia. Newer atypical antipsychotics such as clozapine (Clozaril) are both dopamine and serotonin antagonists. Drug studies have shown that clozapine can dramatically reduce psychotic symptoms and ameliorate the negative signs of schizophrenia (Kane & Marder, 2005).

Researchers are also exploring the possibility that schizophrenia may have three separate symptom complexes or syndromes: hallucinations/delusions, disorganization of thought and behaviour and negative symptoms (Buchanan & Carpenter, 2005). Investigations show that the three syndromes relate to neurobiological differences in the brain. It is postulated that schizophrenia has (these three) subgroups, which may be homogeneous relative to course, pathophysiology and, therefore, treatment.

IMMUNOVIROLOGICAL FACTORS

Popular theories have emerged stating that exposure to a virus, or the body's immune response to a virus, could alter the brain physiology of people with schizophrenia. Although scientists continue to study these possibilities, few findings have validated them.

Cytokines are chemical messengers between immune cells, mediating inflammatory and immune responses. Specific cytokines also play a role in signalling the brain to produce behavioural and neurochemical changes needed in the face of physical or psychological stress, to maintain homeostasis. It is believed that cytokines may have a role in the development of major psychiatric disorders such as schizophrenia (Brown et al., 2005).

Recently, researchers have been focusing on infections in pregnant women as a possible origin for schizophrenia. 'Waves' of schizophrenia in England, Wales, Denmark, Finland and other countries have, it seems, occurred a generation after influenza epidemics. There are also higher rates of schizophrenia among children born in crowded areas in cold weather, conditions that are hospitable to respiratory ailments (Brown et al., 2005).

STRESS VULNERABILITY

Stress vulnerability models in the care and treatment of people experiencing psychosis (Zubin & Spring (1977), Das et al. (2001), Morrison et al. (2004)) emphasise the need for an inclusive approach. The models value biological, interpersonal, social/cultural and psychological explanations of the experience, binding those explanations together in a pragmatic approach and suggesting that 'recovery' is often the result of a number of interlinking factors. The relationship between life-stressors (see Chapter 7) and the experience of psychosis is tackled collaboratively, drawing on problem-solving CBT techniques underpinned with optimism and respect.

CULTURAL CONSIDERATIONS

Awareness of cultural differences is important when assessing for symptoms of schizophrenia. Ideas that are considered delusional in one culture, such as beliefs in sorcery or witchcraft, may be commonly accepted by other cultures. In addition, auditory or visual hallucinations, such as seeing the Virgin Mary or hearing God's voice, may be a normal part of religious experiences in some cultures. The assessment of affect requires sensitivity to differences in eye contact, body language and acceptable emotional expression; these vary widely across cultures (American Psychiatric Association, 2000).

'Psychotic behaviour' observed in countries other than the developed world, or among particular ethnic groups, has been identified as a 'culture-bound' syndrome. Although these episodes exist primarily in certain countries, they may be seen in other places as people visit or immigrate to other countries or areas. Mojtabai (2005) summarized some of these psychotic behaviours:

- *Bouffée délirante,* a syndrome found in West Africa and Haiti, involves a sudden outburst of agitated and aggressive behaviour, marked confusion and psychomotor excitement. It is sometimes accompanied by visual and auditory hallucinations or paranoid ideation.
- *Ghost sickness* is preoccupation with death and the deceased frequently observed among members of some Native American tribes. Symptoms include bad dreams, weakness, feelings of danger, loss of appetite, fainting, dizziness, fear, anxiety, hallucinations, loss of consciousness, confusion, feelings of futility and a sense of suffocation.
- *Locura* refers to a chronic psychosis experienced by Latino people in the US and Latin America. Symptoms include incoherence, agitation, visual and auditory hallucinations, inability to follow social rules, unpredictability and, possibly, violent behaviour.
- *Qi-gong* psychotic reaction is an acute, time-limited episode characterized by dissociative, paranoid or other psychotic symptoms that occur after participating in the Chinese folk health-enhancing practice of *qi-gong*. Especially vulnerable are those who become overly involved in the practice.
- *Zar,* an experience of spirits possessing a person, is seen in Ethiopia, Somalia, Egypt, Sudan, Iran and other North African and Middle Eastern societies. The afflicted person may laugh, shout, wail, bang her or his head on a wall or be apathetic and withdrawn, refusing to eat or carry out daily tasks. Locally, such behaviour is not considered pathological.

Ethnicity may also be a factor in the way a person responds to psychotropic medications. This difference in response is probably the result of the person's genetic make-up. Some people metabolize certain drugs more slowly, so the drug level in the bloodstream is higher than desired.

Table 14.1	ANTIPSYCHOTIC DRUGS AND INCIDENCE OF SIDE-EFFECTS			
Generic (Trade) Name	Sedation	Hypotension	EPS	Anticholinergic
Chlorpromazine (Thorazine)	++++	+++	++	+++
Perphenazine (Fentazin)	++	++++	+	
Fluphenazine (Modecate)	+	+	++++	+
Haloperidol	+	+	++++	+/0
Trifluoperazine (Stelazine)	+	+	++++	+
Clozapine (Clozaril)	++++	++	+/0	++
Risperidone (Risperdal)	+++	++	++	+
Olanzapine (Zyprexa)	++++	+++	+	++
Quetiapine (Seroquel)	+/0	++++	+	+
Aripiprazole (Abilify)	+	++	+	+++

EPS, extrapyramidal side-effects.

++++, very significant; +++, significant; ++, moderate; +, mild; +/0, rare or absent.

Afro-Caribbean and white British people appear to require comparable therapeutic doses of antipsychotic medications. Asian clients, however, often need lower doses of drugs such as haloperidol (Haldol) to obtain the same effects; they would, therefore, be likely to experience more severe side-effects if given the traditional or usual doses.

TREATMENT

Psychopharmacology

The primary medical treatment for schizophrenia has long been psychopharmacology. In the past, electroconvulsive therapy, insulin shock therapy and psychosurgery were used, but since the creation of chlorpromazine (Largactil) in 1952, other treatment modalities have become all but obsolete. Antipsychotic medications, also known as **neuroleptics**, are prescribed primarily for their efficacy in decreasing psychotic symptoms. They do not cure schizophrenia; rather, they are used to manage its symptoms.

The older, or conventional, antipsychotic medications are dopamine antagonists. The newer, or atypical, antipsychotic medications are both dopamine and serotonin antagonists (see Chapter 3). These medications, usual daily dosages, and common side-effects are listed in Table 14.1. The conventional antipsychotics target the positive signs of schizophrenia, such as delusions, hallucinations, disturbed thinking and other psychotic symptoms, but have no observable effect on the negative signs. The atypical antipsychotics not only diminish positive symptoms but also, for many clients, lessen the negative signs of lack of volition and motivation, social withdrawal and anhedonia.

MAINTENANCE THERAPY

Six antipsychotics are available in depot injection forms for maintenance therapy: Haldol, Depixol, Modecate, Piportil, Clopixol and Risperdal Consta.

The vehicle for depot injections is sesame oil; therefore, the medications are absorbed slowly over time into the client's system. The effects of the medications last 2 to 4 weeks, eliminating the need for daily oral antipsychotic medication (see Chapter 3). It may take several weeks of oral therapy with these medications to reach a stable dosing level before the transition to depot injections can be made. Therefore, these preparations are not suitable for the management of acute episodes of psychosis. They are, however, very useful for clients requiring supervised medication concordance over an extended period.

SIDE-EFFECTS

The side-effects of antipsychotic medications are significant and can range from mild discomfort to permanent movement disorders (Kane & Marder, 2005). Because many of these side-effects are frightening and upsetting to clients, they are frequently cited as the primary reason that clients discontinue or reduce the dosage of their medications. Serious neurological side-effects include **extrapyramidal side-effects (EPS)** (acute dystonic reactions, akathisia and parkinsonism), tardive dyskinesia, seizures and neuroleptic malignant syndrome (NMS; discussion to follow). Non-neurological side-effects include weight gain, sedation, photosensitivity and anticholinergic symptoms such as dry mouth, blurred vision, constipation, urinary retention and orthostatic hypotension. Table 14.2 lists the side-effects of antipsychotic medications and appropriate nursing interventions.

Extrapyramidal Side-effects. EPS are reversible movement disorders induced by neuroleptic medication. They include dystonic reactions, parkinsonism and akathisia.

Dystonic reactions to antipsychotic medications appear early in the course of treatment and are characterized by spasms in discrete muscle groups such as the neck muscles (torticollis) or eye muscles (oculogyric crisis). These spasms may also be accompanied by protrusion of the tongue, dysphagia and laryngeal and pharyngeal spasms that can

| Table 14.2 | SIDE-EFFECTS OF ANTIPSYCHOTIC MEDICATIONS AND NURSING INTERVENTIONS |

Side-effect	Nursing Intervention
Dystonic reactions	Administer medications as ordered; assess for effectiveness; reassure client if he or she is frightened
Tardive dyskinesia	Assess using tool such as AIMS; report occurrence or score increase to doctor
Neuroleptic malignant syndrome	Stop all antipsychotic medications; alert doctor immediately
Akathisia	Administer medications as ordered; assess for effectiveness
EPS or neuroleptic-induced parkinsonism	Administer medications as ordered; assess for effectiveness
Seizures	Stop medication; notify doctor; protect client from injury during seizure; provide reassurance and privacy for client after seizure
Sedation	Caution about activities requiring client to be fully alert, such as driving a car
Photosensitivity	Caution client to avoid sun exposure; advise client when in the sun to wear protective clothing and sun-blocking lotion
Weight gain	Encourage balanced diet with controlled portions and regular exercise; focus on minimizing gain
Anticholinergic symptoms	
Dry mouth	Use ice chips or hard sweets for relief
Blurred vision	Assess side-effect, which should improve with time; report to physician if no improvement
Constipation	Increase fluid and dietary fibre intake; client may need a stool softener if unrelieved
Urinary retention	Instruct client to report any frequency or burning with urination; report to doctor if no improvement over time
Orthostatic hypotension	Instruct client to rise slowly from sitting or lying position; wait to ambulate until no longer dizzy or light-headed

Adapted from the British National Formulary Online (2008) http://www.bnf.org/bnf/bnf/55/

compromise the client's airway, causing a medical emergency. Dystonic reactions are extremely frightening and painful for the client. Acute treatment usually consists of procyclidine or benzatropine, given either intramuscularly or intravenously.

Pseudoparkinsonism, or neuroleptic-induced parkinsonism, includes a shuffling gait, mask-like facies, muscle stiffness (continuous) or cogwheeling rigidity (ratchet-like movements of joints), drooling and akinesia (slowness and difficulty initiating movement). These symptoms usually appear in the first few days after starting or increasing the dosage of an antipsychotic medication. Treatment of pseudoparkinsonism and prevention of further dystonic reactions is usually undertaken with antimuscarinic medications such as benzatropine, orphenadrine, procyclidine and trihexyphenidyl (benzhexol).

Akathisia is characterized by restless movement, pacing, inability to remain still and the client's report of inner restlessness. Akathisia usually develops when the antipsychotic is started or when the dose is increased. Clients are very uncomfortable with these sensations and may stop taking the antipsychotic medication to avoid these side-effects. Beta-blockers such as propranolol have been most effective in treating akathisia, whereas benzodiazepines have also proved successful.

The early detection and successful treatment of extrapyramidal side-effects is very important in promoting the client's compliance with medication. The nurse is most often the person who observes these symptoms or the person to whom the client reports symptoms. To provide consistency in assessment among nurses working with the client, a standardized rating scale for extrapyramidal symptoms is useful. The Simpson–Angus scale for extrapyramidal side-effects is one tool that can be used.

Tardive Dyskinesia. **Tardive dyskinesia**, a late-appearing side-effect of antipsychotic medications, is characterized by abnormal, involuntary movements such as lip smacking, tongue protrusion, chewing, blinking, grimacing and choreiform movements of the limbs and feet. These involuntary movements are embarrassing for clients and may cause them to become more socially isolated. Tardive dyskinesia is irreversible once it has appeared, but decreasing or discontinuing the medication can arrest the progression. Clozapine (Clozaril), an atypical antipsychotic drug, has not been found to cause this side-effect, so is often recommended for clients who have experienced tardive dyskinesia while taking conventional antipsychotic drugs.

Screening clients for late-appearing movement disorders such as tardive dyskinesia is important. The **Abnormal Involuntary Movement Scale** (AIMS) can be used to screen for symptoms of movement disorders. The client is observed in several positions, and the severity of symptoms is rated from 0 to 4. The AIMS can be administered every 3 to 6 months. If the nurse detects an increased score on the AIMS, indicating increased symptoms of tardive dyskinesia, he or she should notify the prescriber so that the client's dosage or drug

Box 14.1   ABNORMAL INVOLUNTARY MOVEMENT SCALE (AIMS) EXAMINATION PROCEDURE

Client identification: _____   Date:_____
Rated by: _____

Either before or after completing the examination procedure, observe the client unobtrusively at rest (e.g., in waiting room). The chair to be used in this examination should be a hard, firm one without arms.

After observing the client, he or she may be rated on a scale of 0 (none), 1 (minimal), 2 (mild), 3 (moderate), and 4 (severe) according to the severity of symptoms.

Ask the client if there is anything in his/her mouth (i.e., gum, sweets, etc.) and, if there is, to remove it.

Ask client about the current condition of his/her teeth. Ask client if he/she wears dentures. Do teeth or dentures bother client now?

Ask client whether he/she notices any movement in mouth, face hands, or feet. If yes, ask to describe and to what extent the movements currently bother patient or interfere with his/her activities.

0 1 2 3 4	Have client sit in chair with hands on knees, legs slightly apart and feet flat on floor. (Look at entire body for movements while in this position.)
0 1 2 3 4	Ask client to sit with hands hanging unsupported. If male, hands between legs; if female and wearing a dress, hands hanging over knees. (Observe hands and other body areas.)
0 1 2 3 4	Ask client to open mouth. (Observe tongue at rest within mouth.) Do this twice.
0 1 2 3 4	Ask client to protrude tongue. (Observe abnormalities of tongue movement.) Do this twice.
0 1 2 3 4	Ask client to tap thumb with each finger as rapidly as possible for 10-15 seconds; separately with right hand, then with left hand. (Observe facial and leg movements.)
0 1 2 3 4	Flex and extend client's left and right arms. (One at a time.)
0 1 2 3 4	Ask client to stand up. (Observe in profile. Observe all body areas again, hips included.)
0 1 2 3 4	*Ask client to extend both arms outstretched in front with palms down. (Observe trunk, legs and mouth.)
0 1 2 3 4	*Have client walk a few paces, turn and walk back to chair. (Observe hands and gait.) Do this twice.

*Activated movements.

can be changed to prevent advancement of tardive dyskinesia. The AIMS examination procedure is presented in Box 14.1.

Seizures. Seizures are an infrequent side-effect associated with antipsychotic medications. The incidence is 1% of people taking antipsychotics. The notable exception is clozapine, which has an incidence of 5%. Seizures may be associated with high doses of the medication. Treatment is a lowered dosage or a different antipsychotic medication.

Neuroleptic Malignant Syndrome. NMS is a serious and frequently fatal condition seen in those being treated with antipsychotic medications. It is characterized by muscle rigidity, high fever, increased muscle enzymes (particularly creatine phosphokinase) and leucocytosis (increased leucocytes). It is estimated that 0.1 to 1% of all clients taking antipsychotics develop NMS. Any of the antipsychotic medications can cause NMS, which is treated by stopping the medication. The client's ability to tolerate other antipsychotic medications after NMS varies, but use of another antipsychotic appears possible in most instances.

Agranulocytosis. Clozapine has the potentially fatal side-effect of agranulocytosis (failure of the bone marrow to produce adequate white blood cells). Agranulocytosis develops suddenly and is characterized by fever, malaise, ulcerative sore throat and leucopenia. This side-effect may not be manifested immediately but can occur as long as 18 to 24 weeks after the initiation of therapy. The drug must be discontinued immediately. Clients taking this antipsychotic must have weekly white blood cell counts for the first 6 months of clozapine therapy and every 2 weeks thereafter. Clozapine is dispensed every 7 or 14 days only, and evidence of a white cell count above 3500 cells/mm^3 is required before a refill is furnished.

Psychosocial Approaches to Care and Treatment

In addition to pharmacological treatment, many other modes of care and psychological therapy can help the person diagnosed with schizophrenia. Individual and group therapies, family therapy and family education, stress vulnerability approaches and social skills, relaxation and mindfulness training are all used in both inpatient and community settings.

CBT can offer help in two ways:

1. It can offer a therapeutic alliance that can help develop new ways of thinking, feeling and behaving when responding to symptoms and dealing with the effects of the diagnosis, medication and reduced ability to carry out activities of daily living.
   It can offer a collaborative way of working directly with the 'content' of symptoms such as delusions and hallucinations in order to reduce their grip on the person's life.
2. Individual and group therapy sessions can also be more generally supportive in nature, giving the client an opportunity for social contact and meaningful relationships with other people. Groups that focus on topics of concern, such as medication management, use of community supports and family concerns, have also been beneficial to clients with schizophrenia (Pfammatter *et al.*, 2006).

People with schizophrenia can improve their social confidence with social skills training, which translates into more effective functioning in the community. Basic social skills training involves breaking complex social behaviour down into simpler steps, practising through role-playing, and applying the concepts in the community or real-world setting. Cognitive adaptation training using environmental supports is designed to improve adaptive functioning in the home setting. Individually tailored environmental supports, such as signs, calendars, hygiene supplies and pill containers, can cue the client to perform associated tasks (Velligan *et al.*, 2006).

A new therapy, cognitive enhancement therapy (CET), combines computer-based cognitive training with group sessions that allow clients to practise and develop social skills. This approach is designed to remediate or improve the clients' social and neurocognitive deficits, such as attention, memory and information processing. The experiential exercises help the client to take the perspective of another person, rather than focusing entirely on himself or herself. Positive results of CET include increased mental stamina, active rather than passive information processing and spontaneous and appropriate negotiation of unrehearsed social challenges (Hogarty *et al.*, 2006).

Family education and therapy are known to diminish the negative effects of schizophrenia and reduce the relapse rate (Penn *et al.*, 2005). Although inclusion of the family is a factor that improves outcomes for the client, family involvement is often neglected by health-care professionals. Families frequently have a difficult time coping with the complexities and ramifications of the client's illness. This creates stress among family members that is not beneficial for the client or family members. Family education helps to make family members a central part of the treatment team.

In addition, family members can benefit from a supportive environment that helps them cope with the many difficulties presented when a loved one has schizophrenia. These concerns include continuing as a carer for the child who is now an adult; worrying about who will care for the client when the parents are gone; dealing with the social stigma of 'mental illness'; and possibly facing financial problems, marital discord and social isolation. Such support is available through a variety of national and local support groups. The client's health-care provider can make referrals to meet specific family needs.

APPLICATION OF THE NURSING PROCESS

Assessment

Schizophrenia affects thought processes and content, perception, emotion, behaviour and social functioning; however, it affects each individual differently. The degree of impairment in both the acute or psychotic phase and the chronic or long-term phase varies greatly, and thus so do the needs of, and the nursing interventions for, each affected client. The nurse must never make assumptions about the client's abilities or limitations based solely on a medical diagnosis of schizophrenia: *everyone* has strengths, experience, wisdom, resources and dreams, and everyone is far more than a set of 'symptoms'.

A nurse may care for a client in an acute inpatient setting, who may appear frightened, hearing voices, making no eye contact and mumbling constantly. The nurse would be dealing with the positive, or psychotic, signs of the condition. Another nurse may encounter a client with schizophrenia in a community setting, who is not experiencing psychotic symptoms; rather, this client lacks energy for daily tasks and has feelings of loneliness and isolation (negative signs – perhaps – of schizophrenia). Although both clients have the same broad medical diagnosis and each deserves compassionate, evidence-based care, the approach and interventions that each nurse takes would be very different.

HISTORY

Having established the context and purpose of the conversation, the nurse first elicits information about the client's previous history with schizophrenia, to establish baseline data and to set an agenda of co-operation and the identification of strengths. He or she may ask questions about how the client functioned before the crisis developed, such as 'How do you usually spend your time?' and 'Can you describe what you do each day?'

The nurse might ask the age at onset of schizophrenic-type problems, knowing that poorer outcomes are associated with an earlier age at onset. Learning the client's previous history of hospital admissions and response to hospitalization also is important.

The nurse also assesses the client for previous suicide attempts. The nurse might ask, 'Have you ever attempted suicide?' or 'Have you ever heard voices telling you to hurt yourself?' Likewise, it is important to elicit information about any history of violence or aggression because a history of aggressive behaviour is a strong predictor of future aggression. The nurse might ask, 'What do you do when you are angry, frustrated, upset or scared?'

The nurse assesses whether the client has been using current support systems by asking the client or significant others the following questions:

- Has the client kept in contact with family or friends?
- Has the client been to scheduled groups or therapy appointments?
- Does the client seem to run out of money before payday or before his giro comes through?
- Have the client's living arrangements changed recently?

Finally, the nurse assesses the client's perception of his or her current situation – that is, what the client believes to be significant present events or stressors. The nurse can gather such information by asking, 'What do you see as the main problem now?' or 'What do you need help managing now?'

GENERAL APPEARANCE, MOTOR BEHAVIOUR AND SPEECH

Appearance may vary widely among different people diagnosed with schizophrenia. Some appear 'normal' in terms of being dressed appropriately, sitting in a chair conversing with the nurse and exhibiting no strange or unusual postures or gestures. Others exhibit odd or bizarre behaviour. They may appear dishevelled and unkempt with no obvious concern for their hygiene, or they may wear strange or seemingly inappropriate clothing (for instance, a heavy coat and woolly hat in hot weather).

Overall motor behaviour may also appear odd. The client may be restless and unable to sit still, exhibit agitation and pacing or appear unmoving (**catatonia**). He or she also may demonstrate seemingly purposeless gestures (stereotypical behaviour) and odd facial expressions such as grimacing. The client may imitate the movements and gestures of someone whom he or she is observing (**echopraxia**). Rambling speech that may or may not make sense to the listener is likely to accompany these behaviours.

Conversely, the client may exhibit **psychomotor retardation** (a general slowing of all movements). Sometimes the client may be almost immobile, curled into a ball (fetal position). Clients with the catatonic type of schizophrenia can exhibit '**waxy flexibility**': they maintain any position in which they are placed, even if the position is awkward or uncomfortable.

The client may exhibit an unusual speech pattern. Two typical patterns are **word salad** (jumbled words and phrases

---

Box 14.2 UNUSUAL SPEECH PATTERNS OF CLIENTS WITH SCHIZOPHRENIA

Clang associations are ideas that are related to one another based on sound or rhyming rather than meaning.
   Example: 'I will take a pill if I go up the hill but not if my name is Jill, I don't want to kill.'
Neologisms are words invented by the client.
   Example: 'I'm afraid of grittiz. If there are any grittiz here, I will have to leave. Are you a grittiz?'
Verbigeration is the stereotyped repetition of words or phrases that may or may not have meaning to the listener.
   Example: 'I want to go home, go home, go home, go home.'
Echolalia is the client's imitation or repetition of what the nurse says.
   Example: *Nurse*: 'Can you tell me how you're feeling?' *Client*: 'Can you tell me how you're feeling, how you're feeling?'
Stilted language is use of words or phrases that are flowery, excessive and pompous.
   Example: 'Would you be so kind, as a representative of Florence Nightingale, as to do me the honour of providing just a wee bit of refreshment, perhaps in the form of some clear spring water?'
Perseveration is the persistent adherence to a single idea or topic and verbal repetition of a sentence, phrase or word, even when another person attempts to change the topic.
   Example: *Nurse*: 'How have you been sleeping lately?' *Client*: 'I think people have been following me.' *Nurse*: 'Where do you live?' *Client*: 'At my place people have been following me.' *Nurse*: 'What do you like to do in your free time?' *Client*: 'Nothing because people are following me.'
Word salad is a combination of jumbled words and phrases that are disconnected or incoherent and make no sense to the listener.
   Example: 'Corn, potatoes, jump up, play games, grass, cupboard.'

that are disconnected or incoherent and make no sense to the listener) and **echolalia** (repetition or imitation of what someone else says). Speech may be slowed or accelerated in rate and volume: the client may speak in whispers or hushed tones or may talk loudly or yell. **Latency of response** refers to hesitation before the client responds to questions. This latency or hesitation may last 30 or 45 seconds and usually indicates the client's difficulty with cognition or thought processes. Box 14.2 lists and gives examples of these unusual speech patterns.

MOOD AND AFFECT

Clients with schizophrenia report and demonstrate wide variances in mood and affect. They are often described as having **flat affect** (no facial expression) or **blunted affect** (few observable facial expressions). The typical facial expression often is described as mask-like. The affect also may be described as silly, characterized by giggling for no apparent reason. The client may exhibit an inappropriate expression or emotions incongruent with the context of the situation. This incongruence ranges from mild or subtle to grossly inappropriate. For example, the client may laugh and grin while describing the death of a family member or weep while talking about the weather.

The client may report feeling depressed and having no pleasure or joy in life (**anhedonia**). Conversely, he or she may report feeling all-knowing, all-powerful, and not at all concerned with the circumstance or situation. It is more common for the client to report exaggerated feelings of well-being during episodes of psychotic or delusional thinking and a lack of energy or pleasurable feelings during the chronic, or long-term, phase of the illness.

THOUGHT PROCESS AND CONTENT

Schizophrenia is often referred to as a thought disorder because that may seem to be the primary feature of the disease: thought processes become disordered, and the continuity of thoughts and information processing is disrupted. The nurse can assess thought processes by inferring from what the client says. He or she can assess thought content by evaluating what the client actually says. For example, clients may suddenly stop talking in the middle of a sentence and remain silent for several seconds to 1 minute (**thought blocking**). They may also state that they believe others can hear their thoughts (**thought broadcasting**), that others are taking their thoughts (**thought withdrawal**) or that others are placing thoughts in their mind against their will (**thought insertion**).

Clients also may exhibit tangential thinking, which is veering onto unrelated topics and never answering the original question:

> *Nurse:* '*How have you been sleeping lately?*'
> *Client:* '*Oh, I try to sleep at night. I like to listen to music to help me sleep. I really like reggae music best. What do you like? Can I have something to eat pretty soon? I'm hungry.*'
> *Nurse:* '*Can you tell me how you've been sleeping?*'

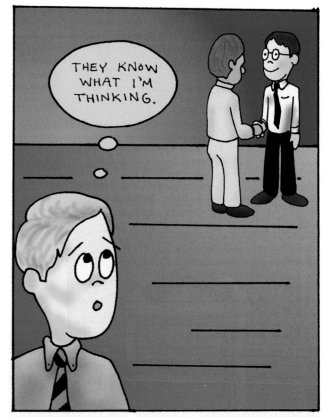

Thought broadcasting

Circumstantiality may be evidenced if the client gives unnecessary details or strays from the topic but eventually provides the requested information:

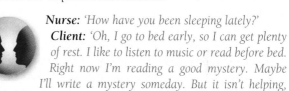

> *Nurse:* '*How have you been sleeping lately?*'
> *Client:* '*Oh, I go to bed early, so I can get plenty of rest. I like to listen to music or read before bed. Right now I'm reading a good mystery. Maybe I'll write a mystery someday. But it isn't helping, reading I mean. I have been getting only 2 or 3 hours of sleep at night.*'

Poverty of content (**alogia**) describes the lack of any real meaning or substance in what the client says:

> *Nurse:* '*How have you been sleeping lately?*'
> *Client:* '*Well, I guess, I don't know, hard to tell.*'

DELUSIONS

Clients diagnosed with schizophrenia frequently experience **delusions** (fixed, false beliefs with no apparent basis in reality) during psychotic phases. A common characteristic of schizophrenic delusions is the direct, immediate and total certainty with which the client holds these beliefs. Because the client believes the delusion, he or she therefore acts accordingly. For example, the client with delusions of persecution is probably suspicious, mistrustful and

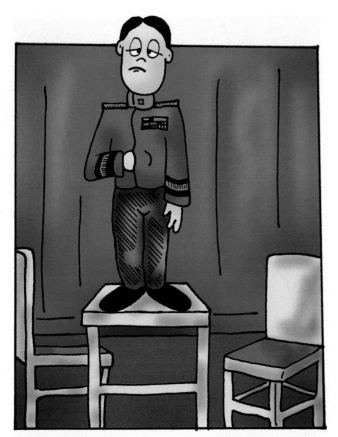

Delusions of grandeur

guarded about disclosing personal information; he or she may examine the room periodically or speak in hushed, secretive tones.

The theme or content of the delusions may vary. Box 14.3 describes and provides examples of the various types of delusions. External contradictory information or 'facts' cannot alter these delusional beliefs. If asked why he or she believes such an unlikely idea, the client often replies, 'I just know it.'

Initially, the nurse assesses the content and depth of the delusion to know what behaviours to expect and to try to establish an agreed reality with the client. When eliciting information about the client's delusional beliefs, the nurse must be careful not to support or challenge them. The nurse might ask the client to explain what he or she believes by saying, 'Please explain that to me,' or 'Tell me what you're thinking about that.'

SENSORY AND INTELLECTUAL PROCESSES

One hallmark symptom of schizophrenic psychosis is **hallucinations** (false sensory perceptions, or perceptual experiences that do not exist in reality). Hallucinations can involve the five senses and bodily sensations. They can be threatening and frightening for the client; less frequently, clients report hallucinations as pleasant. Initially, the client perceives hallucinations as real, but later in the illness, he or she may recognize them as hallucinations.

Hallucinations are distinguished from *illusions*, which are misperceptions of actual environmental stimuli. For example, while walking through the woods, a person might believe he sees a snake at the side of the path. On closer examination, however, he discovers it is only a curved stick. Reality or factual information corrected this illusion. Hallucinations, however, have no such basis in reality.

The following are the various types of hallucinations (Kirkpatrick & Tek, 2005):

- *Auditory hallucinations*, the most common type, involve hearing sounds, most often voices, talking to or about the client. There may be one or multiple voices; a familiar or unfamiliar person's voice may be speaking. **Command hallucinations** are voices demanding that the client take action, often to harm self or others, and need to be considered as potentially dangerous.
- *Visual hallucinations* involve seeing images that do not exist at all, such as lights or a dead person, or distortions such as seeing a frightening monster instead of the nurse. They are the second most common type of hallucination.
- *Olfactory hallucinations* involve smells. They may be a specific scent such as urine or faeces or a more general scent such as a rotten or rancid smell. In addition to clients with schizophrenia, this type of hallucination often occurs with dementia, seizures or cerebrovascular accidents.
- *Tactile hallucinations* refer to sensations such as electricity running through the body or bugs crawling on the skin. Tactile hallucinations are found most often in clients undergoing alcohol withdrawal; they rarely occur in clients with schizophrenia.
- *Gustatory hallucinations* involve a taste lingering in the mouth or the sense that food tastes like something else. The taste may be metallic or bitter or may be represented as a specific taste.
- *Coenesthetic hallucinations* involve the client's report that he or she feels bodily functions that are usually undetectable. Examples would be the sensation of urine forming or impulses being transmitted through the brain.
- *Kinesthetic hallucinations* occur when the client is motionless but reports the sensation of bodily movement. Occasionally, the bodily movement is something unusual, such as floating above the ground.

During episodes of psychosis, clients are commonly disoriented to time and sometimes place. The most extreme form of disorientation is **depersonalization**, in which the client feels detached from his or her behaviour. Although the client can state his or her name correctly, he or she feels as if his or her body belongs to someone else or that his or her spirit is detached from the body.

Assessing the intellectual processes of a client with schizophrenia is difficult if he or she is experiencing psychosis. The client usually demonstrates poor intellectual functioning as a result of disordered thoughts. Nevertheless,

Box 14.3 TYPES OF DELUSIONS

Persecutory/paranoid delusions involve the client's belief that 'others' are planning to harm the client or are spying, following, ridiculing or belittling the client in some way. Sometimes the client cannot define who these 'others' are.
Examples: The client may think that food has been poisoned or that rooms are bugged with listening devices.
Sometimes the 'persecutor' is the government, MI5 or another powerful organization. Occasionally, specific individuals, even family members, may be named as the 'persecutor'.

Grandiose delusions are characterized by the client's claim to association with famous people or celebrities, or the client's belief that he or she is famous or capable of great feats.
Examples: The client may claim to be engaged to a famous movie star or related to some public figure, such as claiming to be the daughter of the Prime Minister, or he or she may claim to have found a cure for cancer.

Religious delusions often centre around the second coming of Christ or another significant religious figure or prophet. These religious delusions appear suddenly as part of the client's psychosis and are not part of his or her religious faith or that of others.
Examples: Client claims to be the Messiah or some prophet sent from God; believes that God communicates directly to him or her, or that he or she has a 'special' religious mission in life or special religious powers.

Somatic delusions are generally vague and unrealistic beliefs about the client's health or bodily functions. Factual information or diagnostic testing does not change these beliefs.
Examples: A male client may say that he is pregnant, or a client may report decaying intestines or worms in the brain.

Referential delusions or ideas of reference involve the client's belief that television broadcasts, music or newspaper articles have special meaning for him or her.
Examples: The client may report that Gordon Brown was speaking directly to him on a news broadcast or that special messages are sent through newspaper articles.

---

the nurse should not assume that the client has limited intellectual capacity based on impaired thought processes. It may be that the client cannot focus, concentrate or pay adequate attention to demonstrate his or her intellectual abilities accurately. The nurse is more likely to obtain accurate assessments of the client's intellectual abilities when the client's thought processes are clearer.

Clients often have difficulty with abstract thinking and may respond in a very literal way to other people and the environment. For example, when asked to interpret the proverb, 'A stitch in time saves nine,' the client may explain it by saying, 'I need to sew up my clothes.' The client may not understand what is being said and can easily misinterpret instructions. This can pose serious problems during medication administration. For example, the nurse may tell the client, 'It is always important to take all your medications.' The client may misinterpret the nurse's statement and take the entire supply of medication at one time.

JUDGEMENT AND INSIGHT

Judgement is frequently impaired in the client with schizophrenia. Because judgement is based on the ability to interpret the environment correctly, it follows that the client with disordered thought processes and environmental misinterpretations will have great difficulty with judgement.

At times, lack of judgement is so severe that clients cannot meet their needs for safety and protection and place themselves in harm's way. This difficulty may range from failing to wear warm clothing in cold weather to failing to seek medical care even when desperately ill. The client also may fail to recognize the need for sleep or food.

Insight can also be severely impaired, especially early on, when the client, family and friends do not understand what is happening. Over time, some clients can learn about the 'illness', anticipate problems and seek appropriate assistance as needed.

SELF-CONCEPT

Deterioration of the concept of self is a major problem in schizophrenia. The phrase *loss of ego boundaries* describes the client's lack of a clear sense of where his or her own body, mind and influence end, and where those aspects of other animate and inanimate objects begin. This lack of ego boundaries is evidenced by depersonalization, derealization (environmental objects become smaller or larger or seem unfamiliar) and **ideas of reference**. Clients may believe they are fused with another person or object, may not recognize body parts as their own or may fail to know whether they are male or female. These difficulties are the source of many bizarre behaviours such as public undressing or masturbating, speaking about oneself in the third person or physically clinging to objects in the environment. Body image distortion also may occur.

ROLES AND RELATIONSHIPS

Social isolation is prevalent in clients with schizophrenia, partly as a result of positive signs such as delusions, hallucinations and loss of ego boundaries. Relating to others is difficult when one's self-concept is not clear. Clients also have problems with trust and intimacy, which interfere with the ability to establish satisfactory relationships. Low self-esteem, one of the negative signs of schizophrenia, further complicates the client's ability to interact with others and the environment. These clients lack confidence, feel strange or different from other people and do not believe they are worthwhile. The result is avoidance of other people.

People diagnosed with schizophrenia may experience great frustration in attempting to fulfil roles in the family and community. Success in school or at work can be severely compromised because the client has difficulty thinking clearly, remembering, paying attention and concentrating. Subsequently, he or she lacks motivation. Clients who develop schizophrenia at a younger age have more difficulties than those whose illness developed later in life because they did not have the opportunity to succeed in these areas before the illness.

Fulfilling family roles, such as that of son or daughter or sibling, is difficult for these clients. Often, their erratic or unpredictable behaviour frightens or embarrasses family members, who become unsure what to expect next. Families may also feel guilty or responsible, believing they somehow failed to provide a loving, supportive home life. These clients also may believe they have disappointed their families because they cannot become independent or successful.

PHYSIOLOGICAL AND SELF-CARE CONSIDERATIONS

Clients with schizophrenia may have significant self-care deficits. Inattention to hygiene and grooming needs is common, especially during psychotic episodes. The client can become so preoccupied with delusions or hallucinations that he or she fails to perform even basic activities of daily living.

Clients may also fail to recognize sensations such as hunger or thirst, and food or fluid intake may be inadequate. This can result in malnourishment and constipation. Constipation is also a common side-effect of antipsychotic medications, compounding the problem. Paranoia or excessive fears that food and fluids have been poisoned are common and may interfere with eating. If the client is agitated and pacing, he or she may be unable to sit down long enough to eat.

Occasionally, clients develop **polydipsia** (excessive water intake), which leads to water intoxication. Serum sodium levels can become dangerously low, leading to seizures. Polydipsia is usually seen in clients who have had severe and persistent mental health problems for many years as

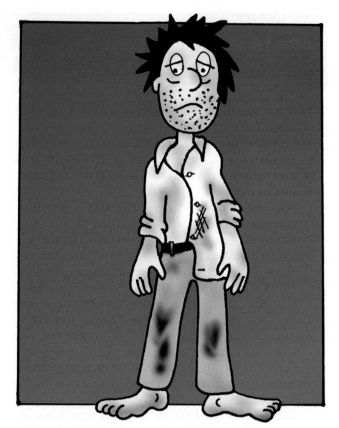

Self-care deficits

well as long-term therapy with antipsychotic medications. Polydipsia may be caused by the behavioural state itself or may be precipitated by the use of antidepressant or antipsychotic medications (Reynolds *et al.*, 2004).

Sleep problems are common. Hallucinations may stimulate clients, resulting in insomnia. Other times, clients are suspicious and believe harm will come to them if they sleep. As in other self-care areas, the client may not correctly perceive or acknowledge physical cues such as fatigue.

To assist the client with community living, the nurse needs to assess daily living skills and functional abilities. Such skills – having a bank account and paying bills, buying food and preparing meals and using public transportation – are often difficult tasks for the client with schizophrenia. He or she might never have learned such skills or may be unable to accomplish them consistently.

Data Analysis

The nurse must analyse assessment data with clients with schizophrenia to determine priorities and establish an effective plan of care. Not all clients have the same problems and needs, nor is it likely that any individual client has all the problems that can accompany schizophrenia. Levels of family and community support and available services also vary, all of which influence the client's care and outcomes.

The analysis of assessment data generally falls into two main categories: data associated with the positive signs of the disease and data associated with the negative signs. Nursing formulations based on the assessment of psychotic symptoms or *positive* signs may be as follows:

- Risk for violence to others
- Risk of suicide
- Disturbed thought processes
- Disturbed sensory perception
- Disturbed personal identity
- Impaired verbal communication.

Nursing formulations based on the assessment of *negative* signs and functional abilities include the following:

- Self-care deficits
- Social isolation
- Inadequate activity
- Ineffective maintenance of health
- Ineffective medication management.

Outcome Identification

It is likely that the client with an acute psychotic episode of schizophrenia will receive treatment in an intensive setting such as an inpatient hospital unit or under the supervision of a crisis team or AOT. During this phase, the focus of care is on stabilizing the client's thought processes and reality orientation as well as ensuring safety. This is also the time to evaluate resources, make referrals and begin planning for the client's re-integration into the community.

Examples of outcomes appropriate to the acute, psychotic phase of treatment are as follows:

1. The person will not injure self or others.
2. The person will re-establish contact with 'reality' in a way that allows him or her to pursue his or her goals.
3. The person will feel safe and not threatened by others or by aspects of self or own behaviour.
4. The person will interact constructively with others in the environment.
5. The person will express thoughts and feelings in a safe and socially acceptable manner.
6. The person will participate as agreed in therapeutic interventions, including, if necessary, medication.

Once the crisis or the acute, psychotic symptoms have been stabilized, the focus is on developing the client's ability to live as independently and successfully as possible in the community. This usually requires continued follow-up care and participation of the client's family in community support services. Prevention and early recognition and treatment of relapse symptoms are important parts of successful rehabilitation. Dealing with the negative signs of schizophrenia, which medication generally does not affect, is a major challenge for the client, family and friends and professionals. Examples of treatment outcomes for continued care after the stabilization of acute symptoms are as follows:

1. The client will work constructively with the agreed CPA plan of care (including medication and follow-up appointments).
2. The client will maintain adequate routines for sleeping and food and fluid intake.
3. The client will demonstrate independence in self-care activities.
4. The client will communicate effectively with others in the community to meet his or her needs.
5. The client will seek or accept assistance to meet his or her needs when indicated.

The nurse must appreciate the severity of schizophrenia and the profound and sometimes devastating effects it has on the lives of clients and their families. It is equally important to avoid treating the client as a 'hopeless case', someone who no longer is capable of having a meaningful and satisfying life. It is not helpful to expect either too much or too little from the client. Careful ongoing assessment is necessary so that appropriate treatment and interventions address the client's needs and difficulties while helping the client to reach his or her optimal level of functioning.

Intervention

PROMOTING THE SAFETY OF CLIENT AND OTHERS

Safety for both the client and the nurse is the first priority when providing care for the client diagnosed with schizophrenia. The client may be paranoid and suspicious of the nurse and the environment, and may feel threatened and intimidated. Although the client's behaviour may be threatening to the nurse, the client is also feeling unsafe and may believe his or her well-being to be in jeopardy. Therefore, the nurse must approach the client in a non-threatening manner. Making demands or being authoritative only increases the client's fears. Giving the client ample personal space usually enhances his or her sense of security.

A fearful or agitated client has the potential to harm themselves or others. The nurse must observe for signs of building agitation or escalating behaviour, such as increased intensity of pacing, loud talking or yelling and hitting or kicking objects. The nurse must institute interventions to protect the client, nurse and others in the environment. This may involve administering medication, moving the client to a quiet, less-stimulating environment and, in extreme situations, temporarily using seclusion or restraints. See Chapter 10 for a discussion of how to deal with anger and hostility and Chapter 15 for how to work with people who are suicidal.

ESTABLISHING A THERAPEUTIC RELATIONSHIP

Establishing trust between the client and nurse also helps to allay the fears of a frightened client. Initially, the client may tolerate only 5 or 10 minutes of contact at one time. Establishing an effective short-term therapeutic alliance may take time, and the nurse must be patient. The nurse should provide explanations that are clear, direct and easy to understand. Body language should include eye contact but not staring, a relaxed body posture and facial expressions that convey genuine interest and concern. Telling the client one's name and calling the client by name are helpful in establishing trust as well as reality orientation.

The nurse must assess carefully the client's response to the use of touch. Sometimes gentle touch conveys caring and concern. At other times, the client may misinterpret the nurse's touch as threatening and therefore undesirable. As the nurse sits near the client, does he or she move or look away? Is the client frightened or wary of the nurse's presence? If so, that client may not be reassured by touch but frightened or threatened by it.

USING THERAPEUTIC COMMUNICATION

Communicating with clients experiencing psychotic symptoms can be difficult and frustrating. The nurse tries to understand and make sense of what the client is saying, but this can be difficult if the client is hallucinating, withdrawn from reality or relatively mute. The nurse must maintain non-verbal communication with the client, especially when verbal communication is not very successful. This involves spending time with the client, perhaps through fairly lengthy periods of silence. The presence of the nurse is a contact with reality for the client and also can demonstrate the nurse's genuine interest and caring to the client. Calling the client by name, making references to the day and time and commenting on the environment are all helpful ways to continue to make contact with a client who is having problems with reality orientation and verbal communication. Clients who are left alone for long periods can become more deeply entrenched in their psychosis, so frequent contact and time spent with a client are important, even if the nurse is unsure that the client is aware of the nurse's presence.

Active listening is an important skill for the nurse trying to communicate with a client whose verbalizations seem disorganized or nonsensical. Rather than dismissing what the client says because it is not clear, the nurse must make efforts to determine the meaning the client is trying to convey. Listening for themes or recurrent statements, asking clarifying questions and exploring the meaning of the client's statements are all useful techniques to increase understanding.

The nurse must let the client know when his or her meaning is not clear. It is never useful to pretend to understand or just to agree or go along with what the client is saying: this is dishonest and violates trust between client and nurse.

Nurse: *'How are you feeling today?'* (using a broad opening statement)
Client: *'Invisible.'*
Nurse: *'Can you explain that to me?'* (seeking clarification)
Client: *'Oh, it doesn't matter.'*
Nurse: *'I'm interested in how you feel; I'm just not sure I understand.'* (offering self/seeking clarification)

Client: *'It doesn't mean much.'*
Nurse: *'Let me see if I can understand. Do you feel like you're being ignored, that no-one is really listening?'* (verbalizing the implied)

IMPLEMENTING INTERVENTIONS FOR DELUSIONAL THOUGHTS

The client experiencing delusions utterly believes them and cannot easily be convinced they are false or untrue. Such delusions powerfully influence the client's behaviour. For example, if the client's delusion is that he or she is being poisoned, he or she will be suspicious, mistrustful and probably resistant to providing information and taking medications.

The nurse must avoid openly confronting the delusion or arguing with the client about it: aggressive denial of a person's subjective reality is abusive, confining and potentially destructive. The nurse must also avoid reinforcing the delusional belief by excessively 'playing along' with what the client says. It is the nurse's responsibility to present and maintain reality by making simple statements, such as

'That sounds really frightening, but I haven't seen any evidence of that myself' (presenting reality)

or

'It doesn't seem that way to me, but I can see how scary that must be for you.' (casting doubt).

As antipsychotic medications and/or psychological interventions begin to have a therapeutic effect, it may become increasingly possible for the nurse to discuss the delusional ideas with the client and identify ways in which the delusions interfere with the client's daily life.

The nurse can also help the client minimize the effects of delusional thinking. Distraction techniques, such as listening to music, watching television, writing or talking to friends, are useful. Direct action, such as engaging in positive self-talk and positive thinking and ignoring the delusional thoughts, may be beneficial as well.

IMPLEMENTING INTERVENTIONS FOR HALLUCINATIONS

Intervening when the client experiences hallucinations requires the nurse to focus on what is real and to help – if possible – shift the client's response toward reality. Work here, as in other areas of mental health nursing, involves maintaining a delicate balance between conversational strategies of validation (of a person's own perspective, thoughts and feelings) and conversations about change (towards a life of meaning and purpose for the person). Initially, the nurse must determine what the client is experiencing – that is, what the voices are saying or what the client is seeing. Doing so increases the nurse's understanding of the nature of the client's feelings and behaviour and can help validate and accept the client as a person. In command hallucinations, the client hears voices directing him or her to do something, often to hurt self or someone else. For this reason, the nurse must elicit a description of the content of the hallucination so that people involved in care can take precautions to protect the client and others as necessary. The nurse might say,

 'I don't hear any voices; what are you hearing?' (presenting reality/seeking clarification).

This also can help the nurse understand how to relieve the client's fears or paranoia. For example, the client might be seeing ghosts or monster-like images, and the nurse could respond,

 'I don't see anything, but you must be frightened. You're safe here in the hospital' (presenting reality/translating into feelings).

This acknowledges the client's fear but reassures the client that no harm will come to him or her.

Clients do not always report or identify hallucinations. At times, the nurse must infer from the client's behaviour that hallucinations are occurring. Examples of behaviour that indicate hallucinations include alternately listening and then talking when no one else is present, laughing inappropriately for no observable reason and mumbling or mouthing words with no audible sound.

A helpful strategy for intervening with hallucinations is to engage the client in a 'reality-based' activity such as playing cards, participating in occupational therapy or listening to music. It is difficult for the client to pay attention to hallucinations and reality-based activity at the same time, so this technique of distracting the client is often useful.

It may also be useful to work with the client to identify certain situations or a particular frame of mind that may precede or trigger auditory hallucinations. Intensity of hallucinations is often related to anxiety levels; therefore, monitoring and intervening to lower a client's anxiety may decrease the intensity of hallucinations. Clients who recognize that certain moods or patterns of thinking precede the onset of voices may eventually be able to manage or control the hallucinations by learning to manage or avoid particular states of mind. This may involve learning to relax when voices occur, engaging in diversions, correcting negative self-talk and seeking out or avoiding social interaction. Exceptions – times when the client experiences the voices as less threatening, feels less inclined to act on them or feels less distressed by them – can usefully be identified as an aid to helping assessment and as clues to possible constructive solutions.

Teaching the client to talk back to the voices forcefully also may help him or her manage auditory hallucinations. The client should do this in a relatively private place rather than in public. There is an international self-help movement of 'voice-hearer groups', developed to assist people

to manage auditory hallucinations. One group devised the strategy of carrying a mobile phone (fake or real) to cope with voices when in public places. With mobiles, members can carry on conversations with their voices in the street – and tell them to shut up – while avoiding ridicule by looking like a normal part of the street scene (Hagen & Mitchell, 2001). Being able to verbalize resistance can help the client feel empowered and capable of dealing with the hallucinations.

COPING WITH SOCIALLY INAPPROPRIATE BEHAVIOURS

People diagnosed with schizophrenia often experience a blurring of identity and boundaries, which can pose enormous difficulties for themselves and others. Behaviours can – rarely – include touching others without warning or invitation, intruding into others' living spaces, talking to or caressing inanimate objects and engaging in such socially inappropriate behaviours as undressing, masturbating or urinating in public. Clients may approach others and make provocative, insulting or sexual statements. The nurse must, of course, attempt to balance the needs of others with the needs of clients in these situations.

Protecting the client is a primary nursing responsibility and includes protecting the client from retaliation by others who experience the client's intrusions and socially unacceptable behaviour. Redirecting the client away from situations or others can interrupt the undesirable behaviour and keep the client from further intrusive behaviours. The nurse must also try to protect the client's right to privacy and dignity. Taking the client to his or her room or to a quiet area with less stimulation and fewer people often helps. Engaging the client in appropriate activities also is indicated. For example, if the client is undressing in front of others, the nurse might say,

 'Let's go to your room and you can put your clothes back on' (encouraging **collaboration**/redirecting to appropriate activity).

If the client is making verbal statements to others, the nurse might ask the client to go for a walk or move to another area to listen to music. The nurse should deal with socially inappropriate behaviour non-judgementally and matter-of-factly. This means making factual adult–adult statements with no overtones of scolding and not talking to the client as if he or she were a naughty child.

Some behaviours may be so offensive or threatening that others respond by yelling at, ridiculing or even taking aggressive action against the client. Although providing physical protection for the client is the nurse's first consideration, helping others affected by the client's behaviour is also important. Usually, the nurse can offer simple and factual statements to others that do not violate the client's confidentiality. The nurse might make statements such as

'You really didn't do anything to provoke that. Sometimes people's mental health problems cause them to act in strange ways. I think it's important not to laugh at things that are part of someone's mental health problems' (presenting reality/giving information).

The nurse reassures the client's family that these behaviours are part of the client's 'illness' and not personally directed at them. Such situations present an opportunity to educate family members about schizophrenia and to help allay their feelings of guilt, shame or responsibility.

Re-integrating the client into the treatment milieu as soon as possible is essential. The client should not feel shunned or punished for inappropriate behaviour. Professionals should introduce limited stimulation gradually. For example, when the client is comfortable and demonstrating appropriate behaviour with the nurse, one or two other people can be engaged in a semi-structured activity with the client. The client's involvement is gradually increased to small groups and then to larger, less-structured groups as he or she can tolerate the increased level of stimulation without 'decompensating' (regressing to previous, less effective coping behaviours).

TEACHING CLIENT AND FAMILY

Coping with a diagnosis of schizophrenia is a major adjustment for both clients and their families. Understanding the 'illness', the need for continuing medication, care co-ordination and/or psychotherapy and the uncertainty of the prognosis or recovery are key issues. Clients and families need help to cope with the emotional upheaval that schizophrenia causes (see Client/Family Education for Schizophrenia for education points).

Identifying and managing one's own health needs are primary concerns for everyone, but this is a particular challenge for clients with schizophrenia because their health needs can be complex and their ability to manage them may be impaired. The nurse helps the client to manage his or her illness and health needs as independently as possible. This can be accomplished only through education and ongoing support.

Teaching the client and family members to prevent or manage relapse is an essential part of a comprehensive plan of care. This includes providing facts about schizophrenia, identifying the early signs of relapse and teaching health practices to promote physical and psychological well-being. Early identification of relapse signs (Box 14.4) has been found to reduce the frequency of relapse (Birchwood *et al.* (2000) and van Meijel *et al.* (2004)); when relapse cannot be prevented, early identification provides the foundation for interventions to manage the relapse. For example, if the nurse finds that the client is tired or exhausted or lacks adequate sleep or proper nutrition, interventions to promote rest and nutrition may prevent a relapse or minimize its intensity and duration.

CLIENT/FAMILY EDUCATION FOR SCHIZOPHRENIA

- How to manage self and symptoms
- Recognizing early warning signs
- Developing a plan to address relapse signs
- Importance of maintaining prescribed medication regime and regular follow-up
- Avoiding alcohol and other drugs
- Self-care and proper nutrition
- Teaching social skills through education, role modelling and practice
- Seeking assistance to avoid or manage stressful situations
- Counselling and education of family/significant others about the possible causes and clinical course of schizophrenia and the need for ongoing support
- Importance of maintaining contact with community and participating in supportive organizations and care

The nurse can use the list of relapse risk factors in several ways. He or she can include these risk factors in discharge teaching before the client leaves the inpatient setting, so that the client and family know what to watch

Box 14.4   EARLY SIGNS OF RELAPSE (PROFESSIONALS' CHECKLIST)

- Impaired cause-and-effect reasoning
- Impaired information processing
- Poor nutrition
- Lack of sleep
- Lack of exercise
- Fatigue
- Poor social skills, social isolation, loneliness
- Interpersonal difficulties
- Lack of control, irritability
- Mood swings
- Ineffective medication management
- Low self-concept
- Looks and acts different
- Hopeless feelings
- Loss of motivation
- Anxiety and worry
- Disinhibition
- Increased negativity
- Neglecting appearance
- Forgetfulness

for and when to seek assistance. The nurse can also use the list when assessing the client in a community setting. The nurse can provide teaching to ancillary personnel who may work with the client, so they know when to contact a mental health professional. Taking medications as prescribed, keeping regular follow-up appointments and avoiding alcohol and other drugs have been associated with fewer and shorter hospital stays. In addition, clients who can identify and avoid stressful situations are less likely to suffer frequent relapses. Using a list of relapse risk factors ('early warning signs') is one way to assess the client's progress in the community.

Families experience a wide variety of responses to the 'illness' of their loved one. Some family members might be ashamed or embarrassed or frightened of the client's strange or threatening behaviours. They worry about a relapse. They may feel guilty for having these feelings or fear for their own mental health or well-being. If the client experiences repeated and profound problems with schizophrenia, the family members may become emotionally exhausted or even alienated from the client, feeling they can no longer deal with the situation. Family members need ongoing support and education, including reassurance that they are not the cause of schizophrenia. Participating in organizations such as Rethink (known as Hafal in Wales), SANE or MIND may help families significantly.

Teaching Self-care and Proper Nutrition. Because of apathy or lack of energy over the course of their experiences, poor personal hygiene can be a problem for clients with schizophrenia. When the client is psychotic, he or she may pay little attention to hygiene or may be unable to sustain the attention or concentration required to complete grooming tasks. The nurse may need to direct the client through the necessary steps for bathing, shampooing, dressing and so forth. The nurse gives directions in short, clear statements to enhance the client's ability to complete the tasks. The nurse should allow ample time for grooming and performing hygiene and does not attempt to rush or hurry the client. In this way, the nurse encourages the client to become more independent as soon as possible – that is, when he or she is better oriented to reality and better able to sustain the concentration and attention needed for these tasks.

If the client has deficits in hygiene and grooming resulting from apathy or lack of energy for tasks, the nurse may vary the approach used to promote the client's independence in these areas. The client is most likely to perform tasks of hygiene and grooming if they become a part of his or her daily routine. The client who has an established structure that incorporates his or her preferences has a greater chance for success than the client who waits to decide about hygiene tasks or performs them randomly. For example, the client may prefer to shower and wash their hair on Monday, Wednesday and Friday when getting up in the morning. This nurse can assist the client to incorporate this plan into the client's daily routine, which leads to it becoming a habit. The client thus avoids making daily decisions about whether or not to shower or whether he or she feels like showering on a particular day.

Adequate nutrition and fluids are essential to the client's physical and emotional well-being. Careful assessment of the client's eating patterns and preferences allows the nurse to determine whether the client needs assistance in these areas. As with any type of self-care deficit, the nurse provides assistance as long as needed and then gradually promotes the client's independence as soon as the client is capable.

When the client is in the community, factors other than the client's 'illness' may contribute to inadequate nutritional intake. Examples include lack of money to buy food, lack of knowledge about a nutritious diet, inadequate transportation or limited abilities to prepare food.

Teaching Social Skills. Clients may be isolated from others for a variety of reasons. The bizarre behaviour or statements of the client who is delusional or hallucinating may frighten or embarrass family or community members. Clients who are suspicious or mistrustful may avoid contact with others. Other times, clients may lack the social or conversation skills they need to make and maintain relationships with others. A significant stigma remains attached to mental health problems, particularly for clients for whom medication and/or psychotherapy fail to relieve the positive signs.

The nurse can help the client develop social skills through education, role modelling and practice. The client may not discriminate between the topics suitable for sharing with the nurse and those suitable for initiating a conversation on a bus. The nurse can help the client learn neutral social topics appropriate to any conversation, such as the weather or local events. The client can also benefit from learning that he or she should share certain details of his or her illness, such as the content of delusions or hallucinations, only with a health-care provider.

Modelling and practising social skills with the client can help him or her experience greater success in social interactions. Specific skills such as eye contact, attentive listening and taking turns talking can increase the client's abilities and confidence in socializing.

Medication Management. Maintaining the medication regime is vital to a successful outcome for many clients with schizophrenia. Failing to take medications as prescribed is one of the most frequent reasons for recurrence of psychotic symptoms and hospital admission (Kane & Marder, 2005). Many clients who respond well to, and maintain, an antipsychotic medication regime may lead satisfying lives with only basic input from services. Some people who do not respond well to antipsychotic agents may face a lifetime of dealing with delusional ideas and hallucinations, negative signs and marked impairment. Many clients find themselves somewhere between these two extremes (see Client Education for Medication Management: Antipsychotics).

There are many reasons why clients may not maintain the medication regime. The nurse must determine the barriers

Nursing Care Plan *Client with Delusions*

Nursing Formulation

Disturbed Thought Processes: *Disruption in cognitive operations and activities*

ASSESSMENT DATA

- Thinking not apparently based in reality
- Disorientation
- Labile affect
- Short attention span
- Impaired judgement
- Distractibility

EXPECTED OUTCOMES

Immediate
The client will
- Be free of injury
- Demonstrate decreased anxiety level
- Respond to reality-based interactions initiated by others

Medium-term
The client will
- Interact on 'reality-based' topics
- Sustain attention and concentration to complete tasks or activities

Longer-term
The client will
- Verbalize recognition of delusional thoughts if they persist
- Be free from delusions or demonstrate the ability to function without responding to persistent delusional thoughts

IMPLEMENTATION

Nursing Interventions *denotes collaborative interventions

Nursing Interventions	Rationale
Be sincere and honest when communicating with the client. Avoid vague or evasive remarks.	Delusional clients are extremely sensitive about others and can recognize insincerity. Evasive comments or hesitation reinforces mistrust or delusions.
Be consistent in setting expectations, enforcing rules and so forth.	Clear, consistent limits provide a secure structure for the client.
Do not make promises that you cannot keep.	Broken promises reinforce the client's mistrust of others.
Encourage the client to talk with you, but do not pry for information.	Probing increases the client's suspicion and interferes with the therapeutic relationship.
Explain procedures, and try to be sure the client understands the procedures before carrying them out.	When the client has full knowledge of procedures, he or she is less likely to feel tricked by the staff.
Give positive feedback for the client's successes.	Positive feedback for genuine success enhances the client's sense of well-being and helps to make non-delusional reality a more positive situation for the client.
Recognize the client's 'delusions' as his or her perception of the environment.	Recognizing the client's perceptions can help you understand the feelings he or she is experiencing.
Initially, do not argue with the client or try to convince the client that delusions are false or unreal.	Logical argument does not dispel delusional ideas and can interfere with the development of trust.
Interact with the client on the basis of real things; do not dwell on the delusional material.	Interacting about reality is healthy for the client.

Nursing Care Plan: for a Client witt Delusions, cont.

IMPLEMENTATION

Nursing Interventions *denotes collaborative interventions	**Rationale**
Engage the client in one-to-one activities at first, then activities in small groups and gradually activities in larger groups.	A distrustful client can best deal with one person initially. Gradual introduction of others as the client tolerates is less threatening.
Recognize and support the client's accomplishments (projects completed, responsibilities fulfilled, interactions initiated).	Recognizing the client's accomplishments can lessen anxiety and the need for delusions as a source of self-esteem.
Show empathy regarding the client's feelings; reassure the client of your presence and acceptance.	The client's delusions can be distressing. Empathy conveys your caring, interest and acceptance of the client.
Do not be judgemental or belittle or joke about the client's beliefs.	The client's delusions and feelings are not funny to him or her. The client may not understand or may feel rejected by attempts at humour.
Never convey to the client that you accept the delusions as reality.	Indicating belief in the delusions reinforces the delusion (and the client's illness).
Directly interject doubt regarding delusions as soon as the client seems ready to accept this (e.g. 'I find that hard to believe.'). Do not argue but present a factual account of the situation as you see it.	As the client begins to trust you, he or she may become willing to doubt the delusion if you express your doubt.
Ask the client if he or she can see that the delusions interfere with or cause problems in his or her life.	Discussion of the problems caused by the delusions is a focus on the present and is reality based.

Adapted from Schultz, J. M. & Videbeck, S. L. (2005). *Lippincott's manual of psychiatric nursing care plans* (7th edn). Philadelphia: Lippincott Williams & Wilkins.

to concordance for each client. Sometimes clients intend to take their medications as prescribed but have difficulty remembering when and if they did so. They may find it difficult to adhere to a routine schedule for medications. Several methods are available to help clients remember when to take medications. One is using a pill box with compartments for days of the week and times of the day. After the box has been filled, perhaps with assistance from the nurse or case manager, the client often has no more difficulties. It is also helpful to make a chart of all administration times so that the client can cross off each time he or she has taken the medications.

Clients may have practical barriers to medication concordance, such as financial restrictions, lack of transport or knowledge about how to obtain repeat prescriptions or inability to plan ahead to get new prescriptions before current supplies run out. Clients can usually overcome all these obstacles once they have been identified.

Sometimes clients decide to decrease or discontinue their medications because they don't fully understand the rationale for the prescription or because of uncomfortable or embarrassing side-effects.

Unwanted side-effects are frequently reported as the reason clients stop taking medications (Kane & Marder, 2005). Interventions, such as eating a proper diet and drinking enough fluids, using a stool softener to avoid constipation, sucking on a sweet to minimize dry mouth or using sunscreen to avoid sunburn, can help to control some of these uncomfortable side-effects (see Table 14.2). Some side-effects, such as dry mouth and blurred vision, improve with time or with lower doses of medication. Medication may be warranted to combat common neurological side-effects such as extrapyramidal side-effects or akathisia.

Some side-effects, such as those affecting sexual functioning, are embarrassing for the client to report, and the client may confirm these side-effects only if the nurse directly enquires about them. This may require discussion with the prescriber in order to obtain a prescription for a different type of antipsychotic.

Sometimes a client discontinues medications because he or she dislikes taking them or believes he or she does not need them. The client may have been willing to take the medications when experiencing psychotic symptoms but may believe that medication is unnecessary when he or she feels well. By refusing to take the medication, the client may be denying the existence or severity of their mental health problem. These issues of non-concordance are much more difficult to resolve. The nurse can work with the client in understanding their experiences of schizophrenia and the importance of medications in managing symptoms and preventing recurrence. For example, the nurse could say, 'This medication should help you think more clearly' or 'Taking this medication should make it less likely that you'll hear troubling voices in your mind again.'

Even after collaborative exchange of information, some clients continue to refuse to take medication; they may understand the connection between medication and prevention of relapse only after experiencing a return of psychotic symptoms. A few clients still do not understand the importance of consistently taking medication and, even after numerous relapses, continue to experience psychosis and hospital admission fairly frequently; some fail to respond to medication at all.

Evaluation

The nurse must consider evaluation of the plan of care in the context of each client and family. Ongoing assessment provides data to determine whether the client's individual outcomes were achieved. The client's perception of the success of treatment also plays a part in evaluation. Even if all outcomes are achieved, the nurse must ask if the client is comfortable or satisfied with the quality of life.

In a global sense, evaluation of the treatment of schizophrenia is based on the following:

• Have the client's psychotic symptoms disappeared? If not, can the client carry out his or her daily life despite the persistence of some psychotic symptoms?
• Does the client understand the prescribed medication regime? Is he or she committed to adherence to the regime?
• Does the client possess the necessary functional abilities for satisfying community living?
• Are community resources adequate to help the client live successfully in the community?
• Is there a sufficient after-care or crisis plan in place to deal with recurrence of symptoms or difficulties encountered in the community?
• Are the client and family adequately knowledgeable about schizophrenia?
• Does the client believe that he or she has a satisfactory quality of life?

CONSIDERATIONS IN NURSING OLDER PEOPLE DIAGNOSED WITH SCHIZOPHRENIA

Late-onset schizophrenia refers to its development after the age of 45; schizophrenia is not initially diagnosed in elder clients. Psychotic symptoms that appear in later life are usually associated with depression or dementia, not schizophrenia. People with schizophrenia do survive into old age, with a variety of long-term outcomes. Jeste *et al.* (2004) reported that about 20% to 30% of the clients experienced dementia, resulting in a steady, deteriorating decline in health; 20% to 30% actually had a reduction in positive symptoms, somewhat like a remission; and schizophrenia remained mostly unchanged in the remaining clients.

CLIENT EDUCATION FOR MEDICATION MANAGEMENT: ANTIPSYCHOTICS

• Drink sugar-free fluids and eat sugar-free sweets to ease the anticholinergic effects of dry mouth.
• Avoid calorie-laden drinks and sweets because they promote dental caries, contribute to weight gain and do little to relieve dry mouth.
• Constipation can be prevented or relieved by increasing intake of water and bulk-forming foods in the diet and by exercising.
• Stool softeners are permissible, but laxatives should be avoided.
• Use sunscreen to prevent burning. Avoid long periods of time in the sun, and wear protective clothing. Photosensitivity can cause you to burn easily.
• Rising slowly from a lying or sitting position prevents falls from orthostatic hypotension or dizziness due to a drop

in blood pressure. Wait until any dizziness has subsided before you walk.
• Monitor the amount of sleepiness or drowsiness you experience. Avoid driving a car or performing other potentially dangerous activities until your response time and reflexes seem normal.
• If you forget a dose of antipsychotic medication, take it if the dose is only 3 to 4 hours late.
• If the missed dose is more than 4 hours late or the next dose is due, omit the forgotten dose.
• If you have difficulty remembering your medication, use a chart to record doses when taken, or use a pill box labelled with dosage times and/or days of the week to help you remember when to take medication.

COMMUNITY-BASED CARE

Clients with schizophrenia are no longer hospitalized for long periods. Most live in the community with assistance provided by family and support services. Clients may live with family members, independently, or in a residential programme such as a group home where they can receive needed services without being admitted to the hospital. Assertive outreach programmes have shown success in reducing the rate of hospital admissions by managing symptoms and medications; assisting clients with social, recreational and vocational needs; and providing support to clients and their families. The CMHN is a member of the multidisciplinary team that works with clients in a variety of community treatment programmes, focusing on psychological support and therapy, the management of medications and their side-effects and the promotion of health and wellness, and is usually the person undertaking the role of care co-ordinator. Recovery-focused care is, as mentioned, also expanding, with nurses providing care to people diagnosed with schizophrenia (as well as other mental health problems) using an holistic, optimistic and collaborative approach to people in the community.

Community mental health teams are an important link in helping people with schizophrenia and their families. The care co-ordinator should provide assistance in handling the wide variety of challenges that the client in community settings faces, and will link with other members of the multidisciplinary team to ensure that the person is receiving appropriate psychiatric, psychological and social support.

CMHT work often includes helping the client with housing and transportation, money management and keeping appointments, as well as with socialization and recreation. Frequent face-to-face and telephone contact with clients in the community helps to address clients' immediate and longer-term concerns and to avoid relapse and rehospitalization. Common concerns of clients include difficulties with treatment and after-care, dealing with psychiatric symptoms, environmental stresses and financial issues. Although the support of professionals in the community is vital, the nurse must not overlook the client's need for autonomy and potential abilities to manage his or her own health.

MENTAL HEALTH RECOVERY AND HEALTH PROMOTION

The principle of 'recovery' has an underlying philosophy for work with clients with major mental health problems that goes well beyond symptom control and medication management (see Chapter 4) and old ideas of health promotion and 'rehabilitation'. Working with people as equals to manage their own lives, make effective care and treatment decisions

NURSING INTERVENTIONS FOR CLIENTS DIAGNOSED WITH SCHIZOPHRENIA

- Promoting safety of client and others and right to privacy and dignity
- Establishing therapeutic relationship by establishing trust
- Using therapeutic communication (clarifying feelings and statements when speech and thoughts are disorganized or confused)
- Interventions for delusions:
  Do not openly confront the apparent delusion or argue with the client.
  Establish and maintain reality for the client.
  Use distracting techniques.
  Teach the client positive self-talk, positive thinking and to ignore delusional beliefs.
- Interventions for hallucinations:
  Help present and maintain reality by frequent respectful contact and communication with client.
  Elicit description of hallucination to protect client and others. The nurse's understanding of the hallucination helps him or her know how to calm or reassure the client.

  Engage client in reality-based activities such as card playing, occupational therapy or listening to music.
- Coping with socially inappropriate behaviours:
  Redirect client away from problem situations.
  Deal with inappropriate behaviours in a non-judgemental and matter-of-fact manner; give factual statements; do not scold or 'tell off'.
  Reassure others that the client's inappropriate behaviours or comments are not his or her fault (without violating client confidentiality).
  Try to reintegrate the client into the treatment milieu as soon as possible.
  Do not make the client feel punished or shunned for inappropriate behaviours.
  Teach social skills through education, role modelling and practice.
- Client and family teaching
- Establishing community support systems and care

and have an improved quality of life which has purpose and meaning are central components of the approach. Recovery principles involve optimism, hope and a genuine desire to collaborate with people and understand the meaning of their experiences. Mental health promotion within this approach, therefore, involves strengthening the client's ability to bounce back from adversity and to manage the inevitable obstacles encountered in life. Strategies included fostering self-efficacy and empowering the client to have control over his or her life; improving the client's resilience, or ability to bounce back emotionally from stressful events; and improving the client's ability to cope with the problems, stress and strains of everyday living. (see Chapter 7 for a full discussion of resilience and self-efficacy, ideas which overlap with recovery principles.)

SELF-AWARENESS ISSUES

Working with clients diagnosed with schizophrenia can present many challenges for the nurse. Clients have many experiences that may be difficult for the nurse to relate to, such as delusions and hallucinations. Suspicious or paranoid behaviour on the client's part may make the nurse feel as though he or she is not trustworthy, or that his or her integrity is being questioned. The nurse must recognize this type of behaviour as part of the illness and not interpret or respond to it as a personal affront. Taking the client's statements or behaviour as a personal accusation only causes the nurse to respond defensively, which is counterproductive to the establishment of a therapeutic relationship.

The nurse may also be genuinely frightened or threatened if the client's behaviour is hostile or aggressive. The nurse must acknowledge these feelings and take measures to ensure his or her safety without appearing to be rejecting of the client. This may involve talking to the client in an open area rather than in a more isolated location, or having an additional staff person present rather than being alone with the client. If the nurse pretends to be unafraid, the client may sense the fear anyway and feel less secure, leading to a greater potential for the client to lose personal control.

As with many mental health problems, the nurse may become frustrated if the client does not follow the medication regime, fails to keep needed appointments or experiences repeated relapses. The nurse may feel as though a great deal of hard work has been wasted or that the situation is futile or hopeless. Schizophrenia can be a debilitating condition, and clients may suffer numerous relapses and hospital admissions. The nurse must not take complete responsibility for the success or failure of treatment efforts or view the client's status as a personal success or failure.

Nurses should look to their colleagues for helpful support, supervision and discussion of these self-awareness issues.

Points to Consider When Working With Clients Diagnosed With Schizophrenia

- Remember that although some people with the diagnosis of schizophrenia may suffer numerous relapses and return for repeated hospital stays, most return to living and functioning well in the community. Focusing on the amount of time the client is outside the hospital setting may help decrease the frustration that can result when working with clients with seemingly long-term problems.
- Everyone has strengths, experience, resources and wisdom: work with people to identify theirs.
- Visualize the client not at his or her worst but as he or she gets better and symptoms become less severe.
- Remember that a client's hostile or paranoid remarks are not usually directed at you personally but are more likely a by-product of the disordered and confused thinking that schizophrenia causes. Nevertheless, don't dismiss a person's thoughts and feelings as merely a 'symptom': work with people to make sense of their views and beliefs about themselves, other people and the world.
- Discuss these issues with a more experienced nurse and in clinical supervision for suggestions on how to deal with your feelings and actions toward these clients. You are *not* expected to have all the answers.

KEY POINTS

- Schizophrenia is one of a number of conditions or disorders that can involve psychotic experiences.

Critical Thinking Questions

1. Clients who fail to take medication regularly or engage fully with services can often end up being admitted repeatedly, and this can become quite expensive. How do you reconcile the client's rights (to refuse treatment or medications) with the need to curtail avoidable health-care costs? What other legal or ethical issues are involved in this process?

2. If a client with schizophrenia who experiences frequent relapses has a young child, should the child remain with the parent? What factors influence this decision? Who should be able to make such a decision?

3. How does the nurse maintain a positive but honest relationship with a client's family if the client does not respond well to the care and treatment offered by the multidisciplinary team?

- Schizophrenia remains an area of great debate and controversy.
- Depression is common in people diagnosed with schizophrenia.
- One in 10 people with the diagnosis kill themselves.
- Schizophrenia can be something with which people live happily and satisfyingly.
- Schizophrenia is considered a clinical syndrome, often apparently involving brain changes that affect a person's planning and memory functions, thoughts, perceptions, emotions, movements and behaviours.
- Schizophrenia can require long-term care and management strategies and the development of new coping skills.
- The effects of schizophrenia on the client may be profound, involving all aspects of his or her life: social interactions, emotional health and ability to work and function in the community.
- Schizophrenia is conceptualized in terms of positive signs such as delusions, hallucinations and disordered thought processes, as well as negative signs such as social isolation, apathy, anhedonia and lack of motivation and volition.
- The clinical picture, prognosis and outcomes for clients diagnosed with schizophrenia vary widely. It is, therefore, important that each client is carefully and individually assessed regularly, in a collaborative, respectful way, with appropriate needs and interventions determined and agreed.
- Careful assessment of, and with, each client as an individual is essential to planning an effective plan of care.
- Families of clients diagnosed with schizophrenia may experience fear, embarrassment and guilt in response to their family member's condition. Families must be educated about the disorder, the course of the disorder and how it can be controlled.
- Failure to comply with treatment and the medication regime and the use of alcohol and other drugs are associated with poorer outcomes in the treatment of schizophrenia.
- For clients with psychotic symptoms, key nursing interventions include helping to protect the client's safety and right to privacy and dignity, dealing with socially inappropriate behaviours in a non-judgemental and matter-of-fact manner, helping present and maintain

reality for the client by frequent contact and communication and ensuring appropriate psychological therapy and medication administration.
- For the client whose condition is 'stabilized' with psychosocial support approaches and medication, key nursing interventions include continuing to maintain a supportive, non-confrontational therapeutic alliance, ensuring trust and trying to clarify the client's feelings and statements when speech and thoughts are disorganized or confused.
- Effective nursing also includes helping to develop social skills by modelling and practising, and helping to educate the client and family about schizophrenia and the importance of maintaining a therapeutic regime and other self-care behaviours.
- Self-awareness issues for the nurse working with clients with schizophrenia include the difficulties of maintaining optimism, dealing with psychotic symptoms, fear for personal safety and frustration as a result of relapses and repeated hospital admissions.

REFERENCES

American Psychiatric Association. (2000). *Diagnostic and statistical manual of mental disorders* (4th edn, text revision). Washington, DC: American Psychiatric Association.

Arseneault, L., Cannon, M., Witton, J., & Murray, R. (2004). Causal association between cannabis and psychosis: examination of the evidence. *British Journal of Psychiatry, 184*, 110–117.

Bechdolf, A., Phillips, L. J., Francey, S. M., *et al.* (2006a). Recent approaches to psychological interventions for people at risk of psychosis. *European Archives of Psychiatry and Clinical Neuroscience, 256*(3), 159–173.

Bechdolf, A., Ruhrmann, S., Wagner, M., *et al.* (2006b). Interventions in the prodromal states of psychosis in Germany: Concept and recruitment. *British Journal of Psychiatry, 48*(Suppl.), s45–48.

Bentall, R. (2004). *Madness explained: psychosis and human nature.* London: Penguin.

Birchwood, M., Spenser, E. & McGovern, D. (2000). Schizophrenia: early warning signs. *Advances in psychiatric treatment, 6*, 93–101.

Borgmann-Winter, K., Calkins, M. E., Kniele, K., & Gur, R. E. (2006). Assessment of adolescents at risk for psychosis. *Current Psychiatry Reports, 8*(4), 313–321.

Brown, A. S., Bresnahan, M., & Susser, E. S. (2005). Schizophrenia: environmental epidemiology. In B. J. Sadock & V. A. Sadock (Eds.), *Comprehensive textbook of psychiatry, Vol.1* (8th edn, pp. 1371–1380). Philadelphia: Lippincott Williams & Wilkins.

INTERNET RESOURCES

RESOURCES	INTERNET ADDRESS
HEARING VOICES NETWORK	http://www.hearing-voices.org/
CAMPAIGN FOR THE ABOLITION OF THE SCHIZOPHRENIA LABEL	http://www.caslcampaign.com/
RETHINK	www.rethink.org/
SANE	http://www.sane.org.uk/
VIRTUAL WARD: RECOVERY	http://www.virtualward.org.uk/recovery.html

Buchanan, R. W. & Carpenter, W. T. (2005). Concept of schizophrenia. In B. J. Sadock & V. A. Sadock (Eds.), *Comprehensive textbook of psychiatry, Vol. 1* (8th edn, pp. 1329–1345). Philadelphia: Lippincott Williams & Wilkins.

Care Services Improvement Partnership, Royal College of Psychiatrists and Social Care Institute for Excellence. (2007). *A common purpose: Recovery in future mental health services.* Available: http://www.scie.org.uk/publications/positionpapers/pp08.pdf

Carter, C. S. (2006). Editorial: Understanding the glass ceiling for functional outcome in schizophrenia. *American Journal of Psychiatry, 163*(3), 356–358.

Clinical Standards Board For Scotland. (2001). *Clinical standards: Schizophrenia.* Available: http://www.nhshealthquality.org/nhsqis/files/Schizophrenia%20jan%2001.pdf

Das, S.K., Malhotra, S., Basu, D., Malhotra, R. (2001). Testing the stress-vulnerability hypothesis in *ICD-10*-diagnosed acute and transient psychotic disorders. *Acta Psychiatry Scand*, 104, 56–58.

Department of Health. (2006). *From values to action: The Chief Nursing Officer's review of mental health nursing.* Available: http://www.dh.gov.uk/en/Publicationsandstatistics/Publications/PublicationsPolicyAndGuidance/DH_4133839

Gopal, Y. & Variand, H. (2005). First-episode schizophrenia: review of cognitive deficits and cognitive remediation. *Advances in Psychiatric Treatment, 11,* 38–44.

Hafner, H. & Maurer, K. (2006). Early detection of schizophrenia: current evidence and future perspectives. *World Psychiatry, 5*(3), 130–138.

Hagen, B. F. & Mitchell, D. L. (2001). Might within the madness: solution-focused therapy and thought-disordered clients. *Archives of Psychiatric Nursing, XV*(2), 86–93.

Hogarty, G. E., Greenwald, D. P., & Eack, S. M. (2006). Durability and mechanism of effects of cognitive enhancement therapy. *Psychiatric Services, 57*(12), 1751–1757.

Jeste, D. V., Dunn, L. B., & Lindamer, L. A. (2004). Psychoses. In J. Sadavoy, L. F. Jarvik, G. T. Grossberg, *et al.* (Eds.), *Comprehensive textbook of geriatric psychiatry* (3rd edn, pp. 655–685). New York: W. W. Norton.

Kane, J. M. & Marder, S. R. (2005). Schizophrenia: somatic treatment. In B. J. Sadock & V. A. Sadock (Eds.), *Comprehensive textbook of psychiatry, Vol. 1* (8th edn, pp. 1467–1476). Philadelphia: Lippincott Williams & Wilkins.

Kirkpatrick, B. & Tek, C. (2005). Schizophrenia: clinical features and psychopathology concepts. In B. J. Sadock & V. A. Sadock (Eds.), *Comprehensive textbook of psychiatry, Vol. 1* (8th edn, pp. 1416–1436). Philadelphia: Lippincott Williams & Wilkins.

Laing, R.D. (1990). The divided self: an existential study in sanity and madness. London: Penguin.

Marshall, M. & Rathbone, J. (2006). Early intervention for psychosis. *Cochrane Database of Systematic Review* [online], 4(CD004718).

Mojtabai, R. (2005). Culture-bound syndromes with psychotic features. In B. J. Sadock & V. A. Sadock (Eds.), *Comprehensive textbook of psychiatry, Vol. 1* (8th edn, pp. 1538–1541). Philadelphia: Lippincott Williams & Wilkins.

Morrison, A.P, Renton, J.C., Dunn, H., *et al.* (2004). Cognitive therapy for psychosis. A formulation-based approach. Hove: Brunner Routledge.

Morrison, A., Renton, J., French, P., & Bentall, R. (2008). *Think you're crazy? Think again: A resource book for cognitive therapy for psychosis.* London: Routledge

Mulholland, C. & Cooper, S. (2000). The symptom of depression in schizophrenia and its management. *Advances in Psychiatric Treatment, 6,* 169–177.

NICE. (2002). *Schizophrenia: core interventions in the treatment and management of schizophrenia in primary and secondary care.* Available: http://www.nice.org.uk/guidance/index.jsp?action=byID&r=true&o=10916

Penn, D. L., Wldheter, E. J., Perkins, D. O., Mueser, K. T., & Lieberman, J. A. (2005). Psychosocial treatment for first-episode psychosis: a research update. *American Journal of Psychiatry, 162*(12), 2220–2232.

Pfammatter, M., Junghan, U. M., & Brenner, H. D. (2006). Efficacy of psychological therapy in schizophrenia: Conclusions from meta-analysis. *Schizophrenia Bulletin, 32*(Suppl. 1), S64–S80.

RETHINK (2006). *Schizophrenia factsheet.* Available: http://www.mental-healthshop.org/products/rethink_publications/schizophrenia_factsh.html

Reynolds, S. A., Schmid, M., & Broome, M. E. (2004). Polydipsia screening tool. *Archives of Psychiatric Nursing, XVIII*(2), 49–59.

Riley, B. P. & Kendler, K. S. (2005). Schizophrenia: genetics. In B. J. Sadock & V. A. Sadock (Eds.), *Comprehensive textbook of psychiatry, Vol. 1* (8th edn, pp. 1354–1371). Philadelphia: Lippincott Williams & Wilkins.

Sass, L. (1993). *The paradoxes of delusion: Wittgenstein, Schreber, and the schizophrenic.* New York: Cornell University Press.

Sass, L. (1998). Schizophrenia, self-consciousness, and the modern mind. *Journal of Consciousness Studies, 5*(23), 543–565.

Savilla, K., Kettler, L., & Galletly, C. (2008). Relationships between cognitive deficits, symptoms and quality of life in schizophrenia. *Australian and New Zealand Journal of Psychiatry, 42*(6), 496–504.

Schneider-Axmann, T., Kamer, T.; Moroni, M., *et al.* (2006). Relation between cerebrospinal fluid, gray matter and white matter changes in families with schizophrenia. *Journal of Psychiatric Research, 40*(7), 646–655.

Scottish Government. (2006). *Rights, relationships and recovery: National review of mental health nursing.* Available: http://www.scotland.gov.uk/Publications/2006/04/18164814/0

SIGN. (1998). *Psychosocial interventions in the management of schizophrenia.* Available: http://www.sign.ac.uk/guidelines/fulltext/30/index.html

Simon, A. E., Dvorsky, D., Boesch, J., *et al.* (2006). Defining subjects at risk for psychosis: a comparison of two approaches. *Schizophrenia Research, 81*(1), 83–90.

Singh, S. & Fisher, H. (2005). Early intervention in psychosis: obstacles and opportunities. *Advances in Psychiatric Treatment, 11,* 71–78.

Szasz, T. (1984). The myth of mental illness: foundations of a theory of personal contact. Harper Perenniel.

van Meijel, B., van der Gaag, M., Kahn Sylvain, R. and Grypdonck, M. (2004). Recognition of early warning signs in patients with schizophrenia: a review of the literature. *International Journal of Mental Health Nursing, 13*(2), 107–116.

Velligan, D. I., Mueller, J., Wang, M., *et al.* (2006). Use of environmental supports among patients with schizophrenia. *Psychiatric Services, 57*(2), 219–224.

Wykes, T., Reader, C., Landau, S., *et al.* (2007). Cognitive remediation therapy in schizophrenia: randomised controlled trial. *British Journal of Psychiatry, 190,* 421–427.

Zubin, J. & Spring, B. (1977). Vulnerability – a new view of schizophrenia. *J of Advanced Psychology, 86*(2), 103–126.

ADDITIONAL READING

Hunt, I. M., Kapur, N., Windfuhr, K., *et al.* (2006). Suicide in schizophrenia: Findings from a national clinical survey. *Journal of Psychiatric Practice, 12*(3), 139–147.

Kane, J. M. (2006). Utilization of long-acting antipsychotic medication in patient care. *CNS Spectrums, 11*(Suppl. 12):14, 1–8.

Klam, J., McLay, M., & Grabke, D. (2006). Personal empowerment program: Addressing health concerns in people with schizophrenia. *Journal of Psychosocial Nursing, 44*(8), 20–28.

Kopelwicz, A., Liberman, R. P., & Zarate, R. (2006). Recent advances in social skills training for schizophrenia. *Schizophrenia Bulletin, 32*(Suppl. 1), S12–23.

NIMHE. (2004). *Emerging best practices in recovery.* Available: http://www.virtualward.org.uk/silo/files/emerging-best-practice-in-recoverypdf.pdf

Repper, J. & Perkins, R. (2003). *Social inclusion and recovery: A model for mental health practice.* Oxford: Bailliere Tindall.

Watkins, P. (2007). *Recovery: A guide for mental health practitioners.* Oxford: Butterworth-Heinemann.

Chapter Study Guide

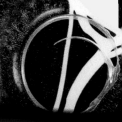

MULTIPLE-CHOICE QUESTIONS

Select the best answer for each of the following questions.

1. Which of the following are considered the positive signs of schizophrenia?
   a. Delusions, anhedonia, ambivalence
   b. Hallucinations, illusions, ambivalence
   c. Delusions, hallucinations, disordered thinking
   d. Disordered thinking, anhedonia, illusions

2. The family of a client with schizophrenia asks the nurse about the difference between conventional and atypical antipsychotic medications. The nurse's answer is based on which of the following?
   a. Atypical antipsychotics are newer medications but act in the same ways as conventional antipsychotics.
   b. Conventional antipsychotics are dopamine antagonists; atypical antipsychotics inhibit the reuptake of serotonin.
   c. Conventional antipsychotics have serious side-effects; atypical antipsychotics have virtually no side-effects.
   d. Atypical antipsychotics are dopamine and serotonin antagonists; conventional antipsychotics are only dopamine antagonists.

3. The nurse is planning a pre-discharge conversation with a client about taking clozapine (Clozaril). Which of the following is essential to include?
   a. Caution the client not to be outdoors in the sunshine without protective clothing.
   b. Remind the client of the importance of having blood taken and staying in contact with the care co-ordinator.
   c. Instruct the client about dietary restrictions.
   d. Give the client a chart to record a daily pulse rate.

4. Which of the following statements would indicate that family teaching about schizophrenia had been effective?
   a. 'If our son takes his medication properly, he won't have another psychotic episode.'
   b. 'I guess we'll have to face the fact that our daughter will eventually be in care permanently.'
   c. 'It's a relief to find out that we did not cause our son's schizophrenia.'
   d. 'It is a shame our daughter will never be able to have children.'

5. When the client describes fear of leaving his flat as well as the desire to get out and meet others, it is called
   a. Ambivalence
   b. Anhedonia
   c. Alogia
   d. Avoidance

6. The client who hesitates 30 seconds before responding to any question is described as having
   a. Blunted affect
   b. Latency of response
   c. Paranoid delusions
   d. Poverty of speech

7. The overall goal of working with someone with a diagnosis of schizophrenia should be:
   a. Control of symptoms
   b. Freedom from hospitalization
   c. Establishing a full, satisfying life
   d. Recovery from the illness

FILL-IN-THE-BLANK QUESTIONS

Identify the type of speech pattern exhibited for each of the following client statements.

_____ 1. 'Do you have any phletz here? I like phletz.'

_____ 2. 'It's time to eat, to eat, to eat.'

_____ 3. 'Mountains, tigers, pie, singing, spring.'

_____ 4. 'Is that clock or a sock, can the door lock, tick tock.'

GROUP DISCUSSION TOPICS

Discuss:

1. The concept of 'optimism' in working with people with schizophrenia: how realistic is it?

2. 'Insight': are any of us ever fully insightful?

3. Would you take a drug that got rid of tormenting voices but affected the way you walked and talked?

For each of the following client statements, agree a response the nurse might make and the rationale for the nurse's response.

4. 'I can't live in my flat anymore because it's bugged by MI5.'

5. 'Have they told you why I'm here in the hospital?'

6. 'I can feel my stomach rotting away.'

7. 'I must do what God tells me to do.'

CLINICAL EXAMPLE

John Jones, 33, has been admitted to the hospital for the third time with a diagnosis of paranoid schizophrenia. John had been taking haloperidol (Haldol) but stopped taking it 2 weeks ago, telling his CPN it was 'the poison that's making me sick'. Yesterday, John was brought to the hospital after neighbours called the police because he had been up all night yelling loudly in his apartment. Neighbours reported him saying, 'I can't do it! They don't deserve to die!' and similar statements.

John appears guarded and suspicious and has very little to say to anyone. His hair is matted, he has a strong body odour and he is dressed in several layers of heavy clothing even though the temperature is warm. So far, John has been refusing any offers of food or fluids. When the nurse approaches John with a dose of haloperidol, he said, 'Do you want me to die?'

1. What additional assessment data does the nurse need to plan care for John?

2. Identify the three priorities, nursing formulations and expected outcomes for John's care, with your rationales for the choices.

3. Identify at least two nursing interventions for the three priorities listed above.

4. What community referrals or supports might be beneficial for John when he is discharged?

Chapter

15

Mood Disorders

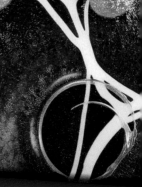

Key Terms

- affect
- anergia
- anhedonia
- automatic thoughts
- clinical supervision
- collaboration
- core beliefs
- electroconvulsive therapy (ECT)
- cognitive-behavioural therapy (CBT)
- engagement
- euthymic
- flight of ideas
- hypertensive crisis
- hypomania
- kindling
- labile emotions
- latency of response
- mania
- mindfulness-based cognitive therapy
- mood disorders
- non-judgemental
- pressured speech
- psychomotor agitation
- psychomotor retardation
- ruminations
- seasonal affective disorder (SAD)
- suicidal ideation
- suicide
- suicide precautions
- validation

Learning Objectives

After reading this chapter, you should be able to:

1. Be more aware of the impact of mood disorders on people.

2. Discuss aetiological theories of depression and bipolar disorder.

3. Describe safety and risk factors for, and the characteristics of, mood disorders.

4. Apply the nursing process to the care of clients and families with mood disorders.

5. Work psycho-educationally with clients, families, carers and the general public to increase knowledge and understanding of mood disorders.

6. Identify people and populations at risk of suicide.

7. Apply the nursing process to the care of a suicidal person.

8. Evaluate your feelings, beliefs and attitudes regarding mood disorders and suicide.

Everyone occasionally feels sad, low and tired, with the desire to stay in bed and shut out the world. These episodes are often accompanied by **anergia** (lack of energy), exhaustion, agitation, noise intolerance and slowed thinking processes, all of which make decisions difficult. Work, family and social responsibilities drive most of us to get on with our daily routines, even when nothing seems to be going right and our irritability or low mood is obvious to all. Such periods usually pass in a few days, and energy returns. Fluctuations in mood are so common to the human condition that we think nothing of hearing someone say, 'I'm feeling depressed – everything seems to be going wrong at the moment.' Yet this everyday use of the word *depressed* doesn't necessarily mean the person is *clinically* depressed but, rather, that the person is experiencing a temporary shift in thoughts, feelings and behaviour that is a 'normal' part of life. Sadness in mood can also be a response to loss or perceived trauma: death of a friend or relative, financial problems or loss of a job may cause a person to grieve (see Chapter 12).

At the other end of the mood spectrum are episodes of exaggeratedly energetic behaviour. The person has absolute confidence that he or she can take on any task or relationship. In an elated mood, stamina for work, family and social events is untiring. This feeling of being 'on top of the world' also usually recedes in a few days to a **euthymic** mood (average affect and activity). Happy events can stimulate this joy and short-term enthusiasm and these mood alterations are again normal, do not interfere meaningfully with the person's life and are not a sign of 'disorder'.

Mood disorders, also called affective disorders, on the other hand, are *pervasive* alterations in emotions that are manifested by depression, mania or both. They interfere with a person's life, plaguing him or her with drastic and long-term sadness, agitation or elation. Accompanying self-doubt, guilt and anger alter life activities, especially those that involve self-esteem, occupation and relationships.

From early history, people have suffered from mood disturbances. Archaeologists have found holes drilled into ancient skulls to relieve the 'evil humors' of those suffering from sad feelings and strange behaviours. Babylonians and ancient Hebrews believed that overwhelming sadness and extreme behaviour were sent to people through the will of God or other divine beings. Biblical notables – King Saul, King Nebuchadnezzar and Moses – suffered overwhelming 'grief of heart', 'unclean spirits' and 'bitterness of soul', all of which could be seen as symptoms of depression. Both Abraham Lincoln and Queen Victoria had recurrent episodes of depression. Other famous people who've experienced mood disorders include Britney Spears, Sylvia Plath, Jim Carrey, Stephen Fry, George Frideric Handel, Kate Moss, Amy Winehouse, Vincent Van Gogh, Friedrich Nietzsche.

Until the mid-1950s, treatment available to help people with serious depression or mania was *ad hoc*, scattered, poorly evidenced and dependent on income. People often suffered alone through their altered moods, thinking they were hopelessly weak for succumbing to these devastating symptoms. Families and mental health professionals tended to agree, seeing sufferers as egocentric, self-indulgent or simply viewing life negatively: they should just 'snap out of it'.

Over the past few decades, more effective and focused treatments – psychotherapeutic and pharmacological – for both depression and mania have, thankfully, become available.

Mood disorders are the most common psychiatric diagnoses associated with suicide; depression is one of the most important risk factors for it (Sudak, 2005). For that reason, this chapter focuses on major depression, bipolar disorder *and* suicide. It is important to note that clients with schizophrenia, substance use disorders, antisocial and borderline personality disorders and panic disorders are also at increased risk of suicide and suicide attempts. We should recognize, also, that depression (like so many mental health problems) rarely manifests in a 'pure' form: anxiety is frequently a common part of the experience of people diagnosed as 'depressed'. According to the Office for National Statistics (2001), 'mixed anxiety and depression is the most common mental disorder in Britain, with almost 9% of people meeting criteria for diagnosis'.

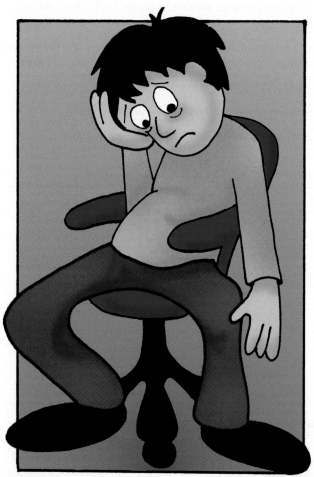

Anergia

CATEGORIES OF MOOD DISORDER

The primary mood disorders are depression and bipolar affective disorder (formerly called manic-depressive illness or manic depression).

Depression

In the UK, depression is frequently referred to as 'mild', 'moderate' or 'severe', in line with *ICD-10* (Box 15.1). In typical mild, moderate, or severe depressive episodes, the patient suffers from lowering of mood, reduction of energy and decrease in activity. Capacity for enjoyment, interest and concentration is reduced, and marked tiredness after even minimum effort is common. Sleep is usually disturbed and appetite diminished. Self-esteem and self-confidence are almost always reduced and, even in the mild form, some ideas of guilt or worthlessness are often present. The lowered mood varies little from day to day, is unresponsive to circumstances and may be accompanied by so-called 'somatic' symptoms, such as loss of interest and pleasurable feelings, waking in the morning several hours before the usual time, depression worst in the morning, marked psychomotor retardation, agitation, loss of appetite, weight loss and loss of libido. Depending upon the number and severity of the symptoms, a depressive episode may be specified as mild, moderate or severe.

Bipolar Affective Disorder

Bipolar affective disorder is a disorder characterized by two or more episodes in which the patient's mood and activity levels are significantly disturbed, this disturbance consisting, on some occasions, of an elevation of mood and increased energy and activity (hypomania or mania) and, on others, of a lowering of mood and decreased energy and activity (depression). Repeated episodes of hypomania or mania only are also classified as bipolar.

According to *ICD-10*, **mania** occurs when 'mood is elevated out of keeping with the patient's circumstances and may vary from carefree joviality to almost uncontrollable excitement. Elation is accompanied by increased energy, resulting in overactivity, pressure of speech and a decreased need for sleep. Attention cannot be sustained, and there is often marked distractibility. Self-esteem is often inflated with grandiose ideas and overconfidence. Loss of normal social inhibitions may result in behaviour that is reckless, foolhardy or inappropriate to the circumstances and out of character'. Some people also exhibit delusions and hallucinations during a manic episode (in which case *ICD-10* refers to 'mania with psychotic symptoms' rather than 'mania without psychotic symptoms').

Hypomania is 'a disorder characterized by a persistent mild elevation of mood, increased energy and activity, and usually marked feelings of well-being and both physical and mental efficiency. Increased sociability, talkativeness, over-familiarity, increased sexual energy and a decreased need for sleep are often present but not to the extent that they lead to severe disruption of work or result in social rejection. Irritability, conceit and boorish behaviour may take the place of the more usual euphoric sociability. The disturbances of mood and behaviour are not accompanied by hallucinations or delusions' (http://www.who.int/classifications/apps/icd/icd10online/).

RELATED DISORDERS

Postnatal Disorders

Postnatal (or 'postpuerperal') disorders that involve changes in mood include the following:

- '*Baby blues*' are a frequent, normal experience after delivery of a baby. They are characterized by labile mood and affect, crying spells, sadness, insomnia and anxiety. Symptoms begin approximately 1 day after delivery, usually peak in 3–7 days and disappear rapidly with no medical treatment (Sit *et al.*, 2006).

Box 15.1 DEPRESSIVE EPISODE

Over a period of at least 2 weeks:

F32.0 **Mild depressive episode:** Two or three of the above symptoms are usually present. The patient is usually distressed by these but will probably be able to continue with most activities.

F32.1 **Moderate depressive episode:** Four or more of the above symptoms are usually present and the patient is likely to have great difficulty in continuing with ordinary activities.

F32.2 **Severe depressive episode without psychotic symptoms:** An episode of depression in which several of the above symptoms are marked and distressing, typically loss of self-esteem and ideas of worthlessness or guilt. Suicidal thoughts and acts are common and a number of 'somatic' symptoms are usually present.

F32.3 **Severe depressive episode with psychotic symptoms:** An episode of depression as described in F32.2, but with the presence of hallucinations, delusions, psychomotor retardation or stupor so severe that ordinary social activities are impossible; there may be danger to life from suicide, dehydration or starvation. The hallucinations and delusions may or may not be mood-congruent.

Adapted from http://www.who.int/classifications/apps/icd/icd10online/

- As well as the *ICD-10* and *DSM-IV* definitions, a number of 'looser' working definitions of postnatal depression are used. Broadly, in the UK, 'postnatal depression' is seen as a depression that meets all the criteria for clinical depression but with an onset within 6–12 weeks of delivery. An additional, and hugely significant, element in postnatal depression is, often, guilt about the mother's ability to look after or to bond with the baby.
- Affecting between 1 in 500 and 1 in 1000 mothers, postnatal (or 'postpartum') psychosis is a potentially life-threatening psychotic episode developing within 3 weeks of delivery and beginning with fatigue, sadness, emotional lability, poor memory and confusion, and progressing to delusions, hallucinations, poor insight and judgement and loss of contact with reality. This psychiatric emergency requires immediate treatment: the disorder can lead to harm to baby, mother or both (Sit *et al.*, 2006).

Seasonal Affective Disorder

Seasonal affective (or **'seasonal depressive'**) **disorder (SAD)** is a disorder in which depression seems to occur seasonally – usually beginning in late autumn and becoming worse in the winter and improving in spring and the summer.

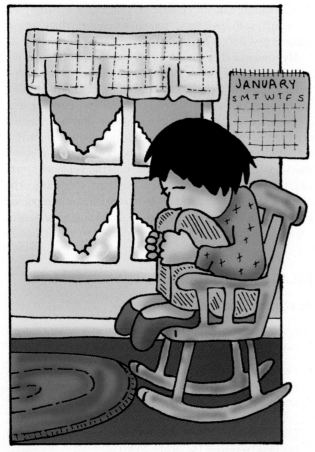

Anergia

AETIOLOGY

Various theories for the aetiology of mood disorders exist. Most recent research focuses on chemical biological imbalances as the cause. Nevertheless, psychosocial stressors and interpersonal events appear to trigger certain physiological and chemical changes in the brain, which significantly alter the balance of neurotransmitters (Akiskal, 2005). It is important to note that – where there is a chemical imbalance in the brain – there are a number of ways in which balance can be restored.

There seems little doubt that psychological treatments – in particular **cognitive-behavioural therapy (CBT)** and **mindfulness-based cognitive therapy** – have an increasingly impressive evidence base for their efficacy in depression. There is some evidence that – in terms of preventing relapse – they have a clear advantage over pharmacological approaches (Teasdale *et al.*, 2000; Segal *et al.*, 2002; Ma & Teasdale, 2004; NICE, 2007).

Effective treatment addresses both the biological *and* psychosocial components of mood disorders, and nurses need a sound knowledge of both perspectives when working with clients experiencing these disorders.

Biological Theories

GENETIC THEORIES

Genetic studies implicate the transmission of major depression in first-degree relatives, who have twice the risk for developing depression compared with the general population (American Psychiatric Association, 2000). First-degree relatives of people with bipolar disorder have a 3% to 8% risk of developing bipolar disorder, compared with a 1% risk in the general population. For all mood disorders, monozygotic (identical) twins have a concordance rate (both twins having the disorder) two to four times higher than that of dizygotic (fraternal) twins. Although heredity is a significant factor, the concordance rate for monozygotic twins is not 100%, so genetics alone do not account for all mood disorders (Kelsoe, 2005).

NEUROCHEMICAL THEORIES

Neurochemical influences of neurotransmitters (chemical messengers) focus on serotonin and noradrenaline as the two major biogenic amines implicated in mood disorders. Serotonin has many roles in behaviour: mood, activity, aggressiveness and irritability, cognition, pain, biorhythms and neuroendocrine processes (i.e. growth hormone, cortisol and prolactin levels are abnormal in depression). Deficits of serotonin, its precursor tryptophan or a metabolite (5-hydroxyindole acetic acid, or 5-HIAA) of serotonin found in the blood or cerebrospinal fluid occur in people with depression. Positron emission tomography demonstrates reduced metabolism in the prefrontal cortex, which may promote depression (Tecott & Smart, 2005).

Noradrenaline levels may be deficient in depression and increased in mania. This catecholamine energizes the body to mobilize during stress and inhibits kindling. **Kindling** is the process by which seizure activity in a specific area of the brain is initially stimulated by reaching a threshold of the cumulative effects of stress, low amounts of electric impulses or chemicals such as cocaine that sensitize nerve cells and pathways. These highly sensitized pathways respond by no longer needing the stimulus to induce seizure activity, which now occurs spontaneously. It is theorized that kindling may underlie the cycling of mood disorders as well as addiction. Anticonvulsants inhibit kindling; this may explain their efficacy in the treatment of bipolar disorder (Akiskal, 2005).

Dysregulation of acetylcholine and dopamine also are being studied in relation to mood disorders. Cholinergic drugs alter mood, sleep, neuroendocrine function and the electroencephalographic pattern; therefore, acetylcholine seems to be implicated in depression and mania. The neurotransmitter problem may not be as simple as under-production or depletion through overuse during stress. Changes in the sensitivity, as well as the number, of receptors are being evaluated for their roles in mood disorders (Tecott & Smart, 2005).

NEUROENDOCRINE INFLUENCES

Hormonal fluctuations are being studied in relation to depression. Mood disturbances have been documented in people with endocrine disorders, such as those of the thyroid, adrenal, parathyroid and pituitary. Elevated glucocorticoid activity is associated with the stress response, and evidence of increased cortisol secretion is apparent in about 40% of clients with depression, with the highest rates found among older clients. Postpartum hormone alterations precipitate mood disorders such as postpartum depression and psychosis. About 5% to 10% of people with depression have thyroid dysfunction, notably an elevated thyroid-stimulating hormone. This problem must be corrected with thyroid treatment, or treatment for the mood disorder is affected adversely (Thase, 2005).

Cognitive-Behavioural Theories

- The concept of 'an invalidating environment' – one in which children grow up in a world that ignores or punishes them for any display of emotion, which involves an absence of, or an unpredictability or uncertainty about, attention from and security provided by adults, in which there is direct and indirect neglect and abuse (emotional, physical and/or sexual) – is used to describe one of the key foundations for susceptibility for a number of mental health problems, including depression.
- Beck, Linehan and others see depression as resulting from specific cognitive distortions in susceptible people. Early invalidating experiences shape these distorted ways of thinking – **core beliefs** – about one's self, the world

and the future; these distortions involve magnification of negative events, traits and expectations and the simultaneous minimization of anything positive. Such thinking affects behaviour and affect, and a vicious cycle of low mood, avoidance and reinforcement develops, trapping people in an approach to themselves and others that embeds the depression further.

Psychodynamic Theories

- Freud looked at the self-deprecation of people with depression and attributed that self-reproach to anger turned inward, related to either a real or perceived loss. Feeling abandoned by this loss, people became angry while both loving and hating the lost object.
- Bibring believed that one's ego (or self) aspired to be ideal (i.e. good and loving, superior or strong) and that to be loved and worthy, one must achieve these high standards. Depression results when, in reality, the person is not able to achieve these ideals all the time.
- Jacobson compared the state of depression to a situation in which the ego is a powerless, helpless child victimized by the superego, much like a powerful and sadistic mother who takes delight in torturing the child.
- Most psychoanalytical theories of mania view manic episodes as a 'defence' against underlying depression, with the id taking over the ego and acting as an undisciplined hedonistic being (child).
- Meyer viewed depression as a reaction to a distressing life experience.
- Horney believed that children raised by rejecting or unloving parents were prone to feelings of insecurity and loneliness, making them susceptible to depression and helplessness.

CULTURAL CONSIDERATIONS

Other behaviours considered 'age-appropriate' can mask depression, which makes the disorder difficult to identify and diagnose in certain age groups. Children with depression often appear irritable and difficult. They may have school phobia, hyperactivity, learning disorders, failing grades and antisocial behaviours. Adolescents with depression may abuse substances, join gangs, engage in risky behaviour, be underachievers or drop out of school. In adults, manifestations of depression can include substance abuse, eating disorders, compulsive behaviours such as being a workaholic and gambling, and hypochondriasis. Older adults who are 'cranky' and argumentative may actually be depressed.

Many somatic ailments (physiological ailments) accompany depression. This manifestation varies among cultures and is more apparent in cultures that avoid verbalizing emotions. For example, some Asian people who are anxious or depressed are more likely to have somatic complaints of headache, backache or other symptoms; people from some Latin cultures may complain of 'nerves' or headaches; some people from Middle Eastern cultures complain of heart problems (Andrews & Boyle, 2003).

DEPRESSION

Clinical depression affects around one person in five in their lifetime and is roughly twice as common in women as men. According to the Mental Health Foundation (2008) '1 in 4 women will require treatment for depression at some time, compared to 1 in 10 men . . . It has also been suggested that depression in men may have been under-diagnosed because they present to their GP with different symptoms'. Between 8% and 12% of the UK population experience depression in any year (Office for National Statistics, 2001).

There is a 1.5 to 3 times greater incidence in first-degree relatives than in the general population. Incidence of depression may decrease with age in women and increase with age in men. The highest risk groups for depression are separated men, widowed men, separated women and divorced women. The lowest risk groups are married men, followed by married women. Depression is high amongst the homeless, the unemployed, prisoners and those with drug and alcohol problems.

Onset and Clinical Course

An untreated episode of depression can last 6 to 24 months before remitting. Fifty to sixty per cent of people who have one episode of depression will have another. After a second episode of depression, there is a 70% chance of recurrence. Depressive symptoms can vary from mild to severe. The degree of depression is comparable with the person's sense of helplessness and hopelessness (American Psychiatric Association, 2000).

Care, Treatment and Prognosis

The NICE guideline on depression (NICE, 2007) recommends that for mild and moderate depression, psychological treatments specifically focused on depression (such as problem-solving therapy, CBT and counselling) can be as effective as drug treatments, and should be offered as treatment options.

The guideline also recommends that:

- Antidepressants should not be used for the initial treatment of mild depression, because the risk–benefit ratio is poor.
- When an antidepressant is prescribed for moderate or severe depression it should be a SSRI, because SSRIs are as effective as tricyclic antidepressants and their use is less likely to be discontinued because of side-effects.
- All patients prescribed antidepressants should be informed that, although the drugs are not associated with tolerance and craving, discontinuation/withdrawal symptoms may occur on stopping or missing doses or, occasionally, on reducing the dose of the drug.
- Screening should be carried out for all high-risk groups; for example, those with a past history of depression, significant physical illnesses causing disability or other mental health problems such as dementia.
- For severe depression, psychological treatment (specifically CBT) should be used in combination with antidepressant medication.

CLINICAL VIGNETTE: DEPRESSION

'Just get out! I don't want any food – I'm not interested in it,' said Chris to her husband, Matt, who had come into their bedroom to invite her to the dinner he and their daughters had prepared. 'Can't they just leave me alone?' she thought to herself as she miserably pulled the covers over her shoulders. Yet she felt guilty about the way she'd snapped at Matt. She knew she was constantly rejecting her family's efforts to help, but she couldn't stop.

She was physically and emotionally exhausted. 'I can't remember when I felt well . . . maybe last year sometime – maybe never,' she thought, fretfully. She'd always worked hard to get things done; lately, she couldn't do anything at all except complain. Kathy, her 13-year-old, accused her of hating everything and everybody, including her family. Linda, 11 years old, said, 'Everything has to be your way, Mum. You snap at us for every little thing. You never listen anymore.' Matt had long ago withdrawn from her moodiness, her acid tongue and her disinterest in sex.

One day, she overheard Matt tell his brother that Chris was 'grumpy, agitated, and self-centred and if it wasn't for the girls, I don't know what I'd do. I've tried to get her to go to a doctor, but she says it's all our fault, then she sulks for days. What's our fault? I don't know what to do for her. I feel as if I am living in a minefield and never know what will set off an explosion. I try to remember the love we had together, but her behaviour is getting old.'

Chris has lost 12 pounds in the past 2 months, has difficulty sleeping, and is hostile, angry and guilty about it. She has no desire for any pleasure. 'Why bother? There's nothing to enjoy. Life is so bleak.' She feels stuck, worthless, hopeless and helpless. Hoping against hope, Chris thinks to herself, 'I wish I were dead. I'd never have to do anything again.'

PSYCHOPHARMACOLOGY

It is important to be aware of the findings of Kirsch *et al.* (2008), referred to in Chapter 3: their large review of SSRI clinical trial data concluded that, in all but the most severe cases, antidepressants were no more effective than placebos. Nurses need to stay aware of this research and subsequent findings and be able to advise clients accordingly.

Major categories of antidepressants include cyclic antidepressants, MAOIs, SSRIs and atypical antidepressants. Chapter 3 details biological treatments. The choice of which antidepressant to use is based on the client's symptoms, age and physical health needs; drugs that have or have not worked in the past, or that have worked for a blood relative with depression; and other medications that the client is taking.

Researchers believe that levels of neurotransmitters, especially noradrenaline and serotonin, are decreased in depression. Usually, presynaptic neurons release these neurotransmitters to allow them to enter synapses and link with postsynaptic receptors. Depression results if too few neurotransmitters are released, if they linger too briefly in synapses, if the releasing presynaptic neurons reabsorb them too quickly, if conditions in synapses do not support linkage with postsynaptic receptors or if the number of postsynaptic receptors has decreased. The goal is to increase the efficacy of available neurotransmitters and the absorption by postsynaptic receptors. To do so, antidepressants establish a blockade for the reuptake of noradrenaline and serotonin into their specific nerve terminals. This permits them to linger longer in synapses and to be more available to postsynaptic receptors. Antidepressants also increase the sensitivity of the postsynaptic receptor sites (Rush, 2005).

In clients who have acute depression with psychotic features, an antipsychotic is often used in combination with an antidepressant. The antipsychotic treats the psychotic features; several weeks into treatment, the client is reassessed to determine whether the antipsychotic can be withdrawn and the antidepressant maintained.

There is some evidence that antidepressant therapy should continue for longer than the 3 to 6 months originally believed necessary. Fewer relapses seem to occur in people with depression who receive 18 to 24 months of antidepressant therapy.

NICE guidelines suggest that SSRIs should normally be the first drug intervention in moderate and severe

Table 15.1 SELECTIVE SEROTONIN REUPTAKE INHIBITOR (SSRI) ANTIDEPRESSANTS*

Generic (Trade) Name	Possible Side-effects (not exclusive: others possible)	Nursing Implications
Fluoxetine (Prozac)	Headache, nervousness, anxiety, sedation, tremor, sexual dysfunction, anorexia, constipation, nausea, diarrhoea, weight gain or weight loss, rash	Administer in AM (if nervous) or PM (if drowsy) Monitor for hyponatremia Encourage adequate fluids Report sexual difficulties to doctor If rash: discontinue
Sertraline (Lustral)	Dizziness, sedation, headache, insomnia, tremor, sexual dysfunction, diarrhoea, dry mouth and throat, nausea, vomiting, sweating	Administer in PM if client is drowsy Encourage use of sugar-free beverages or hard sweets Drink adequate fluids Monitor hyponatremia; report sexual difficulties to doctor
Paroxetine (Seroxat)	Dizziness, sedation, headache, insomnia, weakness, fatigue, constipation, dry mouth and throat, nausea, vomiting, diarrhoea, sweating	Administer with food Administer in PM if client is drowsy Encourage use of sugar-free hard sweets or beverages Encourage adequate fluids
Citalopram (Cipramil)	Drowsiness, sedation, insomnia, nausea, vomiting, weight gain, constipation, diarrhoea	Monitor for hyponatraemia Administer with food Administer dose at 6 PM or later Promote balanced nutrition and exercise
Escitalopram (Cipralex)	Drowsiness, dizziness, weight gain, sexual dysfunction, restlessness, dry mouth, headache, nausea, diarrhoea	Check orthostatic blood pressure Assist client to rise slowly from sitting position Encourage use of sugar-free beverages or hard sweets Administer with food
Fluvoxamine (Faverin)	As above; palpitations, tachycardia	Monitor blood pressure

*Less sedating and have fewer antimuscarinic and cardiotoxic effects than tricyclic antidepressants.
Adapted from British National Formulary Online. (2008). http://www.bnf.org/bnf/bnf/55/

depression, though venlafaxine, at a dose of 150 mg or greater, may also be more effective than SSRIs for major depression of at least moderate severity (British National Formulary Online, 2008).

As a rule, antidepressants should be tapered before being discontinued.

Selective Serotonin Reuptake Inhibitors. SSRIs, the newest category of antidepressants (Table 15.1), are effective for most clients. Their action is specific to serotonin reuptake inhibition; these drugs produce few sedating, anticholinergic and cardiovascular side-effects, which make them safer for use in older adults. Because of their low side-effects and relative safety, people using SSRIs are more apt to be compliant with the treatment regime than clients using more troublesome medications. Insomnia should decrease in 3 to 4 days, appetite return to a more normal state in 5 to 7 days and energy return in 4 to 7 days. In 7 to 10 days, mood, concentration and interest in life should improve.

Fluoxetine (Prozac) produces a slightly higher rate of mild agitation and weight loss but less somnolence. It has a half-life of more than 7 days, which differs from the 25-hour half-life of other SSRIs.

Cyclic Antidepressants. Tricyclics, first introduced for the treatment of depression in the mid-1950s, are the oldest antidepressants. They can relieve symptoms of hopelessness, helplessness, anhedonia, inappropriate guilt, suicidal ideation and daily mood variations (feeling bad in the morning and better in the evening). Other indications include panic disorder, OCD and eating disorders. Each drug has a different degree of efficacy in blocking the activity of noradrenaline and serotonin or increasing the sensitivity of postsynaptic receptor sites. Tricyclic and heterocyclic antidepressants have a lag period of 10 to 14 days before reaching a serum level that begins to alter symptoms; they take 6 weeks to reach full effect. Because they have a long serum half-life, there is a lag period of 1 to 4 weeks before steady plasma levels are reached and the client's symptoms begin to lessen. They cost less primarily because they have been around longer and generic forms are available.

Table 15.2	TRICYCLIC ANTIDEPRESSANT MEDICATIONS	
Generic (Trade) Name	**Side-effects**	**Nursing Implications**
Amitriptyline	Dizziness, orthostatic hypotension, tachycardia, sedation, headache, tremor, blurred vision, constipation, dry mouth and throat, weight gain, urinary hesitancy, sweating	Assist client to rise slowly from sitting position Administer at bedtime Encourage use of sugar-free drinks and hard sweets Ensure adequate fluids and balanced nutrition Encourage exercise Monitor cardiac function
Clomipramine (Anafranil)	Dizziness, orthostatic hypotension, sedation, insomnia, constipation, dry mouth and throat, rashes	Assist client to rise slowly from sitting position Administer at bedtime if client is sedated Ensure adequate fluids Encourage use of sugar-free drinks and hard sweets Report rashes to doctor
Doxepin (Sinepin)	Dizziness, orthostatic hypotension, tachycardia, sedation, blurred vision, constipation, dry mouth and throat, weight gain, sweating	Assist client to rise slowly from sitting position Administer at bedtime if client is sedated Ensure adequate fluids and balanced nutrition Encourage use of sugar-free drinks and hard sweets Encourage exercise
Imipramine (Tofranil)	Dizziness, orthostatic hypotension, weakness, fatigue, blurred vision, constipation, dry mouth and throat, weight gain	Assist client to rise slowly from sitting or supine position Ensure adequate fluids and balanced nutrition Encourage use of sugar-free drinks and hard sweets Encourage exercise
Nortriptyline (Allegron)	Cardiac dysrhythmias, tachycardia, confusion, excitement, tremor, constipation, dry mouth and throat	Monitor cardiac function Administer in AM if stimulated Ensure adequate fluids Encourage use of sugar-free drinks and hard sweets Report confusion to doctor

Adapted from British National Formulary Online. (2008). http://www.bnf.org/bnf/bnf/55/

Tricyclic antidepressants are contraindicated in severe impairment of liver function and in myocardial infarction (acute recovery phase). They cannot be given concurrently with MAOIs. Because of their anticholinergic side-effects, tricyclic antidepressants must be used cautiously in clients who have glaucoma, benign prostatic hypertrophy, urinary retention or obstruction, diabetes mellitus, hyperthyroidism, cardiovascular disease, renal impairment or respiratory disorders (Table 15.2).

Overdosage of tricyclic antidepressants occurs over several days and results in confusion, agitation, hallucinations, hyperpyrexia and increased reflexes. Seizures, coma and cardiovascular toxicity can occur with ensuing tachycardia, decreased output, depressed contractility and atrioventricular block. Because many older adults have concomitant health problems, cyclic antidepressants are used less often in the geriatric population than newer types of antidepressants that have fewer side-effects and fewer drug interactions.

Atypical Antidepressants. Atypical antidepressants are used when the client has an inadequate response to, or side-effects from, SSRIs. Atypical antidepressants vary widely chemically, in their action and in their side-effects, although have some elements in common (see Table 15.3). Venlafaxine, for example, a serotonin and noradrenaline reuptake inhibitor (SNRI), is less sedative than tricyclics although clients can experience distressing withdrawal effects if they stop taking the drug too quickly. Mirtazapine also has a possible withdrawal syndrome associated with it: it is a 'tetracyclic' antidepressant which increases central noradrenergic and serotonergic neurotransmission. Duloxetine, which inhibits both serotonin and noradrenaline reuptake, can produce withdrawal effects if stopped rapidly, while reboxetine is a selective inhibitor of noradrenaline reuptake which can cause weight loss and postural hypotension, among other side-effects. Flupentixol is used as an antipsychotic in higher doses, an antidepressant

Table 15.3 ATYPICAL ANTIDEPRESSANTS

Generic (Trade) Name	Indicative Side-effects	Nursing Implications
Venlafaxine (Efexor)	Increased blood pressure and pulse, nausea, vomiting, headache, dizziness, drowsiness, dry mouth, sweating; can alter many lab tests, e.g. AST, ALT, alkaline phosphatase, creatinine, glucose, electrolytes	Administer with food Ensure adequate fluids Give in PM Encourage use of sugar-free drinks or hard sweets
Duloxetine (Cymbalta)	Increased blood pressure and pulse, nausea, vomiting, drowsiness or insomnia, headache, dry mouth, constipation, lowered seizure threshold, sexual dysfunction	Administer with food Ensure adequate fluids Encourage use of sugar-free drinks or hard sweets
Reboxetine (Edronax)	Nausea, dry mouth, constipation, anorexia, tachycardia, palpitation, vasodilation, postural hypotension, headache, insomnia, dizziness, chills, impotence, urinary retention, impaired visual accommodation, sweating	Give with food Ensure adequate fluids Administer dose in AM Ensure balanced nutrition and exercise
Tryptophan (Optimax)	Drowsiness, nausea, headache, lightheadedness, suicidal behaviour	Give with food; monitor closely for suicidal thoughts/feelings
Mirtazapine (Zispin)	Sedation, dizziness, dry mouth and throat, weight gain, sexual dysfunction, constipation	Administer in PM Encourage use of sugar-free drinks and hard sweets Ensure adequate fluids and balanced nutrition Report sexual difficulties to doctor Clients must be encouraged to report any fever, sore throat, stomatitis or other signs of infection during treatment; a blood count should be performed and drug stopped immediately if blood dyscrasia (cellular abnormalities) is suspected
Flupentixol (Fluanxol)	Restlessness, insomnia; hypomania reported; rarely dizziness, tremor, visual disturbances, headache, hyperprolactinaemia, extrapyramidal symptoms; suicidal behaviour	Should not be taken in the evenings – can have an alerting effect

ALT, alanine aminotransferase; AST, aspartate aminotransferase.

Adapted from British National Formulary Online. (2008). http://www.bnf.org/bnf/bnf/55/

Table 15.4	MONOAMINE OXIDASE INHIBITOR (MAOI) ANTIDEPRESSANTS	
Generic (Trade) Name	**Side-effects**	**Nursing Implications**
Isocarboxazid (Marplan) Phenelzine (Nardil) Tranylcypromine (Parnate)	Drowsiness, dry mouth, overactivity, insomnia, nausea, anorexia, constipation, urinary retention, orthostatic hypotension	Assist client to rise slowly from sitting position Administer in AM Administer with food Ensure adequate fluids Perform essential teaching on importance of low tyramine diet

Adapted from British National Formulary Online. (2008). http://www.bnf.org/bnf/bnf/55/

in lower. Tryptophan is sometimes used for the adjunctive treatment of depression when other antidepressants have proved ineffective, but it can cause eosinophilia-myalgia syndrome, a rare but sometimes fatal neurological condition, and so needs to be initiated under specialist supervision (British National Formulary Online, 2008).

Monoamine Oxidase Inhibitors. This class of antidepressants is used infrequently because of potentially fatal side-effects and interactions with numerous drugs, both prescription and over-the-counter preparations (Table 15.4). The most serious side-effect is **hypertensive crisis** a life-threatening condition that can result when a client taking MAOIs ingests tyramine-containing foods (see Chapter 3, Box 3.1) and fluids or other medications. Symptoms are occipital headache, hypertension, nausea, vomiting, chills, sweating, restlessness, nuchal rigidity, dilated pupils, fever and motor agitation. These can lead to hyperpyrexia, cerebral haemorrhage and death. The MAOI–tyramine interaction produces symptoms within 20 to 60 minutes after ingestion. For hypertensive crisis, transient antihypertensive agents such as phentolamine mesilate are given to dilate blood vessels and decrease vascular resistance (Facts and Comparisons, 2007).

There is a 2 to 4-week lag period before MAOIs reach therapeutic levels. Because of the lag period, adequate washout periods of 5 to 6 weeks are recommended between the times that the MAOI is discontinued and another class of antidepressant is started.

WARNING ● Hyponatraemia and Antidepressant Therapy

Hyponatraemia (usually in the elderly and possibly due to inappropriate secretion of antidiuretic hormone) has been associated with all types of antidepressants; however, it has been reported more frequently with SSRIs than with other antidepressants. The Committee on Safety of Medicines (CSM) has advised that hyponatraemia should be considered in all patients who develop drowsiness, confusion or convulsions while taking an antidepressant.

WARNING ● Suicidal Behaviour and Antidepressant Therapy

The use of antidepressants has been linked with suicidal thoughts and behaviour. Where necessary, patients should be monitored for suicidal behaviour, self-harm or hostility, particularly at the beginning of treatment or if the dose is changed. Depressed clients who begin taking an antidepressant may have a continued or increased risk for suicide in the first few weeks of therapy. They may experience an increase in energy from the antidepressant but remain depressed. This increase in energy may make clients more likely to act on suicidal ideas and able to carry them out. Also, because antidepressants take several weeks to reach their peak effect, clients may become discouraged, and act on suicidal ideas because they believe the medication is not helping them. For these reasons, it is extremely important to monitor the suicidal ideation of depressed clients until the risk has subsided.

Drug Alert!

Serotonin Syndrome

Serotonin syndrome occurs when there is an inadequate washout period between taking MAOIs and SSRIs, or high doses of, or combinations of, a variety of drugs that can lead to excessive serotonergic activity, including lithium, carbamazepine, buspirone, amphetamines, cocaine, ecstasy, LSD, antiemetics, antimigraine drugs, cough and cold remedies, herbal remedies and St. John's wort. Symptoms of serotonin syndrome include:

- Change in mental state: confusion, agitation
- Neuromuscular excitement: muscle rigidity, weakness, sluggish pupils, shivering, tremors, myoclonic jerks, collapse, muscle paralysis
- Autonomic abnormalities: hyperthermia, tachycardia, tachypnoea, hypersalivation, diaphoresis.

ANTIDEPRESSANTS AND CHILDREN

Only fluoxetine has been shown to have any clinical effect in trials with depression in the under-18 age-group. According to the British National Formulary, careful monitoring is essential because of a small risk of increased self-harm and suicidal thoughts.

OTHER MEDICAL TREATMENTS

Electroconvulsive Therapy. Psychiatrists may – with certain legal restrictions (see Chapter 9) and after full multidisciplinary team discussion – elect to use **electroconvulsive therapy (ECT)** as a short-term intervention to treat depression in selected groups, such as severely depressed and/or actively suicidal clients who do not respond to antidepressants, or those who experience intolerable side-effects at therapeutic doses (this may be particularly true for older adults). It is also sometimes used in mania, schizophrenia and catatonia (Box 15.2). According to the UK ECT Review Group (2003), 'bilateral' ECT is more effective than unilateral, and high-dose more effective than low-dose.

ECT involves the application of electrodes to the head of the client to deliver an electrical impulse to the brain; this causes a seizure. It is believed that the shock stimulates brain chemistry to correct the chemical imbalance of depression. Historically, clients did not receive any anaesthetic or other medication before ECT, and they had full-blown grand mal seizures that often resulted in injuries ranging from biting the tongue to breaking bones. ECT fell out of favour for a period and was seen as 'barbaric'. Today, although ECT is administered in a safe and humane way with almost no injuries, there are still many critics of the treatment and the nature of the evidence for its effectiveness still unconvincing. Short-term memory loss can be a major problem.

Clients are usually given a series of 6 to 12 treatments, scheduled one a day for up to three times a week. Physical preparation of a client for ECT is similar to preparation for any outpatient minor surgical procedure. The client receives nothing by mouth after midnight, removes any fingernail polish and excretes and urinates just before the procedure. An intravenous line is started for the administration of medication.

Drug Alert !

Overdose of MAOI and Cyclic Antidepressants

Both the cyclic compounds and MAOIs are potentially lethal when taken in overdose. To decrease this risk, depressed or impulsive clients who are taking any antidepressants in these two categories may need to have prescriptions and refills in limited amounts.

Drug Alert !

MAOI Drug Interactions

Other antidepressants should **not** be started for 2 weeks after treatment with MAOIs has been stopped (3 weeks if starting clomipramine or imipramine). Some psychiatrists use selected tricyclics in conjunction with MAOIs but this is hazardous, indeed potentially lethal, except in experienced hands, and there is no evidence that the combination is more effective than when either constituent is used alone. The combination of tranylcypromine with clomipramine is particularly **dangerous**.

Conversely, an MAOI should not be started until at least 7–14 days after a tricyclic or related antidepressant (3 weeks in the case of clomipramine or imipramine) has been stopped. In addition, an MAOI should not be started for at least 2 weeks after a previous MAOI has been stopped (then started at a reduced dose).

From British National Formulary Online. (2008). Available: http://www.bnf.org/bnf/

Initially, the client receives a short-acting anaesthetic so he or she is not awake during the procedure. Next, he or she receives a muscle relaxant/paralytic, usually succinylcholine, which relaxes all muscles to reduce greatly the outward signs of the seizure (e.g. clonic–tonic muscle contractions). Electrodes are placed on the client's head: one on either

---

Box 15.2   ELECTROCONVULSIVE THERAPY

ECT is used only to achieve rapid and short-term improvement of severe symptoms after an adequate trial of other treatment options has proven ineffective and/or when the condition is considered to be potentially life-threatening, in individuals with:

• Severe depressive illness
• Catatonia
• A prolonged or severe manic episode.

The current state of the evidence does not allow the general use of ECT in the management of schizophrenia to be recommended.

National Institute for Health and Clinical Excellence (NICE). (2003). TA59. Guidance on the use of electroconvulsive therapy. London: NICE. Available: www.nice.org.uk/TA59. Reproduced with permission.

side (bilateral) or both on one side (unilateral). The electrical stimulation is delivered, which causes seizure activity in the brain, which is monitored by an electroencephalogram (EEG). The client receives oxygen and is assisted to breathe with an Ambu-bag. He or she generally begins to waken after a few minutes. Vital signs are monitored and the client is assessed for the return of a gag reflex.

After ECT treatment, the client may be mildly confused or briefly disoriented. He or she is very tired and often has a headache. The symptoms are just like those of anyone who has had a grand mal seizure. In addition, the client will have some short-term memory impairment. After a treatment, the client may eat as soon as he or she is hungry and usually sleeps for a period. Headaches are treated symptomatically.

Unilateral ECT may result in less memory loss for the client, but more treatments may be needed to see sustained improvement. Bilateral ECT may result in more rapid improvement but with increased short-term memory loss.

The literature continues to be divided about the effectiveness of ECT (Challiner & Griffiths, 2000; NICE, 2003). Some studies report that ECT is as effective as medication for depression, whereas other studies report only short-term improvement. Likewise, some studies report that memory loss side-effects of ECT are short-lived, whereas others report they are serious and long term (Fenton *et al.*, 2006; Ross, 2006).

ECT is also used for relapse prevention in depression. Clients may continue to receive treatments, such as one per month, to maintain their mood improvement. Kellner *et al.* (2006) found that maintenance ECT had limited ability to prevent relapse, whereas other studies found it to be effective in relapse prevention (Frederikse *et al.*, 2006).

THE NURSING ROLE IN ECT

1. Provide emotional and educational support to the patient and family/carer.
2. Assess the pre-treatment plan and the patient's behaviour, memory and functional ability prior to ECT.
3. Prepare and monitor the patient during the actual procedure.
4. Support the recovering patient, observing and interpreting patient responses to ECT, with recommendations for changes in the treatment plan as appropriate.

These elements of nursing care should be reflected in the nursing care plan for patients receiving ECT.

From Royal College of Nursing:
http://www.rcn.org.uk/development/communities/specialisms/mental_health/good_practice/new_guidance_on_ect_21_apr_2005. © 2007/08 Royal College of Nursing.

Box 15.3 ECT: NURSING OBLIGATIONS

Prior to educating any client about the benefits and risks of ECT, the MHN needs to understand not only the implications for ECT based on empirical data, but also the importance of the client's right to refuse this type of treatment, regardless of how well informed he or she is. The nurse must acknowledge the client's feelings, give the appropriate information and respect the client's decision. The MHN must also act as a consultant, collaborating in the decision making regarding the appropriateness of ECT, and weighing the risks and benefits.

From Heffern, W. (2000). Psychopharmacological and electroconvulsive treatment of anxiety and depression in the elderly. *Journal of Psychiatric and Mental Health Nursing*, 7(3), 199–204.

Nurses have an obligation to express fully any reservations based on knowledge of an individual patient and of the evidence-base about any medical or psychological procedure (Box 15.3).

Investigational Treatments. Other treatments for depression are being tested. These include transcranial magnetic stimulation (TMS), magnetic seizure therapy, deep brain stimulation and vagal nerve stimulation. TMS is the closest to approval for clinical use. These novel brain stimulation techniques seem to be safe, but efficacy in relieving depression needs to be established (Eitan & Lerer, 2006).

PSYCHOTHERAPY

Psychotherapy. NICE guidelines suggest that a combination of psychotherapy (specifically CBT) and medication may be the most effective treatment for depressive disorders (see http://www.nice.org.uk/nicemedia/pdf/CG23quickrefguideamended.pdf). The goals of combined therapy are symptom remission, psychosocial restoration, prevention of relapse or recurrence and reduced secondary consequences such as marital discord or occupational difficulties.

Table 15.5 and Box 15.4 describe the 'unhelpful thinking styles' that are one of the focuses of CBT in depression. CBT (as mentioned before) targets these distortions and the concomitant feelings and behaviour in the context of the person's life, working collaboratively and in a structured way toward effecting change at an affective, cognitive and behavioural level.

Many other approaches – including DBT, psychodynamic psychotherapies, solution-focused therapies and supportive counselling approaches – have also been found to be helpful. Above all, focused, compassionate help in the context of

Table 15.5	DISTORTIONS ADDRESSED BY COGNITIVE THERAPY

Cognitive Distortion	Definition
Absolute, dichotomous thinking	Tendency to view everything in polar categories, i.e. all or none, black or white
Arbitrary inference	Drawing a specific conclusion without sufficient evidence, i.e. jumping to (negative) conclusions
Specific abstraction	Focusing on a single (often minor) detail while ignoring other, more significant aspects of the experience, i.e. concentrating on one small (negative) detail while discounting positive aspects
Over-generalization	Forming conclusions based on too little or too narrow experience, i.e. if one experience was negative, then all similar experiences will be negative
Magnification and minimization	Over- or undervaluing the significance of a particular event, i.e. one small negative event is the end of the world or a positive experience is totally discounted
Personalization	Tendency to self-reference external events without basis, i.e. believing that events are directly related to one's self, whether they are or not

a trusting, mutually respectful relationship can make a huge difference to people struggling with low mood.

APPLICATION OF THE NURSING PROCESS: DEPRESSION

Assessment

HISTORY

The nurse can collect tentative assessment data from the client and family or significant others, previous information in notes, and others involved in the support or care. It may take several short periods to complete the assessment because clients who are severely depressed often feel exhausted and overwhelmed. It can take time for them to process any questions asked and to formulate a response. It is important that the nurse does not try to rush clients because doing so leads to frustration – and incomplete assessment data.

To assess the client's perception of the problem, the nurse asks about behavioural, thinking and affective changes: when they started, what was happening when they began, their duration and what the client has tried to do about them. Assessing the history is important as part of the engagement process and to determine any previous episodes of depression, treatment and the client's response to treatment. The nurse should also ask about family history of mood disorders, suicide or attempted suicide.

Box 15.4 THE UNHELPFUL THINKING STYLES

People with depressed and anxious thinking tend to show certain common characteristics:

- They overlook their strengths, become very self-critical and have a bias against themselves, thinking that they cannot tackle difficulties.
- They unhelpfully dwell on past, current or future problems; they put a negative slant on things, using a negative mental filter that focuses only on their difficulties and failures.
- They have a gloomy view of the future and get things out of proportion; they make negative predictions about how things will work out and jump to the very worst conclusion (catastrophize) that things have gone or will go very badly wrong.
- They mind-read and second-guess that others think badly of them, rarely checking whether this is true.
- They unfairly feel responsible if things do not turn out well (bearing all responsibility) and take things to heart.
- They make extreme statements and have unhelpfully high standards that are almost impossible to meet; they hold rules such as 'I should/must/ought/have got to . . .'
- Overall, thinking becomes extreme, unhelpful and out of proportion.

From Williams, C. & Garland, A. (2002). A cognitive–behavioural therapy assessment model for use in everyday clinical practice. *Advances in Psychiatric Treatment*, 8, 172–179, with permission. © 2009 The Royal College of Psychiatrists.

GENERAL APPEARANCE AND MOTOR BEHAVIOUR

Many people with depression look sad; sometimes they just look ill. The posture is often slouched with head down, and they may make minimal eye contact. They may have **psycho-motor retardation** (slow body movements, slow cognitive processing and slow verbal interaction). Responses to questions may be minimal, with only one or two words. **Latency of response** is seen when clients take up to 30 seconds to respond to a question. They may answer some questions with 'I don't know' because they are simply too fatigued and overwhelmed to think of an answer or respond in any detail. People may also exhibit signs of agitation or anxiety, such as wringing their hands and having difficulty sitting still. These people are said to have 'psychomotor agitation' (increased body movements and thoughts), which includes pacing, accelerated thinking and argumentativeness.

MOOD AND AFFECT

Clients with depression may describe themselves as feeling hopeless, helpless, down, pissed-off or anxious. They also may say they are a burden on others or are a failure at life, or they may make other similar statements. They are easily frustrated, are angry at themselves and can be angry at others. They may experience **anhedonia**, losing any sense of pleasure from activities they formerly enjoyed. Clients may be apathetic, that is, not caring about self, activities or much of anything.

Their **affect** is sad or depressed, or may be flat with no emotional expressions. Typically, depressed clients sit alone, staring into space or lost in thought. When addressed, they interact minimally with a few words or a gesture. They are overwhelmed by noise and people who might make demands on them, so they withdraw from the stimulation of interaction with others.

THOUGHT PROCESS AND CONTENT

People with depression experience slowed thinking processes: their thoughts seem to occur in slow motion. With severe depression, they may not respond verbally to questions. They tend to be negative and pessimistic in their thinking, that is, they believe that they will always feel this bad, things will never get any better and nothing will help. People might make self-deprecating remarks, criticizing themselves harshly and focusing only on failures or negative attributes. They tend to ruminate, which is repeatedly going over the same thoughts. Those who experience psychotic symptoms may experience delusions; they often believe they are responsible for all the tragedies and miseries in the world.

Often people with depression have thoughts of dying or committing suicide. It is important to assess suicidal ideation by asking about it directly. The nurse may ask, 'Are you thinking about suicide?' or 'What suicidal thoughts are you having?' Most clients readily admit to suicidal thinking. Suicide is discussed more fully later in this chapter.

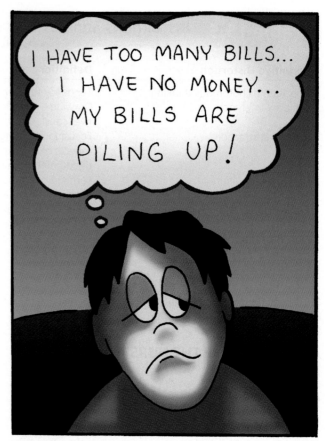

Rumination

SENSORY AND INTELLECTUAL PROCESSES

Some clients with depression are oriented to person, time and place; others experience difficulty with orientation, especially if they experience psychotic symptoms or are withdrawn from their environment. Assessing general knowledge is difficult because of their limited ability to respond to questions. Memory impairment is common. People may have extreme difficulty concentrating or paying attention. If psychotic, clients may hear degrading and belittling voices, or they may even have command hallucinations that order them to commit suicide.

JUDGEMENT AND INSIGHT

People with depression experience impaired judgement because they cannot use their cognitive abilities to solve problems or to make decisions. They often cannot make decisions or choices because of their extreme apathy or their negative belief that it 'doesn't matter anyway'.

'Insight' may be intact, especially if they have been depressed previously. Others have very limited insight and are totally unaware of their behaviour, feelings or even their illness.

SELF-CONCEPT

Sense of self-esteem is greatly reduced; clients often use phrases such as 'good for nothing' or 'just worthless' to describe themselves. They feel guilty about not being able to function and often personalize events or take responsibility for incidents over which they have no control. They believe that others would be better off without them, a belief that leads to suicidal thoughts.

ROLES AND RELATIONSHIPS

Clients with depression have difficulty fulfilling roles and responsibilities. The more severe the depression, the greater the difficulty. They have problems going to work or school; when there, they seem unable to carry out their responsibilities. The same is true with family responsibilities. Clients are less able to cook, clean or care for children. In addition to the inability to fulfil roles, clients become even more convinced of their 'worthlessness' for being unable to meet life responsibilities.

Depression can cause great strain in relationships. Family members who have limited knowledge about depression may believe clients should 'just get on with it'. Clients often avoid family and social relationships because they feel overwhelmed, experience no pleasure from interactions and feel unworthy. As clients withdraw from relationships, the strain increases.

PHYSIOLOGICAL AND SELF-CARE CONSIDERATIONS

Clients with depression often experience pronounced weight loss because of lack of appetite or disinterest in eating. Sleep disturbances are common: either clients cannot sleep, or they feel exhausted and unrefreshed no matter how much time they spend in bed. They lose interest in sexual activities, and men often experience impotence. Some clients neglect personal hygiene because they lack the interest or energy. Constipation commonly results from decreased food and fluid intake as well as from inactivity. If fluid intake is severely limited, clients also may be dehydrated.

DEPRESSION RATING SCALES

Clients complete some rating scales for depression; mental health professionals administer others. These assessment tools, along with evaluation of behaviour, thought processes, history, family history and situational factors, help to create a diagnostic picture. Self-rating scales of depressive symptoms include the Zung Self-Rating Depression Scale and the Beck Depression Inventory. Self-rating scales are used for case-finding in the general public and may be used over the course of treatment to determine improvement from the client's perspective.

The Hamilton Rating Scale for Depression (Box 15.5) is a clinician-rated depression scale used like a clinical interview. The clinician rates the range of the client's behaviours, such as depressed mood, guilt, suicide and insomnia. There is also a section to score diurnal variations, depersonalization (sense of unreality about the self), paranoid symptoms and obsessions.

Data Analysis

The nurse analyses assessment data to determine priorities and to establish a plan of care. Nursing formulations commonly established for the client with depression include the following:

- Risk of suicide
- Imbalanced nutrition: less than body requirements
- Anxiety
- Ineffective coping
- Hopelessness
- Ineffective role performance
- Self-care deficit
- Chronic low self-esteem
- Disturbed sleep pattern
- Impaired social interaction.

Outcome Identification

Outcomes for clients with depression relate to how the depression is manifested – for instance, whether or not the person is slow or agitated, sleeps too much or too little or eats too much or too little. Examples of outcomes for a client with the psychomotor retardation form of depression include the following:

- The client will not injure himself or herself.
- The client will independently carry out activities of daily living (showering, changing clothing, grooming).
- The client will establish a balance of rest, sleep and activity.
- The client will establish a balance of adequate nutrition, hydration and elimination.
- The client will evaluate self-attributes realistically.
- The client will socialize with staff, peers and family/friends.
- The client will return to occupation or school activities.
- The client will understand benefits and side-effects of medication.
- The client will verbalize symptoms of a recurrence.

Intervention

ENSURING SAFETY

The first priority is to determine whether a client with depression is suicidal. If a client has suicidal ideation or hears voices commanding him or her to commit suicide, measures to provide a safe environment are necessary. If the client has a suicide plan, the nurse asks additional questions to determine the lethality of the intent and plan. The nurse reports this information to the team. Teams should follow local policies and procedures for instituting **suicide precautions** (e.g. if in hospital already, removal of harmful items, increased supervision; if in the community, appropriate urgent crisis intervention). A thorough discussion is presented later in this chapter.

Box 15.5   HAMILTON RATING SCALE FOR DEPRESSION

For each item select the 'cue' that best characterizes the patient.

1: Depressed mood (sadness, hopeless, helpless, worthless)
   0 Absent
   1 These feeling states indicated only on questioning
   2 These feeling states spontaneously reported verbally
   3 Communicates feeling states non-verbally, i.e. through facial expression, posture, voice and tendency to weep
   4 Patient reports VIRTUALLY ONLY these feeling states in his spontaneous verbal and non-verbal communication

2: Feelings of guilt
   0 Absent
   1 Self-reproach, feels he has let people down
   2 Ideas of guilt or rumination over past errors or sinful deeds
   3 Present illness is a punishment. Delusions of guilt
   4 Hears accusatory or denunciatory voices and/or experiences threatening visual hallucinations

3: Suicide
   0 Absent
   1 Feels life is not worth living
   2 Wishes he were dead or any thoughts of possible death to self
   3 Suicide ideas or gesture
   4 Attempts at suicide (any serious attempt rates 4)

4: Insomnia early
   0 No difficulty falling asleep
   1 Complains of occasional difficulty falling asleep, i.e. more than ¼ hour
   2 Complains of nightly difficulty falling asleep

5: Insomnia middle
   0 No difficulty
   1 Patient complains of being restless and disturbed during the night
   2 Waking during the night – any getting out of bed rates 2 (except for purpose of voiding)

6: Insomnia late
   0 No difficulty
   1 Waking in early hours of the morning but goes back to sleep
   2 Unable to fall asleep again if gets out of bed

7: Work and activities
   0 No difficulty
   1 Thoughts and feelings of incapacity, fatigue or weakness related to activities, work or hobbies

2 Loss of interest in activity, hobbies or work – either directly reported by patient, or indirect in listlessness, indecision and vacillation (feels he has to push self to work or activities)
3 Decrease in actual time spent in activities or decrease in productivity. In hospital, rate 3 if patient does not spend at least 3 hours a day in activities (hospital job or hobbies) exclusive of ward chores
4 Stopped working because of present illness. In hospital, rate 4 if patient engages in no activities except ward chores, or if patient fails to perform ward chores unassisted

8: Retardation (slowness of thought and speech; impaired ability to concentrate; decreased motor activity)
   0 Normal speech and thought
   1 Slight retardation at interview
   2 Obvious retardation at interview
   3 Interview difficult
   4 Complete stupor

9: Agitation
   0 None
   1 'Playing with' hands, hair, etc.
   2 Hand wringing, nail biting, hair pulling, biting of lips

10: Anxiety psychic
   0 No difficulty
   1 Subjective tension and irritability
   2 Worrying about minor matters
   3 Apprehensive attitude apparent in face or speech
   4 Fears expressed without questioning

11: Anxiety somatic

0	Absent	Physiologic concomitants of anxiety, such as:
1	Mild	Gastrointestinal – dry mouth, wind, indigestion, diarrhoea, cramps, belching
2	Moderate	Cardiovascular – palpitations, headaches
3	Severe	Respiratory – hyperventilation, sighing
4	Incapacitating	Urinary frequency, sweating

12: Somatic symptoms gastrointestinal
   0 None
   1 Loss of appetite but eating without staff encouragement. Heavy feelings in abdomen.
   2 Difficulty eating without staff urging. Requests or requires laxatives or medication for bowels or medication for GI symptoms

continued ┄┄➤

Box 15.5: Hamilton Rating Scale for Depression, cont.

13: Somatic symptoms general
- 0 None
- 1 Heaviness in limbs, back or head. Backaches, headache, muscle aches. Loss of energy and fatigability
- 2 Any clear-cut symptom rates 2

14: Genital symptoms
- 0 Absent   Symptoms such as:
- 1 Mild   Loss of libido
- 2 Severe   Menstrual disturbances

15: Hypochondriasis
- 0 Not present
- 1 Self-absorption (bodily)
- 2 Preoccupation with health
- 3 Frequent complaints, requests for help, etc.
- 4 Hypochondriacal delusions

16: Loss of weight

A: When rating by history
- 0 No weight loss
- 1 Probable weight loss associated with present illness
- 2 Definite (according to patient) weight loss

B: On weekly ratings by staff, when actual weight changes are measured
- 0 Less than 1 lb weight loss in week
- 1 Greater than 1 lb weight loss in week
- 2 Greater than 2 lb weight loss in week

17: Insight
- 0 Acknowledges being depressed and ill
- 1 Acknowledges illness but attributes cause to bad food, climate, overwork, virus, need for rest, etc.
- 2 Denies being ill at all

18: Diurnal variation

AM	PM	If symptoms are worse in the
0	0 Absent	morning or evening, note which
1	1 Mild	it is and rate severity of variation
2	2 Severe	

19: Depersonalization and derealization
- 0 Absent
- 1 Mild   Such as:
- 2 Moderate   Feelings of unreality
- 3 Severe   Nihilistic ideas
- 4 Incapacitating

20: Paranoid symptoms
- 0 None
- 1
- 2 Suspiciousness
- 3 Ideas of reference
- 4 Delusions of reference and persecution

21: Obsessional and compulsive symptoms
- 0 Absent
- 1 Mild
- 2 Severe

22: Helplessness
- 0 Not present
- 1 Subjective feelings that are elicited only by enquiry
- 2 Patient volunteers his helpless feelings
- 3 Requires urging, guidance and reassurance to accomplish ward chores or personal hygiene
- 4 Requires physical assistance for dress, grooming, eating, bedside tasks or personal hygiene

23: Hopelessness
- 0 Not present
- 1 Intermittently doubts that 'things will improve' but can be reassured
- 2 Consistently feels 'hopeless' but accepts reassurances
- 3 Expresses feelings of discouragement, despair, pessimism about future, which cannot be dispelled
- 4 Spontaneously and inappropriately perseverates 'I'll never get well' or its equivalent

24: Worthlessness (ranges from mild loss of esteem, feelings of inferiority, self-depreciation to delusional notions of worthlessness)
- 0 Not present
- 1 Indicates feelings of worthlessness (loss of self-esteem) only on questioning
- 2 Spontaneously indicates feelings of worthlessness (loss of self-esteem)
- 3 Different from 2 by degree. Patient volunteers that he is 'no good', 'inferior', etc.
- 4 Delusional notions of worthlessness, i.e. 'I am a heap of garbage' or its equivalent

Reprinted with permission from Hamilton, M. (1960). A rating scale for depression. *Journal of Neurology, Neurosurgery and Psychiatry*, 23, 56.

PROMOTING A THERAPEUTIC RELATIONSHIP

It is vital to have meaningful contact with clients who are depressed and to begin a therapeutic alliance regardless of the state of depression. Some people are quite open in describing their feelings of sadness, hopelessness, helplessness or agitation. They may be unable to sustain a long interaction, so several shorter conversations help the nurse to assess status and to establish a therapeutic relationship.

NURSING INTERVENTIONS FOR DEPRESSION

- Ensure the safety of the client and others.
- Institute suicide precautions if indicated.
- Begin a therapeutic alliance by spending non-demanding time with the client.
- Promote completion of activities of daily living by assisting – or facilitating others to assist – the client only as necessary.
- Establish adequate nutrition and hydration.
- Promote sleep and rest.
- Engage the client in activities.
- Encourage the client to verbalize and describe emotions and begin to identify goals.
- Work with the client to manage medications and side-effects.
- Work psychotherapeutically towards identified goals.

The nurse may find it difficult to interact with these clients because he or she empathizes with such sadness and depression. The nurse also may feel unable to 'do anything' for clients with limited responses. Clients with psychomotor retardation (slow speech, slow movement, slow thought processes) are very non-communicative or may even be mute. The nurse can sit with such clients for a few minutes at intervals throughout the day. The nurse's presence conveys genuine interest and caring. It is not necessary for the nurse to talk to clients the entire time; rather, silence can convey that people are worthwhile even if they are not interacting.

'My name's Marri. I'm your nurse today. I'm going to sit with you for a few minutes. If you need anything, or if you'd like to talk, please tell me.'

After time has elapsed, the nurse would say the following:

'I'm going now. I'll be back in an hour to see you again.'

It is also important that the nurse avoids being overly cheerful or trying to 'cheer up' clients. It is impossible to coax or to humour clients out of their depression. In fact, an overly cheerful approach may make clients feel worse or convey a lack of understanding of their despair.

PROMOTING ACTIVITIES OF DAILY LIVING AND PHYSICAL CARE

The ability to perform daily activities is related to the level of psychomotor retardation. To assess ability to perform activities of daily living independently, the nurse first asks the client to perform the global task. For example, in a ward setting:

'Martin, it's time to get dressed.' (global task)

If a client cannot respond to the global request, the nurse breaks the task into smaller segments. Clients with depression can become overwhelmed easily with a task that has several steps. The nurse can use success in small, concrete steps as a basis to increase self-esteem and to build competency for a slightly more complex task the next time. If clients cannot choose between articles of clothing, the nurse selects the clothing and directs clients to put them on. For example,

'Here are your grey trousers. Try and put them on.'

This still allows clients to participate in dressing. If this is what clients are capable of doing at this point, this activity will reduce dependence on staff. This request is concrete, and if clients cannot do this, the nurse has information about the level of psychomotor retardation.

If a client cannot put on his trousers, the nurse assists by saying,

'Let me help you with your trousers, Martin.'

The nurse helps clients to dress only when they cannot perform any of the above steps. This allows clients to do as much as possible for themselves and to avoid becoming dependent on a professional. The nurse can carry out this same process with clients when they eat, take a shower and perform routine self-care activities.

Because abilities change over time, the nurse must assess them on an ongoing basis. This continual assessment takes more time than simply helping clients to dress. Nevertheless, doing so promotes independence and provides dynamic assessment data about psychomotor abilities.

Often, clients decline to engage in activities because they're too fatigued or have no interest. The nurse can validate these feelings yet still promote participation. For example,

'I know you feel like staying in bed, but it's time to get up for breakfast.'

Often, clients may want to stay in bed until they 'feel like getting up' or engaging in activities of daily living. The nurse can let clients know they must become more active to feel better, rather than waiting passively for improvement. It may be helpful to avoid asking 'yes-or-no' questions. Instead of asking, *'Do you want to get up now?'* the nurse might say, *'It's time to get up now.'*

Re-establishing balanced nutrition can be challenging when clients have no appetite or don't feel like eating. The nurse can explain that beginning to eat helps stimulate appetite. Food offered frequently and in small amounts can prevent overwhelming clients with a large meal that they feel unable to eat. Sitting quietly with clients during meals can promote eating. Monitoring food and fluid intake may be necessary until clients are consuming adequate amounts.

Promoting sleep may include the short-term use of a sedative or giving medication in the evening if drowsiness or sedation is a side-effect. It is also important to encourage clients to remain out of bed and active during the day to facilitate sleeping at night. It is important to monitor the number of hours clients sleep as well as whether they feel refreshed on awakening.

USING THERAPEUTIC COMMUNICATION

Clients with depression are often overwhelmed by the intensity of their emotions. Talking about these feelings can be beneficial. Initially, the nurse encourages clients to describe in detail how they are feeling. Sharing the burden with another person can provide some relief. At these times, the nurse can listen attentively, encourage clients and validate the intensity of their experience. For example,

Nurse: *'How are you feeling today?'* (broad opening)
Client: *'I feel so awful . . . terrible.'*
Nurse: *'Tell me more. What's that like for you?'* (using a general lead; encouraging description)
Client: *'I don't feel like myself. I don't know what to do.'*
Nurse: *'That must be really frightening.'* (validating)

It is important at this point that the nurse does not attempt to 'fix' the client's difficulties or offer clichés such as 'Things will get better' or 'But you know your family really needs you.' Although the nurse may have good intentions, remarks of this type belittle the client's feelings or make the client feel more guilty and worthless.

As clients begin to improve, the nurse can help them to learn or rediscover more effective coping strategies such as talking to friends, spending leisure time relaxing, taking positive steps to deal with stressors and so forth. Improved coping skills may not prevent depression but may assist clients to deal with the effects of depression more effectively.

MANAGING MEDICATION

The increased activity and improved mood that antidepressants may produce can provide the energy for suicidal clients to carry out the act. Thus, the nurse must assess suicide risk even when clients are receiving antidepressants.

It is also important to ensure that clients actually swallow the medication and are not saving it in an attempt to commit suicide. On a ward, as clients become ready for discharge, careful assessment of suicide potential is important because they will have a supply of antidepressant medication at home. SSRIs are rarely fatal in overdose, but cyclic and MAOI antidepressants are potentially fatal. Prescriptions may need to be limited to only a 1-week supply at a time if concerns linger about overdose.

An important component of client care is management of side-effects. The nurse must make careful observations and ask clients pertinent questions to determine how they are tolerating medication. Tables 15.1–15.4 give specific interventions to manage side-effects of antidepressant medications.

Clients and family must learn how to manage any medication regime because clients may need to take these medications for months, years or even a lifetime. Collaborative, transparent information-exchange promotes concordance.

PROVIDING CLIENT AND FAMILY TEACHING

Teaching clients and family about depression is important. They must understand that depression is a debilitating mental health difficulty, not merely a lack of willpower or motivation. Learning about the beginning symptoms of relapse may assist clients to seek treatment early and avoid a lengthy recurrence.

Clients and family should know that treatment outcomes are often best when psychotherapy and antidepressants are combined. Psychotherapy helps clients to explore anger, dependence, guilt, hopelessness, helplessness, object loss, interpersonal issues and irrational beliefs. The goal is to reverse negative views of the future, improve self-image, and help clients gain competence and self-mastery. If not providing it herself, the nurse can refer to an appropriate therapist.

CLIENT/FAMILY EDUCATION FOR DEPRESSION

- Teach about depression: possible causes, treatments and outcomes.
- Identify early signs of relapse.
- Discuss the importance of support groups and assist in locating resources.
- Teach the client and family about the benefits of therapy and follow-up appointments.
- Encourage participation in support groups.
- Teach the action, side-effects and special instructions regarding medications.
- Discuss methods to manage side-effects of medication.

Support group participation also helps some clients and their families. People can receive support and encouragement from others who struggle with depression, and family members can offer support to one another. The Depression Alliance is one leading organization that can help clients and families connect with each other.

Evaluation

Evaluation of the plan of care is based on achievement of individual client outcomes. It is essential that clients feel safe and are not experiencing uncontrollable urges to commit suicide. Participation in therapy and medication concordance produce more favourable outcomes for clients with depression. Being able to identify signs of relapse and to seek treatment immediately can significantly decrease the severity of a depressive episode.

BIPOLAR AFFECTIVE DISORDER

Bipolar affective disorder involves extreme mood swings from episodes of mania to episodes of depression (it was formerly known as manic depression). During manic phases, clients are euphoric, grandiose, energetic and sleepless. They may have poor judgement and rapid thoughts, actions and speech. During depressed phases, mood, behaviour and thoughts are the same as in people diagnosed with clinical depression (see previous discussion). In fact, if a person's first episode of bipolar disorder is a depressed phase, he or she might be diagnosed with depression; a diagnosis of bipolar affective disorder may not be made until the person experiences a manic episode. To increase awareness about bipolar affective disorder, health-care professionals can use tools such as the Mood Disorder Questionnaire (Box 15.6).

Bipolar affective disorder ranks second only to depression as a cause of worldwide disability. The lifetime risk for bipolar disorder is at least 1.2%, with a risk of completed suicide for 15%. Young men early in the course of their illness seem to be at highest risk of suicide, especially those with a history of suicide attempts or alcohol abuse, as are those recently discharged from hospital (Rihmer & Angst, 2005).

Whereas a person with depression may slowly slide into depression that can last for 6 months to 2 years, the person with bipolar affective disorder cycles between depression and normal behaviour (bipolar depressed) or mania and normal behaviour (bipolar manic). A person with bipolar mixed episodes alternates between depressive and manic episodes interspersed with periods of normal behaviour. Each mood may last for weeks or months before the pattern begins to descend or ascend once again. Figure 15.1 shows the three categories of bipolar cycles.

Bipolar affective disorder seems to occur almost equally among men and women. It is probably more common in highly educated people. Because some people deny their mania, prevalence rates may actually be higher than reported.

Onset and Clinical Course

The mean age for a first manic episode is the early twenties; some people experience onset in adolescence, whereas others start experiencing symptoms when they are older than 50 (American Psychiatric Association, 2000). Currently, debate exists about whether or not some children diagnosed with ADHD actually have a very early onset of bipolar disorder. Manic episodes typically begin suddenly, with rapid escalation of symptoms over a few days, and they last from a few weeks to several months. They tend to be briefer and to end more suddenly than depressive episodes. Adolescents are more likely to have psychotic manifestations.

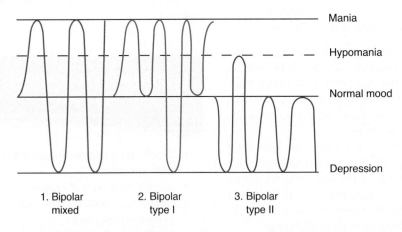

1. Bipolar mixed—Cycles alternate between periods of mania, normal mood, depression, normal mood, mania and so forth.

2. Bipolar type I—Manic episodes with at least one depressive episode.

3. Bipolar type II—Recurrent depressive episodes with at least one hypomanic episode.

Figure 15.1. Graphic depiction of mood cycles.

Box 15.6 MOOD DISORDER QUESTIONNAIRE

The following questionaire can be used as a starting point to help you recognize the signs/symptoms of bipolar disorder but is not meant to be a substitute for a full medical evaluation. Bipolar disorder is complex and **an accurate, thorough diagnosis can be made through a personal evaluation by your doctor.** However, a positive screening may suggest that you might benefit from seeking such an evaluaiton from your doctor. Regardless of the questionnaire results, if you or your family has concerns about your mental health, please contact your physician and/or other health-care professional.

When completed, you may want to print out your responses.

Instructions: Please answer each question as best you can.

	YES	NO
1. Has there ever been a period of time when you were not your usual self and . . .		
. . . you felt so good or so hyper that other people thought you were not your normal self or you were so hyper that you got into trouble?	☐	☐
. . . you were so irritable that you shouted at people or started fights or arguments?	☐	☐
. . . you felt much more self-confident than usual?	☐	☐
. . . you got much less sleep than usual and found you didn't really miss it?	☐	☐
. . . you were much more talkative or spoke much faster than usual?	☐	☐
. . . thoughts raced through your head or you couldn't slow your mind down?	☐	☐
. . . you were so easily distracted by things around you that you had trouble concentrating or staying on track?	☐	☐
. . . you had much more energy than usual?	☐	☐
. . . you were much more active or did many more things than usual?	☐	☐
. . . you were much more social or outgoing than usual, for example, you telephoned friends in the middle of the night?	☐	☐
. . . you were much more interested in sex than usual?	☐	☐
. . . you did things that were unusual for you or that other people might have thought were excessive, foolish or risky?	☐	☐
. . . spending money got you or your family into trouble?	☐	☐
2. If you checked YES to more than one of the above, have several of these ever happened during the same period of time?	☐	☐

3. How much of a problem did any of these cause you—like being unable to work; having family, money or legal troubles; getting into arguments or fights? Please select one response only.

[☐] No   [☐] Minor   [☐] Moderate   [☐] Serious
problem   problem   problem   problem

4. Have any of your blood relatives (children, siblings, parents, grandparents, aunts, uncles) had manic-depressive illness or bipolar disorder?	☐	☐
5. Has a healthcare professional ever told you that you have manic-depressive illness or bipolar disorder?	☐	☐

Hirschfeld, R. M. A., Williams, J. B., Spitzer, R. L., *et al.* (2000). Development and validation of a screening instrument for bipolar spectrum disorder: The Mood Disorder Questionnaire, *American Journal of Psychiatry 157(11)*, 1873–1875.

Clients often do not understand how their disorder affects others. They may stop taking medication because they like the euphoria and feel burdened by the side-effects, blood tests and visits needed to maintain treatment. Family members are concerned and exhausted by their loved ones' behaviours; they often stay up late at night for fear the manic person may do something impulsive and dangerous.

Treatment

PSYCHOPHARMACOLOGY

Treatment for bipolar disorder often involves a lifetime regime of medications: either an antimanic agent such as lithium or anticonvulsant medications used as mood stabilizers (see Chapter 3). Once thought to help reduce manic behaviour only, lithium and the anticonvulsants also seem to protect against the effects of bipolar depressive cycles. If a client in the acute stage of mania or depression exhibits psychosis (disordered thinking as seen with delusions, hallucinations and illusions), an antipsychotic agent is administered in addition to the bipolar medications. Some clients keep taking both bipolar medications and antipsychotics.

Lithium. Lithium salts such as lithium carbonate are used as mood stabilizers. Once believed to be helpful for bipolar mania only, investigators quickly realized that lithium could also partially or completely mute the cycling toward bipolar depression. The response rate to lithium therapy in acute mania is 70% to 80%. In addition to treating the range of bipolar behaviours, lithium also can stabilize bipolar disorder by reducing the degree and frequency of cycling or eliminating manic episodes (Freeman et al., 2006).

Lithium not only competes for salt receptor sites but also affects calcium, potassium and magnesium ions as well as glucose metabolism. Its mechanism of action is unknown, but it is thought to work in the synapses to hasten destruction of catecholamines (dopamine, noradrenaline), inhibit neurotransmitter release and decrease the sensitivity of postsynaptic receptors (Facts and Comparisons, 2007).

Lithium's action peaks in 30 minutes to 4 hours for regular forms and in 4 to 6 hours for the slow-release form. It crosses the blood–brain barrier and placenta and is distributed in sweat and breast milk. Lithium use during pregnancy is not recommended because it can lead to first-trimester developmental abnormalities. Onset of action is 5 to 14 days; with this lag period, antipsychotic or antidepressant agents are used carefully in combination with lithium to reduce symptoms in acutely manic or acutely depressed clients. The half-life of lithium is 20 to 27 hours (Facts and Comparisons, 2007).

Anticonvulsant Drugs. Lithium is effective in about 75% of people with bipolar affective disorder. The rest do not respond, or have difficulty taking lithium because of side-effects, problems with the treatment regime, drug interactions or medical conditions, such as renal disease, that contraindicate use of lithium. Several anticonvulsants traditionally used to treat seizure disorders have proved helpful in stabilizing the moods of people with bipolar illness. These drugs are sometimes categorized as miscellaneous anticonvulsants. Their mechanism of action is largely unknown, but they may raise the brain's threshold for dealing with stimulation; this prevents the person from being bombarded with external and internal stimuli (Table 15.6).

Carbamazepine (Tegretol), which had been used for grand mal and temporal lobe epilepsy as well as for trigeminal neuralgia, was the first anticonvulsant found to have mood-stabilizing properties, but the threat of agranulocytosis is of great concern. Clients taking carbamazepine need to have drug serum levels checked regularly to monitor for toxicity and to determine whether the drug has reached therapeutic levels, which are generally 4 to 12 mg/l (Ketter et al., 2006). Baseline and periodic laboratory testing must also be done to monitor for suppression of white blood cells.

Valproic acid (Depakote), also known as sodium valproate, is an anticonvulsant used for simple absence and mixed seizures, migraine prophylaxis and mania. The mechanism of action is unclear. Therapeutic levels are monitored periodically to maintain at 50 to 125 mg/l, as are baseline and ongoing liver function tests, including serum ammonia levels and platelet and bleeding times (Bowden, 2006).

PSYCHOTHERAPY

Psychotherapy (including CBT) can be useful in the mildly depressive or normal portion of the bipolar cycle. It is not necessarily useful during acute manic stages because the person's attention span is brief and he or she can gain little

Table 15.6	ANTICONVULSANTS USED AS MOOD STABILIZERS	
Generic (Trade) Name	**Side-effects**	**Nursing Implications**
Carbamazepine (Tegretol)	Dizziness, hypotension, ataxia, sedation, blurred vision, leucopenia, rashes	Assist client to rise slowly from sitting position. Monitor gait and assist as necessary. Report rashes to doctor.
Valproic acid (Depakote)	Ataxia, drowsiness, weakness, fatigue, menstrual changes, dyspepsia, nausea, vomiting, weight gain, hair loss	Monitor gait and assist as necessary. Provide rest periods. Give with food. Establish balanced nutrition.

Adapted from British National Formulary Online (2008) http://www.bnf.org/bnf/bnf/55/

CLINICAL VIGNETTE: MANIC EPISODE

'Everyone is stupid! What's the matter? Have you all taken dumb pills? Dumb pills, rum pills, shlummy shlum lum pills!' Mitch screamed as he waited for his staff to snap to attention and get with the programme. He had started the Well Bread Co. 10 years ago and now had a thriving business, baking and delivering organic breads.

He knew how to do everything in this place and, running from person to person to watch what each was doing, he didn't like what he saw. It was 8 AM, and he'd already fired the supervisor, who had been with him for 5 years.

By 8:02 AM, Mitch had fired six baking assistants because he did not like the way they looked. Then he threw pots and spoons at them because they weren't leaving fast enough. Rich, his brother, walked in during this melee and quietly asked everyone to stay, then invited Mitch outside for a walk.

'Are you nuts?' Mitch screamed at his brother. 'Everyone here is out of control. I have to do everything.' Mitch was trembling, shaking. He hadn't slept in 3 days and didn't need to. The

only time he'd left the building in these 3 days was to have sex with any woman who had agreed. He felt euphoric, supreme, able to leap tall buildings in a single bound. He glared at Rich. 'I feel good! What are you bugging me for?' He slammed out the door, shrilly reciting, 'Rich and Mitch! Rich and Mitch! Well Bread rich!'

'Rich and Mitch, Rich and Mitch. With dear old auntie, now we're rich.' Mitch couldn't stop talking and speed walking. Watching Mitch, Rich gently said, 'Jen called me last night. She says you're manic again. When did you stop taking your lithium?'

'Manic? Who's manic? I'm just feeling good. Who needs that stuff? I like to feel good. It's wonderful, marvellous, stupendous. I'm not manic,' shrieked Mitch as he swerved around to face his brother. Rich, weary and sad, said, 'I'm taking you to see the Crisis Team. If you don't agree to go, I'll call the police. I know you don't see this in yourself, but you're out of control and getting dangerous.'

WARNING ● Lithium

Overdosage, usually with serum lithium concentration of over 1.5 mmol/l, may be fatal, and toxic effects include tremor, ataxia, dysarthria, nystagmus, renal impairment and convulsions. If these potentially hazardous signs occur, treatment should be stopped, serum lithium concentrations redetermined and steps taken to reverse lithium toxicity. In mild cases, withdrawal of lithium and administration of generous amounts of sodium salts and fluid will reverse the toxicity. A serum lithium concentration in excess of 2 mmol/l requires urgent treatment.

From British National Formulary Online (2008) http://www.bnf.org/bnf/

insight during times of accelerated psychomotor activity: psychotherapeutic interventions therefore have to be significantly adjusted. Psychotherapy combined with medication can reduce the risk of suicide and injury, provide support to the client and family and help the client to accept the diagnosis and treatment plan (Griswold & Pessar, 2000).

APPLICATION OF THE NURSING PROCESS: MANIA IN BIPOLAR AFFECTIVE DISORDER

The focus of this discussion is on the client experiencing a manic episode of bipolar disorder. The reader should review the Application of the Nursing Process: Depression to examine nursing care of the client experiencing a depressed phase of bipolar affective disorder.

Assessment

HISTORY

Taking a history with a client in the manic phase often proves difficult. The client may jump from subject to subject, which makes it difficult for the nurse to follow. Obtaining data in several short sessions, as well as talking to family members, may be necessary. The nurse can obtain much information, however, by watching and listening.

GENERAL APPEARANCE AND MOTOR BEHAVIOUR

Clients with mania experience **psychomotor agitation** and seem to be in perpetual motion; sitting still is difficult. This continual movement has many ramifications: clients can become exhausted or injure themselves.

In the manic phase, the client may wear clothes that reflect the elevated mood: brightly coloured, flamboyant, attention-seeking and perhaps sexually suggestive. For example, a woman in the manic phase may wear a lot of jewellery and hair ornaments, or her make-up may be garish and heavy, whereas a male client may wear a tight shirt and trousers or go bare-chested.

Clients experiencing a manic episode think, move and talk quickly. **Pressured speech**, one of the hallmark symptoms, is evidenced by unrelentingly rapid and often loud speech without pauses. Those with pressured speech interrupt and cannot listen to others. They ignore verbal and non-verbal cues indicating that others wish to speak, and they continue with constant intelligible or unintelligible speech, turning from one listener to another or speaking to no one at all. If interrupted, clients with mania often start over from the beginning.

MOOD AND AFFECT

Mania is reflected in periods of euphoria, exuberant activity, grandiosity and false sense of well-being. Projection of an all-knowing and all-powerful image may be an unconscious defence against underlying low self-esteem. Some clients manifest mania with an angry, verbally aggressive tone and are sarcastic and irritable, especially when others set limits on their behaviour. Clients' mood is quite labile, and they may alternate between periods of loud laughter and episodes of tears.

THOUGHT PROCESS AND CONTENT

Cognitive ability or thinking is confused and jumbled, with thoughts racing one after another, which is often referred to as **flight of ideas**. Clients cannot connect concepts, and they jump from one subject to another. Circumstantiality and tangentiality also characterize thinking. At times, clients may be unable to communicate thoughts or needs in ways that others understand.

These clients start many projects at one time but cannot carry any to completion. There is little true planning, but clients talk non-stop about plans and projects to anyone and everyone, insisting on the importance of accomplishing these activities. Sometimes they try to enlist help from others in one or more activities. They do not consider risks or personal experience, abilities or resources. Clients start these activities as they occur in their thought processes. Examples of these multiple activities are going on shopping sprees, using credit cards excessively while unemployed and broke, starting several business ventures at once, having promiscuous sex, gambling, taking impulsive trips, embarking on illegal endeavours, making risky investments, talking with many people and speeding (American Psychiatric Association, 2000).

Some clients experience psychotic features during mania; they express grandiose delusions involving importance, fame, privilege and wealth. Some may claim to be the Prime Minister, a famous film star, or even God or a prophet.

SENSORY AND INTELLECTUAL PROCESSES

Clients may be oriented to person and place but rarely to time. Intellectual functioning, such as fund of knowledge, is difficult to assess during the manic phase. Clients may claim to have many abilities they do not possess. The ability to concentrate or to pay attention is grossly impaired. Again, if a client is psychotic, he or she may experience hallucinations.

JUDGEMENT AND INSIGHT

People in the manic phase are easily angered and irritated and strike back at what they perceive as censorship by others because they impose no restrictions on themselves. They are impulsive and rarely think before acting or speaking, which makes their judgement poor. Insight is limited because they believe they are 'fine' and have no problems. They blame any difficulties on others.

SELF-CONCEPT

Clients with mania often have exaggerated self-esteem; they believe they can accomplish anything. They rarely discuss their self-concept realistically. Nevertheless, a false sense of well-being masks difficulties with chronic low self-esteem.

ROLES AND RELATIONSHIPS

Clients in a manic phase can rarely fulfil role responsibilities. They have trouble at work or school (if they are even attending) and are too distracted and hyperactive to pay attention to children or activities of daily living. Although they may begin many tasks or projects, they complete few.

These clients have a great need to socialize but little understanding of their excessive, overpowering and confrontational social interactions. Their need for socialization often leads to promiscuity. Clients invade the intimate space and personal business of others. Arguments result when others feel threatened by such boundary invasions. Although the usual mood of manic people is elation, emotions are unstable and can fluctuate (**labile emotions**) readily between euphoria and hostility. Clients with mania can become hostile to others whom they perceive as standing in the way of desired goals. They cannot postpone or delay gratification. For example, a manic client tells his wife, 'You are the most wonderful woman in the world. Give me £50 so I can buy you a ticket to the opera.' When she refuses, he snarls and accuses her of being tight and selfish and may even hit her.

PHYSIOLOGICAL AND SELF-CARE CONSIDERATIONS

Clients with mania can go for days without sleep or food and not even realize they are hungry or tired. They may be on the brink of physical exhaustion but are unwilling or unable to stop, rest or sleep. They often ignore personal hygiene as 'boring' when they have 'more important things' to do. Clients may throw away possessions or destroy valued items. They may even physically injure themselves and tend to ignore or be unaware of health needs that can worsen.

Data Analysis

The nurse analyses assessment data to determine priorities and to establish a plan of care. Nursing formulations commonly established for clients in the manic phase are as follows:

- Risk for other-directed violence
- Risk of injury
- Imbalanced nutrition: less than body requirements

- Ineffective coping
- Non-concordance with medication
- Ineffective role performance
- Self-care deficit
- Chronic low self-esteem
- Disturbed sleep pattern.

Outcome Identification

Examples of outcomes appropriate to mania are as follows:

- The client will not injure self or others.
- The client will establish a balance of rest, sleep and activity.
- The client will establish adequate nutrition, hydration and elimination.
- The client will participate in self-care activities.
- The client will evaluate personal qualities realistically.
- The client will engage in socially appropriate, reality-based interaction.
- The client will verbalize knowledge of his or her illness and treatment.

Intervention

PROVIDING FOR SAFETY

Because of the safety risks that clients in the manic phase take, safety plays a primary role in care, followed by issues related to self-esteem and socialization. A primary nursing responsibility is to provide a safe environment for clients and others. The nurse assesses clients directly for suicidal ideation and plans or thoughts of hurting others. In addition, clients in the manic phase have little insight into their anger and agitation and how their behaviours affect others. They often intrude into others' space, take others' belongings without permission or appear aggressive in approaching others. This behaviour can threaten or anger people who then retaliate. It is important to monitor the clients' whereabouts and behaviours frequently if they are on the ward.

A ward nurse should also tell clients that staff members will help them control their behaviour if clients cannot do so alone. For clients who feel out of control, the nurse must establish external controls empathetically and non-judgementally. These external controls provide long-term comfort to clients, although their initial response may be aggression. People in the manic phase have labile emotions; it is not unusual for them to hit staff members who have set limits in a way clients dislike.

These clients invade boundaries physically and psychologically. It is necessary to set limits when they cannot set limits on themselves. For example, the nurse might say,

'John, you are too close to my face. Please stand back a couple of feet.'

or

'It's not OK to hug other clients. You can talk to others, but please don't touch them.'

When setting limits, it is important to clearly identify the unacceptable behaviour and the expected, appropriate behaviour. All staff must consistently set and enforce limits for those limits to be effective.

MEETING PHYSIOLOGICAL NEEDS

Clients with mania may get very little rest or sleep, even if they are on the brink of physical exhaustion. Medication may be helpful, though clients may resist taking it. Decreasing environmental stimulation may assist clients to relax. The nurse provides a quiet environment without noise, television or other distractions. Establishing a bedtime routine, such as a tepid bath, may help clients to calm down enough to rest.

Nutrition is another area of concern. Manic clients may be too 'busy' to sit down and eat, or they may have such poor concentration that they fail to stay interested in food for very long. 'Finger foods' or things clients can eat while moving around are the best options to improve nutrition. Such foods should also be as high in calories and protein as possible. For example, celery and carrots are finger foods, but they supply little nutrition. Sandwiches, protein bars and fortified drinks are better choices. Clients with mania also benefit from food that is easy to eat without much preparation. Meat that must be cut into bite sizes or plates of spaghetti are not likely to be successful options. Having snacks available between meals, so clients can eat whenever possible, is also useful.

The nurse needs to monitor food and fluid intake and hours of sleep until clients routinely meet these needs without difficulty. Observing and supervising clients at meal times are also important to prevent clients from taking food from others.

PROVIDING THERAPEUTIC COMMUNICATION

People with mania have short attention spans, so the nurse should use clear, simple sentences when communicating. They may not be able to handle a lot of information at once, so the nurse breaks information into many small segments. It helps to ask clients to repeat brief messages to ensure they have heard and incorporated them.

Clients may need to undergo baseline and follow-up blood tests. A brief explanation of the purpose of each test allays anxiety. The nurse gives printed information to reinforce verbal messages, especially those related to rules, schedules, legal rights, treatment, staff names and client education.

The speech of manic clients may be pressured: rapid, circumstantial, rhyming, noisy or intrusive with flights of ideas. Such disordered speech indicates thought processes

NURSING INTERVENTIONS FOR MANIA

Provide for client's physical safety and safety of those around client.

- Set limits on client's behaviour when necessary.
- Remind the client to respect distances between self and others.
- Use short, simple sentences to communicate.
- Clarify the meaning of client's communication.
- Frequently provide finger foods that are high in calories and protein.
- Promote rest and sleep.
- Protect the client's dignity when inappropriate behaviour occurs.
- Channel client's need for movement into socially acceptable motor activities.

that are flooded with thoughts, ideas and impulses. The nurse must keep channels of communication open with clients, regardless of speech patterns. The nurse can say,

'Please speak more slowly. I'm having trouble following you.'

This puts the responsibility for the communication difficulty on the nurse rather than on the client. The nurse patiently and frequently repeats this request during conversation because clients will return to rapid speech.

Clients in the manic phase often use pronouns when referring to people, making it difficult for listeners to understand who is being discussed and when the conversation has moved to a new subject. While clients are agitatedly talking, they are usually thinking and moving just as quickly, so it is a challenge for the nurse to follow a coherent story. The nurse can ask clients to identify each person, place or thing being discussed.

When speech includes flight of ideas, the nurse can ask clients to explain the relationship between topics; for example,

'What happened then?'

or

'Was that before you got married?'

The nurse also assesses and documents the coherence of messages.

Clients with pressured speech rarely let others speak. Instead, they talk non-stop until they run out of steam or just stand there looking at the other person before moving away. Those with pressured speech do not respond to others' verbal or non-verbal signals that indicate a desire to speak. The nurse avoids becoming involved in power struggles over who will dominate the conversation. Instead, the nurse may talk to clients away from others so there is no 'competition' for the nurse's attention. The nurse also sets limits regarding taking turns speaking and listening, as well as giving attention to others when they need it. Clients with mania cannot have all requests granted immediately even though that may be what they want.

PROMOTING APPROPRIATE BEHAVIOURS

These clients need to be protected from their pursuit of socially unacceptable and/or risky behaviours. The nurse can direct their need for movement into socially acceptable, large motor activities such as arranging chairs for a community meeting or walking. In acute mania, clients lose the ability to control their behaviour and engage in risky activities. Because acutely manic clients feel extraordinarily powerful, they place few restrictions on themselves. They act out impulsive thoughts, have inflated and grandiose perceptions of their abilities, are demanding and need immediate gratification. This can affect their physical, social, occupational or financial safety, as well as that of others. Clients may make purchases that exceed their ability to pay. They may give away money or jewellery or other possessions. The nurse may need to monitor a client's access to such items until his or her behaviour is less impulsive.

In an acute manic episode, clients also may lose sexual inhibitions, resulting in provocative and risky behaviours. Clothing may be flashy or revealing, or clients may undress in public areas. They may engage in unprotected sex with virtual strangers. Clients may ask staff members or other clients (of the same or opposite sex) for sex, graphically describe sexual acts or display their genitals. The nurse handles such behaviour in a matter-of-fact, **non-judgemental** manner. For example,

'Mary, let's go to your room and find a sweater.'

It is important to treat clients with dignity and respect despite their inappropriate behaviour. It is not helpful to 'scold' or chastise them; they are not children engaging in wilful misbehaviour.

In the manic phase, clients cannot understand personal boundaries, so it is the staff's role to keep clients in view for intervention as necessary. For example, a staff member who sees a client invading the intimate space of others can say,

'Jeffrey, I'd really appreciate your help in set-ting up a circle of chairs in the group therapy room.'

This large motor activity distracts Jeffrey from his inappropriate behaviour, appeals to his need for heightened physical activity, is non-competitive and is socially acceptable. The staff's vigilant redirection to a more socially appropriate activity protects clients from the hazards of unprotected sex and reduces embarrassment over such behaviours when they return to normal behaviour.

MANAGING MEDICATIONS

Lithium is not metabolized; rather, it is reabsorbed by the proximal tubule of the kidney and excreted in the urine. Periodic serum lithium levels are used to monitor the client's safety and to ensure that the dose given has increased the serum lithium level to a treatment level or reduced it to a maintenance level. There is a narrow range of safety between maintenance levels (0.4 to 1 mmol/l) and toxic levels (1.5 mmol/l and above). It is important to assess for signs of toxicity and to ensure that clients and their families have this information before discharge (Table 15.7). Older adults can have symptoms of toxicity at lower serum levels. Lithium is potentially fatal in overdose.

Clients should drink adequate water (approximately 2 litres/day) and continue with the usual amount of dietary table salt. Having too much salt in the diet because of unusually salty foods or the ingestion of salt-containing antacids can reduce receptor availability for lithium and increase lithium excretion, so the lithium level will be too low. If there is too much water, lithium is diluted and the lithium level will be too low to be therapeutic. Drinking too little water or losing fluid through excessive sweating, vomiting or diarrhoea increases the lithium level, which may result in toxicity. Monitoring daily weight and the balance between intake and output, and checking for dependent oedema, can be helpful in monitoring fluid balance. A medical assessment needs to be undertaken urgently if the client has diarrhoea, fever, flu or any condition that leads to dehydration.

Thyroid function tests are usually ordered as a baseline and every 6 months during treatment with lithium. In 6 to 18 months, one-third of clients taking lithium have an increased level of thyroid-stimulating hormone, which can cause anxiety, labile emotions and sleeping difficulties. Decreased levels are implicated in fatigue and depression.

Because most lithium is excreted in the urine, baseline and periodic assessments of renal status are necessary to assess renal function. The reduced renal function in older adults necessitates lower doses. Lithium is contraindicated in people with compromised renal function or urinary retention and those taking low-salt diets or diuretics. Lithium is also contraindicated in people with brain or cardiovascular damage.

PROVIDING CLIENT AND FAMILY TEACHING

Educating clients about the dangers of risky behaviour is necessary; however, clients with acute mania largely fail to heed such teaching because they have little patience or capacity to listen, understand and see the relevance of this information. Clients with euphoria may not see why the behaviour is a problem because they believe they can do

Table 15.7 SYMPTOMS OF AND INTERVENTIONS IN LITHIUM TOXICITY

Serum Lithium Level	Symptoms of Lithium Toxicity	Interventions
1.5–2 mmol/l	Nausea and vomiting, diarrhoea, reduced co-ordination, drowsiness, slurred speech, muscle weakness	Withhold next dose; call doctor. Serum lithium levels are ordered and doses of lithium are usually suspended for a few days or the dose is reduced
2–3 mmol/l	Ataxia, agitation, blurred vision, tinnitus, giddiness, choreoathetoid movements, confusion, muscle fasciculation, hyperreflexia, hypertonic muscles, myoclonic twitches, pruritus, maculopapular rash, movement of limbs, slurred speech, large output of dilute urine, incontinence of bladder or bowel, vertigo	Withhold future doses, call doctor, order serum lithium levels immediately. Gastric lavage may be used to remove oral lithium; IV containing saline and electrolytes used to ensure fluid and electrolyte function and maintain renal function
3.0 mmol/l and above	Cardiac arrhythmia, hypotension, peripheral vascular collapse, focal or generalized seizures, reduced levels of consciousness from stupor to coma, myoclonic jerks of muscle groups and spasticity of muscles	All preceding interventions plus lithium ion excretion is augmented with use of aminophylline, mannitol or urea. Haemodialysis may also be used to remove lithium from the body. Respiratory, circulatory, thyroid and immune systems are monitored and assisted as needed

Adapted from British National Formulary Online (2008) http://www.bnf.org/bnf/bnf/55/

anything with impunity. As they begin to cycle toward a more balanced mood, however, risky behaviour lessens, and clients become ready and able for teaching.

Manic clients start many tasks, create many goals and try to carry them out all at once. The result is that they usually cannot complete any. They move readily between these goals while sometimes obsessing about the importance of one over another, but the goals can quickly change. Clients may invest in a business in which they have no knowledge or experience, go on spending sprees, impulsively travel, speed, make new 'best friends' and take the centre of attention in any group. They are egocentric and have little concern for others except as listeners, sexual partners or the means to achieve one of their poorly conceived goals.

Education and collaborative information-exchange about the cause of bipolar affective disorder, medication management, ways to deal with behaviours and potential problems that manic people can encounter is important for family members. Education reduces the guilt, blame and shame that accompany mental health problems; increases client safety; enlarges the support system for clients and the family members; and promotes concordance. Education takes the 'mystery' out of treatment for mental health problems by providing a proactive view: this is what we know, this is what can be done and this is what you can do to help.

Family members often say they know clients have stopped taking their medication when, for example, clients become more argumentative, talk about buying expensive items that they cannot afford, hotly deny anything is wrong or demonstrate any other signs of escalating mania. People sometimes need permission to act on their observations, so a family education session is an appropriate place to give this permission and to set up interventions for various behaviours.

Working with partners of people diagnosed with bipolar affective disorder can be especially useful. Financial mismanagement and sexual promiscuity can place immense strain on relationships: educational and supportive counselling interventions can help with the distress that behaviours like this can cause.

Clients should learn the potential benefits of adhering to the established dosage of lithium and not to omit doses or change dosage intervals; unprescribed dosage alterations interfere with maintenance of serum lithium levels. Clients should know about the many drugs that interact with lithium and should tell each doctor or nurse they consult that they are taking lithium. When a client taking lithium seems to have increased manic behaviour, lithium levels should be checked to determine whether there is lithium toxicity. Periodic monitoring of serum lithium levels is necessary to ensure the safety and adequacy of the treatment regimen. Persistent thirst and diluted urine can indicate the need to call a doctor and have the serum lithium level checked to see if the dosage needs to be reduced.

Clients and family members should know the symptoms of lithium toxicity and interventions to take, including

CLIENT/FAMILY EDUCATION FOR MANIA

- Teach about bipolar affective disorder and ways to manage the disorder.
- Teach about medication management, including the need for periodic blood tests and management of side-effects.
- For clients taking lithium, teach about the need for adequate salt and fluid intake.
- Teach the client and family about signs of toxicity and the need to seek medical attention immediately.
- Educate the client and family about risk-taking behaviour and how to avoid it.
- Teach about behavioural signs of relapse and how to seek treatment in early stages.

backup plans if the physician is not immediately available. The nurse should give these in writing and explain them to clients and family.

MDF, The Bipolar Organization, runs a pragmatic online and face-to-face programme called STEADY for young people (aged 18–25) diagnosed with bipolar affective disorder: this programme helps people develop the knowledge and necessary tools needed to cope with swings in mood and the impact on self and others.

Evaluation

Evaluation of the treatment of bipolar affective disorder includes, but is not limited to, the following:

- Safety issues
- Comparison of mood and affect between start of treatment and present
- Adherence to a treatment regimen of medication and psychotherapy
- Changes in client's perception of quality of life
- Achievement of specific goals of treatment, including new coping methods.

SUICIDE

Suicide is the intentional act of killing oneself. As we've seen, suicidal thoughts and behaviours are common in people with a wide range of mental health problems, including bipolar disorder and depression.

UK and Irish strategies such as The National Suicide Prevention Strategy for England, launched in 2002 (Department of Health, 2002) have had some small success: in England, reducing both overall suicide rates and those in young men and in mental-health inpatients – groups particularly at risk. Nevertheless, 4187 men and 1706 women killed themselves in the UK and Ireland in 2005.

The higher suicide rates for men are partly the result of the method chosen (e.g. shooting, hanging, jumping from a high place): women are more likely to overdose on medication. Men, young women, whites and separated and divorced people are at increased risk for suicide. Adults older than age 65 years compose 10% of the population but account for 25% of suicides. Suicide is the second leading cause of death (after accidents) among people between 15 and 24 years of age, and the rate of suicide is increasing most rapidly in this age group (Andreasen & Black, 2006).

Clients diagnosed with psychiatric disorders, especially depression, bipolar disorder, schizophrenia, substance abuse, PTSD and borderline personality disorder, are at increased risk of suicide (Rihmer, 2007). Chronic medical illnesses associated with increased risk of suicide include cancer, HIV or AIDS, diabetes, cerebrovascular accidents and head and spinal cord injury. Environmental factors that increase suicide risk include isolation, recent loss, lack of social support, unemployment, critical life events and family history of depression or suicide. Behavioural factors that increase risk include impulsivity, erratic or unexplained changes from usual behaviour and unstable lifestyle (Swann et al., 2005; Valente & Saunders, 2005).

'Suicidal ideation' is a common term meaning thinking about killing oneself. *Active* suicidal ideation is when a person thinks about and seeks ways to commit suicide. *Passive* suicidal ideation is when a person thinks about wanting to die or wishes he or she were dead but has no plans to cause his or her death. People with active suicidal ideation are considered more potentially lethal.

Attempted suicide is a suicidal act that either failed or was incomplete. In an incomplete suicide attempt, the person did not finish the act because (1) someone recognized the suicide attempt as a 'cry for help' and responded; or (2) the person was discovered and rescued (Sudak, 2005).

Suicide involves ambivalence (Shea, 2002). Many fatal accidents may be impulsive suicides. It is impossible to know, for example, whether the person who drove into a telephone pole did this intentionally. Hence, keeping accurate statistics on suicide is difficult. There are also many myths and misconceptions about suicide, of which the nurse should be aware. The nurse must know the facts and warning signs for those at risk for suicide, as described in Box 15.7.

Assessment

A history of previous suicide attempts increases risk of suicide. The first 2 years after an attempt represent the highest risk period, especially the first 3 months. Those with a relative who committed suicide are at increased risk for suicide: the closer the relationship, the greater the risk. One possible explanation is that the relative's suicide offers a sense of 'permission' or acceptance of suicide as a method

of escaping a difficult situation. This familiarity and acceptance is also believed to contribute to 'copycat suicides' by teenagers, who are greatly influenced by their peers' actions (Sudak, 2005).

Many people with depression who have suicidal ideation lack the energy to implement suicide plans. The natural energy that accompanies increased sunlight in spring is believed to explain why most suicides occur in April. Most suicides happen on Monday mornings, when most people return to work (another energy spurt). Research has shown that antidepressant treatment can actually give clients with depression the energy to act on suicidal ideation (Sudak, 2005).

WARNINGS OF SUICIDAL INTENT

Most people with suicidal ideation send either direct or indirect signals to others about their intent to harm themselves. The nurse *never* ignores any hint of suicidal ideation regardless of how trivial or subtle it seems and the client's intent or emotional status. Often, people contemplating suicide have ambivalent and conflicting feelings about their desire to die; they frequently reach out to others for help. For example, a client might say,

 'I keep thinking about taking my entire supply of medications to end it all' (direct) or *'I just can't take it anymore'* (indirect).

Box 15.8 provides more examples of client statements about suicide, and effective responses from the nurse.

Asking clients directly about thoughts of suicide is important. Assessment interview forms routinely include such questions. It is also standard practice to enquire about suicide or self-harm thoughts in any setting where people seek treatment for emotional problems.

RISKY BEHAVIOURS

A few people who commit suicide give no warning signs. Some artfully hide their distress and suicide plans. Others act impulsively by taking advantage of a situation to carry out the desire to die. Some suicidal people in treatment describe placing themselves in risky or dangerous situations such as speeding in a blinding rainstorm or when intoxicated. This 'Russian roulette' approach carries a high risk for harm to clients and innocent bystanders alike. It allows clients to feel brave by repeatedly confronting death and surviving.

LETHALITY ASSESSMENT

When a client admits to having a 'death wish' or suicidal thoughts, the next step is to determine potential lethality. This assessment involves asking the following questions:

- Does the client have a plan? If so, what is it? Is the plan specific?

Box 15.7   MYTHS AND FACTS ABOUT SUICIDE

Myths	Facts
People who talk about suicide never commit suicide.	Suicidal people often send out subtle or not-so-subtle messages that convey their inner thoughts of hopelessness and self-destruction. Both subtle and direct messages of suicide should be taken seriously with appropriate assessments and interventions.
Suicidal people only want to hurt themselves, not others.	Although the self-violence of suicide demonstrates anger turned inward, the anger can be directed toward others in a planned or impulsive action. *Physical harm:* Psychotic people may be responding to inner voices that command the individual to kill others before killing the self. A depressed person who has decided to commit suicide with a gun may impulsively shoot the person who tries to grab the gun in an effort to thwart the suicide. *Emotional harm:* Often, family members, friends, healthcare professionals, and even police involved in trying to avert a suicide, or those who did not realize the person's depression and plans to commit suicide, feel intense guilt and shame because of their failure to help, and are 'stuck' in a never-ending cycle of despair and grief. Some people, depressed after the suicide of a loved one, will rationalize that suicide was a 'good way out of the pain' and plan their own suicide to escape pain. Some suicides are planned to engender guilt and pain in survivors; for example, as someone who wants to punish another for rejecting or not returning love.
There is no way to help someone who wants to kill himself or herself.	Nearly all suicidal people have mixed feelings about their wish to die, wish to kill others, or to be killed. This ambivalence often prompts the cries for help evident in overt or covert cues. Intervention can help the suicidal individual get help from situational supports, choose to live, learn new ways to cope and move forward in life.
Do not mention the word *suicide* to a person you suspect to be suicidal, because this could give him or her the idea to commit suicide. Ignoring verbal threats of suicide or challenging a person to carry out his or her suicide plans will reduce the individual's use of these behaviours.	Suicidal people have already thought of the idea of suicide and may have begun plans. Asking about suicide does not cause a non-suicidal person to become suicidal. Suicidal gestures are a potentially lethal way to act out. Threats should not be ignored or dismissed, nor should a person be challenged to carry out suicidal threats. All plans, threats, gestures or cues should be taken seriously, and immediate help given that focuses on the problem about which the person is suicidal. When asked about suicide, it is often a relief for the client to know that his or her cries for help have been heard and that help is on the way.
Once a suicide risk, always a suicide risk.	Although it is true that most people who successfully commit suicide have made attempts at least once before, most people with suicidal ideation can have positive resolution to the suicidal crisis. With proper support, finding new ways to resolve the problem helps these individuals become emotionally secure and have no further need for suicide as a way to resolve a problem.

- Are the means available to carry out this plan? (For example, if the person plans to shoot himself, does he have access to a gun and ammunition?)
- If the client carries out the plan, is it likely to be lethal? (For example, a plan to take 10 aspirin is probably not lethal; a plan to take a 2-week supply of a tricyclic antidepressants is.)
- Has the client made preparations for death, such as giving away prized possessions, writing a suicide note or talking to friends one last time?
- Where and when does the client intend to carry out the plan?
- Is the intended time a special date or anniversary that has meaning for the client?

Box 15.8   SUICIDAL IDEATION: CLIENT STATEMENTS AND NURSE RESPONSES

Client Statement	Nurse Responses
'I just want to go to sleep and not think any more.'	'Can you tell me exactly how you're planning to sleep and not think anymore?' 'By "sleep", do you mean "die"?' 'What is it you don't want to think of anymore?' 'I'm wondering if you're thinking about suicide?'
'I want it to be all over.'	'What is it you specifically want to be over?' 'Are you planning to end your life?'
'It will just be the end of the story.'	'How do you plan to end your story?'
'You have been a good friend.' 'Remember me.'	'You sound as if you're saying goodbye. Are you?' 'Are you planning to commit suicide?' 'What is it you really want me to remember about you?'
'Here is my chess set that you have always admired.'	'What's going on that you're giving away things to remember you by?'
'If there is ever any need for anyone to know this, my will and insurance papers are in the top drawer of my dresser.'	'I appreciate you trusting me. However, I think there's maybe a message you're giving me. Are you thinking of ending your life?'
'I can't stand the pain anymore.'	'How do you plan to end the pain?' 'Tell me about the pain.' 'Sounds like you are planning to harm yourself.'
'Everyone will feel bad soon.' 'I just can't bear it anymore.'	'Who is the person you want to feel bad by killing yourself?' 'What is it you can't bear?' 'How do you see an end to this?'
'Everyone would be better off without me.'	'Who is one person you believe would be better off without you?' 'How do you plan to eliminate yourself, if you think everyone would be better off without you?' 'What is one way you perceive others would be better off without you?'
Non-verbal change in behaviour from agitated to calm, anxious to relaxed, depressed to smiling, hostile to benign, from being without direction to appearing to be goal-directed	'You seem different today. What's that about?' 'I sense you've reached a decision. Tell me about it.'

Specific and positive answers to these questions all increase the client's likelihood of committing suicide. It is important to consider whether or not the client believes her or his method is lethal even if it is not. Believing a method to be lethal poses a significant risk.

Outcome Identification

Suicide prevention frequently involves intensive psychological input alongside treating any underlying disorder, such as mood disorder or psychosis, with psychoactive agents. The overall goals are first to keep the client safe and later to help him or her to develop new coping skills that do not involve self-harm. Other outcomes may relate to activities of daily living, sleep and nourishment needs, and problems specific to the crisis, such as stabilization of symptoms.

Examples of outcomes for a suicidal person include the following:

- The client will be safe from harming self or others.
- The client will engage in a therapeutic relationship.
- The client will establish a no-suicide contract.
- The client will create a list of positive attributes.
- The client will generate, test and evaluate realistic plans to address underlying issues.

Intervention

USING AN AUTHORITATIVE ROLE

Intervention for suicide or suicidal ideation becomes the first priority of nursing care. The nurse assumes a nurturing, parental and authoritative role to help clients stay safe. In this crisis situation, clients see few or no alternatives to

Nursing Care Plan *Depression*

Nursing Formulation

Ineffective Coping: *Inability to form a valid appraisal of external and internal stressors, and/or inability to use available resources.*

ASSESSMENT DATA

- Suicidal ideas or behaviour
- Slowed mental processes
- Disordered thoughts
- Feelings of despair, hopelesssness and worthlessness
- Guilt
- Anhedonia (inability to experience pleasure)
- Diorientation
- Generalized restlessness or agitation
- Sleep disturbances: early waking, insomnia or excessive sleeping
- Anger or hostility (may not be overt)
- Rumination
- Delusions, hallucinations or other psychotic symptoms
- Diminished interest in sexual activity
- Fear of intensity of feelings
- Anxiety

EXPECTED OUTCOMES

Immediate
The client will
- Be free from self-inflicted harm
- Engage in satisfying, reality-based interactions
- Be oriented to person, place and time
- Express anger or hostility outwardly in a safe manner

Medium term
The client will
- Express feelings directly with congruent verbal and non-verbal messages
- Be free from psychotic symptoms
- Demonstrate functional level of psychomotor activity

Longer term
The client will
- Demonstrate concordance with and knowledge of medications, if any
- Demonstrate an increased ability to cope with anxiety, stress or frustration
- Verbalize or demonstrate acceptance of loss or change, if any
- Identify a support system in the communities

IMPLEMENTATION

Nursing Interventions *denotes collaborative interventions

Provide a safe environment for the client.

Continually assess the client's potential for suicide. Remain aware of this suicide potential at all times.

Observe the client closely, especially under the following circumstances:
- After antidepressant medication begins to raise the client's mood.
- In first weeks after discharge.
- After significant life change.
- Unstructured time on the unit or times when the number of staff on the unit is limited.
- After any dramatic behavioural change (sudden cheerfulness, relief or giving away personal belongings).

Rationale

Physical safety of the client is a priority. Many common items may be used in a self-destructive manner.

Depressed clients may have a potential for suicide that may or may not be expressed, and that may change with time.

You must be aware of the client's activities at all times when there is a potential for suicide or self-injury. Risk for suicide increases as the client's energy level is increased by medication, when the client's time is unstructured and when observation of the client decreases. These changes may indicate that the client has come to a decision to commit suicide.

continued ⋯⟩

Nursing Care Plan: Depression, cont.

IMPLEMENTATION

Nursing Interventions *denotes collaborative interventions	**Rationale**
Reorient the client to person, place and time as indicated (call the client by name, tell the client your name, tell the client where he or she is and so forth).	Repeated presentation of reality is concrete reinforcement for the client.
Spend time with the client.	Your physical presence is reality.
If the client is ruminating, tell him or her that you will talk about reality or about the client's feelings, but limit the attention given to repeated expressions of rumination.	Minimizing attention may help decrease rumination. Providing reinforcement for reality orientation and expression of feelings will encourage these behaviours.
Initially assign the same staff members to work with the client whenever possible.	The client's ability to respond to others may be impaired. Limiting the number of new contacts initially will facilitate familiarity and trust. However, the number of people interacting with the client should increase as soon as possible, to minimize dependency and to facilitate the client's abilities to communicate with a variety of people.
When approaching the client, use a moderate, level tone of voice. Avoid being overly cheerful.	Being overly cheerful may indicate to the client that being cheerful is the goal and that other feelings are not acceptable.
Use silence and active listening when interacting with the client. Let the client know that you are concerned and that you consider the client a worthwhile person.	The client may not communicate if you are talking too much. Your presence and use of active listening will communicate your interest and concern.
When first communicating with the client, use simple, direct sentences; avoid complex sentences or directions.	The client's ability to perceive and respond to complex stimuli is impaired.
Avoid asking the client many questions, especially questions that require only brief answers.	Asking questions and requiring only brief answers may discourage the client from expressing feelings.
Be comfortable sitting with the client in silence. Let the client know you are available to converse, but do not require the client to talk.	Your silence will convey your expectation that the client will communicate and your acceptance of the client's difficulty with communication.
Allow (and encourage) the client to cry. Stay with and support the client if he or she desires. Provide privacy if the client desires and it is safe to do so.	Crying is a healthy way of expressing feelings of sadness, hopelessness and despair. The client may not feel comfortable crying and may need encouragement or privacy.
Do not cut off interactions with cheerful remarks or platitudes (e.g. 'No one really wants to die,' or 'You'll feel better soon'). Do not belittle the client's feelings. Accept the client's verbalizations of feelings as real, and give support for expressions of emotions, especially those that may be difficult for the client (like anger).	You may be uncomfortable with certain feelings the client expresses. If so, it is important for you to recognize this and discuss it with another staff member rather than directly or indirectly communicating your discomfort to the client. Proclaiming the client's feelings to be inappropriate or belittling them is detrimental.
Encourage the client to ventilate feelings in whatever way is comfortable – verbal and non-verbal. Let the client know you will listen and accept what is being expressed.	Expressing feelings may help relieve despair, hopelessness and so forth. Feelings are not inherently good or bad. You must remain non-judgemental about the client's feelings and express this to the client.

continued ⋯⟶

Nursing Care Plan: Depression, cont.

IMPLEMENTATION

Nursing Interventions *denotes collaborative interventions	**Rationale**
Interact with the client on topics with which he or she is comfortable. Do not probe for information.	Topics that are uncomfortable for the client and probing may be threatening and discourage communication. After trust has been established, the client may be able to discuss more difficult topics.
Teach the client about the problem-solving process: explore possible options, examine the consequences of each alternative, select and implement an alternative and evaluate the results.	The client may be unaware of a systematic method for solving problems. Successful use of the problem-solving process facilitates the client's confidence in the use of coping skills.
Provide positive feedback at each step of the process. If the client is not satisfied with the chosen alternative, assist the client to select another alternative.	Positive feedback at each step will give the client many opportunities for success, encourage him or her to persist in problem solving and enhance confidence. The client also can learn to 'survive' making a mistake.

Adapted from Schultz, J. M. & Videbeck, S. L. (2005). *Lippincott's manual of psychiatric nursing care plans* (7th edn). Philadelphia: Lippincott Williams & Wilkins.

resolve their problems. The nurse lets clients know their safety is the primary concern and takes precedence over other needs or wishes. For example, a client may want to be alone in her room to think privately but this is not allowed while she is at increased risk of suicide.

PROVIDING A SAFE ENVIRONMENT

Inpatient units have policies for general environmental safety. Some policies are more liberal than others, but most usually deny clients access to cleaning materials their own medications, sharp scissors and penknives. For suicidal clients, staff members remove any item they can use to commit suicide, such as sharp objects, shoelaces, belts, lighters, matches, pencils, pens and even clothing with drawstrings.

Institutional policies for suicide precautions vary. Observation must always consider the need for continued **engagement** and **collaboration**: it can be therapy as well as containment. For clients with very high apparent risk, one-to-one (or 'special') supervision by one or more staff may need to be initiated. This will mean that staff are at arms length of the client at all times. This may be frustrating or upsetting (and potentially counterproductive), so staff members need to explain the purpose and duration of such supervision, more than once if necessary. It is vital that this observation be combined, wherever possible, with active therapeutic engagement, that its purpose be clearly explained to clients and others (and agreed to if at all possible), that it be seen as a temporary measure – designed as empowering rather than disempowering – and that it be carried out only by appropriately trained staff.

A second level of observation – constant (or 'close') observation – necessitates an allocated member of staff being constantly aware of the exact whereabouts of a patient, either seeing them or hearing them, at all times. (A third level, 'general observation', involves staff being aware of the general whereabouts of all patients at all times.)

Appleby *et al.* (2006) emphasize the need for special observation and close observation to be strictly adhered to when agreed. Bowers and Simpson (2007) found that the more intermittent observations (regular checks at intervals), *alongside* close observation, special observation and general observation, the less self-harm there seemed to be: in addition, the presence of qualified nursing staff and patient activity also seemed to reduce such incidents.

Community environments are – clearly – far harder to make safe, and professionals need to be continually engaging, continually making assessments, taking into account all the time organizational policy, and balancing risk with therapeutic need. CMHTs, crisis teams, AOTs and others who work with people at risk need to have clear risk-assessment and risk-management protocols and excellent communication systems within the team and between teams.

INITIATING A NO-SUICIDE CONTRACT

The nurse can implement a no-suicide contract at home as well as in an inpatient setting. In such contracts, clients agree to keep themselves safe and to notify staff at the first impulse to harm themselves (at home, clients agree to notify their carers; the contract must identify backup people in case carers are unavailable). The urge to commit suicide

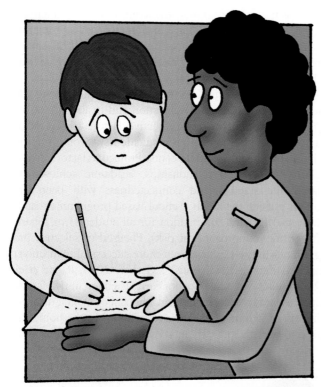

No-suicide contract

may return suddenly, so someone must always be available for support. A list of support people who agree to be readily available should be generated.

Many suicidal people are happy to adhere to no-suicide contracts because they appeal to the will to live. These contracts, however, are not a guarantee of safety. Fallow and O'Brien (2003) questioned whether a suicidal person is truly able to give informed consent to enter into such a contract. Potter and associates (2005) reported that contracts do not prevent self-harm behaviours, but they may assist the nurse in client assessment, and promote interaction about safety issues. At no time should a nurse assume that a client is safe just because a contract is in place.

CREATING A SUPPORT SYSTEM LIST

Suicidal clients often lack social support systems, such as relatives and friends or religious, occupational and community support groups. This lack may result from social withdrawal, behaviour associated with a mental health or medical disorder or movement of the person to a new area because of school, work or change in family structure or financial status. The nurse needs to assess support systems and the type of help each person or group can give a client. CMHTs, hotlines, crisis services, student health services, church groups, support and self-help groups are all potential parts of the community support system.

The nurse makes a list of specific names and agencies that clients can call for support; he or she obtains client consent to avoid breach of confidentiality. Many

suicidal people do not have to be admitted to a hospital and can be treated successfully in the community with the help of effective assertive intervention and care co-ordination.

Family Response

Suicide can be seen as the ultimate rejection of family and friends. Implicit in the act of suicide is the message to others that their help was incompetent, irrelevant or unwelcome. Some suicides are done to place blame on a certain person – even to the point of planning how that person will be the one to discover the body. Most suicides are efforts to escape untenable situations. Even if a person believes love for family members prompted his or her suicide – as in the case of someone who commits suicide to avoid lengthy legal battles or to save the family the financial and emotional cost of a lingering death – relatives still grieve and may feel guilt, shame and anger.

Significant others may feel guilty for not knowing how desperate the suicidal person was, angry because the person did not seek their help or trust them, ashamed that their loved one ended his or her life with a socially unacceptable act and sad about being rejected. Suicide is newsworthy, and there may be whispered gossip and even news coverage. The one death may also rarely spark 'copycat suicides' among family members or others, who may believe they have been 'given permission' to do the same: families and communities can disintegrate after a suicide.

Nurse's Response

When dealing with a client who has suicidal ideation or behaviour, the nurse's attitude must indicate unconditional positive regard – not for the act itself but for the person and his or her desperation. Regardless of diagnosis, the ideas or attempts are serious signals of a desperate emotional state. The nurse must convey the belief that the person can be helped and can grow and change.

Trying to make clients feel guilty for thinking of or attempting suicide is not helpful; they already feel incompetent, hopeless and helpless. The nurse does not blame clients or act judgementally when asking about the details of a planned suicide, rather he or she uses a non-judgemental tone of voice and monitors his or her body language and facial expressions to make sure not to convey disgust or blame.

As nurses, we believe that one person can make a difference in another's life. We must convey this belief when caring for suicidal people. Nevertheless, we must also realize that no matter how competent and caring our interventions are, some people will still commit suicide. A client's suicide can be devastating to the staff members who treated him or her, especially if they have grown to know the person and his or her family well over time. Even with therapy, staff members may end up leaving the particular team or the profession as a result.

CONSIDERATIONS IN OLDER PEOPLE

Alexopoulos (2004) reported that depression is common among the elderly and is markedly increased when elders are medically ill. Older people tend to have psychotic features, particularly delusions, more frequently than younger people with depression. Suicide rates among people older than age 65 are double those of people younger than 65. Late-onset bipolar disorders are rare.

Older people are treated for depression with ECT more frequently than younger people. Older people have increased intolerance of side-effects of antidepressant medications and may not be able to tolerate doses high enough to treat the depression effectively. Also, ECT produces a more rapid response than medications, which may be desirable if the depression is compromising the medical health of the older person. Because suicide risk among the elderly is increased, the most rapid response to treatment becomes even more important (Kellner *et al.*, 2004).

COMMUNITY-BASED CARE CONSIDERATIONS

Nurses in any area of practice in the community are frequently the first health-care professionals to recognize behaviours consistent with mood disorders. In some cases, a family member may mention distress about a client's withdrawal from activities; difficulty thinking, eating and sleeping; complaints of being tired all the time; sadness; and agitation (all symptoms of depression). They might also mention cycles of euphoria, spending binges, loss of inhibitions, changes in sleep and eating patterns and loud clothing styles and colours (all symptoms of the manic phase of bipolar disorder). Documenting and reporting such behaviours can help these people to receive treatment. In the US, estimates are that nearly 40% of people who have been diagnosed with a mood disorder do not receive treatment (Akiskal, 2005). Contributing factors may include the stigma still associated with mental disorders, the lack of understanding about the disruption to life that mood disorders can cause, confusion about treatment choices or a more compelling medical diagnosis; these combine with the reality of limited time that health-care professionals devote to any one client.

People with depression and bipolar disorders can be treated successfully in the community by CMHTs, AOTs and crisis teams. The clinician who treats a person with bipolar disorder must understand psychological approaches, the drug treatment, dosages, desired effects, therapeutic levels and potential side-effects, so that he or she can answer questions and promote understanding of, and agreement with, a plan of care.

MENTAL HEALTH PROMOTION

Many studies have been conducted to determine how to prevent mood disorders and suicide, but prediction of suicide risk in clinical practice remains difficult (Carter *et al.*, 2005). Programmes that use an educational approach designed to address the unique stressors that contribute to the increased incidence of depressive illness in women have had some success. These programmes focus on increasing self-esteem and reducing loneliness and hopelessness, which in turn decrease the likelihood of depression.

Because suicide is a leading cause of death among adolescents, prevention, early detection and treatment are very important. Strengthening protective factors (those factors associated with a reduction in suicide risk) would improve the mental health of adolescents. Protective factors include close parent–child relationships, academic achievement, family-life stability and connectedness with peers and others outside the family. School-based programmes can be universal (general information for all students) or focused (targeting young people at risk). Focused or selective programmes in the US have been more successful than universal programmes (Horowitz & Garber, 2006; Rapee *et al.*, 2006). Likewise, screening for early detection of risk factors, such as family strife, parental alcoholism or mental disorder, history of fighting and access to weapons in the home, can lead to referral and early intervention.

SELF-AWARENESS ISSUES

Nurses working with clients who are depressed often empathize with them and may themselves begin to feel sad or agitated. They may unconsciously start to avoid contact with these clients to escape such feelings. The nurse must monitor his or her feelings and reactions closely when dealing with clients with depression to be sure he or she fulfils the responsibility to establish a therapeutic nurse–client relationship.

People with depression may be negative, pessimistic and unable to generate new ideas easily. They can feel hopeless and incompetent. The nurse can easily become consumed with suggesting ways to fix the problems. Clients may find some reason why the nurse's solutions will not work: 'I have tried that,' 'It would never work,' 'I don't have the time to do that,' or 'You just don't understand,' Rejection of suggestions can make the nurse feel incompetent and question his or her professional skill. Unless a client is suicidal or is experiencing a crisis, the nurse does not try to solve the client's problems. Instead, the nurse uses therapeutic techniques to encourage clients to generate their own solutions. Studies have shown that clients tend to act on plans or solutions they generate rather than those that others offer (Schultz & Videbeck, 2005). Finding and acting on their own solutions gives clients renewed competence and self-worth.

Working with clients who are manic can be exhausting. They are so hyperactive that the nurse may feel spent or tired after caring for them. The nurse may feel frustrated because these clients engage in the same behaviours repeatedly, such as being intrusive with others, undressing, singing, rhyming and dancing. It takes hard work to remain patient and calm with the manic client, but it is essential for the nurse to provide limits and redirection in a calm manner until the client can control his or her own behaviour independently.

Some health-care professionals consider suicidal people to be failures, immoral or unworthy of care. These negative attitudes may result from several factors. They may reflect society's negative view of suicide. Health-care professionals may feel inadequate and anxious dealing with suicidal clients, or they may be uncomfortable about their own mortality. Many of us have had thoughts about 'ending it all', even if for a fleeting moment when life is not going well. The scariness of remembering such flirtations with suicide causes anxiety. If this anxiety is not resolved, the staff person can demonstrate avoidance, demeaning behaviour and superiority to suicidal clients. Therefore, to be effective, the nurse must be aware of his or her own feelings and beliefs about suicide.

Points to Consider When Working With Someone Who May Be Suicidal

- Do I feel that suicide is a sign of weakness in which people should feel shame?
- Do I feel that suicide is immoral or a sin?
- Do I feel that the topic of suicide is taboo? (Have I ever asked someone I know outside of my professional work, such as a family member or close friend, whether he or she is having suicidal ideation? If the answer is 'No', there is a good chance the topic is personally taboo at some level.)
- Do I feel that suicide is essentially illogical and that someone would have to be pretty crazy to ever consider it seriously?
- Do I tend to overreact to the conveyance of suicidal ideation? Do I tend to admit such patients to the hospital too quickly? (Has a supervisor ever commented that I admit too readily? Have I ever placed 'forensic fears' above patient care?)

Adapted from Shea (2002).

Points to Consider When Working With Clients With Mood Disorders

- Remember that clients with mania may appear outwardly happy, but they may also be really suffering internally.
- For clients with mania, delay client education until the acute manic phase is resolving.
- Schedule specific, short periods with depressed or agitated clients to eliminate unconscious avoidance of them.
- Do not try to fix a client's problems. Use therapeutic techniques to help him or her find solutions.
- Use a journal to deal with frustration, anger or personal needs.
- If a particular client's care is troubling, talk with another professional – informally or in **clinical supervision** – about the plan of care, how it is being carried out and how it is working.

Critical Thinking Questions

1. Is it possible for someone to make a 'rational' decision to commit suicide? Under what circumstances?
2. Should suicide have ever been legalized?
3. A person with bipolar disorder frequently discontinues taking medication when out of the hospital, becomes manic and engages in risky behaviour such as speeding, drinking and driving and incurring large debts. How do you reconcile the client's right to refuse medication with public or personal safety? Who should make such a decision? How could it be enforced?

KEY POINTS

- Studies have found a genetic component to some mood disorders. The incidence of depression is up to three times greater in first-degree relatives of people with diagnosed depression. People with bipolar affective disorder often have a blood relative with bipolar disorder.
- Some 9% of people with mood disorders exhibit psychosis.
- Clinical depression is a mood disorder that robs the person of joy, self-esteem and energy. It interferes with relationships and occupational productivity.
- Symptoms of depression include sadness, disinterest in previously pleasurable activities, crying, lack of motivation, asocial behaviour and psychomotor retardation (slowed thinking, talking and movement). Sleep disturbances, somatic complaints, loss of energy, change in weight and a sense of worthlessness are other common features.
- Several antidepressants are used to treat depression. SSRIs, the newest type, have the fewest side-effects. Tricyclic antidepressants are older and have a longer lag period before reaching adequate serum levels; they are the least expensive type. MAOIs are used least: clients are at risk of a hypertensive crisis if they ingest tyramine-rich foods and fluids while taking these drugs. MAOIs also have a lag period before reaching adequate serum levels.
- People with bipolar affective disorder cycle between mania, 'normality' and depression. They may also cycle only between mania and normality or between depression and euthymia.
- Clients with mania may have labile mood, be grandiose and manipulative, have high self-esteem and believe they are capable of anything. They sleep little, are always in frantic motion, invade others' boundaries, cannot sit still and start many tasks. Speech is rapid and pressured, reflects rapid thinking and may be circumstantial and tangential with features of rhyming, punning and flight of ideas. Clients show

poor judgement with little sense of safety needs and take physical, financial, occupational or interpersonal risks.

- Lithium is used to treat bipolar affective disorder. It is helpful for bipolar mania and can partially or completely eradicate cycling toward bipolar depression. Lithium is effective in 75% of clients but has a narrow range of safety; thus, ongoing monitoring of serum lithium levels is necessary to establish efficacy while preventing toxicity. Clients taking lithium must ingest adequate salt and water to avoid overdosing or underdosing because lithium salt uses the same postsynaptic receptor sites as does sodium chloride. Other antimanic drugs include sodium valproate, carbamazepine, other anticonvulsants and clonazepam, which is also a benzodiazepine.
- For clients with mania, the nurse must monitor food and fluid intake, rest and sleep and behaviour, with a focus on safety, until medications reduce the acute stage and clients resume responsibility for themselves.
- People with increased rates of suicide include single adults, divorced men, adolescents, older adults, the very poor or very wealthy, urban dwellers, migrants, students, whites, people with mood disorders, substance abusers, people with medical or personality disorders and people with psychosis.
- The nurse must be alert to clues to a client's suicidal intent – both direct (making threats of suicide) and indirect (giving away prized possessions, putting his or her life in order, making vague goodbyes).
- Conducting a suicide lethality assessment involves determining the degree to which the person has planned his or her death, including time, method, tools, place, person to find the body, reason and funeral plans.
- Nursing interventions for a client at risk for suicide involve keeping the person safe by ensuring focused, empathic, one-to-one engagment, instituting a no-suicide contract, ensuring close supervision and removing objects that the person could use to commit suicide.

REFERENCES

Akiskal, H. S. (2005). Mood disorders: Historical introduction and conceptual overview. In B. J. Sadock & V. A. Sadock (Eds.), *Comprehensive textbook of psychiatry, Vol. 1* (8th edn, pp. 1559–1575). Philadelphia: Lippincott Williams & Wilkins.

Alexopoulos, G. S. (2004). Late-life mood disorders. In J. Sadavoy, L. F. Jarvik, G. T. Grossberg, *et al.* (Eds.), *Comprehensive textbook of geriatric psychiatry* (3rd edn, pp. 609–653). New York: W. W. Norton and Company.

American Psychiatric Association. (2000). *Diagnostic and statistical manual of mental disorders* (4th edn, text revision). Washington, DC: American Psychiatric Association.

Andreasen, N. C. & Black, D. W. (2006) *Introductory textbook of psychiatry* (4th edn). Washington DC: American Psychiatric Publishing.

Andrews, M. M. & Boyle, J. S. (2003). *Transcultural concepts in nursing care* (4th edn). Philadelphia: Lippincott Williams & Wilkins.

Appleby, L., Shaw, L., Kapur, N., & Windfur, K. (2006). *Avoidable deaths: five year report by the National Confidential Inquiry into Suicide and Homicide by People with Mental Illness.* Available: www.medicine.manchester.ac.uk/suicideprevention/nci/Useful/avoidable_deaths_full_report.pdf

Bowden, C. L. (2006). Valproate. In A. F. Schatzberg & C. B. Nemeroff (Eds.), *Essentials of clinical pharmacology* (2nd edn, pp. 355–366). Washington DC: American Psychiatric Publishing.

Bowers, L. & Simpson, A. (2007). Observing and engaging: new ways to reduce self-harm and suicide. *Mental Health Practice, 10,* 10

British National Formulary Online. (2008). Available: http://www.bnf.org/bnf/

Carter, G., Reith, D. M., Whyte, I. M., & McPherson, M. (2005). Repeated self-poisoning: increasing severity of self-harm as a predictor of subsequent suicide. *British Journal of Psychiatry, 186,* 253–257.

Challiner, V. & Griffiths, L. (2000). Electroconvulsive therapy: a review of the literature. *Journal of Psychiatric and Mental Health Nursing, 7*(3), 191–198.

Department of Health. (2002). *National suicide prevention strategy.* Available: http://www.dh.gov.uk/en/Publicationsandstatistics/Publications/PublicationsPolicyAndGuidance/DH_4009474

Eitan, R. & Lerer, B. (2006). Nonpharmacological, somatic treatments of depression: electroconvulsive therapy and novel brain stimulation modalities. *Dialogues in Clinical Neuroscience, 8*(2), 241–258.

Facts and Comparisons. (2007). *Drug facts and comparisons* (61st edn). St. Louis: Facts and Comparisons: A Wolters Kluwer Company.

Fallow, T. L. & O'Brien, A. J. (2003). No-suicide contracting in psychiatric inpatient settings. *Archives of Psychiatric Nursing, 15*(3), 99–106.

Fenton, L., Fasula, M., Ostroff, R., & Sanacora, G. (2006). Can cognitive behavioural therapy reduce relapse rates of depression after ECT? A preliminary study. *Journal of ECT, 22*(3), 196–198.

Frederikse, M., Petrides, G., & Kellner, C. (2006). Continuation and maintenance electroconvulsive therapy for the treatment of depressive illness: A response to the National Institute for Clinical Excellence report. (2006). *Journal of ECT, 22*(1), 13–17.

Freeman, M. P., Wiegand, C., & Gelenberg, A. J. (2006). Lithium. In A. F. Schatzberg & C. B. Nemeroff (Eds.), *Essentials of clinical pharmacology* (2nd edn, pp. 335–354). Washington DC: American Psychiatric Publishing.

Griswold, K. S. & Pessar, L. F. (2000). Management of bipolar disorder. *American Family Physician, 62*(6), 1343–1353.

INTERNET RESOURCES

RESOURCES	INTERNET ADDRESS
Manic Depression Fellowship	http://www.mdf.org.uk
Depression Alliance	www.depressionalliance.org
Samaritans	http://www.samaritans.org/
Supportline	http://www.supportline.org.uk/problems/suicide.php

Horowitz, J. L. & Garber, J. (2006). The prevention of depressive symptoms in children and adolescents: A meta-analytic review. *Journal of Consulting and Clinical Psychology, 74*(3), 401–415.

Kellner, C. H., Coffey, C. E., & Greenberg, R. M. (2004). Electroconvulsive therapy. In J. Sadavoy, L. F. Jarvik, G. T. Grossberg, *et al.* (Eds.), *Comprehensive textbook of geriatric psychiatry* (3rd edn, pp. 845–901). New York: W. W. Norton and Company.

Kellner, C. H., Knapp, R. G., Petrides, G., *et al.* (2006). Continuation electro-convulsive therapy vs pharmacotherapy for relapse prevention in major depression: A multisite study from the consortium for research in electroconvulsive therapy (CORE). *Archives of General Psychiatry, 63*(12), 1337–1344.

Kelsoe, J. R. (2005). Mood disorders: genetics. In B. J. Sadock & V. A. Sadock (Eds.), *Comprehensive textbook of psychiatry, Vol. 1* (8th edn, pp. 1582–1594). Philadelphia: Lippincott Williams & Wilkins.

Ketter, T. A., Wang, P. W., & Post, R. M. (2006). Carbamazepine and oxcarbazepine. In A. F. Schatzberg & C. B. Nemeroff (Eds.), *Essentials of clinical pharmacology* (2nd edn, pp. 367–393). Washington DC: American Psychiatric Publishing.

Kirsch, I., Deacon, B.J., Huedo-Medina, T.B., *et al.* (2008) Initial severity and antidepressant benefits: a meta-analysis of data submitted to the Food and Drug Administration. *PLoS Medicine, 5*(2): e45.

Ma, H. & Teasdale, J. D. (2004). Mindfulness-based cognitive therapy for depression: Replication and exploration of differential relapse prevention effects. *Journal of Consulting and Clinical Psychology, 72*, 31–40.

Mental Health Foundation. (2008). *Statistics on mental health.* Available: http://www.mentalhealth.org.uk/information/mental-health-overview/statistics/

NICE. (2003). *Electroconvulsive therapy.* Available: http://www.nice.org.uk/TA059

NICE. (2007). *Depression: management of depression in primary and secondary care.* Available: http://www.nice.org.uk/nicemedia/pdf/CG23quickrefguideamended.pdf

Office for National Statistics. (2001). *Psychiatric morbidity report.* Available http://www.statistics.gov.uk/STATBASE/Product.asp?vlnk=8258

Potter, M. L., Vitale-Nolen, R., & Dawson, A. M. (2005). Implementation of safety agreements in an acute psychiatric facility. *Journal of the American Psychiatric Nurses Association, 11*(3), 144–155.

Rapee, R. M., Wignall, A., Sheffield, J., *et al.* (2006). Adolescents' reactions to universal and indicated prevention programs for depression: perceived stigma and consumer satisfaction. *Prevention Science, 7*(2), 167–177.

Rihmer, Z. (2007). Suicide risk in mood disorders. *Current Opinion in Psychiatry, 20*(1), 17–22.

Rihmer, Z. & Angst, J. (2005). Mood disorders: epidemiology. In B. J. Sadock & V. A. Sadock (Eds.), *Comprehensive textbook of psychiatry, Vol. 1* (8th edn, pp. 1575–1582). Philadelphia: Lippincott Williams & Wilkins.

Ross, C. A. (2006). The sham ECT literature: implications for consent to ECT. *Ethical Human Psychology and Psychiatry, 8*(1), 17–28.

Rush, A. J. (2005). Mood disorders: treatment of depression. In B. J. Sadock & V. A. Sadock (Eds.), *Comprehensive textbook of psychiatry, Vol. 1* (8th edn, pp. 1652–1661). Philadelphia: Lippincott Williams & Wilkins.

Schultz, J. M. & Videbeck, S. (2005). *Lippincott's manual of psychiatric nursing care plans* (7th edn). Philadelphia: Lippincott Williams & Wilkins.

Segal, Z., Williams, M., & Teasdale, J. (2002). *Mindfulness-based cognitive therapy for depression: a new approach to preventing relapse.* New York: Guilford Press.

Shea, S. (2002). *The practical art of suicide assessment: a guide for mental health professionals and substance abuse counsellors.* Chichester: Wiley.

Sit, D., Rothschild, A. J., & Wisner, K. L. (2006). A review of postpartum psychosis. *Journal of Women's Health, 15*(4), 352–368.

Sudak, H. S. (2005). Suicide. In B. J. Sadock & V. A. Sadock (Eds.), *Comprehensive textbook of psychiatry, Vol. 2* (8th edn, pp. 2442–2453). Philadelphia: Lippincott Williams & Wilkins.

Swann, A. C., Dougherty, D. M., Pazzaglia, P. J., *et al.* (2005). Increased impulsivity associated with severity of suicide attempt history in patients with bipolar disorder. *American Journal of Psychiatry, 162*(9), 1680–1687.

Teasdale, J. T., Segal, Z. V., Williams, J. M. G., Ridgeway, V., Soulsby, J., & Lau, M. (2000). Prevention of relapse–recurrence in major depression by mindfulness-based cognitive therapy. *Journal of Consulting and Clinical Psychology, 68*, 615–623.

Tecott, L. H. & Smart, S. L. (2005). Monoamine neurotransmitters. In B. J. Sadock & V. A. Sadock (Eds.), *Comprehensive textbook of psychiatry, Vol. 1* (8th edn, pp. 49–60). Philadelphia: Lippincott Williams & Wilkins.

Thase, M. E. (2005). Mood disorders: neurobiology. In B. J. Sadock & V. A. Sadock (Eds.), *Comprehensive textbook of psychiatry, Vol. 1* (8th edn, pp. 1594–1603). Philadelphia: Lippincott Williams & Wilkins.

UK ECT Review Group. (2003). Efficacy and safety of electroconvulsive therapy in depressive disorders: a systematic review and meta-analysis. *Lancet, 361*, 799–808.

Valente, S. M. & Saunders, J. (2005). Screening for depression and suicide: Self-report instruments that work. *Journal of Psychosocial Nursing, 43*(11), 22–31.

Williams, C. & Garland, A. (2002). A cognitive–behavioural therapy assessment model for use in everyday clinical practice. *Advances in Psychiatric Treatment, 8*, 172–179.

ADDITIONAL READING

Crocker, L., Clare, L., & Evans, K. (2006). Giving up or finding a solution? The experience of attempted suicide in later life. *Aging and Mental Health, 10*(6), 638–647.

D'Augelli, A. R., Grossman, A. H., Saiter, N. P., *et al.* (2005). Predicting the suicide attempts of lesbian, gay, and bisexual youth. *Suicide and Life-threatening Behaviour, 35*(6), 646–660.

Gorlyn, M. (2005). Impulsivity in the prediction of suicidal behaviour in adolescent populations. *International Journal of Adolescent Medicine and Health, 17*(3), 205–209.

Greenberger, D. & Padesky, C. (1995). *Mind over mood: Change how you feel by changing the way you think.* New York: Guilford.

Lurie, S. J., Gawinski, B., Pierce, D., & Rousseau, S. J. (2006). Seasonal affective disorder. *American Family Physician, 74*(9), 1521–1524.

NHS Scotland Clinical Resource and Audit Group. (2002). *Engaging people – observation of people with acute mental health problems: a Good Practice statement.* Available: http://www.crag.scot.nhs.uk/topics/mhealth/opmh.pdf

Royal College of Psychiatrists. (2005). *The ECT handbook.* Available: http://www.rcpsych.ac.uk/files/pdfversion/cr128.pdf

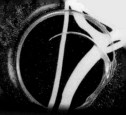

Chapter Study Guide

MULTIPLE-CHOICE QUESTIONS

Select the best answer for each of the following questions.

1. The nurse observes that a client with bipolar disorder is pacing in the corridor, talking loudly and rapidly and using elaborate hand gestures. The nurse concludes that the client is demonstrating which of the following?
   a. Aggression
   b. Anger
   c. Anxiety
   d. Psychomotor agitation

2. A client with bipolar disorder begins taking lithium carbonate (lithium), 300mg four times a day. After 3 days of therapy, the client says, 'My hands are shaking.' The best response by the nurse is
   a. 'Fine motor tremors are an early effect of lithium therapy that usually subsides in a few weeks.'
   b. 'It is nothing to worry about unless it continues for the next month.'
   c. 'Tremors can be an early sign of toxicity, but we'll keep monitoring your lithium level to make sure you're okay.'
   d. 'You can expect tremors with lithium. You seem very concerned about such a small tremor.'

3. What are the most common types of side-effects from SSRIs?
   a. Dizziness, drowsiness, dry mouth
   b. Convulsions, respiratory difficulties
   c. Diarrhoea, weight gain
   d. Jaundice, agranulocytosis

4. The nurse observes that a client with depression sat at a table with two other clients during lunch. The best feedback the nurse could give the client is
   a. 'Do you feel better after talking with others during lunch?'
   b. 'I'm so happy to see you interacting with other clients.'
   c. 'I see you were sitting with others at lunch today.'
   d. 'You must feel much better than you were a few days ago.'

5. Which of the following typifies the speech of a person in the acute phase of mania?
   a. Flight of ideas
   b. Psychomotor retardation
   c. Hesitant
   d. Mutism

6. What is the rationale for a person taking lithium to have enough water and salt in his or her diet?
   a. Salt and water are necessary to dilute lithium to avoid toxicity.
   b. Water and salt convert lithium into a usable solute.
   c. Lithium is metabolized in the liver, necessitating increased water and salt.
   d. Lithium is a salt that has greater affinity for receptor sites than sodium chloride.

7. Identify the serum lithium level for maintenance and safety.
   a. 0.1 to 1.0 mmol/l
   b. 0.5 to 1.5 mmol/l
   c. 10 to 50 mmol/l
   d. 50 to 100 mmol/l

8. A client says to the nurse, 'You are the best nurse I've ever met. I want you to remember me.' What is an appropriate response by the nurse?
   a. 'Thank you. I think you're special too.'
   b. 'I suspect you want something from me. What is it?'
   c. 'You probably say that to all your nurses.'
   d. 'Thanks – but I'm wondering – are you thinking about suicide?'

9. A client with mania begins dancing around the day room. When she twirled her skirt in front of the male clients, it was obvious she had no knickers on. The nurse distracts her and takes her to her room to put on knickers. The nurse acted as she did to
   a. Minimize the client's embarrassment about her present behaviour.
   b. Keep her from dancing with other clients.
   c. Avoid embarrassing the male clients who are watching.
   d. Teach her about proper attire and hygiene.

GROUP DISCUSSION TOPICS

1. Identify four areas that must be included in a teaching plan for a client starting lithium treatment.

2. Identify four client statements that might indicate a subtle message about suicidal ideation.

3. Discuss a person's right to take their own life.

CLINICAL EXAMPLE

June, 46 years old, is divorced with three children: 10, 13, and 16 years of age. She works for the county council and has called in sick four times in the past 2 weeks. June has lost 17 pounds in the past 2 months, is spending a lot of time in bed, but still feels exhausted 'all the time'. During the admission interview, June looks overwhelmingly sad, is tearful, has her head down and makes little eye contact. She answers the nurse's questions with one or two words. The nurse considers postponing the remainder of the interview because June seems unable to provide much information.

1. What assessment data are crucial for the nurse to obtain before ending the interview?

2. Identify three nursing formulations based on the available data.

3. Identify a short-term outcome for each of the nursing formulations.

4. Discuss nursing interventions that would be helpful for June in the longer term.

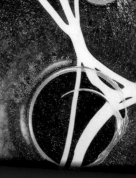

Key Terms

- **abuse**
- **antisocial personality disorder**
- **avoidant personality disorder**
- **borderline personality disorder**
- **character**
- **clinical supervision**
- **cognitive restructuring**
- **compassion**
- **confrontation**
- **decatastrophizing**
- **dependent personality disorder**
- **depressive personality disorder**
- **dialectical behaviour therapy (DBT)**
- **dysphoria**
- **histrionic personality disorder**
- **limit setting**
- **mindfulness**
- **narcissistic personality disorder**
- **no-self-harm contract**
- **obsessive-compulsive personality disorder**
- **paranoid personality disorder**
- **passive-aggressive personality disorder**

- **personality**
- **personality disorders**
- **positive self-talk**
- **schizoid personality disorder**
- **schizotypal personality disorder**

- **self-harm**
- **suicide**
- **temperament**
- **thought stopping**
- **time-out**

Learning Objectives

After reading this chapter, you should be able to:

1. Describe 'personality disorders' in terms of a person's difficulty in perceiving, relating to, and thinking about self, others and the environment.

2. Discuss factors thought to influence the development of 'personality disorders'.

3. Apply the nursing process to the care and treatment of people diagnosed with a personality disorder.

4. Provide education to clients, families and community members to increase their knowledge and understanding of personality disorders.

5. Evaluate personal feelings, attitudes and responses to clients diagnosed with personality disorders.

In 2003, the Department of Health produced a guidance document for developing services for people with 'personality disorders', optimistically entitled 'Personality disorder: no longer a diagnosis of exclusion'. Services for people with the label – in the main staffed by mental health nurses – have been poor and almost invariably excluding rather than including. This sometimes extremely challenging group of people have often felt ostracized, patronized and marginalized throughout their lives. Those feelings have often been compounded by their contact with mental health services.

The difficulties mental health workers – and society as a whole – have with working effectively and compassionately with many people who live with the problems covered in this chapter have been further highlighted by the ongoing battles over the inclusion or exclusion of a treatability clause in the 2007 Mental Health Act and by the 'new' diagnosis of 'dangerous and severe personality disorder': the controversy continues.

This chapter aims to help the reader make sense of 'personality disorders' and to work effectively and compassionately with people with the diagnosis.

Personality can be defined as an ingrained, enduring pattern of behaving and relating to self, others and the environment; it includes perceptions, attitudes and emotions. These behaviours and characteristics are consistent across a broad range of situations and do not change easily. Many factors influence personality: some stem from biological and genetic make-up, whereas some are acquired as a person develops and interacts with the environment and other people.

Personality disorders are diagnosed when personality traits become inflexible and maladaptive, and significantly interfere with how a person functions in society or cause the person emotional distress. They are usually not diagnosed until adulthood, when personality is more completely formed. Nevertheless, maladaptive behavioural patterns can often be traced to early childhood or adolescence. Although there can be great variation among people diagnosed with personality disorders, many experience significant impairment in fulfilling family, academic, employment and other functional roles.

Caring for clients with personality disorders occurs primarily in community settings. Acute settings, such as hospitals and intensive home-treatment, are useful for safety concerns for short periods and tend to be used for those diagnosed with antisocial or borderline personality disorder.

Nurses use therapeutic skills to deal with clients who have personality disorders in primary-care settings, CMHTs, in people's own homes and many other settings. Often, the personality disorder is not the initial focus of attention; rather, the client may be seeking treatment for a physical condition or for another mental health problem. There is a complex overlap between mental disorders such as depression, schizophrenia and bipolar affective disorder and personality disorder, complicated further by misuse of alcohol or drugs: rarely do people fit nice, neat textbook categories!

Most people diagnosed with personality disorders are treated in group or individual therapy settings, community support programmes or self-help groups. Others will not seek treatment for their personality disorder but may be treated for a major mental disorder. Wherever the nurse encounters people with personality disorders or with characteristics of them, including in his or her own personal relationships, the interventions discussed in this chapter can prove useful.

Diagnosis is made when the person exhibits enduring behavioural patterns that deviate from cultural expectations in two or more of the following areas:

- Ways of perceiving and interpreting self, other people and events (cognition)
- Range, intensity, lability and appropriateness of emotional response (affect)
- Interpersonal functioning
- Ability to control impulses or express behaviour at the appropriate time and place (impulse control).

Personality disorders are longstanding because personality characteristics do not change easily. Thus, clients diagnosed with personality disorders, like most of us, continue to behave in their same familiar ways even when these behaviours cause them difficulties or distress. No specific medication alters personality as such, and therapy designed to help clients make changes is often long term, with very slow progress. Some people diagnosed with personality disorders believe their problems stem from others or the world in general; they may not recognize their own behaviour as part of the source of difficulty. At the same time, people around them – including professionals – often see them as solely responsible for their problems, neglecting their lack of skills and the invalidating environment in which they've grown up and are continuing to live. Winship and Hardy (2007) point out that personality disorders are, in the absence of clear biological pathways, often seen as 'not genuine': people struggling to cope with them are often judged (by professionals as well as by the general public) as lacking enough moral fibre, will, self-control or desire to make changes. There are also difficulties in diagnosing and treating clients with personality disorders because of similarities, overlaps and subtle differences between categories or types. 'Types' often overlap and lack concrete validity, and many people diagnosed with personality disorders also have coexisting mental disorders such as depression, bipolar affective disorder or anxiety disorders. 'Personality disorder' in itself is a contested and controversial term and one which, unfortunately, is often used by professionals as a label to dismiss or belittle someone whose behaviour is challenging.

For all these reasons, people with personality disorders are difficult to work with and may be frustrating for the nurse and other professionals, as well as for family and friends: they require commitment, **compassion** and real desire from those around them. It is vital that all nursing interventions with people diagnosed as 'personality disordered' are underpinned with validation, respect, hope and optimism, and that people are seen as individuals first and foremost: people who, like everyone else, have flaws, strengths, desires, dreams and regrets.

CATEGORIES OF PERSONALITY DISORDERS

The *DSM-IV-TR* (American Psychiatric Association, 2000) lists 'personality disorders' as a separate and distinct category from other major mental 'illnesses'. They are on axis II of the multi-axial classification system (see Chapter 1). The *DSM-IV-TR* classifies personality disorders into 'clusters', or categories, based on the predominant or identifying features (Box 16.1):

• Cluster A includes people whose behaviour appears odd or eccentric and includes paranoid, schizoid and schizotypal personality disorders.
• Cluster B includes people who appear dramatic, emotional or erratic, and includes antisocial, borderline, histrionic and narcissistic personality disorders.
• Cluster C includes people who appear anxious or fearful and includes avoidant, dependent and obsessive-compulsive personality disorders.

The *ICD-10* classification is also used in the UK: there are, as with other groups of mental disorder, significant elements in common as well as some differences. This said, *DSM-IV* terms are used more commonly in clinical practice and will be used here, with the proviso that comments about the difficulty of diagnosis (previously mentioned) and the potential problems caused by diagnosis (to be discussed later) are borne in mind throughout.

In mental health care, nurses will probably most often encounter clients diagnosed with the Cluster B 'antisocial' and 'borderline' personality disorders. These two disorders are, therefore, the primary focus of this chapter. Clients with a diagnosis of (or perceived as having elements of) **antisocial personality disorder** – often overlapping with depressive or psychotic symptoms and/or substance misuse – may enter the mental health system as part of specialized forensic or drug and alcohol services or in acute inpatient, crisis or home-treatment settings. People diagnosed with **borderline personality disorder** are still often hospitalized – despite evidence that it can be counter-productive and policy drives to reduce the practice and develop more comprehensive and intensive community services – because their emotional instability can lead to **self-harm** and suicidal ideation and behaviour. Both groups of people present massive challenges to organizations, teams and individuals: they require high levels of support and intervention, an emotionally literate, honest and reflective nursing approach and a willingness to work co-operatively and collaboratively within and across teams. Historically vilified and excluded, and frequently presenting with a lifetime of interpersonal difficulties, people diagnosed with a personality disorder require well-trained, highly skilled and well-supervised nursing.

This chapter discusses the other 'personality disorders' briefly. The majority of Cluster C-type clients are only rarely treated in acute-care settings – much more frequently in primary care – although there are often overlaps between people with behaviours and subjective experiences typical of Cluster A (and B) 'personality disorders' and people diagnosed as depressed, anxious, with a bipolar affective disorder or with schizophrenia.

ONSET AND CLINICAL COURSE

According to the Department of Health (2003), 'personality disorders' are relatively common, occurring in 10% to 13% of the general population. The incidence is even higher for people in lower socioeconomic groups and unstable or disadvantaged populations. Estimates of the prevalence of personality disorders in psychiatric hospital populations vary, but range between 36% and 67%. Forty to 45% of those with a primary diagnosis of major mental disorder also have a coexisting personality disorder that significantly complicates treatment. People with personality disorders have a higher death rate, especially as a result of **suicide**; they also have higher rates of suicide attempts, accidents and emergency department visits, and increased rates of separation, divorce and involvement in legal proceedings regarding child custody (Svrakic & Cloninger, 2005). Personality disorders have been correlated highly with criminal behaviour (a recent study indicated that the prevalence of personality disorder in the prison population was as high as 78%, with antisocial personality disorder being the most common presentation; Department of Health, 2003), alcoholism (60% to 70% of alcoholics have personality disorders) and drug

---

Box 16.1 | *DSM-IV-TR* PERSONALITY DISORDER CATEGORIES

Cluster A: Individuals whose behaviour appears odd or eccentric (paranoid, schizoid and schizotypal personality disorders)

Cluster B: Individuals who appear dramatic, emotional or erratic (antisocial, borderline, histrionic and narcissistic personality disorders)

Cluster C: Individuals who appear anxious or fearful (avoidant, dependent and obsessive-compulsive personality disorders)

Proposed personality disorder categories: depressive and passive–aggressive personality disorders

Adapted from American Psychiatric Association. (2000). *DSM-IV-TR: Diagnostic and Statistical Manual of Mental Disorders* (4th edn, text revision). Washington, DC: APA.

abuse (70% to 90% of those who abuse drugs have a personality disorder) (Svrakic & Cloninger, 2005). Antisocial personality disorder has a prevalence of between 2% and 3%, and is more common in men, younger people, those of low socioeconomic status, single individuals and in those who have been poorly educated.

People with personality disorders are often described as 'difficult' or 'treatment resistant'. This is not surprising, considering that personality characteristics, behavioural patterns and ways of relating to others are deeply ingrained – for all of us. It's difficult to change one's 'personality'; if such changes occur, they almost always evolve slowly. The slow course of treatment can thus be very frustrating for family, friends and practitioners.

Another barrier to treatment is that many clients with personality disorders do not necessarily perceive their dysfunctional or maladaptive behaviours as a problem; indeed, sometimes these behaviours are a source of pride. For example, a belligerent or aggressive person may perceive himself or herself as having a strong personality and being someone who can't be taken advantage of or pushed around. Clients with personality disorders frequently fail to understand the need to change their behaviour and may view changes as a threat.

The difficulties associated with personality disorders persist throughout young and middle adulthood but tend to diminish in the 40s and 50s. Those with antisocial personality disorder are less likely to engage in criminal behaviour, although problems with substance abuse and disregard for the feelings of others persist. Clients with borderline personality disorder tend to demonstrate decreased impulsive behaviour, increased adaptive behaviour and more stable relationships by 50 years of age. This increased stability and improved behaviour can occur even without treatment. Some personality disorders, such as schizoid, schizotypal, paranoid, avoidant and obsessive-compulsive, tend to remain consistent throughout life (Seivewright et al., 2002).

AETIOLOGY

Biological Theories

'Personality' develops through the interaction of hereditary dispositions and environmental influences. '**Temperament**' refers to the biological processes of sensation, association and motivation that underlie the integration of skills and habits based on emotion. Genetic differences seem to account for about 50% of the variances in temperament traits.

The 'four temperament traits' are harm avoidance, novelty seeking, reward dependence and persistence. Each of these four genetically influenced traits affects a person's automatic responses to certain situations. These response patterns are ingrained by 2 to 3 years of age (Svrakic & Cloninger, 2005).

People with high *harm avoidance* exhibit fear of uncertainty, social inhibition, shyness with strangers, rapid fatigability

and pessimistic worry in anticipation of problems. Those with low harm avoidance are carefree, energetic, outgoing and optimistic. High harm-avoidance behaviours may result in maladaptive inhibition and excessive anxiety. Low harm-avoidance behaviours may result in unwarranted optimism and unresponsiveness to potential harm or danger.

A high *novelty-seeking* temperament results in someone who is quick-tempered, curious, easily bored, impulsive, extravagant and disorderly. He or she may be easily bored and distracted with daily life, prone to angry outbursts and fickle in relationships. The person low in novelty seeking is slow-tempered, stoic, reflective, frugal, reserved, orderly and tolerant of monotony; he or she may adhere to a routine of activities.

Reward dependence defines how a person responds to social cues. People high in reward dependence are tenderhearted, sensitive, sociable and socially dependent. They may become overly dependent on approval from others and readily assume the ideas or wishes of others without regard for their own beliefs or desires. People with low reward dependence are practical, tough-minded, cold, socially insensitive, irresolute and indifferent to being alone. Social withdrawal, detachment, aloofness and disinterest in others can result.

Highly *persistent* people are hardworking and ambitious overachievers who respond to fatigue or frustration as a personal challenge. They may persevere even when a situation dictates they should change or stop. People with low persistence are inactive, indolent, unstable and erratic. They tend to give up easily when frustrated and rarely strive for higher accomplishments.

These four genetically independent temperament traits occur in all possible combinations. Some of the previous descriptions of high and low levels of traits correspond closely with the descriptions of the various personality disorders. For example, people with antisocial personality disorder are low in harm-avoidance traits and high in novelty-seeking traits, whereas people with dependent personality disorder are high in reward-dependence traits and harm-avoidance traits.

Psychodynamic Theories

Although temperament is largely inherited, social learning, culture and random life events unique to each person influence character. **Character** consists of concepts about the self and the external world. It develops over time as a person comes into contact with people and situations, and confronts challenges. Three major character traits have been distinguished: self-directedness, co-operativeness and self-transcendence. When fully developed, these character traits define a mature personality (Svrakic & Cloninger, 2005).

Self-directedness is the extent to which a person is responsible, reliable, resourceful, goal oriented and self-confident. Self-directed people are realistic and effective and can adapt their behaviour to achieve goals. People low in self-directedness may be blaming, helpless, irresponsible and unreliable. They cannot set and pursue meaningful goals.

Co-operativeness refers to the extent to which a person sees himself or herself as an integral part of human society. Highly co-operative people can be described as empathic, tolerant, compassionate, supportive and principled. People with low co-operativeness are self-absorbed, intolerant, critical, unhelpful, revengeful and opportunistic; that is, they look out for themselves without regard for the rights and feelings of others.

Self-transcendence describes the extent to which a person considers himself or herself to be an integral part of the universe. Self-transcendent people are spiritual, unpretentious, humble and fulfilled. These traits are helpful when dealing with suffering, illness or death. People low in self-transcendence are practical, self-conscious, materialistic and controlling. They may have difficulty accepting suffering, loss of control, personal and material losses and death.

Character matures in stepwise stages from infancy through late adulthood. Chapter 2 discusses psychological development according to Freud, Erikson and others. Each stage has an associated developmental task that the person must perform for mature personality development. Failure to complete a developmental task jeopardizes the person's ability to achieve future developmental tasks. For example, if the task of basic trust is not achieved in infancy, mistrust results and subsequently interferes with achievement of all future tasks.

Experiences with family, peers and others can significantly influence psychosocial development. Social education in the family creates an environment that can support or oppress specific character development. For example, a family environment that does not value and demonstrate co-operation with others (compassion, tolerance) fails to support the development of that trait in its children. Likewise, the person with non-supportive or difficult peer relationships growing up may have lifelong difficulties relating to others and forming satisfactory relationships.

In summary, personality develops in response to inherited dispositions (temperament) and environmental influences (character), which are experiences unique to each person. Personality disorders result when the combination of temperament and character development produces maladaptive, inflexible ways of viewing self, coping with the world and relating to others.

Dialectical-Behavioural Theories

Dialectical-behavioural theories draw on ideas from biological, psychodynamic and cognitive-behavioural theories, and Eastern theories of **mindfulness** in order to understand the 'personality' of the client and the ways in which he or she interacts with others. People with 'borderline personality disorder' in particular are seen as growing up with both a biological predisposition to emotional difficulties and within an 'invalidating' environment (often, although not always, involving physical, emotional and/or sexual **abuse**), both of which have combined to lead to current difficulties. Emotional vulnerability is worsened by a skills deficit: the

invalidating environment – sexual, physical and/or emotional abuse in childhood – has meant that the necessary skills to deal with others, with distress, with crises, with experiencing the here-and-now, have never been fully integrated into someone's way of dealing with themselves, with others and with the world.

CULTURAL CONSIDERATIONS

Judgements about personality functioning must involve a consideration of the person's ethnic, cultural and social background (American Psychiatric Association, 2000; Department of Health, 2003). Members of minority groups, immigrants, political refugees and people from different ethnic backgrounds may display guarded or defensive behaviour as a result of language barriers or previous negative experiences; this should not be confused with, say, paranoid personality disorder. Equally, people with religious or spiritual beliefs, such as clairvoyance, speaking in tongues or evil spirits as a cause of disease, could be misinterpreted as having schizotypal personality disorder.

There is also a difference in how some cultural groups view avoidance or dependent behaviour, particularly for women. An emphasis on deference, passivity and politeness should not be confused with a dependent personality disorder. Cultures that value work and productivity may produce citizens with a strong emphasis in these areas; this should not be confused with obsessive-compulsive personality disorder.

Certain personality disorders – for example, antisocial and schizoid personality disorders – are diagnosed more often in men. Borderline and histrionic personality disorders are diagnosed more often in women. Social stereotypes about typical gender roles and behaviours can influence diagnostic decisions if clinicians are unaware of such biases, although this is not to say that the influence of gender does not have a real impact on 'personality' and behaviour.

TREATMENT

Care and treatment of individuals with a personality disorder often focuses on mood stabilization, decreasing impulsivity and developing social and relationship skills. Hayward *et al.* (2006) studied clients with personality disorders in terms of their perceptions of their unmet needs. They found that clients perceived unmet needs in five areas: self-care (keeping clean and tidy); sexual expression (dissatisfaction with sex life); budgeting (managing daily finances); psychotic symptoms; and psychological distress. Although psychotic symptoms and psychological distress are usually addressed by mental health professionals, the other three areas are not. This suggests that dealing with those areas in the treatment of a client might result in a greater sense of well-being and improved health.

Several treatment strategies are used with clients with personality disorders; these strategies are, in part, based on the type and severity of the disorder or the amount of distress or functional impairment the client experiences. Combinations of group and individual therapies and medication (Boxes 16.2 and 16.3) are more likely to be effective than is any single treatment (Department of Health, 2003; Svrakic & Cloninger, 2005). Not all people with personality disorders seek treatment, however, even when significant others urge them to do so. Typically, people diagnosable with paranoid, schizoid, schizotypal, narcissistic and passive-aggressive personality disorders are least likely to engage or remain in any treatment. They tend to see other people, rather than their own behaviour, as the cause of their problems.

Psychopharmacology

Pharmacological treatment of clients with personality disorders focuses on the client's symptoms rather than the particular subtype. The four symptom categories that underlie personality disorders are cognitive-perceptual distortions, including psychotic symptoms; affective symptoms and mood dysregulation; aggression and behavioural dysfunction; and anxiety. These four symptom categories can be related to the underlying temperaments that distinguish the *DSM-IV-TR* clusters of personality disorders:

- Low reward dependence and Cluster A disorders correspond to the categories of affective dysregulation, detachment and cognitive disturbances.
- High novelty-seeking and Cluster B disorders correspond to the target symptoms of impulsiveness and aggression.
- High harm-avoidance and Cluster C disorders correspond to the categories of anxiety and depression symptoms.

Box 16.2 PERSONALITY DISORDERS: PSYCHOTHERAPY

DYNAMIC PSYCHOTHERAPY

- This is based on a developmental model of personality.
- Treatment is generally long term.
- The aim of therapy is to understand the way in which the past influences the present with the use of interpretation.
- Treatment focuses on the therapeutic alliance between patient and therapist, the individual's emotional life and defences.
- Therapy uses the relationship between patient and therapist (transference) as a way to understand how the internal world of the individual affects relationships.

COGNITIVE ANALYTICAL THERAPY

- Postulates that a set of partially dissociated 'self-states' account for the clinical features of borderline personality disorder.
- Rapid switching between these self-states leads to dyscontrol of emotions including intense expression and virtual absence (depersonalization).
- Therapy aims to formulate these processes collaboratively, examining them as they occur in treatment as well as in life experiences.

COGNITIVE THERAPY

- This is a modification of standard cognitive and behaviour therapy that is goal directed and focused more on altering underlying belief structures rather than reduction of symptoms.

- It is likely to take up to 30 sessions of treatment, of which the initial ones help to define the areas of intervention by identifying what are the fundamental structures of past, present and future experiences.
- The therapist and patient maintain a collaborative therapeutic alliance throughout treatment which includes homework and testing of core beliefs and structures.

DIALECTICAL BEHAVIOUR THERAPY (DBT)

- This is a special adaptation of cognitive therapy, originally used for the treatment of women with borderline personality disorder who harmed themselves repeatedly.
- DBT is a manualized therapy including functional analysis of behaviour, skills training and support (empathy, validation of feelings, management of trauma).
- Directed at reducing self-harm.

THERAPEUTIC COMMUNITY TREATMENTS

- Therapeutic communities provide intensive psychosocial treatment which may include a variety of therapies but where the therapeutic environment itself is seen as the primary agent of change.
- They include democratic and concept types, the former including members of the community as decision makers.
- External control is kept to a minimum: members of the community take a significant role in decision making and the everyday running of the unit.

From Department of Health. (2003). *Personality disorder: No longer a diagnosis of exclusion*. http://www.dh.gov.uk/en/Publicationsandstatistics/Publications/PublicationsPolicyAndGuidance/DH_4009546. © 2003 Crown Copyright.

Box 16.3   MEDICATION FOR PERSONALITY DISORDERS

ANTIPSYCHOTIC DRUGS

- These have shown variable results in controlled trials.
- Reduction in hostility and impulsivity are claimed but not always reliably achieved.
- 'Schizotypal' features are helped most.
- Atypical neuroleptics may offer advantages but results are preliminary.

ANTIDEPRESSANT DRUGS

- Both tricyclic antidepressants and SSRIs have been recommended in the treatment of borderline personality disorder.
- Improvement in borderline patients may be linked to depressive symptoms rather than personality pathology.
- Impulsiveness is particularly improved and SSRIs may offer advantages in this respect.

MOOD STABILIZERS

- Lithium, carbamazepine and sodium valproate have all been used to treat symptoms of mood disorder in those with personality disorder.
- There is weak support for the notion that Cluster B (antisocial, borderline, histrionic and impulsive) personality disorders may be helped by mood stabilizers.

Cognitive-perceptual disturbances include magical thinking, odd beliefs, illusions, suspiciousness, ideas of reference and low-grade psychotic symptoms. These chronic symptoms may respond well to low-dose antipsychotic medications (Simeon & Hollander, 2006).

Several types of aggression have been described in people with personality disorders. Aggression may occur in impulsive people (some with a normal electroencephalogram, some with an abnormal one); people who exhibit predatory or cruel behaviour; or people with organic-like impulsivity, poor social judgement and emotional lability. Lithium, anticonvulsant mood stabilizers and benzodiazepines are used most often to treat aggression. Low-dose neuroleptics may be useful in modifying predatory aggression (Simeon & Hollander, 2006).

Mood dysregulation symptoms include emotional instability, emotional detachment, depression and **dysphoria**. Emotional instability and mood swings respond favourably to lithium, carbamazepine (Tegretol), valproate (Depakote) or low-dose neuroleptics such as haloperidol (Haldol). Emotional detachment, cold and aloof emotions and disinterest in social relations often respond to SSRIs or atypical

antipsychotics such as risperidone (Risperdal), olanzapine (Zyprexa) and quetiapine (Seroquel). Atypical depression is often treated with SSRIs, MAOI antidepressants or low-dose antipsychotic medications (Simeon & Hollander, 2006).

Anxiety seen with personality disorders may be chronic cognitive anxiety, chronic somatic anxiety or severe acute anxiety. Chronic cognitive anxiety responds to SSRIs and MAOIs, as does chronic somatic anxiety or anxiety manifested as multiple physical complaints. Episodes of severe acute anxiety are best treated with MAOIs or low-dose antipsychotic medications.

These drugs, including side-effects and nursing considerations, are discussed in detail in Chapter 3.

Individual and Group Psychotherapy

Therapy helpful to clients with personality disorders varies according to the type and severity of symptoms and the person's particular 'disorder'. Inpatient hospitalization may be indicated when safety is a serious concern; for example, when a person with a diagnosed personality disorder has suicidal or homicidal ideation or engages in life-threatening self-injury, or behaviours putting others at risk. Hospitalization may also be necessary if the severity of a concurrent mental disorder – psychosis, mood disorder or substance misuse problem, for example – warrants it. Hospitalization may be life-saving; it may also be counterproductive, stripping people with a 'personality disorder' of their autonomy, minimizing their strengths, achievements and personal qualities and producing a debilitating dependence.

Individual and group psychotherapy goals for clients with personality disorders focus on building trust, teaching basic living skills, providing support, acknowledgement and validation, decreasing distressing symptoms such as anxiety and improving interpersonal relationships and the capacity to deal with distress and crisis. Relaxation or meditation techniques can, as an example, help manage anxiety for clients with Cluster C personality disorders. Improvement in basic living skills through the relationship with a case manager or therapist can improve the functional skills of people with schizotypal and schizoid personality disorders. Assertiveness training groups can assist people with dependent and passive-aggressive personality disorders to have more satisfying relationships with others and to build self-esteem.

CBT has been particularly helpful for many clients with personality disorders (Harvard Medical School Health, 2002; Department of Health, 2003). Several cognitive restructuring techniques are used to change the way the client thinks about self and others: thought stopping, in which the client stops negative thought patterns; positive self-talk, designed to change negative self-messages; and decatastrophizing, which teaches the client to view life events more realistically and not as catastrophes. Examples of these techniques are presented later in this chapter.

| Table 16.1 | SUMMARY OF CHARACTERISTICS AND NURSING INTERVENTIONS FOR PERSONALITY DISORDERS | |

Personality Disorder	Characteristics	Nursing Interventions
Paranoid	Mistrust and suspicions of others; guarded, restricted affect	Serious, straightforward approach; help client to validate ideas before taking action; involve client in treatment planning; CBT
Schizoid	Detached from social relationships; restricted affect; involved with things more than people	Improve client's functioning in the community; assist client to find appropriate resources; CBT
Schizotypal	Acute discomfort in relationships; cognitive or perceptual distortions; eccentric behaviour	Develop self-care skills; improve community functioning; social skills training; CBT
Antisocial	Disregard for rights of others, rules and laws	Limit setting; confrontation; teach client to solve problems effectively and manage emotions of anger or frustration; CBT
Borderline	Unstable relationships, self-image and affect; impulsivity; self-harm	Promote safety; help client to cope and control emotions; DBT and cognitive restructuring techniques; structure time; teach social skills
Histrionic	Excessive emotionality and attention seeking	Teach social skills; provide factual feedback about behaviour; CBT
Narcissistic	Grandiose; lack of empathy; need for admiration	Matter-of-fact approach; gain co-operation with needed treatment; teach client any needed self-care skills; CBT
Avoidant	Social inhibitions; feelings of inadequacy; hypersensitive to negative evaluation	Support and reassurance; CBT; cognitive restructuring techniques; promote self-esteem
Dependent	Submissive and clinging behaviour; excessive need to be taken care of	Foster client's self-reliance and autonomy; teach problem-solving and decision-making skills; cognitive restructuring techniques; CBT
Obsessive-compulsive	Preoccupation with orderliness, perfectionism and control	Encourage negotiation with others; assist client to make timely decisions and complete work; cognitive restructuring techniques; CBT
Depressive	Pattern of depressive cognitions and behaviours in a variety of contexts	Assess self-harm risk; provide factual feedback; promote self-esteem; increase involvement in activities; CBT
Passive-aggressive	Pattern of negative attitudes and passive resistance to demands for adequate performance in social and occupational situations	Help client to identify feelings and express them directly; assist client to examine own feelings and behaviour realistically; CBT

CBT, cognitive-behavioural therapy; DBT, dialectical behavioural therapy.

As mentioned previously, **dialectical behaviour therapy (DBT)** was designed for clients with borderline personality disorder (Linehan, 1993) and has, in recent years, become increasingly used in the UK. Table 16.1 summarizes the symptoms of, and nursing interventions for, personality disorders.

Cluster A: Personality Disorders

PARANOID PERSONALITY DISORDER

Clinical Picture

Paranoid personality disorder is characterized by pervasive mistrust and suspiciousness of others. Clients diagnosed with this disorder interpret others' actions as potentially harmful. During periods of stress, they may develop transient psychotic symptoms. Incidence is estimated to be 0.5% to 2.5% of the general population; the disorder is more common in men than in women. Data about prognosis and long-term outcomes are limited because most people with paranoid personality disorder do not readily seek or remain in treatment (American Psychiatric Association, 2000).

In an inpatient setting, clients can appear aloof and withdrawn, and may remain a considerable physical distance from the nurse; they view this as necessary for their protection. Clients may also appear guarded or hypervigilant; they may survey the room and its contents, look behind furniture or doors and generally appear alert to any impending danger. They may choose to sit near the door to have ready access to an exit, or with their backs against the wall to prevent anyone from sneaking up behind them.

They may have a restricted affect and may be unable to demonstrate warm or empathic emotional responses such as 'You look nice today,' or 'I'm sorry you're having a bad day.' Mood may be labile, quickly changing from quietly suspicious to angry or hostile. Responses may become sarcastic for no apparent reason. The constant mistrust and suspicion that clients feel toward others and the environment distorts thoughts, thought processing and content. Clients frequently see malevolence in the actions of others when none exists. They may spend a disproportionate amount of time examining and analysing the behaviour and motives of others to discover hidden and threatening meanings. Clients often feel attacked by others and may devise elaborate plans or fantasies for protection.

In psychodynamic terms, these clients use the defence mechanism of *projection*, which is blaming other people, institutions or events for their own difficulties. It is common for such clients to blame the government for personal problems. For example, a client who gets a parking ticket may say it is part of a plot by the police to drive him out of the neighbourhood. He may engage in fantasies of retribution or devise elaborate and sometimes violent plans to get even. Although most clients do not carry out such plans, there is a potential danger.

Conflict with authority figures at work is common; clients may even resent being given directions from a supervisor. Paranoia may extend to feelings of being singled out for menial tasks, treated as stupid or more closely monitored than other employees.

Nursing Interventions

Forming an effective working relationship with paranoid or suspicious clients is difficult. The nurse must remember that these clients frequently take everything seriously and are particularly sensitive to the reactions and motivations of others. Therefore, the nurse needs to approach these clients in a formal, business-like manner and refrain from social chit-chat or jokes. Being on time, keeping commitments and being particularly straightforward are essential to the success of the nurse–client relationship.

Because these clients need to feel in control, it is important to involve them in formulating their plans of care. The nurse asks what the client would like to accomplish in concrete terms, such as minimizing problems at work or getting along with others. Clients are more likely to engage in the therapeutic process if they believe they have something to gain. One of the most effective interventions is helping clients to learn to validate ideas before taking action; however, this requires the ability to trust and to listen to one person. The rationale for this intervention is that clients can avoid problems if they can refrain from taking action until they have validated their ideas with another person. This helps prevent clients from acting on paranoid ideas or beliefs. It also assists them to start basing decisions and actions on reality.

SCHIZOID PERSONALITY DISORDER
Clinical Picture

Schizoid personality disorder is characterized by a pervasive pattern of detachment from social relationships and a restricted range of emotional expression in interpersonal settings. It occurs in approximately 0.5% to 7% of the general population and is more common in men than in women. People with schizoid personality disorder avoid treatment as much as they avoid other relationships, unless their life circumstances change significantly (American Psychiatric Association, 2000).

Clients with schizoid personality disorder display a constricted affect and little, if any, emotion. They are aloof and indifferent, appearing emotionally cold, uncaring or unfeeling. They report no leisure or pleasurable activities because they rarely experience enjoyment. Even under stress or adverse circumstances, their response appears passive and disinterested. There is marked difficulty experiencing and expressing emotions, particularly anger or aggression. Oddly, clients do not report feeling distressed about this lack of emotion; it is more distressing to family members. Clients usually have a rich and extensive fantasy life, although they may be reluctant to reveal that information to the nurse or anyone else. The ideal relationships that occur in the client's fantasies are rewarding and gratifying; these fantasies, though, are in stark contrast to real-life experiences. The fantasy relationship often includes someone the client has met only briefly. Nevertheless, these clients can distinguish fantasies from reality, and no disordered or delusional thought processes are evident.

People with these difficulties are generally accomplished intellectually and often involved with computers or electronics in hobbies or work. They may spend long hours solving puzzles or mathematical problems, although they see these pursuits as useful or productive rather than fun.

They may be indecisive and lack future goals or direction. They see no need for planning and really have no aspirations. They have little opportunity to exercise judgement or decision making because they rarely engage in these activities. Insight might be described as impaired, at least by the social standards of others: these clients do not see their situation as a problem and fail to understand why their lack of emotion or social involvement troubles others. They are self-absorbed and loners in almost all aspects of daily life. Given an opportunity to engage with other people, these clients turn it down. They are also indifferent to praise or criticism and are relatively unaffected by the emotions or opinions of others. They also experience significant dissociation from bodily or sensory pleasures. For example, the client has little reaction to beautiful scenery, a sunset or a walk on the beach.

Clients have a pervasive lack of desire for involvement with others in all aspects of life. They do not have or desire friends, rarely date or marry and have little or no sexual contact. They may have some connection with a first-degree relative, often a parent. Clients may remain in the parental home well into adulthood if they can maintain adequate separation and distance from other family members. They have few social skills, are oblivious to the social cues or overtures of others and do not engage in social conversation. They may succeed in vocational areas, provided they value their jobs and have little contact with others in work, which may typically involve things like computers or electronics.

Nursing Interventions

Nursing interventions focus on improved functioning in the community and developing the capacity to relate to others in a way that doesn't increase anxiety. If a client needs housing or a change in living circumstances, the CMHN, for example, may make referrals to social services or appropriate local agencies for assistance. The nurse can help people find suitable housing that accommodates the client's desire and need for solitude. For example, the client with a schizoid personality disorder would function best in accommodation which provides meals and a laundry service but requires little social interaction. Facilities designed to actively promote socialization through group activities may be less desirable.

If the client has an identified family member as his or her primary relationship, the nurse must ascertain whether that person can continue in that role. If that person cannot, the client may need to establish at least a working relationship with a single worker or care co-ordinator in the community. The professional can then help the client to obtain services and health care, manage finances and so on. The client has a greater chance of success if he or she can relate his or her needs to just one person (as opposed to neglecting important areas of daily life).

SCHIZOTYPAL PERSONALITY DISORDER

Clinical Picture

Schizotypal personality disorder is characterized by a pervasive pattern of social and interpersonal deficits marked by acute discomfort with, and reduced capacity for, close relationships, as well as by cognitive or perceptual distortions and behavioural eccentricities. Incidence is about 3% to 5% of the population; the disorder is slightly more common in men than in women. Clients may experience transient psychotic episodes in response to extreme stress. An estimated 10% to 20% of people with schizotypal personality disorder eventually develop schizophrenia (American Psychiatric Association, 2000).

Clients often have an odd appearance that causes others to notice them. They may be unkempt and dishevelled, and their clothes are often ill-fitting, do not match and may be stained or dirty. They may wander aimlessly and, at times, become preoccupied with some environmental detail. Speech is coherent but may be loose, digressive or vague. Clients often provide unsatisfactory answers to questions and may be unable to specify or to describe information clearly. They frequently use words incorrectly, which makes their speech sound bizarre. For example, in response to a question about sleeping habits, the client might respond, 'Sleep is slow, the REMs don't flow.' These clients have a restricted range of emotions; that is, they lack the ability to experience and to express a full range of emotions such as anger, happiness and pleasure. Affect is often flat and sometimes is silly or inappropriate.

Cognitive distortions include ideas of reference, magical thinking, odd or unfounded beliefs and a preoccupation with parapsychology, including extrasensory perception and clairvoyance. Ideas of reference usually involve the client's belief that events have special meaning for him or her; however, these ideas are not firmly fixed and delusional, as may be seen in clients diagnosed with schizophrenia. In magical thinking, which is normal in small children, a client believes he or she has special powers – that by thinking about something, he or she can make it happen. In addition, clients may express ideas that indicate paranoid thinking and suspiciousness, usually about the motives of other people.

Clients experience great anxiety around other people, especially those who are unfamiliar. This does not improve with time or repeated exposures; rather, the anxiety may intensify. This results from the belief that strangers cannot be trusted. Clients do not view their anxiety as a problem that arises from a threatened sense of self. Interpersonal relationships are troublesome; therefore, clients may have only one significant relationship, usually with a first-degree relative. They may remain in their parents' home well into the adult years. They have a limited capacity for close relationships, even though they may be unhappy being alone.

Clients cannot respond to normal social cues and hence cannot engage in superficial conversation. They may have skills that could be useful in a vocational setting, but they are not often successful in employment without support or assistance. Mistrust of others, bizarre thinking and ideas and unkempt appearance can make it difficult for these clients to get and to keep jobs.

Nursing Interventions

The focus of nursing care for clients with schizotypal personality disorder is development of self-care and social skills and improved functioning in the community. The nurse encourages clients to establish a daily routine for hygiene and grooming. Such a routine is important because it does not depend on the client to decide when hygiene and grooming tasks are necessary. It may be preferable for clients to have an appearance that is not bizarre or dishevelled: stares or comments from others can increase discomfort. Because these clients are uncomfortable around others and this is unlikely to change in the short term, the nurse must help them function in the community with minimal discomfort. It may help to ask clients to prepare a list of people in the community with whom they must have contact, such as a landlord, shop assistant or pharmacist. The nurse can then role-play interactions that clients would have with each of these people; this allows clients to practise clear and logical requests to obtain services or to conduct personal business. Because face-to-face contact is more uncomfortable, clients may be able to make written requests or to use the telephone for business. Social skills training may help clients to talk clearly with others and to reduce bizarre conversations. It helps to identify one person with whom clients can discuss unusual or bizarre beliefs, such as a CMHN or family member. Given an acceptable outlet for these topics, clients may be able to refrain from these conversations with people who might react negatively.

Cluster B: Personality Disorders

ANTISOCIAL PERSONALITY DISORDER

Antisocial personality disorder is characterized by a pervasive pattern of disregard for, and violation of, the rights of others – and with the central characteristics of deceit and manipulation. This pattern has also been referred to as 'psychopathy', 'sociopathy' or 'dyssocial personality disorder'. It occurs in about 3% of the general population and is three to four times more common in men than in women. In some studies of prison populations, about 50% are diagnosed with antisocial personality disorder. Antisocial behaviours tend to peak in the 20s and diminish significantly after 45 years of age (American Psychiatric Association, 2000).

APPLICATION OF THE NURSING PROCESS: ANTISOCIAL PERSONALITY DISORDER

Assessment

Clients are often skilful at deceiving themselves and others, so during assessment, it may help to check and to validate information from other sources.

HISTORY

Onset is in childhood or adolescence, although formal diagnosis is not made until the client is 18 years of age. Childhood histories of enuresis, sleepwalking and acts of cruelty toward people or animals are characteristic predictors. In adolescence, clients may have engaged in lying, truancy, sexual promiscuity, cigarette smoking, substance use and illegal activities that brought them into contact with police (McGue & Iacono, 2005). Families have high rates of depression, substance abuse, antisocial personality disorder, poverty and divorce. Erratic, neglectful, harsh or even abusive parenting frequently marks the childhoods of these clients.

GENERAL APPEARANCE AND MOTOR BEHAVIOUR

Appearance is usually normal; these clients may be quite engaging and even charming. Depending on the circumstances of the interview, they may exhibit signs of mild or moderate anxiety, especially if another person or agency arranged the assessment.

MOOD AND AFFECT

Clients often display false emotions chosen to suit the occasion or to work to their advantage. For example, a client who is forced to seek treatment instead of going to jail may appear engaging or try to evoke sympathy by sadly relating a story of his or her 'terrible childhood'. The client's actual emotions may be quite shallow. It is important to realize, however, that it is likely the person did indeed experience such a childhood: he has learnt to deal with others in a 'manipulative' way precisely because of this.

These clients frequently cannot empathize with the feelings of others, which enables them to exploit others without guilt. Usually, they feel remorse only if they are caught breaking the law or exploiting someone.

THOUGHT PROCESS AND CONTENT

Clients do not experience disordered thoughts, but their view of the world is narrow and distorted. Because coercion

---

CLINICAL VIGNETTE: ANTISOCIAL PERSONALITY DISORDER

Steve found himself in jail again after being arrested for burglary. He had told the police it wasn't breaking and entering; he had his friend's permission to use his parents' home, but they'd just forgotten to leave the key. Steve has a long juvenile record of truancy, fighting and drug use, which he blames on 'having the wrong friends'. This is his third arrest, and Steve claims the police are picking on him ever since an elderly lady in the community gave him £5000 when he was out of work. He intends to pay her back when his ship comes in. Steve's wife of 3 years left him recently, claiming he couldn't hold a decent job and was running up bills they couldn't pay. Steve was tired of her nagging and was ready for a new relationship anyway, he says. He wishes he could win the lottery and find a beautiful girl to love him. He's tired of people demanding that he grow up, get a job and settle down. They just don't understand that he's got more exciting things to do.

DSM-IV-TR DIAGNOSTIC CRITERIA: SYMPTOMS OF ANTISOCIAL PERSONALITY DISORDER

- Violation of the rights of others
- Lack of remorse for behaviour
- Shallow emotions
- Lying
- Rationalization of own behaviour
- Poor judgement
- Impulsivity
- Irritability and aggressiveness
- Lack of insight
- Thrill-seeking behaviours
- Exploitation of people in relationships
- Poor work history
- Consistent irresponsibility

Adapted from American Psychiatric Association. (2000). *Diagnostic and Statistical Manual of Mental Disorders* (4th edn, text revision). Washington, DC: American Psychiatric Association.

and personal profit motivate them, they tend to believe that others are similarly governed. They view the world as cold and hostile, and therefore rationalize their behaviour. Clichés such as 'It's a dog-eat-dog world' represent their viewpoint. Clients believe that they are only taking care of themselves because no one else will.

SENSORY AND INTELLECTUAL PROCESSES

Clients are oriented, have no sensory-perceptual alterations and have average or above-average IQs.

JUDGEMENT AND INSIGHT

These clients generally exercise poor judgement for various reasons. They pay little attention to the legality of their actions and do not consider morals or ethics when making decisions. Their behaviour is determined primarily by what they want, and they perceive their needs as immediate. In addition to seeking immediate gratification, these clients also are impulsive. Such impulsivity ranges from simple failure to use normal caution (waiting for a green light to cross a busy street) to extreme thrill-seeking behaviours such as driving recklessly.

Clients lack 'insight' and almost never see their actions as the cause of their problems. It is always someone else's fault: some external source is responsible for their situation or behaviour.

SELF-CONCEPT

Superficially, clients appear confident, self-assured and accomplished, perhaps flip or arrogant. They feel fearless, disregard their own vulnerability and usually believe they cannot be caught in lies, deceit or illegal actions. They may be described as egocentric (believing the world revolves around them), but actually the self is quite shallow and empty; these clients seem devoid of personal emotions. They realistically appraise their own strengths and weaknesses.

ROLES AND RELATIONSHIPS

Clients manipulate and exploit those around them. They view relationships as serving their needs and pursue others only for personal gain. They never think about the repercussions of their actions to others. For example, a client is caught conning an older person out of her entire life savings. The client's only comment when caught is 'Can you believe that's all the money I got? I was cheated! There should have been more.'

These clients are often involved in many relationships, sometimes simultaneously. They may marry and have children, but they cannot sustain long-term commitments. They are usually unsuccessful as partners and parents and leave others abandoned and disappointed. They may obtain employment readily with their adept use of superficial social skills, but over time their work history is poor. Problems may result from absenteeism, theft or embezzlement, or they may simply quit out of boredom.

Data Analysis

People with antisocial personality disorder generally do not seek treatment voluntarily unless they perceive some personal gain from doing so. For example, a client may choose a treatment setting as an alternative to prison or to gain sympathy from an employer; they may cite stress as a reason for absenteeism or poor performance. Inpatient treatment settings are not necessarily effective for these clients and may, in fact, bring out their worst qualities.

Nursing formulations commonly used when working with these clients include the following:

- Ineffective coping
- Ineffective role performance
- Risk of violence toward others.

Outcome Identification

The treatment focus is often, at least initially, behavioural change. Short-term treatment is unlikely to affect the client's insight or view of the world and others, but it is possible to make changes in behaviour. Treatment outcomes may include the following:

- The client will demonstrate non-destructive ways to express feelings and frustration.
- The client will identify ways to meet his or her own needs that do not infringe on the rights of others.
- The client will achieve or maintain satisfactory role performance (e.g. at work, as a parent).

Intervention

FORMING A THERAPEUTIC RELATIONSHIP AND PROMOTING RESPONSIBLE BEHAVIOUR

This group of people can be exceptionally challenging to nurses, eliciting feelings of fear, hostility and sometimes even love or admiration. The nurse must provide validation, honesty and structure in the therapeutic relationship, identify acceptable and expected behaviours and be consistent in those expectations. The nurse must minimize attempts by these clients to manipulate and to control the relationship; he or she must ensure he or she is aware of – and can discuss honestly with a supervisor or colleague – his or her own affective and cognitive response to the person.

Limit setting is an effective technique that involves three steps:

1. Stating the behavioural limit (describing the unacceptable behaviour).
2. Identifying the consequences if the limit is exceeded.
3. Identifying the expected or desired behaviour.

Consistent limit setting in a matter-of-fact non-judgemental manner is crucial to success. For example, a client may approach the nurse flirtatiously and attempt to gain personal information. The nurse could use limit setting by saying,

> *'It's really not OK for you to ask personal questions. If you carry on, I'll have to stop this conversation. I think we need to use the time we've got to look at solving your problems about your job.'*

The nurse should try not to display anger or respond to the client harshly or punitively.

Confrontation is another technique designed to manage manipulative or deceptive behaviour. The nurse points out a client's problematic behaviour while remaining neutral and matter-of-fact; he or she avoids accusing the client. The nurse can also use confrontation to keep clients focused on the topic and in the present. The nurse can focus on the behaviour itself rather than on attempts by clients to justify it. For example:

> **Nurse:** *'You've said you're interested in learning to manage angry outbursts, but you've missed the last three group meetings.'*
> **Client:** *'Well, I can tell no one in the group likes me. Why should I bother?'*
> **Nurse:** *'The group meetings are designed to help you and the others, but you can't work on issues if you're not there.'*

HELPING CLIENTS SOLVE PROBLEMS AND CONTROL EMOTIONS

Clients diagnosed with antisocial personality disorder have an established pattern of reacting impulsively when confronted with problems. The nurse can teach problem-solving skills and help clients to practise them. Problem-solving

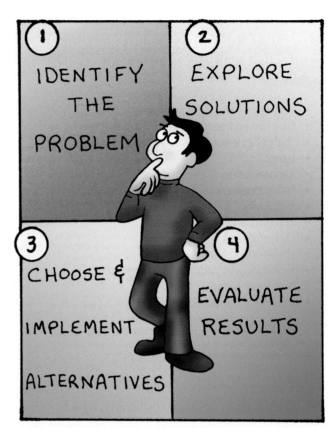

Problem-solving skills

skills include identifying the problem, exploring alternative solutions and related consequences, choosing and implementing an alternative and evaluating the results. Although these clients have the cognitive ability to solve problems, they need to learn a step-by-step approach to deal with them. For example, a client's car isn't running, so he stops going to work. The problem is transportation to work; alternative solutions might be taking the bus, asking a co-worker for a ride and getting the car fixed. The nurse can help the client to discuss the various options and choose one so that he can go back to work.

Managing emotions, especially anger and frustration, can be a major problem. When clients are calm and not upset, the nurse can encourage them to identify sources of frustration, how they respond to it and the consequences. In this way, the nurse assists clients to anticipate stressful situations and to learn ways to avoid negative future consequences. Taking a **time-out** or leaving the area and going to a neutral place to regain internal control is often a helpful strategy. Time-outs help clients to avoid impulsive reactions and angry outbursts in emotionally charged situations, regain control of emotions and engage in constructive problem solving. Techniques such as mindfulness, meditation and yoga can be helpful.

ENHANCING ROLE PERFORMANCE

The nurse helps clients to identify specific problems at work or home that are barriers to success in fulfilling roles.

Assessing use of alcohol and other drugs is essential when examining role performance because many clients use or abuse these substances. These clients tend to blame others for their failures and difficulties, and the nurse must redirect them to examine the source of their problems realistically. Referrals to vocational or job programmes may be indicated.

Evaluation

As with work with all mental health clients, the nurse evaluates the effectiveness of care and treatment based on attainment of, or progress toward, outcomes that have been agreed with the client and with significant others. After a lifetime of creating chaos and damaging relationships, if a

---

Nursing Care Plan *Antisocial Personality Disorder*

Nursing Formulation

Ineffective Coping: *Inability to form a valid appraisal of the stressors, inadequate choices of practised responses and/or inability to use available resources.*

ASSESSMENT DATA

- Low frustration tolerance
- Impulsive behaviour
- Inability to delay gratification
- Poor judgement
- Conflict with authority
- Difficulty following rules and obeying laws
- Lack of feelings of remorse
- Socially unacceptable behaviour
- Dishonesty
- Ineffective interpersonal relationships
- Manipulative behaviour
- Failure to learn or change behaviour based on past experience or punishment
- Failure to accept or handle responsibility

EXPECTED OUTCOMES

Inpatient
The client will
- Reduce harm to self or others
- Identify behaviours leading to crisis
- Function within limits demanded by unit, family and community

Stabilization
The client will
- Demonstrate non-destructive ways to deal with stress and frustration
- Identify ways to meet own needs that do not infringe on the rights of others

Community
The client will
- Achieve or maintain satisfactory work and social performance
- Meet own needs without exploiting or infringing on the rights of others

IMPLEMENTATION

Nursing Interventions *denotes collaborative interventions

On Ward:
Encourage the client to identify the actions that precipitated hospitalization (e.g. debts, marital problems, criminal activity).

Give positive feedback for honesty. The client may try to avoid responsibility by acting as though he or she is 'sick' or helpless.

Identify unacceptable behaviours, either general (stealing others' possessions) or specific (embarrassing Ms X by telling lewd jokes).

Rationale

These clients frequently deny responsibility for consequences of their own actions.

Honest identification of the consequences of the client's behaviour is necessary for future behaviour change.

You must supply clear, concrete limits when the client is unable or unwilling to do so.

continued ⋯⟩

Nursing Care Plan: Antisocial Personality Disorder, cont.

IMPLEMENTATION

Nursing Interventions *denotes collaborative interventions	**Rationale**
Develop specific consequences for unacceptable behaviours (e.g. the client may not watch television).	Unpleasant consequences may help decrease or eliminate unacceptable behaviours. To be effective, the consequences must be related to something the client enjoys.
Avoid any discussion about why requirements exist. State the requirement in a matter-of-fact manner. Avoid arguing with the client.	The client may attempt to bend the rules 'just this once' with numerous excuses and justifications. Your refusal to be manipulated or charmed will help decrease manipulative behaviour.
Inform the client of unacceptable behaviours and the resulting consequences in advance of their occurrence.	The client must be aware of expectations and consequences.
*Communicate and document in the client's care plan all behaviours and consequences in specific terms.	The client may attempt to gain favour with individual staff members or play one staff member against another. ('Last night the nurse told me I could do that.') If all team members follow the written plan, the client will not be able to manipulate changes.
Avoid discussing another staff member's actions or statements unless the other staff member is present.	The client may try to manipulate staff members or focus attention on others to decrease attention to himself or herself.
*Be consistent and firm with the care plan. Do not make independent changes in rules or consequences. Any change should be made by the staff as a group and conveyed to all staff members working with this client. (You may designate a primary staff person to be responsible for minor decisions and refer all questions to this person.)	Consistency is essential. If the client can find just one person to make independent changes, any plan will become ineffective.
Avoid trying to coax or convince the client to do the 'right thing'.	The client must decide to accept responsibility for his or her behaviour and its consequences.
When the client exceeds a limit, provide consequences immediately after the behaviour in a matter-of-fact manner.	Consequences are most effective when they closely follow the unacceptable behaviour. Do not react to the client in an angry or punitive manner. If you show anger toward the client, the client may take advantage of it. It is better to get out of the situation if possible and let someone else handle it.
Point out the client's responsibility for his or her behaviour in a non-judgemental manner.	The client needs to learn the connection between behaviour and the consequences, but blame and judgement are not appropriate.
Provide immediate positive feedback or reward for acceptable behaviour.	Immediate positive feedback will help to increase acceptable behaviour. The client must receive attention for positive behaviours, not just unacceptable ones.
Gradually, require longer periods of acceptable behaviour and greater rewards, and inform the client of changes as decisions are made.	This gradual progression will help to develop the client's ability to delay gratification. This is necessary if the client is to function effectively in society.

continued ⋯⋗

Nursing Care Plan: Antisocial Personality Disorder, cont.

IMPLEMENTATION

Nursing Interventions *denotes collaborative interventions	**Rationale**
Encourage the client to identify sources of frustration, how he or she dealt with it previously and any unpleasant consequences that resulted.	This may facilitate the client's ability to accept responsibility for his or her own behaviour.
Explore alternative, socially and legally acceptable methods of dealing with identified frustrations.	The client has the opportunity to learn to make alternative choices.
Help the client to try alternatives as situations arise. Give positive feedback when the client uses alternatives successfully.	The client can role-play alternatives in a non-threatening environment.
*Discuss job seeking, work attendance, court appearances and so forth when working with the client in anticipation of discharge.	Dealing with consequences and working are responsible behaviours. The client may have had little or no successful experience in these areas and may benefit from assistance.

Adapted from Schultz, J. M. & Videbeck, S. L. (2005). *Lippincott's manual of psychiatric nursing care plans* (7th edn). Philadelphia: Lippincott Williams & Wilkins.

NURSING INTERVENTIONS FOR ANTISOCIAL PERSONALITY DISORDER

- Promoting responsible behaviour
  Limit setting
  State the limit.
  Identify consequences of exceeding the limit.
  Identify expected or acceptable behaviour.
  Consistent adherence to rules and treatment plan
  Confrontation
  Point out problem behaviour.
  Keep client focused on self.
- Helping clients solve problems and control emotions
  Effective problem-solving skills
  Decreased impulsivity
  Expressing negative emotions such as anger or frustration
  Taking a time-out from stressful situations
- Enhancing role performance
  Identifying barriers to role fulfilment
  Decreasing or eliminating use of drugs and alcohol

CLIENT/FAMILY EDUCATION FOR ANTISOCIAL PERSONALITY DISORDER

- Avoiding use of alcohol and other drugs
- Appropriate social skills
- Effective problem-solving skills
- Managing emotions such as anger and frustration
- Taking a time-out to avoid stressful situations

BORDERLINE PERSONALITY DISORDER

BPD is characterized by a pervasive pattern of unstable interpersonal relationships, self-image and affect, as well as marked impulsivity. About 2% to 3% of the general population has borderline personality disorder; it is five times more common in those with a first-degree relative with the diagnosis. Borderline personality disorder is the most common personality disorder found in clinical settings. It is three times more common in women than in men. Under stress, transient psychotic symptoms are common. Eight per cent to 10% of people with this diagnosis commit suicide, and many more suffer permanent damage from self-harming injuries such as cutting or burning (American Psychiatric Association, 2000; Department of Health, 2003). Typically, recurrent self-harming may be a desperate attempt to ask for help, an expression of intense anger or helplessness or

client can maintain a job with acceptable performance and some personal satisfaction, meet basic interpersonal responsibilities and avoid committing illegal or abusive acts, then treatment could be seen to be successful.

a form of self-punishment. The resulting physical pain is also a means to block emotional pain. Clients who engage in self-mutilation may do so to reinforce that they are still alive; they seek to experience physical pain in the face of emotional numbing (Paris, 2005).

APPLICATION OF THE NURSING PROCESS: BORDERLINE PERSONALITY DISORDER

First, it needs to be said that the diagnosis of borderline personality disorder itself (while accepted, even celebrated by some clients) can be problematic: it can be seen as pejorative, judgemental or critical. It can, in other words, reinforce the beliefs people with the diagnosis have about themselves and what others have been telling them throughout their life. Horn *et al.* (2007) found that many users of services themselves felt that an understanding, an agreed formulation of specific problems and an ongoing, collaborative search for knowledge was far more helpful than clinging to a static, reducing label: what they wanted from clinicians was clarity, purpose and empathy.

Yet this is not easy. Working with clients who are diagnosed with borderline personality disorder can be immensely frustrating and emotionally demanding. They can be bright, funny, wise, insightful and engaging, able to hold down a high-pressure job, be creative and imaginative and gifted in the arts. The dynamics between someone diagnosed with BPD and someone working therapeutically with them are frequently infused with a whole range of contradictory thoughts, desires and feelings – on both sides. People with the diagnosis are – in almost every way – harder to see as 'different', as 'ill', as 'one of them' than people with almost any other diagnosis: paradoxically, the temptation for clinicians is to then reject them as a way of protecting against the uncomfortable truths that they – consciously or unconsciously – are pointing out to us about ourselves. The majority of nurses will, if honest, recognize themselves (at least at one point in their life) in more than one of the *DSM-IV-TR* diagnostic criteria listed in the box below.

The sheer intensity of relationships for someone diagnosed with BPD, the feelings of not being good enough, the need to be loved, the need to hold on to people and the terror of losing them, the need to trust and the dread of doing so: these are all mirrored in most of our own lives. When we come across someone who expresses these things openly, dramatically, in a way that can't be ignored, we can find it hard to cope, especially if we lack an awareness of our own needs, fears and desires. Unravelling what is 'mine' and what is 'yours' (reducing 'projections'), recognizing when a client reminds us of someone important to us, or reminds us of ourselves ('transference' and 'counter-transference'), noticing 'splitting' – within us, between us and the client, between ourselves and other members of the team: all these processes can help us work effectively with people diagnosed with BPD and help us maintain compassion. Exploration of the processes can also help clients understand themselves and their own relationships.

People diagnosed with BPD may cling and ask for help one minute and then become angry, 'act out' and reject all offers of help in the next minute. They may attempt to manipulate people to gain immediate gratification of needs and, at times, sabotage their own treatment plans by failing to do what they have agreed. Their labile mood, unpredictability and diverse destructive behaviours can make it feel as if the clinician is always 'back to square one' with them.

Self-harming behaviours may be an attempt to regain a sense of control, to reduce unbearable thoughts and emotions, to escape the numbness and alienation of an empty life – 'feeling something rather than nothing'; on occasion, they can be an unconscious attempt to re-enact symbolically abusive encounters with others, often from childhood. Understanding this – and not dismissing self-harm as 'manipulative' or 'attention-seeking' or 'acting-out' – is essential.

Assessment

HISTORY

Many people report disturbed early relationships with their parents that often begin at 18 to 30 months of age. Commonly, early attempts by these clients to achieve developmental independence were met with punitive responses from parents or threats of withdrawal of parental support and approval. At least 50% of these clients have experienced childhood sexual abuse; others have experienced physical and verbal abuse and parental alcoholism (Meissner, 2005). Clients tend to use transitional objects (e.g. teddy bears,

---

DSM-IV-TR DIAGNOSTIC CRITERIA: SYMPTOMS OF BORDERLINE PERSONALITY DISORDER

- Fear of abandonment, real or perceived
- Unstable and intense relationships
- Unstable self-image
- Impulsivity or recklessness
- Recurrent self-mutilating behaviour or suicidal threats or gestures
- Chronic feelings of emptiness and boredom
- Labile mood
- Irritability
- Polarized thinking about self and others ('splitting')
- Impaired judgement
- Lack of insight
- Transient psychotic symptoms such as hallucinations demanding self-harm

Adapted from American Psychiatric Association. (2000). *Diagnostic and Statistical Manual of Mental Disorders* (4th edn, text revision). Washington, DC: American Psychiatric Association.

pillows, blankets, dolls) extensively; this may continue into adulthood. Transitional objects are often similar to favourite items from childhood that the client used for comfort or security.

GENERAL APPEARANCE AND MOTOR BEHAVIOUR

Clients experience a wide range of dysfunction – from severe to mild. Initial behaviour and presentation may vary widely, depending on a client's present status. When dysfunction is severe, clients may appear dishevelled and may be unable to sit still, or they may display very labile emotions. In other cases, initial appearance and motor behaviour may seem normal. The client seen in A&E threatening suicide or self-harm may seem out of control, whereas a client seen at home may appear calm and rational.

MOOD AND AFFECT

The pervasive mood is usually **dysphoric**, involving unhappiness, restlessness and malaise. Clients often report intense loneliness, boredom, frustration and feeling 'empty'. They rarely experience periods of satisfaction or well-being. Although there is a pervasive depressed affect, it is unstable and erratic. Clients may become irritable, even hostile or sarcastic and complain of episodes of panic anxiety. They experience intense emotions such as anger and rage, but rarely express them productively or usefully. They usually are hypersensitive to others' emotions, which can easily trigger reactions. Minor changes may precipitate a severe emotional crisis, for example, when an

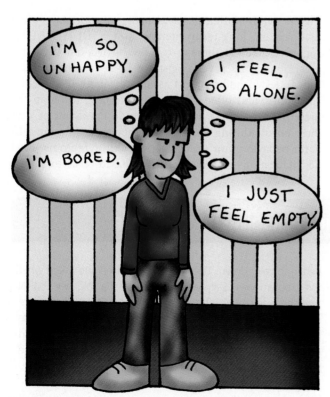

Unstable, unhappy affect of borderline personality disorder

appointment must be changed from one day to the next. Commonly, these clients can experience major emotional trauma when their key worker or care co-ordinator takes a holiday.

THOUGHT PROCESS AND CONTENT

Thinking about self and others is often polarized and extreme: this is sometimes referred to as *splitting*. Clients tend to adore and idealize other people even after a brief acquaintance, but then quickly devalue them if these others do not meet their expectations in some way. They can have excessive and chronic fears of abandonment even in normal situations; this reflects their intolerance of being alone. They may also engage in obsessive rumination about almost anything, regardless of the issue's relative importance.

Clients may experience dissociative episodes (periods of wakefulness when they are unaware of their actions). Self-harming behaviours often occur during these dissociative episodes, although at other times clients may be fully aware of injuring themselves. As stated earlier, under extreme stress, clients may develop transient psychotic symptoms such as delusions or hallucinations.

SENSORY AND INTELLECTUAL PROCESSES

Intellectual capacities are intact, and clients are fully oriented to reality. The exception is transient psychotic symptoms; during such episodes, reports of auditory hallucinations encouraging or demanding self-harm are most common. These symptoms usually abate when the stress is relieved. Many clients also report flashbacks of previous abuse or trauma. These experiences are consistent with PTSD, which is common in clients with borderline personality disorder (see Chapter 11).

JUDGEMENT AND INSIGHT

Clients frequently report behaviours consistent with impaired judgement and lack of care and concern for safety, such as gambling, shoplifting and reckless driving. They make decisions based impulsively on emotions rather than facts.

Clients have difficulty accepting responsibility for meeting needs outside a relationship. They see life's problems and failures as a result of others' shortcomings. Because others are always to blame, insight is limited. A typical reaction to a problem is 'I wouldn't have got into this mess if so-and-so had been there.'

SELF-CONCEPT

Clients have an unstable view of themselves that can shift dramatically and suddenly. They may appear needy and dependent one moment and angry, hostile and rejecting the next. Sudden changes in opinions and plans about career, sexual identity, values and types of friends are common. Clients view themselves as inherently bad or evil and often report feeling as if they don't really exist at all.

Suicidal threats, gestures and attempts are common. Self-harm and mutilation, such as cutting, punching or burning, are common. These behaviours must be taken very seriously because these clients are at increased risk for completed suicide, even if numerous previous attempts have not been life threatening. These self-inflicted injuries cause much pain and often require extensive treatment; some result in massive scarring or permanent disability, such as paralysis or loss of mobility from injury to nerves, tendons and other essential structures.

ROLES AND RELATIONSHIPS

People with a diagnosis of BPD often hate being alone, but their erratic, labile and sometimes dangerous behaviours often isolate them. Relationships are unstable, stormy and intense; the cycle repeats itself continually. These clients have extreme fears of abandonment and difficulty believing a relationship still exists once the person is away from them. They engage in many desperate behaviours, even suicide attempts, to gain or to maintain relationships. Feelings for others are often distorted, erratic and inappropriate. For example, they may view someone they have only met once or twice as their best and only friend or the 'love of my life'. If another person does not immediately reciprocate their feelings, they may feel rejected, become hostile and declare him or her to be their enemy. These erratic emotional changes can occur in the space of 1 hour. Often, these situations precipitate self-mutilating behaviour; occasionally, clients may attempt to harm others physically.

People with the diagnosis may have a history of poor school and work performance because of constantly changing career goals and shifts in identity or aspirations, preoccupation with maintaining relationships, and fear of real or perceived abandonment. Clients lack the concentration and self-discipline to follow through on sometimes mundane tasks associated with work or school.

PHYSIOLOGICAL AND SELF-CARE CONSIDERATIONS

In addition to suicidal and self-harm behaviour, clients also may engage in bingeing (excessive overeating) and purging (self-induced vomiting), substance abuse, unprotected sex or reckless behaviour, such as driving while intoxicated. They frequently have difficulty sleeping.

Data Analysis

Nursing formulations for clients with borderline personality disorder may include the following:

- Risk of suicide
- Risk of self-harm
- Risk of violence towards others
- Ineffective coping
- Social isolation.

Outcome Identification

Treatment outcomes may include the following:

- The client will be safe and free of significant injury.
- The client will not harm others or destroy property.
- The client will demonstrate increased control of impulsive behaviour.
- The client will take appropriate steps to meet his or her own needs.
- The client will demonstrate problem-solving skills.
- The client will verbalize greater satisfaction with relationships.

Interventions

Clients with borderline personality disorder are often involved in long-term therapy (often DBT, CBT or cognitive analytic therapy (CAT)) carried out by nurse practitioners, by psychologists or by psychotherapists – sometimes to address past issues of family dysfunction and abuse, and often to begin functioning better in the present. Nurses may be most likely to have contact with these clients during crises, when they are exhibiting self-harm behaviours or transient psychotic symptoms. Brief hospitalizations or intensive home-based crisis treatment

---

CLINICAL VIGNETTE: BORDERLINE PERSONALITY DISORDER

Sally had been calling her CMHN all day, ever since their meeting this morning. But the CMHN hadn't called her back, even though all her messages said this was an emergency. She was sure her CMHN was angry at her and was probably going to drop her as a client. Then she'd have no one; she'd be abandoned by the only person in the world she could talk to. Sally was upset and crying as she began to run the razor blade across her arm. As the blood trickled out, she began to calm down. Then her CMHN called and asked what the problem was. Sally was sobbing as she told her CMHN that she was cutting her arm because the CMHN didn't care anymore, that she was abandoning Sally just like everyone else in her life – her parents, her best friend, every man she had a relationship with. No one was ever there for her when she needed them.

are often used to manage these difficulties and to stabilize the client's condition.

PROMOTING CLIENTS' SAFETY

Clients' physical safety is always a priority. The nurse must always seriously consider suicidal ideation with the presence of a plan, access to means for enacting the plan and self-harm behaviours and institute appropriate interventions (see Chapter 15). Clients often experience chronic suicidality or ongoing intermittent ideas of suicide over months or years. The challenge for the nurse, in concert with clients, is to determine when suicidal ideas are likely to be translated into action.

Clients may enact self-harm urges by cutting, burning or punching themselves, which sometimes causes permanent physical damage. Self-injury can occur when a client is enraged or experiencing dissociative episodes or psychotic symptoms, or it may occur for no readily apparent reason. Helping clients to avoid self-injury can be difficult when antecedent conditions vary greatly. Sometimes, clients may discuss self-harm urges with the nurse if they feel comfortable doing so. The nurse must remain non-judgemental when discussing this topic. The nurse can encourage clients to enter a **no-self-harm contract**, in which a client promises to not engage in self-harm and to report to the nurse when he or she is losing control. The nurse emphasizes that the no-self-harm contract is not a promise to the nurse but is the client's promise to himself or herself to be safe. This distinction is critical to avoid blurring the boundaries between nurse and client.

When clients are relatively calm and thinking clearly, it is helpful for the nurse to explore self-harm behaviour. The nurse avoids sensational aspects of the injury; the focus is on identifying mood and affect, level of agitation and distress and circumstances surrounding the incident. In this way, clients can begin to identify trigger situations, moods or emotions that precede self-harm and to use more effective coping skills to deal with the trigger issues.

If clients do injure themselves, the nurse assesses the injury and need for treatment in a calm, matter-of-fact manner. Lecturing or chastising clients is punitive and has no positive effect on self-harm behaviours. Deflecting attention from the actual physical act may, however, be desirable.

PROMOTING THE THERAPEUTIC RELATIONSHIP

Regardless of the clinical setting, the nurse must provide compassion, security, safety, structure and limit-setting in the therapeutic relationship. In a community setting, this may mean seeing the client for scheduled appointments of a predetermined length rather than whenever the client appears and demands the nurse's immediate attention. In the hospital setting, the nurse might plan to spend a specific amount of time with the client, working on issues or coping strategies, rather than giving the client exclusive access

> ### NURSING INTERVENTIONS FOR BORDERLINE PERSONALITY DISORDER
>
> - Promoting client's safety
>   No-self-harm contract
>   Safe expression of feelings and emotions
> - Helping client to cope and control emotions
>   Identifying feelings
>   Coping with crises
>   Journal entries
>   Moderating emotional responses
>   Decreasing impulsivity
>   Delaying gratification
>   Mindfulness
>   Meditation
> - Cognitive restructuring techniques
>   Thought stopping
>   Decatastrophizing
> - Structuring time
> - Teaching social skills
> - Teaching effective communication skills
> - Therapeutic relationship
>   Limit setting
>   Confrontation

when he or she has exhibited self-damaging behaviour. Limit-setting and confrontation techniques, which have been described earlier, may also be helpful.

ESTABLISHING BOUNDARIES IN RELATIONSHIPS

Clients have difficulty maintaining satisfying interpersonal relationships. Personal boundaries are unclear, and clients often have unrealistic expectations. Erratic patterns of thinking and behaving often alienate them from others. This may be true for both professional and personal relationships. Clients can easily misinterpret the nurse's genuine interest and caring as a personal friendship, and the nurse may feel flattered by a client's compliments. The nurse must be quite clear about establishing the boundaries of the therapeutic relationship to ensure that neither the client's nor the nurse's boundaries are violated. For example:

Client: 'You're better than my family and the psychiatrist. You understand me more than anyone else.'

Nurse: 'I'm interested in helping you get better, just as the other staff members are.' (establishing boundaries)

TEACHING EFFECTIVE COMMUNICATION SKILLS

It may be important to teach basic communication skills such as eye contact, active listening, taking turns talking, validating the meaning of another's communication and using 'I'

CLIENT/FAMILY EDUCATION FOR BORDERLINE PERSONALITY DISORDER

- Teaching social skills
    - Maintaining personal boundaries
    - Realistic expectations of relationships
- Teaching time structuring
    - Making a written schedule of activities
    - Making a list of solitary activities to combat boredom
- Teaching self-management through cognitive restructuring
    - Decatastrophizing situation
    - Thought stopping
    - Positive self-talk
- Mindfulness and meditation
- Using assertiveness techniques such as 'I' statements
- Use of distraction such as walking or listening to music

statements ('I think . . .', 'I feel . . .', 'I need . . .'). The nurse can model these techniques and engage in role-playing with clients. The nurse asks how clients feel when interacting, and gives feedback about non-verbal behaviour, such as 'I noticed you were looking at the floor when discussing your feelings.'

HELPING CLIENTS TO COPE AND TO CONTROL EMOTIONS

Clients often react to situations with extreme emotional responses without actually recognizing their feelings. The nurse can help clients to identify their feelings and learn to tolerate them without exaggerated responses such as destruction of property or self-harm. Keeping a journal often helps clients gain awareness of feelings. The nurse can review journal entries as a basis for discussion.

Another aspect of emotional regulation is decreasing impulsivity and learning to delay gratification. When clients have an immediate desire or request, they must learn that it is unreasonable to expect it to be granted without delay. Clients can use distraction such as taking a walk or listening to music to deal with the delay, or they can think about ways to meet needs themselves. Clients can write in their journals about their feelings when gratification is delayed.

RESHAPING THINKING PATTERNS

People with this diagnosis can often view everything, people and situations, in extremes – totally good or totally bad. **Cognitive restructuring** is a technique useful in changing patterns of thinking by helping clients to recognize negative thoughts and feelings and to replace them with more realistic patterns of thinking. **Thought stopping** is a technique to alter the process of negative or self-critical thought patterns such as 'I'm dumb, I'm stupid, I can't do anything right.'

When the thoughts begin, the client may actually say 'Stop!' in a loud voice to stop the negative thoughts. Later, more subtle means such as forming a visual image of a stop sign will be a cue to interrupt the negative thoughts. The client then learns to replace recurrent negative thoughts of worthlessness with more positive thinking. In **positive self-talk**, the client reframes negative thoughts into positive ones: 'I made a mistake, but it's not the end of the world. Next time, I'll know what to do' (Andreasen & Black, 2006).

Decatastrophizing is a technique that involves learning to assess situations realistically rather than always assuming a catastrophe will happen. The nurse asks, 'So what is the worst thing that could happen?' or 'How likely do you think that is?' or 'How do you suppose other people might deal with that?' or 'Can you think of any exceptions to that?' In this way, the client must consider other points of view and actually think about the situation; in time, his or her thinking may become less rigid and inflexible (Andreasen & Black, 2006).

STRUCTURING THE CLIENTS' DAILY ACTIVITIES

Feelings of chronic boredom and emptiness, fear of abandonment and intolerance of being alone are common problems. Clients are often at a loss about how to manage unstructured time, become unhappy and ruminative and may engage in frantic and desperate behaviours (e.g. self-harm) to change the situation. Minimizing unstructured time by planning activities can help clients to manage time alone. Clients can make a written schedule that includes appointments, shopping, reading the paper and going for a walk. They may be more likely to follow the plan if it is in written form. This can also help clients to plan ahead to spend time with others, instead of frantically calling others when in distress. The written schedule also allows the nurse to help clients to engage in more healthy behaviours, such as exercising, planning meals and cooking nutritious food.

Evaluation

As for people diagnosed with any personality disorder, changes may be small and slow. The degree of functional impairment of clients with borderline personality disorder may vary widely. Clients with severe impairment may be evaluated in terms of their ability to be safe and to refrain from self-injury. Other clients may be employed and enjoy stable interpersonal relationships. Generally, when clients experience fewer crises less frequently over time, treatment can be seen as effective.

HISTRIONIC PERSONALITY DISORDER

Clinical Picture

Histrionic personality disorder is characterized by a pervasive pattern of excessive emotionality and attention seeking. It occurs in 2% to 3% of the general population and in

10% to 15% of the clinical population. It is seen more often in women than in men. Clients usually seek treatment for depression, unexplained physical problems and difficulties in relationships (American Psychiatric Association, 2000).

The tendency of these clients to exaggerate the closeness of relationships or to dramatize relatively minor occurrences can result in unreliable 'data' being provided during assessment. Speech is usually colourful and theatrical, full of superlative adjectives. It becomes apparent, however, that although colourful and entertaining, descriptions are vague and lack detail. Overall appearance is normal, although clients may overdress (e.g. wear an evening dress and high heels for a clinical interview). Clients are overly concerned with impressing others with their appearance and spend inordinate time, energy and money to this end. Dress and flirtatious behaviour are not limited to social situations or relationships but also occur in occupational and professional settings. The nurse may feel that these clients are charming or even seducing him or her.

Clients are emotionally expressive, gregarious and effusive. They often exaggerate emotions inappropriately. For example, a client may say 'He's the most wonderful doctor! He's fantastic! He's changed my life!' when describing a GP she has seen once or twice. In such a case, the client cannot specify why she views the doctor so highly. Expressed emotions, although colourful, are insincere and shallow; this is readily apparent to others but not to clients. They experience rapid shifts in moods and emotions and may be laughing uproariously one moment and sobbing the next. Thus, their displays of emotion may seem phony or forced to observers. Clients are self-absorbed and focus most of their thinking on themselves with little or no thought about the needs of others. They are highly suggestible and will agree with almost anyone to gain attention. They express strong opinions very firmly, but because they base them on little evidence or facts, the opinions often shift under the influence of someone they are trying to impress.

Clients are uncomfortable when they are not the centre of attention and go to great lengths to gain that status. They use their physical appearance and dress to gain attention. At times, they may fish for compliments in unsubtle ways, fabricate unbelievable stories or create public scenes to attract attention. They may even faint, become ill or fall to the floor. They brighten considerably when given attention after some of these behaviours; this leaves others feeling that they have been used. Any comment or statement that could be interpreted as uncomplimentary or unflattering may produce a strong response such as a temper tantrum or crying outburst.

Clients tend to exaggerate the intimacy of relationships. They refer to almost all acquaintances as 'dear, dear friends'. They may embarrass family members or friends by flamboyant and inappropriate public behaviour such as hugging and kissing someone who has just been introduced or sobbing uncontrollably over a minor incident. Clients

may ignore old friends if someone new and interesting has been introduced. People with whom these clients have relationships often describe being used, manipulated or exploited shamelessly.

Clients may have a wide variety of vague physical complaints or relate exaggerated versions of physical illness. These episodes usually involve the attention clients received (or failed to receive) rather than any particular physiological concern.

Nursing Interventions

Once again, nurses may recognize themselves or people they know in these descriptions: it is important that this doesn't get in the way of effective helping.

The nurse should give clients honest but gentle feedback about their social interactions with others, including manner of dress and non-verbal behaviour. Feedback should focus on appropriate alternatives, not merely criticism. For example, the nurse might say,

'When you embrace and kiss other people on first meeting them, they might interpret your behaviour in a sexual way. Maybe it would be better to stand at least 2 feet away from them and to shake hands?'

It may also help to discuss social situations to explore clients' perceptions of others' reactions and behaviour. Teaching social skills and role-playing those skills in a safe, non-threatening environment can help clients to gain confidence in their ability to interact socially. The nurse must be specific in describing and modelling social skills, including establishing eye contact, engaging in active listening and respecting personal space. It also helps to outline topics of discussion appropriate for casual acquaintances, closer friends or family and the nurse only.

Clients may be quite sensitive about discussing self-esteem and may respond with exaggerated emotions. It is important to explore personal strengths and assets and to give specific feedback about positive characteristics. Encouraging clients to use assertive communication, such as 'I' statements, may promote self-esteem and help them to get their needs met more appropriately. The nurse must convey genuine confidence in the client's abilities.

NARCISSISTIC PERSONALITY DISORDER

Clinical Picture

Narcissistic personality disorder is characterized by a pervasive pattern of grandiosity (in fantasy or behaviour), need for admiration and lack of empathy. It occurs in 1% to 2% of the general population and in 2% to 16% of the clinical population. Fifty to 75% of people with this diagnosis are men. Narcissistic traits are common in adolescence and do not necessarily indicate that a personality disorder will develop in adulthood. Individual psychotherapy is the most effective

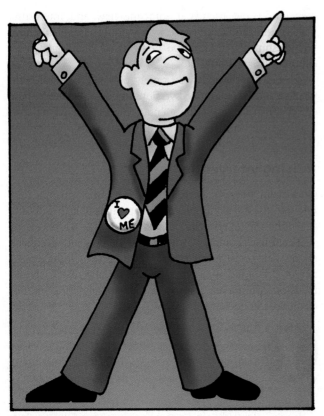

Narcissistic personality

treatment, and hospitalization is rare unless co-morbid conditions exist for which the client requires inpatient treatment (American Psychiatric Association, 2000).

Clients may display an arrogant or haughty attitude. They lack the ability to recognize or to empathize with the feelings of others. They may express envy and begrudge others any recognition or material success, because they believe it rightfully should be theirs. Clients tend to disparage, belittle or discount the feelings of others. They may express their grandiosity overtly, or they may quietly expect to be recognized for their perceived greatness. They are often preoccupied with fantasies of unlimited success, power, brilliance, beauty or ideal love. These fantasies reinforce their sense of superiority. Clients may ruminate about long-overdue admiration and privilege, and compare themselves favourably with famous or privileged people.

Thought-processing is intact, but insight is limited or poor. Clients believe themselves to be superior and special, and are unlikely to consider that their behaviour has any relation to their problems: they view their problems as the fault of others.

Underlying self-esteem is almost always fragile and vulnerable. These clients are hypersensitive to criticism and need constant attention and admiration. They often display a sense of entitlement (unrealistic expectation of special treatment or automatic compliance with wishes). They may believe that only special or privileged people can appreciate their unique qualities or are worthy of their friendship. They

expect special treatment from others and often are puzzled, or even angry, when they do not receive it. They often form and exploit relationships to elevate their own status. Clients assume total concern from others about their welfare. They discuss their own concerns in lengthy detail with no regard for the needs and feelings of others, and often become impatient or contemptuous of those who discuss their own needs and concerns.

At work, these clients may experience some success because they are ambitious and confident. Difficulties are common, however, because they have trouble working with others (whom they consider to be inferior) and have limited ability to accept criticism or feedback. They also are likely to believe they are underpaid and under-appreciated or should have a higher position of authority even though they are not qualified.

Nursing Interventions

Clients with narcissistic personality disorder can present one of the greatest challenges to the nurse. The nurse must use self-awareness skills to avoid the anger and frustration that these clients' behaviour and attitude can engender. Clients may be rude and arrogant, unwilling to wait and harsh and critical of the nurse. The nurse must not internalize such criticism or take it personally. The goal is to gain co-operation of these clients with other treatment as indicated. The nurse may teach about co-morbid medical or mental health conditions, any medication regime and any needed self-care skills in a matter-of-fact manner. He or she may need to set limits on rude or verbally abusive behaviour and explain his or her expectations of the client.

Cluster C: Personality Disorders

AVOIDANT PERSONALITY DISORDER

Clinical Picture

Avoidant personality disorder is characterized by a pervasive pattern of social discomfort and reticence, low self-esteem and hypersensitivity to negative evaluation. It occurs in 0.5% to 1% of the general population and in 10% of the clinical population. It is equally common in men and women. Clients are good candidates for individual psychotherapy (American Psychiatric Association, 2000).

These clients are likely to report being overly inhibited as children and that they often avoid unfamiliar situations and people, with an intensity beyond that expected for their developmental stage. This inhibition, which may have continued throughout upbringing, contributes to low self-esteem and social alienation. Clients are apt to be anxious and may fidget in chairs and make poor eye contact with the nurse. They may be reluctant to ask questions or to make requests. They may appear sad as well as anxious. They describe being shy, fearful, socially awkward and easily devastated by real or perceived criticism. Their usual response to these feelings is to become more reticent and withdrawn.

Clients have very low self-esteem. They are hypersensitive to negative evaluation from others and readily believe themselves to be inferior. Clients are reluctant to do anything perceived as risky, which, for them, is almost anything. They are fearful and convinced they will make a mistake, be humiliated or embarrass themselves and others. Because they are unusually fearful of rejection, criticism, shame or disapproval, they tend to avoid situations or relationships that may result in these feelings. They usually strongly desire social acceptance and human companionship: they wish for closeness and intimacy but fear possible rejection and humiliation. These fears hinder socialization, which makes clients seem awkward and socially inept and reinforces their beliefs about themselves. They may need excessive reassurance of guaranteed acceptance before they are willing to risk forming a relationship.

Clients may report some success in occupational roles because they are so eager to please or to win a supervisor's approval. Shyness, awkwardness or fear of failure, however, may prevent them from seeking jobs that might be more suitable, challenging or rewarding. For example, a client may reject a promotion and continue to remain in a junior position for years even though he or she is well qualified to advance.

Nursing Interventions

These clients require much support and reassurance from the nurse. In the non-threatening context of a focused, compassionate relationship, the nurse can help them to explore positive self-aspects, positive responses from others and possible reasons for self-criticism. Helping clients to practise self-affirmations and positive self-talk may be useful in promoting self-esteem. Other cognitive restructuring techniques, such as reframing and decatastrophizing (described previously), can enhance self-worth. The nurse can teach social skills and help clients to practise them in the safety of the nurse–client relationship. Although these clients have many social fears, those are often counterbalanced by their desire for meaningful social contact and relationships. The nurse must be careful and patient with clients, and not expect them to implement social skills too rapidly.

DEPENDENT PERSONALITY DISORDER

Clinical Picture

Dependent personality disorder is characterized by a pervasive and excessive need to be taken care of, which leads to submissive and clinging behaviour and fears of separation. These behaviours are designed to elicit caretaking from others. The disorder occurs in as much as 15% of the population and is seen three times more often in women than in men. It runs in families and is most common in the youngest child.

People with dependent personality disorder often seek treatment for anxious, depressed or somatic symptoms (American Psychiatric Association, 2000).

Clients are frequently anxious and may be mildly uncomfortable. They are often pessimistic and self-critical; other people hurt their feelings easily. They commonly report feeling unhappy or depressed; this is associated most likely with the actual or threatened loss of support from another. They are preoccupied excessively with unrealistic fears of being left alone to care for themselves. They believe they would fail on their own, so keeping or finding a relationship occupies much of their time. They have tremendous difficulty making decisions, no matter how minor. They seek advice and repeated reassurances about all types of decisions, from what to wear to what type of job to pursue. Although they can make judgements and decisions, they lack the confidence to do so.

Clients perceive themselves as unable to function outside a relationship with someone who can tell them what to do. They are very uncomfortable and feel helpless when alone, even if the current relationship is intact. They have difficulty initiating projects or completing simple daily tasks independently. They believe they need someone else to assume responsibility for them, a belief that far exceeds what is age- or situation-appropriate. They may even fear gaining competence, because doing so would mean an eventual loss of support from the person on whom they depend. They may do almost anything to sustain a relationship, even one of poor quality. This includes doing unpleasant tasks, going places they dislike or, in extreme cases, tolerating abuse. Clients are reluctant to express disagreement for fear of losing the other person's support or approval; they may even consent to activities that are wrong or illegal to avoid that loss.

When these clients do experience the end of a relationship, they urgently and desperately seek another. The unspoken motto seems to be 'Any relationship is better than none at all.'

Nursing Interventions

The nurse must help clients to express feelings of grief and loss over the end of a relationship, while fostering autonomy and self-reliance. Helping clients to identify their strengths and needs is more helpful than encouraging the overwhelming belief that 'I can't do anything alone!' Cognitive restructuring techniques, such as reframing and decatastrophizing, and mindfulness training may be beneficial.

Clients may need assistance in daily functioning if they have little or no past success in this area. Included are such things as planning menus, doing the weekly shopping, budgeting and paying bills. Careful assessment to determine areas of need is essential. Depending on the client's abilities and limitations, referral to agencies for services or assistance may be indicated.

The nurse also may need to teach problem solving and decision making and help clients apply them to daily life.

He or she must refrain from giving advice about problems or making decisions for clients, even though clients may ask the nurse to do so. The nurse can help the client to explore problems, serve as a sounding board for discussion of alternatives and provide support and positive feedback for the client's efforts in these areas.

OBSESSIVE-COMPULSIVE PERSONALITY DISORDER

Clinical Picture

Obsessive-compulsive personality disorder is characterized by a pervasive pattern of preoccupation with perfectionism, mental and interpersonal control and orderliness, at the expense of flexibility, openness and efficiency. It occurs in about 1% to 2% of the population, affecting twice as many men as women. This increases to 3% to 10% in clients in mental health settings. Incidence is increased in oldest children and people in professions involving facts, figures or methodical focus on detail. These people often seek treatment because they recognize that their life is pleasureless or they are experiencing problems with work or relationships. Clients frequently benefit from individual therapy (American Psychiatric Association, 2000).

The demeanour of these clients is usually formal and serious, and they answer questions with precision and much detail. They often report feeling the need to be perfect beginning in childhood. They were expected to be good and to do the right thing to win parental approval. Expressing emotions or asserting independence was probably met with harsh disapproval and emotional consequences. Emotional range is usually quite constricted. They have difficulty expressing emotions, and any emotions they do express are rigid, stiff and formal, lacking spontaneity. Clients can be very stubborn and reluctant to relinquish control, which makes it difficult for them to be vulnerable to others by expressing feelings. Affect is also restricted: they usually appear anxious and fretful, or stiff and reluctant to reveal underlying emotions.

Clients are preoccupied with orderliness and try to maintain it in all areas of life. They strive for perfection as though it were attainable and are preoccupied with details, rules, lists and schedules to the point of often missing 'the big picture'. They become absorbed in their own perspective, believe they are right and do not listen carefully to others because they have already dismissed what is being said. Clients check and recheck the details of any project or activity; often, they never complete the project because of 'trying to get it right'. They have problems with judgement and decision making – specifically actually reaching a decision. They consider and reconsider alternatives, and the desire for perfection prevents reaching a decision. Clients interpret rules or guidelines literally and cannot be flexible or modify decisions based on circumstances. They prefer written rules for each and every activity at work. Insight is limited, and they are often oblivious that their behaviour annoys or frustrates others. If confronted with this annoyance, these clients are stunned, unable to believe that others 'don't want me to do a good job.'

These clients have low self-esteem and are always harsh, critical and judgemental of themselves; they believe that they 'could have done better', regardless of how well the job has been done. Praise and reassurance do not change this belief. Clients are burdened by extremely high and unattainable standards and expectations. Although no one could live up to these expectations, they feel guilty and worthless for being unable to achieve them. They tend to evaluate self and others solely on deeds or actions without regard for personal qualities.

These clients have real difficulties in relationships, often with few friends and little social life. They do not express warm or tender feelings to others; attempts to do so are very stiff and formal and may sound insincere. For example, if a significant other expresses love and affection, a client's response might be a mumbled 'The feeling's mutual.'

Marital and parental–child relationships are often difficult because these clients can be harsh and unrelenting. For example, most clients are frugal, do not give gifts or want to discard old items and insist that those around them do the same. Shopping for something new to wear may seem frivolous and wasteful. Clients cannot tolerate lack of control and hence may organize family outings to the point that no one enjoys them. These behaviours can cause daily strife and discord in family life.

At work, clients may experience some success, particularly in fields when precision and attention to detail are desirable. They may miss deadlines, however, while trying to achieve perfection, or may fail to make needed decisions while searching for more data. They fail to make timely decisions because of continually striving for perfection. They have difficulty working collaboratively, preferring to 'do it myself' so it is done correctly. If clients do accept help from others, they may give such detailed instructions and watch the other person so closely that co-workers are insulted, annoyed and refuse to work with them. Given this excessive need for routine and control, new situations and compromise are also difficult.

Nursing Interventions

Nurses may be able to help clients to view decision making and completion of projects from a different perspective. Rather than striving for the goal of perfection, clients can set a goal of completing the project or making the decision by a specified deadline. Helping clients to accept or to tolerate less-than-perfect work or decisions made on time may alleviate some difficulties at work or home. Clients may benefit from cognitive restructuring techniques. The nurse can ask, 'What is the worst that could happen?' or 'How might your boss (or your wife) see this situation?' These questions may help challenge some rigid and inflexible thinking.

Encouraging clients to take risks, such as letting someone else plan a family activity, may improve relationships. Practising negotiation with family or friends also may help clients to relinquish some of their need for control.

Other Related Disorders

Researchers are studying the following two disorders, depressive personality disorder and passive-aggressive disorder, for inclusion as personality disorders. The *DSM-IV-TR* currently lists and describes these conditions.

DEPRESSIVE PERSONALITY DISORDER

Clinical Picture

Depressive personality disorder is characterized by a pervasive pattern of depressive cognitions and behaviours in various contexts. It occurs equally in men and women and more often in people with relatives who have major depressive disorders. People with depressive personality disorders often seek treatment for their distress and generally have a favourable response to antidepressant medications (American Psychiatric Association, 2000).

Although clients with depressive personality disorder may seem to have similar behaviour characteristics as clients with major depression (e.g. moodiness, brooding, joylessness, pessimism), the personality disorder is much less severe. Clients with depressive personality disorder usually do not experience the severity and long duration of major depression, or the hallmark symptoms of sleep disturbances, loss of appetite, recurrent thoughts of death and total disinterest in all activities. Major depressive episodes are discussed in Chapter 15.

These clients have a sad, gloomy or dejected affect. They express persistent unhappiness, cheerlessness and hopelessness, regardless of the situation. They often report the inability to experience joy or pleasure in any activity; they cannot relax and do not display a sense of humour. Clients may repress or not express anger. They brood and worry over all aspects of daily life. Thinking is negative and pessimistic; these clients rarely see any hope for future improvement. They view this pessimism as 'being realistic'. Regardless of positive outcomes in a given situation, negative thinking continues. Judgement or decision-making skills are usually intact but dominated by pessimistic thinking; clients often blame themselves or others unjustly for situations beyond anyone's control.

Self-esteem is quite low, with feelings of worthlessness and inadequacy even when clients have been successful. Self-criticism often leads to punitive behaviour and feelings of guilt or remorse. Clients may appear overtly quiet and passive; they prefer to follow others rather than be leaders in any work or social situation. Although clients feel dependent on approval from others, they tend to be overly critical and quick to reject others first. These clients, who need and want the approval and attention of others, actually drive others away; this reinforces feelings of being unworthy of anyone's attention.

Nursing Interventions

When working with clients who report depressed feelings, it is always important to assess whether there is risk for self-harm. If a client expresses suicidal ideation or has urges for self-injury, the nurse must provide interventions and plan care as indicated (see Chapter 15).

The nurse explains that the client must take action, rather than wait, to feel better. Encouraging the client to become involved in activities or engaged with others provides opportunities to interrupt the cyclical, negative thought patterns.

Giving factual feedback, rather than general praise, reinforces attempts to interact with others and gives specific positive information about improved behaviours. An example of general praise is

'Oh, you're doing so well today.'

This statement does not identify specific positive behaviours. Allowing the client to identify specific positive behaviours often helps to promote self-esteem. An example of specific praise is

'You talked to Mrs Jones for 10 minutes, even though it was difficult. I know that took a lot of effort.'

This statement gives the client a clear message about what specific behaviour was effective and positive – the client's ability to talk to someone else.

Cognitive restructuring techniques such as thought stopping or positive self-talk (discussed previously) also can enhance self-esteem. Clients learn to recognize negative thoughts and feelings and learn new positive patterns of thinking about themselves.

It may be necessary to teach the client effective social skills such as eye contact, attentive listening and topics appropriate for initial social conversation (e.g. the weather, current events, local news). Even if the client knows these social skills, practising them is important – first with the nurse and then with others. Practising with the nurse is initially less threatening. Another simple but effective technique is to help the client practise giving others compliments. This requires the client to identify something positive rather than negative in others. Giving compliments also promotes receiving compliments, which further enhances positive feelings.

PASSIVE-AGGRESSIVE PERSONALITY DISORDER

Clinical Picture

Passive-aggressive personality disorder is characterized by a negative attitude and a pervasive pattern of passive resistance to demands for adequate social and occupational performance. It occurs in 1% to 3% of the general population and in 2% to 8% of the clinical population. It is thought to be slightly more prevalent in women than in men (American Psychiatric Association, 2000).

These clients may appear co-operative, even ingratiating, or sullen and withdrawn, depending on the circumstances. Their mood may fluctuate rapidly and erratically, and they may be easily upset or offended. They may alternate between hostile self-assertion, such as stubbornness or fault finding, and excessive dependence, expressing contrition and guilt. There is a pervasive attitude that is negative, sullen and defeatist. Affect may be sad or angry. The negative attitude influences thought content: clients perceive and anticipate difficulties and disappointments where none exist. They view the future negatively, believing that nothing good ever lasts. Their ability to make judgements or decisions is often impaired. Clients are frequently ambivalent and indecisive, preferring to allow others to make decisions that these clients then criticize. Insight is also limited: clients tend to blame others for their own feelings and misfortune. Rather than accepting reasonable responsibility for the situation, these clients may alternate blaming behaviour with exaggerated remorse and contrition.

Clients experience intense conflict between dependence on others and a desire for assertion. Self-confidence is low despite the bravado shown. Clients may complain they are misunderstood and unappreciated by others and may report feeling cheated, victimized and exploited. They habitually resent, oppose and resist demands to function at a level expected by others. This opposition occurs most frequently in work situations but also can be evident in social functioning. They express such resistance through procrastination, forgetfulness, stubbornness and intentional inefficiency, especially in response to tasks assigned by authority figures. They also may obstruct the efforts of co-workers by failing to do their share. In social or family relationships, these clients may play the role of the martyr who 'sacrifices everything for others' or who may be aggrieved and misunderstood. These behaviours are sometimes effective in manipulating others to do as clients wish, without clients needing to make a direct request.

These clients often have various vague or generalized somatic complaints and may even adopt a sick role. They then can be angry or bitter, complaining, 'No one can figure out what's wrong with me. I just have to suffer. It's just my bad luck!'

Nursing Interventions

The nurse may encounter much resistance from the client in identifying feelings and expressing them directly. Often, clients do not recognize that they feel angry and may express it indirectly. The nurse can help them examine the relationship between feelings and subsequent actions. For example, a client may intend to complete a project at work but then procrastinates, forgets or becomes 'ill' and misses the deadline. Or the client may intend to participate in a family outing but becomes ill, forgets or has 'an emergency' when it is time. By focusing on the behaviour, the nurse can help the client to see what is so annoying or troubling to others. The nurse also can help the client to learn appropriate ways to express feelings directly, especially negative feelings such as anger. Methods such as having the client write about the feelings or role-play are effective. If the client is unwilling to engage in this process, however, the nurse cannot force him or her to do so.

PERSONALITY DISORDERS: CONSIDERATIONS IN OLDER PEOPLE

Personality disorders are not usually first diagnosed in older people but may persist from young adulthood into older age. Abrams and Sadavoy (2004) suggest that personality disorders from Clusters A and C are more prevalent in older age and are closely correlated with depression. Some people with personality disorders tend to stabilize and experience fewer difficulties in later life. Others are described as 'aging badly', that is, they are unable or unwilling to acknowledge limitations that come with aging, they refuse to accept help when needed and they do not make reasonable decisions about their health care, finances or living situation. These individuals seem chronically angry, unhappy or dissatisfied, resulting in strained relationships and even alienation from family, friends, carers and clinicians.

MENTAL HEALTH PROMOTION

Herrenkohl *et al.* (2005) reported that children who have a greater number of 'protective factors' are less likely to develop antisocial behaviour as adults. These protective factors include school commitment or importance of school, parent or peer disapproval of antisocial behaviour, and being involved in a religious community. Interestingly, the study found that children at risk of abuse *and* children who were not at risk were less likely to have antisocial behaviour as adults if these protective factors were present in their environment. Children lacking these protective factors are much more likely to develop antisocial behaviour as adults.

It seems clear that many people diagnosed with a personality disorder struggle with themselves and other people as a result of abuse and neglect in childhood. Huge social changes are needed – at economic, social, political and cultural levels – to begin to work towards changing a society that can produce people who find living in it so difficult.

SELF-AWARENESS ISSUES

People with a diagnosis of personality disorder can be charming, positive, engaging and pleasant. They can also be difficult, negative, frustrating and self-destructive. They are – in other words – just like us, and this fact can make them incredibly demanding to work with (James & Cowman, 2007).

Because people diagnosed with personality disorders can take a long time to change their behaviours, attitudes or coping skills, nurses working with them can easily become frustrated or angry. Nurses must discuss feelings of anger or frustration with colleagues – in **clinical supervision** and informally – to help them recognize and cope with their own feelings.

The overall appearance of clients with personality disorders can be misleading. Unlike clients who are psychotic or severely depressed, someone diagnosed with a personality disorder can look – and behave – as though they are capable of functioning more effectively than they actually do. The nurse can easily, but mistakenly, believe the client simply lacks motivation or the willingness to make changes, and may feel frustrated or angry. It is easy for the nurse to think, 'Why does he continue to do that? Can't he see it only gets him into difficulties?' This reaction is similar to reactions the client has probably received from others.

Clients with personality disorders also challenge the ability of therapeutic staff to work as a team. For example, clients with antisocial or borderline personalities often manipulate staff members – consciously or, more commonly, unconsciously – by 'splitting' them – that is, causing staff members to disagree or to contradict one another in terms of the limits of the treatment plan. This can be quite disruptive and damaging to clients and to staff. In addition, team members may have differing opinions about individual clients. One staff member may believe that a client needs assistance, whereas another may believe the client is overly dependent: this split between 'the good patient' and 'the bad patient' is at the root of many problems, particularly on acute inpatient units. Open, honest and ongoing communication is necessary to remain firm and consistent about expectations for client care.

Points to Consider When Working With Clients With Personality Disorders

- Talking to colleagues about feelings of frustration – formally and informally – will help you to deal with your emotional responses so you can be more effective with clients.
- Clear, frequent communication with other professionals can help to diminish any 'manipulation' or self-destructive behaviour.
- Do not take undue flattery or harsh criticism personally; it is a 'symptom' of the client's dysfunctional attempts to deal with the lifelong relationship difficulties they have.
- Set realistic goals and remember that behaviour changes in clients with personality disorders can take a long time.

Critical Thinking Questions/ Group Discussion Questions

1. Where do you see *yourself* in relation to the four types of temperament (harm avoidance, novelty seeking, reward dependence and persistence)?
2. Which category of personality disorder is closest to describing you?
3. What has been the most significant influence on *your* development as a person?
4. There is a significant correlation between the diagnosis of antisocial personality disorder and criminal behaviour. The *DSM-IV-TR* includes 'violation of the rights of others' in the definition of this disorder. Is this personality disorder more a social than a mental health problem? If so, why?

KEY POINTS

- People diagnosed with personality disorders have traits that are inflexible and maladaptive and cause either significant functional impairment or subjective distress.
- The overlap with other mental disorders – schizophrenia, bipolar affective disorder, depression – and with drug and alcohol misuse is complex and challenging.
- Personality disorders seem to be relatively common and frequently diagnosed in early adulthood, although some behaviours are evident in childhood or adolescence.
- People diagnosed with a personality disorder, particularly borderline personality disorder, have traditionally been treated poorly by services.
- Clinicians need to be acutely aware of their own thoughts, feelings and behaviour, their own personal histories and their own needs and dreams when working with people with a diagnosis of personality disorder.
- Rapid or substantial changes in personality are relatively rare. This can be a primary source of frustration for family members, friends and health-care professionals.
- Schizotypal personality disorder is characterized by social and interpersonal deficits, cognitive and perceptual distortions and eccentric behaviour.
- People diagnosed with paranoid personality disorders are suspicious, mistrustful and feel threatened by others.
- People diagnosed with depressive personality disorder are sad, gloomy and negative; experience no pleasure; and tend to brood or ruminate about their lives.
- Schizoid personality disorder includes marked detachment from others, restricted emotions, indifference and fantasy.
- People diagnosed with antisocial personality disorder often appear glib and charming, but they are suspicious, insensitive and uncaring, and often exploit others for their own gain.

- People diagnosed with borderline personality disorder have markedly unstable mood, affect, self-image, interpersonal relationships and impulsivity; they often engage in self-harm behaviour.
- People diagnosed with obsessive-compulsive personality disorder are preoccupied with orderliness, perfection and interpersonal control, at the expense of flexibility, openness and efficiency.
- Histrionic personality disorder is characterized by excessive emotionality and dramatic, attention-seeking and seductive or provocative behaviour.
- Narcissistic personality disorder is characterized by grandiosity, need for admiration, a lack of empathy for others and a sense of entitlement.
- Avoidant personality disorder is characterized by social discomfort and reticence in all situations, low self-esteem and hypersensitivity to negative evaluation.
- Dependent personality disorder is characterized by a pervasive and excessive need to be taken care of, which leads to submissive and clinging behaviours and fears of separation and abandonment.
- People diagnosed with passive-aggressive personality disorder demonstrate passive resistance to demands for adequate social and occupational performance, and negativity; they often play the role of a martyr.
- The therapeutic relationship is crucial in caring for clients diagnosed with a personality disorder. Nurses can help people to identify their thoughts, beliefs, feelings and dysfunctional behaviours and to develop appropriate coping skills and positive behaviours. Therapeutic communication and role modelling help to promote appropriate social interactions, which help to improve interpersonal relationships.
- Several therapeutic strategies are effective when working with clients diagnosed with personality disorders. Cognitive restructuring techniques such as thought stopping, positive self-talk and decatastrophizing are useful; mindfulness training and self-help skills aid the client to function better in the community.

- Psychotropic medications are prescribed for clients with personality disorders, based on the type and severity of symptoms the client experiences in aggression and impulsivity, mood dysregulation, anxiety and psychotic symptoms.
- Clients with borderline personality disorder often have self-harm urges that they enact by cutting, burning or punching themselves; this behaviour sometimes causes permanent physical damage. The nurse can encourage the client to enter into a no-self-harm contract in which the client promises to try to keep from harming himself or herself and to report to the nurse when he or she is having self-harm urges.
- Nurses must use self-awareness skills to deal with feelings such as frustration, anger, fear and excessive warmth toward a client.
- Nurses must be aware of their own inadequacies, frailties and needs, and be prepared to tackle these in order to provide high-quality care

REFERENCES

Abrams, R. C. & Sadavoy, J. (2004). Personality disorders. In J. Sadavoy, L. F. Jarvik, G. T. Grossberg, et al. (Eds.), *Comprehensive textbook of geriatric psychiatry* (3rd edn, pp. 701–721). New York: W. W. Norton and Company.

American Psychiatric Association. (2000). *Diagnostic and statistical manual of mental disorders* (4th edn, text revision). Washington, DC: American Psychiatric Association.

Andreasen, N. C. & Black, D. W. (2006). *Introductory textbook of psychiatry* (4th edn). Washington DC: American Psychiatric Publishing.

Department of Health. (2003). *Personality Disorder: No Longer A Diagnosis Of Exclusion.* Available: http://www.dh.gov.uk/en/Publicationsandstatistics/Publications/PublicationsPolicyAndGuidance/DH_4009546

Harvard Medical School Health. (2002). Borderline personality disorder. New recommendations. *Harvard Medical Health Letter, 18*(9), 4–6.

Hayward, M., Slade, M., & Moran, P. A. (2006). Personality disorders and unmet needs among psychiatric inpatients. *Psychiatric Services, 57*(4), 538–543.

Herrenkohl, T. I., Tajima, E. A., Whitney, S. D., & Huang, B. (2005). Protection against antisocial behaviour in children exposed to physically abusive discipline. *Journal of Adolescent Health, 36*(6), 457–465.

Horn, N., Johnstone, L., & Brooke, S. (2007). Some service user perspectives on the diagnosis of Borderline Personality Disorder. *Journal of Mental Health, 16*(2), 255–269.

INTERNET RESOURCES

RESOURCE	INTERNET ADDRESS
National Personality Disorder Website	http://www.personalitydisorder.org.uk/index2.php?page_id=99
National Self-Harm Network	http://www.nshn.co.uk/index2.html
NICE Self-harm guideline	http://www.nice.org.uk/guidance/index.jsp?action=byID&r=true&o=10946
Personality Disorder Institute	http://www.pdinstitute.org.uk/
Royal College of Psychiatrists: Personality Disorder	http://www.rcpsych.ac.uk/mentalhealthinformation/mentalhealthproblems/personalitydisorders.aspx
Young People and Self-Harm	http://www.selfharm.org.uk/default.aspa

James, P. D. & Cowman, S. (2007). Psychiatric nurses' knowledge, experience and attitudes towards clients with borderline personality disorder. *Journal of Psychiatric and Mental Health Nursing, 14,* 670–678.

Linehan, M. M. (1993). *Cognitive-behavioural treatment of borderline personality disorder.* New York: Guilford Press.

McGue, M. & Iacono, W. G. (2005). The association of early adolescent problem behaviour with adult psychopathology. *American Journal of Psychiatry, 162(6),* 1118–1124.

Meissner, W. W. (2005). Classic psychoanalysis. In B. J. Sadock & V. A. Sadock (Eds.). *Comprehensive textbook of psychiatry,* Vol. 1 (8th edn, pp. 701–746). Philadelphia: Lippincott Williams & Wilkins.

Paris, J. (2005). Understanding self-mutilation in borderline personality disorder. *Harvard Review of Psychiatry, 13(3),* 179–185.

Seivewright, H., Tyrer, P., & Johnson, T. (2002). Change in personality status in neurotic disorders. *Lancet, 359(9325),* 2253–2254.

Simeon, D. & Hollander, E. (2006). Treatment of personality disorders. In A. F. Schatzberg & C. B. Nereroff (Eds.), *Essentials of clinical psychopharmacology* (2nd edn, pp. 689–705). Washington DC: American Psychiatric Publishing.

Svrakic, D. M. & Cloninger, C. R. (2005). Personality disorders. In B. J. Sadock & V. A. Sadock (Eds.), *Comprehensive textbook of psychiatry,* Vol. 2 (8th edn, pp. 2063–2104). Philadelphia: Lippincott Williams & Wilkins.

Winship, G. & Hardy, S. (2007). Perspectives on the prevalence and treatment of personality disorder. *Journal of Psychiatric and Mental Health Nursing, 14(2),* 148–154.

ADDITIONAL READING

McQuillan, A., Nicastro, R., Guenot, F., Girard, M., Lissner, C., & Ferrero, F. (2005). Intensive dialectic behaviour therapy for outpatients with borderline personality disorder who are in crisis. *Psychiatric Services, 56(2),* 193–197.

Oldham, J. M. (2006). Borderline personality disorder and suicidality. *American Journal of Psychiatry, 163(1),* 20–26.

Paris, J. (2005). The development of impulsivity in borderline personality disorder. *Development and Psychopathology, 17(4),* 1091–1104.

Swenson, C. R., Torrey, W. C., & Koerner, K. (2002). Implementing dialectical behaviour therapy. *Psychiatric Services, 53(2),* 171–178.

Chapter Study Guide

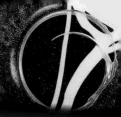

MULTIPLE-CHOICE QUESTIONS

Select the best answer for each of the following questions.

1. When working with a client diagnosed with a paranoid personality disorder, the nurse would use which of the following approaches?
   a. Honest, direct and supportive
   b. Light and flirtatious
   c. Challenging and confronting
   d. Intense and dramatic

2. Which of the following underlying emotions is commonly seen in a passive-aggressive personality disorder?
   a. Anger
   b. Depression
   c. Fear
   d. Guilt

3. Cognitive restructuring techniques include all the following except
   a. Decatastrophizing
   b. Positive self-talk
   c. Reframing
   d. Relaxation

4. Transient psychotic symptoms that occur with borderline personality disorder are most likely treated with which of the following?
   a. Anticonvulsant mood stabilizers
   b. Antipsychotics
   c. Benzodiazepines
   d. Lithium

5. Clients diagnosed with a histrionic personality disorder are most likely to benefit from which of the following nursing interventions?
   a. Facilitating social skills development
   b. Offering structured psychotherapeutic input
   c. Agreeing clear, negotiated goals
   d. All of the above

6. When interviewing any client diagnosed with a personality disorder, the nurse would assess for which of the following?
   a. Ability to charm and manipulate people
   b. Desire for interpersonal relationships
   c. Disruption in some aspects of his or her life
   d. Increased need for approval from others

7. The nurse would assess for which of the following characteristics in a client diagnosed with narcissistic personality disorder?
   a. Entitlement
   b. Fear of abandonment
   c. Hypersensitivity
   d. Suspiciousness

8. The most important short-term goal for the client who tries to manipulate others would be to
   a. Acknowledge own behaviour
   b. Express feelings verbally
   c. Stop initiating arguments
   d. Sustain lasting relationships

FILL-IN-THE-BLANK QUESTIONS

Identify the personality disorder that is described in each of the following.

_____ Unstable relationships, affect and self-image

_____ Disregard for the rights of others

_____ Detachment from social relationships, restricted affect

_____ Social inhibitions, feelings of inadequacy

CLINICAL EXAMPLE

Susan Marks, 25 years old, is diagnosed with borderline personality disorder. She has been attending college sporadically but has only completed one module and has no real career goal. She is angry because her parents have told her she must get a job to support herself. Last week, she met a man in the park and fell in love with him on the first date. She has been calling him repeatedly, but he will not return her calls. Declaring that her parents have deserted her and her boyfriend doesn't love her anymore, she slashes her forearms with a sharp knife. She then calls 999, stating, 'I'm about to die! Please help me!' She is taken by ambulance to A&E and is admitted to the inpatient mental health unit.

1. Identify two priority nursing formulations that would be appropriate for Susan on her admission to the unit.

2. Write an expected outcome for each of the identified nursing formulations.

3. List three nursing interventions for each of the identified nursing formulations.

4. What community resources or referrals would be beneficial for Susan?

Chapter

17

Substance Abuse

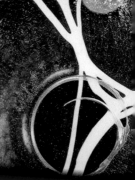

Key Terms

- 12-step programme
- blackout
- co-dependence
- controlled substance
- denial
- detoxification
- dual diagnosis
- flushing
- hallucinogen
- harm reduction/harm minimi-zation
- inhalant
- intoxication
- motivational interviewing
- opioid
- polysubstance abuse
- relapse prevention
- respect
- spontaneous remission
- stimulants
- substance misuse
- substance dependence
- tapering
- tolerance
- tolerance break
- withdrawal

Learning Objectives

After reading this chapter, you should be able to:

1. Explain current trends in substance use and misuse and discuss the need for related health-promotion programmes.

2. Discuss the personal and interpersonal characteristics, risk factors and family dynamics prevalent with substance misuse and dual diagnosis.

3. Describe the principles of a 12-step treatment approach for substance misuse.

4. Describe the principles of cognitive-behavioural and motivational inter-viewing approaches for substance misuse.

5. Describe the principles of a harm minimization approach to substance misuse.

6. Apply the nursing process to the care of clients with substance misuse issues.

7. Provide education to clients, families and community members to increase knowledge and understanding of substance use and abuse and its relationship with mental health and mental disorder.

8. Discuss the nurse's role in dealing with the substance-misusing professional.

9. Evaluate your feelings, attitudes and responses to clients and families with substance use and abuse.

The first part of this Chapter will look at the impact of alcohol and drugs on people, and at appropriate nursing interventions. The second part is dedicated to the concept of '**dual diagnosis**': the complex overlap between mental health problems and substance misuse has become more evident over the past few years and substance misuse has appeared to become the norm amongst people with severe mental health problems (Department of Health, 2002)

Substance misuse and related disorders are major social, economic and health issues in the UK. The actual prevalence of alcohol and other drug misuse is difficult to determine, in part because diagnostic criteria for 'misuse', 'dependence' and 'addiction' vary greatly, in part because the relationship between substance misuse and mental health problems, employment problems and problems of crime and disorder is a complex one; in part because many people meeting criteria for diagnosis fail to seek treatment; and in part because surveys conducted to estimate prevalence are based on self-reported data that may be inaccurate.

This said, there is little doubt that substance misuse causes immense economic, social and personal damage. According to the Cabinet Office (2003) around 2.8 million people in England alone are dependent on alcohol.

In addition, alcohol misuse accounts for somewhere between 2% and 12% of total NHS hospital expenditure (around £3 billion) (Royal College of Physicians, 2001). In a survey of physical and mental illnesses directly attributable to alcohol misuse, the Cabinet Office found that 495,269 bed days, costing £126,239,086, were taken up, including 274,759 by 'mental and behavioural disorders due to use of alcohol'.

Drugscope (2008) reports that, in England and Wales between 2003 and 2004, somewhere between 25,000 and 200,000 people died as a result of alcohol, around 5000 from opiates such as heroin, morphine and methadone, 575 from cocaine, 384 from amphetamines, 227 from ecstasy and 246 from solvents. In Scotland, which uses a different coding system, 137 people died as a result of cocaine use, 93 from ecstasy, 51 from solvents and 1348 from opiates between 1998 and 2004. Around 80% of people who die a drug-related death in the UK are men, around 75% are under 45 and 94% are white (International Centre for Drug Policy, 2008). Between 1950 and 2000, 6 million people in Britain died from tobacco-related diseases. Currently, approximately 82,800 are dying each year, a figure which accounts for a fifth of all UK deaths (Action On Smoking and Health (ASH), 2008a).

The number of infants suffering the physiological and emotional consequences of prenatal exposure to alcohol or drugs (e.g. foetal alcohol syndrome, 'crack babies') appears to be increasing at alarming rates. Chemical abuse also results in increased violence, including domestic abuse, homicide and child abuse and neglect. Children of alcoholics are four times more likely than the general population to develop problems with alcohol (National Institute on Alcohol Abuse and Alcoholism, 2007). Many people in

treatment programmes as adults report having had their first drink of alcohol as a young child, when they were younger than age 10. This first drink was often a taste of the drink of a parent or family member. With the increasing rates of use being reported among young people, some fear this problem could spiral out of control unless great strides can be made through effective programmes for prevention, early detection and effective treatment.

Poor outcomes have been associated with an earlier age at onset, longer periods of substance use and the coexistence of a major mental health disorder. With extended use, the risk of mental and physical deterioration and infectious disease, such as HIV and AIDS, hepatitis and tuberculosis, increases, especially for those with a history of intravenous drug use.

In a Northern Ireland study (Foster, 2001), the risk of suicide was eight times higher in someone with current alcohol misuse or dependence; the National Suicide Prevention Strategy for England Annual Report, 2007 (National Institute for Mental Health in England, 2008) highlights the crucial (but complex) nature of relationships between substance misuse, mental health problems and suicide.

The nursing role in health education, therapy and ongoing support in substance misuse is key.

TYPES OF SUBSTANCE ABUSE

Many substances can be used and abused; some can be obtained legally, others are illegal. This discussion includes alcohol and prescription medications as substances that can be abused. Abuse of more than one substance is sometimes termed **polysubstance abuse**.

Caffeine is the most used (and often abused!) drug in use in the UK, followed by alcohol and then tobacco. When it comes to illegal drugs, the most commonly tried drugs are:

- Cannabis
- Amphetamine
- Nitrites/poppers
- LSD
- Magic mushrooms
- Ecstasy
- Solvents (aerosols, gases and glues)
- Cocaine
- Minor tranquillizers (not prescribed)
- Heroin and crack cocaine.

This chapter describes the specific symptoms of intoxication, overdose, withdrawal and detoxification for each substance, with the exception of caffeine and nicotine. Although caffeine and nicotine abuse can cause significant physiological health problems and result in substance-induced disorders such as sleep disorders, anxiety and withdrawal, treatment of these two substances is not usually (perhaps erroneously) viewed as falling into the mental health arena.

For the purpose of this book, **intoxication** is defined as the use of a substance that results in maladaptive behaviour. **Withdrawal** refers to the syndrome of negative psychological and physical reactions that occurs when use of a substance ceases or dramatically decreases. **Detoxification** is the process of safely withdrawing from a substance. The treatment of other substance-induced disorders, such as psychosis and mood disorders, is discussed in depth in separate chapters.

Substance misuse can be defined as using a drug in a way that is inconsistent with medical or social norms and despite negative consequences. Substance misuse (or abuse) denotes problems in social, vocational or legal areas of the person's life, whereas **substance dependence** also includes problems associated with addiction, such as tolerance, withdrawal and unsuccessful attempts to stop using the substance. This distinction between abuse and dependence is frequently viewed as unclear and unnecessary (Jaffe & Anthony, 2005) because the distinction does not necessarily affect clinical decisions once withdrawal or detoxification has been completed. Hence, the terms *substance misuse* and *substance dependence* or *chemical dependence* can be used interchangeably. In this chapter, the term *substance use* is employed to include both misuse and dependence; it is not meant to refer to the occasional or one-time user.

The term 'addiction' is usually used with reference to people who regularly use heroin, cocaine or alcohol. It is the belief of agencies such as Drugscope that 'drug dependent' is a less judgement-laden term than 'addict'. People can be physically dependent on a drug, psychologically dependent or, frequently, a combination of the two. The degree to which some illicit drugs actually do produce physical dependence is still debated (in particular cocaine, amphetamines, crack and nicotine).

ONSET AND CLINICAL COURSE

Much research on substance use has focused on alcohol because it is legal and more widely used; more is known about the effects of alcohol than those of other drugs. However, a full understanding of alcohol use in general is problematic because, usually, only people actually *seeking treatment* for problems with alcohol are studied.

The early course of alcoholism typically begins with a first episode of intoxication between 15 and 17 years of age (Schuckit, 2005); the first evidence of minor alcohol-related problems is seen in the late teens. These events do not differ significantly from the experiences of people who do not go on to develop alcoholism but a pattern of more severe difficulties for people with alcoholism begins to emerge in the middle 20s to the middle 30s; these difficulties can be the alcohol-related break-up of a significant relationship, an arrest for being drunk and disorderly or drink-driving, evidence of alcohol withdrawal, early alcohol-related health problems or significant interference with functioning at work or school. During this time, the person may experience his or her first blackout,

an episode during which the person continues to function but has no conscious awareness of his or her behaviour at the time, or indeed any later memory of the behaviour.

As the person continues to drink, he or she often develops a **tolerance** for alcohol; that is, he or she needs more alcohol to produce the same effect. After continued heavy drinking, the person experiences a **tolerance break**, which means that very small amounts of alcohol can intoxicate them.

The later course of alcoholism, when the person's functioning is definitely affected, is often characterized by periods of abstinence or temporarily controlled drinking. Abstinence may occur after some legal, social or interpersonal crisis, and the person may then set up rules about drinking, such as drinking only at certain times or drinking only beer. This period of temporarily controlled drinking soon leads to an escalation of alcohol intake, more problems and a subsequent crisis. Without intervention the cycle can repeat continuously (Schuckit, 2005).

The highest rates for successful recovery seem to be for people who abstain from substances, are highly motivated to give up, and have a past history of life success (i.e. satisfactory experiences in coping, work, relationships and so forth).

Evidence shows that some people with alcohol-related problems can modify or give up drinking on their own without a treatment programme; this is sometimes called **spontaneous remission** or natural recovery (Bischof *et al.*, 2005). The abstinence is often in response to a crisis or a promise to a loved one, and is accomplished by engaging

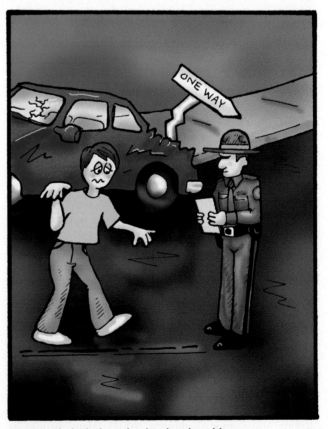

Drugs and alcohol can lead to legal problems

in alternative activities, relying on relationships with family and friends and avoiding alcohol, alcohol users and social cues associated with drinking. Spontaneous remission can occur in as many as 20% of alcoholics, although it is highly unlikely that people in the late stage of alcoholism can recover without treatment (Schuckit, 2005).

RELATED DISORDERS

Substance-induced disorders, such as psychoses, anxiety, mood disorders and dementia, are discussed in other chapters. For instance, Chapter 21 discusses delirium, which may be seen in severe alcohol withdrawal.

AETIOLOGY

The exact causes of drug use, dependence and addiction are not known, but various factors are thought to contribute to the development of substance-related disorders for individuals (Jaffe & Anthony, 2005). Much of the research on biological and genetic factors has been done on alcohol abuse, but psychological, social and environmental studies have examined other drugs as well.

Biological Factors

Children of alcoholic parents seem to be at higher risk of developing alcoholism and drug dependence than are children of non-alcoholic parents. This increased risk is partly the result of environmental factors, but evidence points to the importance of genetic factors as well. Several studies of twins have shown a higher rate of concordance (when one twin misuses alcohol, the other twin does too) among identical than among fraternal twins. Adoption studies have shown higher rates of alcoholism in sons of biological fathers with alcoholism than in those of non-alcoholic biological fathers. These studies led theorists to describe the genetic component of alcoholism as a genetic vulnerability that is then influenced by various social and environmental factors (Jaffe & Anthony, 2005). Dick and Beirut (2006) suggested that 50% to 60% of the variation in causes of alcoholism was the result of genetics, with the remainder caused by environmental influences.

Neurochemical influences on substance use patterns have been studied primarily in animal research (Jaffe & Anthony, 2005). The ingestion of mood-altering substances stimulates dopamine pathways in the limbic system, which produces pleasant feelings or a 'high' that is a reinforcing, or positive, experience. Distribution of the substance throughout the brain alters the balance of neurotransmitters that modulate pleasure, pain and reward responses. Researchers have proposed that some people have an internal alarm that limits the amount of alcohol consumed to one or two drinks, so that they feel a pleasant sensation but go no further. People without this internal signalling mechanism experience the

high initially but continue to drink until central nervous system depression is marked and they become intoxicated.

Psychological Factors

In addition to the genetic links to alcoholism, family dynamics are thought to play a part. Children of alcoholics are four times as likely to develop alcoholism (Schuckit, 2005) compared with the general population. Some theorists believe that inconsistency in the parent's behaviour, poor role modelling and lack of nurturing pave the way for the child to adopt a similar style of maladaptive coping, stormy relationships and substance abuse. Others hypothesize that even children who abhorred the behaviour of the family are likely to abuse substances as adults because they lack adaptive coping skills and cannot form successful relationships (Brown University Digest, 2001).

Some people use alcohol as a coping mechanism or to relieve stress and tension, increase feelings of power, and decrease psychological pain. High doses of alcohol, however, actually increase muscle tension and nervousness (Schuckit, 2005).

Social and Environmental Factors

Cultural factors, social attitudes, peer behaviours, the law, cost and availability all influence initial and continued use of substances (Jaffe & Anthony, 2005). In general, younger experimenters have traditionally used substances that carry less social disapproval, such as alcohol and cannabis, whereas older people have used drugs such as cocaine and opioids that are more costly and rate higher disapproval. Alcohol consumption increases in areas where availability increases, and decreases in areas where costs of alcohol are higher because of increased taxation. Many people view the social use of cannabis, although illegal, as not very harmful; some even advocate legalizing the use of marijuana for social purposes. Urban areas where cocaine and opioids are readily available also tend to have high crime rates, high unemployment and substandard school systems, which contribute to high rates of cocaine and opioid use and low rates of recovery. Thus, environment and social customs can influence a person's use of substances.

CULTURAL CONSIDERATIONS

Attitudes toward substance use, patterns of use and physiological differences to substances vary in different cultural and ethnic groups. Most Muslims do not drink alcohol; wine is an integral part of Jewish religious rites. It is important to be aware of such beliefs when assessing for a substance abuse problem.

Certain ethnic groups have genetic traits that either predispose them to, or protect them from, developing alcoholism. For instance, **flushing**, a reddening of the face and neck as a result of increased blood flow, has been linked to variants of genes for enzymes involved in alcohol metabolism. Even small amounts of alcohol can produce flushing, which may be accompanied by headaches and nausea. The flushing reaction seems to be highest among people of Asian ancestry (Wakabayashi & Masuda, 2006).

Another genetic difference between ethnic groups is found in other enzymes involved in metabolizing alcohol in the liver. In the US, variations have been found in the structure and activity levels of these enzymes among Asian people, African–American people and white people. One enzyme found in people of Japanese descent has been associated with faster elimination of alcohol from the body. Other enzyme variations are being studied to determine their effects on the metabolism of alcohol among various ethnic groups (National Institute on Alcohol Abuse and Alcoholism, 2007).

In Japan, alcohol consumption has quadrupled since 1960. The Japanese traditionally do not regard alcohol as a drug, and there are no religious prohibitions against drinking. Milne (2002) described a traditionally indulgent attitude toward those who drink too much, stating 'In a tightly knit society where concealing emotions and frustrations is a highly developed and necessary part of maintaining consensus, getting drunk is a socially sanctioned safety valve' (Milne, 2002, p. 388).

In Russia, high rates of alcohol abuse, suicide, cigarette smoking, accidents, violence and cardiovascular disease are found in the male population. Life expectancy for Russian males is 60.5 years, whereas it is 74 years for females. This is a trend mirrored across the entire former Soviet Union (Grogan, 2006).

SPECIFIC SUBSTANCES: CARE AND TREATMENT

The classes of mood-altering substances have some similarities and differences in terms of intended effect, intoxication effects and withdrawal symptoms. Treatment approaches after detoxification, however, have more similarities. This section presents a brief overview of seven classes of substances and the effects of intoxication, overdose, withdrawal and detoxification and it highlights important elements of which the nurse should be aware.

It is important that professionals attempt to keep up-to-date with street terms for drugs, as these are used far more frequently than 'official' chemical names. The website FRANK (among others) offers a useful, updated, glossary (see Internet Resources).

Alcohol

INTOXICATION AND OVERDOSE

Alcohol is a central nervous system depressant that is absorbed rapidly into the bloodstream. Initially, the effects are relaxation and loss of inhibitions. With intoxication,

Box 17.1	**PHYSIOLOGICAL EFFECTS OF LONG-TERM ALCOHOL USE**

- Cardiac myopathy
- Wernicke's encephalopathy
- Korsakoff's psychosis
- Pancreatitis
- Oesophagitis
- Hepatitis
- Cirrhosis
- Leucopenia
- Thrombocytopenia
- Ascites

there is slurred speech, unsteady gait, lack of co-ordination and impaired attention, concentration, memory and judgement. Some people become aggressive or display inappropriate sexual behaviour when intoxicated. The person who is intoxicated may experience a **blackout**.

An overdose, or excessive alcohol intake in a short period, can result in vomiting, unconsciousness and respiratory depression. This combination can cause aspiration pneumonia or pulmonary obstruction. Alcohol-induced hypotension can lead to cardiovascular shock and death. Treatment of an alcohol overdose is similar to that for any central nervous system depressant: gastric lavage or dialysis to remove the drug and support of respiratory and cardiovascular functioning in an intensive care unit. The administration of central nervous system stimulants is contraindicated (Lehne, 2006). The physiological effects of repeated intoxication and long-term use are listed in Box 17.1.

WITHDRAWAL AND DETOXIFICATION

Symptoms of withdrawal usually begin 4 to 12 hours after cessation or marked reduction of alcohol intake. Symptoms include coarse hand tremors, sweating, elevated pulse and blood pressure, insomnia, anxiety and nausea or vomiting. Severe or untreated withdrawal may progress to transient hallucinations, seizures or delirium – called delirium tremens, or DTs. Alcohol withdrawal usually peaks on the second day and is over in about 5 days (American Psychiatric Association, 2000). This can vary, however, and withdrawal may take 1 to 2 weeks. Because alcohol withdrawal can be life-threatening, detoxification needs to be accomplished under medical and nursing supervision. If the client's withdrawal symptoms are mild, and he or she can abstain from alcohol, he or she can be treated safely at home. There may, however, be circumstances where inpatient detoxification is necessary (Box 17.2).

Box 17.2 CRITERIA FOR INPATIENT DETOXIFICATION: ALCOHOL

1. History of epileptiform seizures, which are unlikely to be managed safely during community detoxification
2. Severe liver damage with clinical symptoms, e.g. jaundice, ascites, etc.
3. Cardiovascular complications
4. Recent history of mental health symptoms that become unstable during detoxification, e.g. psychotic symptoms
5. Recent history of significant self-harm attempts, either when detoxifying or when alcohol free
6. Unsuitable community environment – absence of a full-time carer does not necessarily indicate a need for admission
7. History of delirium tremens
8. Severe cognitive deficits
9. Multiple failure of community detoxification programmes

From Northampton Drugs and Alcohol Service. (2007). *Inpatient Admission Guidelines*. Available: http://www.northamptonshire.nhs.uk/nht/related/Policies/Medicines_Management_Committee_Guideline_(MMC-G)/MMG022.pdf

Safe withdrawal is usually accomplished with focused, risk-aware nursing care, including the administration of benzodiazepines such as lorazepam (Ativan), chlordiazepoxide (Librium) or diazepam (Valium) to suppress the withdrawal symptoms. Withdrawal can be accomplished by fixed-schedule dosing, known as **tapering** or symptom-triggered dosing, in which the presence and severity of withdrawal symptoms determine the amount of medication needed and the frequency of administration. Often, the protocol used is based on an assessment tool such as the Clinical Institute Withdrawal Assessment of Alcohol Scale, Revised (Box 17.3). Total scores less than 8 indicate mild withdrawal; scores from 8 to 15 indicate moderate withdrawal (marked arousal); and scores greater than 15 indicate severe withdrawal. Clients on symptom-triggered dosing receive medication based on scores of this scale alone, whereas clients on fixed-dose tapers can also receive additional doses depending on the level of scores from this scale. Both methods of medicating clients appear to be safe and effective (Bayard *et al.*, 2004).

'Minor' Tranquillizers: Sedatives, Hypnotics and Anxiolytics

INTOXICATION AND OVERDOSE

This class of drugs includes all central nervous system depressants: barbiturates, non-barbiturate hypnotics and anxiolytics, particularly benzodiazepines. Benzodiazepines and barbiturates are the most frequently abused drugs in this category (Ciraulo & Sarid-Segal, 2005). The intensity of the effect depends on the particular drug. The effects of the drugs, symptoms of intoxication and withdrawal symptoms are similar to those of alcohol. In the usual prescribed doses, these drugs cause drowsiness and reduce anxiety, which is the intended purpose. Intoxication symptoms include slurred speech, lack of co-ordination, unsteady gait, labile mood, impaired attention or memory and even stupor and coma.

Benzodiazepines alone, when taken orally in overdose, are rarely fatal, but the person is usually lethargic and confused. Treatment includes gastric lavage followed by ingestion of activated charcoal and a saline cathartic; dialysis can be used if symptoms are severe (Lehne, 2006). The client's confusion and lethargy normally improve as the drug is excreted.

Barbiturates, in contrast, can be lethal when taken in overdose. They can cause coma, respiratory arrest, cardiac failure and death. Treatment in an intensive care unit is required using lavage or dialysis to remove the drug from the system and to support respiratory and cardiovascular function.

WITHDRAWAL AND DETOXIFICATION

The onset of withdrawal symptoms depends on the half-life of the drug (see Chapter 3). Medications such as lorazepam, the actions of which typically last about 10 hours, produce withdrawal symptoms in 6 to 8 hours; longer-acting medications such as diazepam may not produce withdrawal symptoms for 1 week (American Psychiatric Association, 2000). The withdrawal syndrome is characterized by symptoms that are the opposite of the acute effects of the drug: that is, autonomic hyperactivity (increased pulse, blood pressure, respirations and temperature), hand tremor, insomnia, anxiety, nausea and psychomotor agitation. Seizures and hallucinations occur only rarely in severe benzodiazepine withdrawal (Ciraulo & Sarid-Segal, 2005).

Detoxification from sedatives, hypnotics or anxiolytics is often managed medically by tapering the amount of the drug the client receives over a period of days or weeks, depending on the drug and the amount the client had been using. Tapering, or administering decreasing doses of a medication, is essential with barbiturates to prevent coma and death, which occur if the drug is stopped abruptly. For example, when tapering the dosage of a benzodiazepine, the client may be given Valium, 10mg four times a day; the dose is decreased every 3 days, and the number of times a day the dose is given also is decreased, until the client is safely withdrawn from the drug.

Box 17.3 ADDICTION RESEARCH FOUNDATION CLINICAL INSTITUTE WITHDRAWAL ASSESSMENT FOR ALCOHOL, REVISED (CIWA-AR)

NAUSEA AND VOMITING – Ask 'Do you feel sick to your stomach? Have you vomited?' Observation.
0 no nausea and no vomiting
1 mild nausea with no vomiting
2
3
4 intermittent nausea with dry heaves
5
6
7 constant nausea, frequent dry heaves and vomiting

TREMOR – Arms extended and fingers spread apart. Observation.
0 no tremor
1 not visible, but can be felt fingertip to fingertip
2
3
4 moderate, with patient's arms extended
5
6
7 severe, flapping tremors

PAROXYSMAL SWEATS – Observation.
0 no sweat visible
1 barely perceptible sweating, palms moist
2
3
4 beads of sweat obvious on forehead
5
6
7 drenching sweats

ANXIETY – Ask, 'Do you feel nervous?' Observation.
0 no anxiety, at ease
1 mildly anxious
2
3
4 moderately anxious, or guarded, so anxiety is inferred
5
6
7 equivalent to acute panic states as seen in severe delirium or acute psychotic reactions

AGITATION – Observation.
0 normal activity
1 somewhat more than normal activity
2
3
4 moderately fidgety and restless
5

6
7 paces back and forth during most of the interview, or constantly thrashes about

TACTILE DISTURBANCES – Ask, 'Have you any itching, pins and needles sensations, any burning, any numbness or do you feel bugs crawling on or under your skin?' Observation.
0 none
1 very mild itching, pins and needles, burning or numbness
2 mild itching, pins and needles, burning or numbness
3 moderate itching, pins and needles, burning or numbness
4 moderately severe hallucinations
5 severe hallucinations
6 extremely severe hallucinations
7 continuous hallucinations

AUDITORY DISTURBANCES – Ask, 'Are you more aware of sounds around you? Are they harsh? Do they frighten you? Are you hearing anything that is disturbing to you? Are you hearing things you know are not there?' Observation.
0 not present
1 very mild harshness or ability to frighten
2 mild harshness or ability to frighten
3 moderate harshness or ability to frighten
4 moderately severe hallucinations
5 severe hallucinations
6 extremely severe hallucinations
7 continuous hallucinations

VISUAL DISTURBANCES – Ask, 'Does the light appear too bright? Is its colour different? Does it hurt your eyes? Are you seeing anything that is disturbing to you? Are you seeing things you know are not there?' Observation.
0 not present
1 very mild sensitivity
2 mild sensitivity
3 moderate sensitivity
4 moderately severe hallucinations
5 severe hallucinations
6 extremely severe hallucinations
7 continuous hallucinations

HEADACHE, FULLNESS IN HEAD – Ask, 'Does your head feel different? Does it feel like there is a band around your head?' Do not rate for dizziness or lightheadedness. Otherwise, rate severity. Observation.
0 not present
1 very mild
2 mild

continued ⋯➔

Box 17.3: Addiction Research Foundation Clinical Institute Withdrawal Assessment for Alcohol, Revised (CIWA-AR), cont.

3 moderate
4 moderately severe
5 severe
6 very severe
7 extremely severe

ORIENTATION AND CLOUDING OF SENSORY – Ask, 'What day is this? Where are you? Who am I?' Observation.
0 oriented and can do serial additions

1 cannot do serial additions or is uncertain about date
2 disoriented for date by no more than 2 calendar days
3 disoriented for date by more than 2 calendar days
4 disoriented for place and/or person

Maximum Possible Score 67

> A score of less than 10 usually indicates no need for additional withdrawal medication.

Stimulants (Amphetamines, Cocaine)

Stimulants are drugs that stimulate or excite the central nervous system. Although the *DSM-IV-TR* categorizes amphetamines, cocaine and central nervous system stimulants separately, the effects, intoxication and withdrawal symptoms of these drugs are virtually identical. They are grouped together here for this reason.

Stimulants have limited clinical use (with the exception of stimulants used to treat ADHD; see Chapter 20) and a high potential for abuse. Amphetamines ('uppers') were popular in the past; they were used by people who wanted to lose weight or to stay awake. Cocaine, an illegal drug with virtually no clinical use in medicine, is highly addictive and a popular recreational drug because of the intense and immediate feeling of euphoria it produces.

Methamphetamine is particularly dangerous. It is highly addictive and causes psychotic behaviour. Brain damage related to its use is frequent, primarily as a result of the substances used to make it – that is, liquid agricultural fertilizer.

INTOXICATION AND OVERDOSE

Intoxication from stimulants develops rapidly; effects include the 'high' or euphoric feeling, hyperactivity, hypervigilance, talkativeness, anxiety, grandiosity, hallucinations, stereotypic or repetitive behaviour, anger, fighting and impaired judgement. Physiological effects include tachycardia, elevated blood pressure, dilated pupils, perspiration or chills, nausea, chest pain, confusion and cardiac dysrhythmias. Overdoses of stimulants can result in seizures and coma; deaths are rare (Jaffe *et al.*, 2005). Treatment with chlorpromazine, an antipsychotic, controls hallucinations, lowers blood pressure and relieves nausea (Lehne, 2006).

WITHDRAWAL AND DETOXIFICATION

Withdrawal from stimulants occurs within a few hours to several days after cessation of the drug and is not life-threatening. Marked dysphoria is the primary symptom and is accompanied by fatigue, vivid and unpleasant dreams, insomnia or hypersomnia, increased appetite and psychomotor retardation or agitation. Marked withdrawal symptoms are referred to as 'crashing'; the person may experience depressive symptoms, including suicidal ideation, for several days. Stimulant withdrawal is not treated pharmacologically.

CLINICAL VIGNETTE: DETOXIFICATION

John, 62 years old, was admitted at 5 AM this morning for elective knee replacement surgery. The surgical procedure, including the anaesthetic, went smoothly. John was stabilized in the recovery room in about 3 hours. His blood pressure was 124/82, temperature 98.8°F, pulse 76, respirations 16. John was alert, oriented and verbally responsive, so he was transferred to a room on the orthopaedic unit.

By 10 PM, John is agitated, sweating and saying, 'I have to get out of here!' His blood pressure is 164/98, pulse 98 and respirations 28. His surgical dressing is dry and intact, and he has no complaints of pain. The nurse talks with John's wife and asks about his usual habits of alcohol consumption. John's wife says he consumes three or four drinks each evening after work and has beer or wine with dinner. John did not report his alcohol consumption to his doctor before surgery. John's wife says, 'No one ever asked me about how much he drank, so I didn't think it was important.'

Cannabis (Marijuana)

Cannabis is the most widely used illicit substance in the UK. As well as being a mild sedative, it also has mild hallucinogenic properties, distorting perception and very occasionally causing hallucinations. About 10% of users become psychologically addicted (possibly more with those who take stronger forms). The past few years has seen a rise in the UK in the use of stronger, more powerful forms of cannabis – 'skunk', 'sensimila', 'homegrown' or 'netherweed' – which may make both dependence and any mental health problems worse.

Cannabis sativa is the hemp plant that is widely cultivated for its fibre used to make rope and cloth and for oil from its seeds. It has become widely known for its psychoactive resin (Hall & Degenhardt, 2005). This resin contains more than 60 substances, called cannabinoids, of which delta-9-tetrahydrocannabinol (usually referred to as THC) is thought to be responsible for most of the psychoactive effects. Marijuana refers to the upper leaves, flowering tops and stems of the plant; hashish is the dried resinous exudate from the leaves of the female plant. Cannabis is most often smoked in cigarettes ('joints') and sometimes in pipes but it can also be eaten or taken in tea.

INTOXICATION AND OVERDOSE

Cannabis begins to act less than 1 minute after inhalation. Peak effects usually occur in 20 to 30 minutes and last at least 2 to 3 hours. Users report a high feeling similar to that with alcohol, lowered inhibitions, relaxation, euphoria and increased appetite. Symptoms of intoxication include impaired motor co-ordination, inappropriate laughter, impaired judgement and short-term memory and distortions of time and perception. Anxiety, dysphoria and social withdrawal may occur in some users. Physiological effects, in addition to increased appetite, include conjunctival injection (bloodshot eyes), dry mouth, hypotension and tachycardia. Excessive use of cannabis may produce delirium or, rarely, cannabis-induced psychotic disorder, both of which are treated symptomatically. Overdoses of cannabis do not occur (Hall & Degenhardt, 2005).

WITHDRAWAL AND DETOXIFICATION

Although some people have reported withdrawal symptoms of muscle aches, sweating, anxiety and tremors, no clinically significant withdrawal syndrome has been identified (Lehne, 2006).

Cannabis can produce anxiety, agitation and suspiciousness, lethargy and fatigue, make asthma worse, raise blood pressure (and thus put those with heart conditions at risk), lower men's sperm count, suppress ovulation and harm the unborn child. It is far from the harmless recreational drug it is often portrayed as.

Research has shown that cannabis has short-term effects of lowering intraocular pressure and thus helping people with glaucoma. It has also been studied for its effectiveness in reducing muscle spasms and tremor in people with multiple sclerosis, relieving the nausea and vomiting associated with cancer chemotherapy and in the anorexia and weight loss related to AIDS.

Opioids: Heroin

Opioids are popular drugs of abuse because they desensitize the user to both physiological and psychological pain and induce a sense of euphoria and well-being. Opioid compounds include potent prescription analgesics such as morphine, codeine, oxycodone or methadone, as well as substances such as street heroin and methadone (often used as a heroin substitute). People who abuse opioids spend a great deal of their time obtaining the drugs; they often engage in illegal activity to get them. Health-care professionals who abuse opioids often write prescriptions for themselves or divert prescribed pain medication for clients to themselves (American Psychiatric Association, 2000).

INTOXICATION AND OVERDOSE

Opioid intoxication develops soon after the initial euphoric feeling; symptoms include apathy, lethargy, listlessness, impaired judgement, psychomotor retardation or agitation, constricted pupils, drowsiness, slurred speech and impaired attention and memory. Severe intoxication or opioid overdose can lead to coma, respiratory depression, pupillary constriction, unconsciousness and death. Administration of naloxone – an opioid antagonist – is the treatment of choice because it reverses all signs of opioid toxicity. Naloxone is given every few hours until the opioid level drops to nontoxic; this process may take days (Lehne, 2006).

WITHDRAWAL AND DETOXIFICATION

Opioid withdrawal develops when drug intake ceases or decreases markedly, or it can be precipitated by the administration of an opioid antagonist. Initial symptoms are anxiety, restlessness, aching back and legs and cravings for more opioids (Jaffe & Strain, 2005). Symptoms that develop as withdrawal progresses include nausea, vomiting, dysphoria, lacrimation, rhinorrhoea, sweating, diarrhoea, yawning, fever and insomnia. Symptoms of opioid withdrawal cause significant distress but do not require pharmacological intervention to support life or bodily functions. Short-acting drugs such as heroin produce withdrawal symptoms in 6 to 24 hours; the symptoms peak in 2 to 3 days and gradually subside in 5 to 7 days. Longer-acting substances such as methadone may not produce significant withdrawal symptoms for 2 to 4 days, and the symptoms may take 2 weeks to subside. Methadone can be used as a replacement for the opioid, and the dosage is then decreased over 2 weeks. Substitution of methadone during detoxification may reduce symptoms to no worse than a mild case of

Box 17.4 OPIOID DEPENDENCE

The management of opioid dependence requires medical, social and psychological treatment; access to a multidisciplinary team is valuable. Treatment with opioid substitutes or with naltrexone is best initiated under the supervision of an appropriately qualified physician.

Methadone, an opioid *agonist*, can be substituted for opioids such as diamorphine, preventing the onset of withdrawal symptoms; it is itself addictive and should only be prescribed for those who are physically dependent on opioids. It is administered in a single daily dose, usually as methadone oral solution 1 mg/ml. The dose is adjusted according to the degree of dependence.

Buprenorphine is an opioid partial agonist. Because of its abuse and dependence potential it should be prescribed only for those who are already physically dependent on opioids. It can be used as substitution therapy for patients with moderate opioid dependence. In patients dependent on high doses of opioids, buprenorphine may precipitate withdrawal due to its partial antagonist properties; in these patients, the daily opioid dose should be reduced gradually before initiating therapy with buprenorphine.

Naltrexone, an opioid *antagonist*, blocks the action of opioids and precipitates withdrawal symptoms in opioid-dependent subjects. Because the euphoric action of opioid agonists is blocked by naltrexone, it is given to former addicts as an aid to prevent relapse.

Lofexidine is used for the alleviation of symptoms in individuals whose opioid use is well controlled and who are undergoing opioid withdrawal. It is an alpha-adrenergic agonist and appears to act centrally to produce a reduction in sympathetic tone.

From British National Formulary Online. (2008). http://www.bnf.org/bnf/bnf/56/3698.htm

flu (Lehne, 2006). Withdrawal symptoms such as anxiety, insomnia, dysphoria, anhedonia and drug craving may persist for weeks or months.

Methadone itself (the prescribed version being Subutex (buprenorphine)) can cause amenorrhoea, short-term nausea and constipation, sedation and sleepiness in higher doses and increase the risk of miscarriage and stillbirths. Tolerance and dependence can occur (Box 17.4).

Hallucinogens: LSD, Magic Mushrooms, Ecstasy

Hallucinogens are substances that distort the user's perception of reality and produce symptoms similar to psychosis, including hallucinations (usually visual) and depersonalization. Hallucinogens also cause increased pulse, blood pressure and temperature; dilated pupils; and hyperreflexia. Examples of hallucinogens are ketamine, mescaline, psilocybin, LSD (lysergic acid diethylamide) and 'designer drugs' such as Ecstasy. Phencyclidine (PCP), developed as an anaesthetic, is included in this section because it acts similarly to hallucinogens.

INTOXICATION AND OVERDOSE

Hallucinogen intoxication can be marked by several behavioural or psychological changes: positive effects can be a 'high' (euphoria), a 'buzz' (increased energy, enhanced intensity of perception); negative effects can be anxiety, depression, paranoid ideation, ideas of reference, fear of losing one's mind and potentially dangerous behaviour, such as jumping out of a window in the belief that one can fly (Jones, 2005). Physiological symptoms can include sweating, tachycardia, dehydration, palpitations, blurred vision, tremors and lack of co-ordination. PCP intoxication often involves belligerence, aggression, impulsivity and unpredictable behaviour.

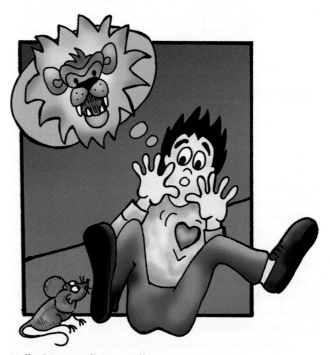

Hallucinogens distort reality

Toxic reactions to hallucinogens (except PCP) are primarily psychological; overdoses as such do not occur. These drugs are not a direct cause of death, although fatalities have occurred from related accidents, aggression and suicide and from the exacerbation of pre-existing physical conditions such as cardiac problems, asthma or epilepsy. Treatment of toxic reactions is supportive. Psychotic reactions are managed best by isolation from external stimuli; restraint may be necessary for the safety of the client and others. PCP toxicity can include seizures, hypertension, hyperthermia and respiratory depression. Medications are used to control seizures and blood pressure. Cooling devices such as hyperthermia blankets are used, and mechanical ventilation is used to support respirations (Lehne, 2006).

Ecstasy has been linked to liver, kidney and heart problems; it can cause panic attacks, confusion and paranoia, dehydration and overheating. When cut with other substances (as it often is) its negative effects are made potentially worse by those substances.

Ketamine can lead to mental health problems such as panic attacks and depression. Its anaesthetic effect can lead to someone being unaware of any injury; in high doses, especially when combined with alcohol, it can dangerously suppress breathing; mixed with ecstasy or amphetamines, it can result in fatal hypertension (Talk To Frank (2008)).

WITHDRAWAL AND DETOXIFICATION

No withdrawal syndrome has been identified for hallucinogens, although some people have reported a craving for the drug. Hallucinogens can produce flashbacks, which are transient recurrences of perceptual disturbances like those experienced with hallucinogen use. These episodes occur even after all traces of the hallucinogen are gone and may persist for a few months up to 5 years.

Solvents/Inhalants/Nitrites

Inhalants are a diverse group of drugs that includes anaesthetics, nitrites and organic solvents that are inhaled for their effects. The most common substances in this category are aliphatic and aromatic hydrocarbons found in gasoline, glue, paint thinner and spray paint. Less frequently used halogenated hydrocarbons include cleaners, correction fluid, spray-can propellants and other compounds containing esters, ketones and glycols (American Psychiatric Association, 2000). Most of the vapours are inhaled from a rag soaked with the compound, from a paper or plastic bag or directly from the container. Inhalants can cause significant brain damage, peripheral nervous system damage and liver disease. Amyl nitrite, butyl nitrite and isobutyl nitrite are all alkyl nitrites available in small bottles and known as 'poppers'; they dilate the blood vessels and are of questionable legal status in the UK – possession is still legal, though supply may not be: some are available in domestic products such as cleaners and air fresheners.

INTOXICATION AND OVERDOSE

Inhalant intoxication involves dizziness, nystagmus, lack of co-ordination, slurred speech, unsteady gait, tremor, muscle weakness and blurred vision. Stupor and coma can occur. Significant behavioural symptoms are belligerence, aggression, apathy, impaired judgement and inability to function. Acute toxicity causes anoxia, respiratory depression, vagal stimulation and dysrhythmias. Death may occur from bronchospasm, cardiac arrest, suffocation or aspiration of the compound or vomitus (Crowley & Sakai, 2005). Treatment consists of supporting respiratory and cardiac functioning until the substance is removed from the body. There are no antidotes or specific medications to treat inhalant toxicity.

WITHDRAWAL AND DETOXIFICATION

There are no withdrawal symptoms or detoxification procedures for inhalants as such, although frequent users report psychological cravings. People who abuse inhalants may suffer from persistent dementia or inhalant-induced disorders, such as psychosis, anxiety or mood disorders, even if the inhalant abuse ceases. These disorders are all treated symptomatically (Crowley & Sakai, 2005).

Tobacco

As we saw earlier, around a fifth of all deaths in the UK can be attributed to smoking tobacco. It causes heart and lung disease, a whole range of cancers and significantly impairs physical and psychological functioning.

Smokers frequently mistakenly link the relief of the cravings associated with a decrease in nicotine levels in the blood with a 'relaxation' afforded by smoking. As with other drugs, increasing levels of nicotine are needed for the addict to feel 'normal' and withdrawal symptoms occur.

There is a complex relationship between depression, anxiety, schizophrenia and smoking, but little doubt that rates are higher in those who have a diagnosed mental health problem. In part because of the association between smoking and the relief of stress, many people with mental health problems find 'kicking the habit' harder than those without. It seems likely that smoking can act as a trigger for mental health problems (Action on Smoking and Health (ASH), 2008b) and is associated with higher suicide risks than for non-smokers.

Pharmacological and cognitive-behavioural approaches used with the general population can be equally effective with those who have a mental health problem, though interactions with other drugs and the impact of the withdrawal of a perceived 'crutch' need to be acknowledged and worked with; as ever, a collaborative approach is necessary.

Box 17.5 SUBSTANCE MISUSE: TYPES OF TREATMENT

ADVICE (non-specialist: e.g. information about drugs, effects, help available)

HARM REDUCTION (specialist: e.g. needle exchange, safe injection, prevention of infection, preventing overdose)

COMMUNITY PRESCRIBING (stabilizing, prescribing by GP, psychiatrists, nurse prescribers)

COUNSELLING/PSYCHOLOGICAL SUPPORT (CBT, motivational interviewing)

STRUCTURED DAY PROGRAMMES

DETOX/ASSISTED WITHDRAWAL (in specialist units, general units, rehab units)

REHAB UNITS (crisis intervention or longer-stay units)

AFTERCARE (maintenance and moving on programmes)

Adapted from National Treatment Agency for Substance Misuse: Types of Treatment. http://www.nta.nhs.uk/about_treatment/Types_of_treatment.aspx

Box 17.6 TWELVE STEPS OF ALCOHOLICS ANONYMOUS

1. We admitted we were powerless over alcohol, that our lives had become unmanageable.
2. Came to believe that a Power greater than ourselves could restore us to sanity.
3. Made a decision to turn our wills and lives over to the care of God as we understood Him.
4. Made a searching and fearless moral inventory of ourselves.
5. Admitted to God, to ourselves and to another human being the exact nature of our wrongs.
6. Were entirely ready to have God remove all these defects of character.
7. Humbly asked Him to remove our shortcomings.
8. Made a list of all persons we had harmed, and became willing to make amends to them all.
9. Made direct amends to such people whenever possible, except when to do so would injure them or others.
10. Continued to take personal inventory and when we were wrong promptly admitted it.
11. Sought through prayer and meditation to improve our conscious contact with God as we understood Him, praying only for knowledge of His will for us and the power to carry that out.
12. Having had a spiritual awakening as a result of these steps, we tried to carry this message to alcoholics and to practise these principles in all our affairs.

TREATMENT AND PROGNOSIS

Traditionally, treatment modalities have been based on the concept of alcoholism (and other addictions) as medical illnesses that are progressive, chronic and characterized by remissions and relapses (Jaffe & Anthony, 2005). Until the 1970s, organized treatment programmes and clinics for substance abuse were scarce. Before 'addiction' and dependence were fully understood, most of society and the medical/nursing community viewed chemical dependency as a personal problem; the user was advised to 'pull yourself together' and 'get control of your problem'. Today, treatment for substance use is available in a variety of community settings (Box 17.5), not all of which involve health professionals. Many independent providers – both charitable and profit-making – provide services.

Therapeutic Approaches

There are a number of differing philosophical and practical approaches to tackling the problems of substance misuse.

TWELVE-STEP APPROACHES

Alcoholics Anonymous (AA) was founded in the 1930s by people with alcohol problems. This self-help group developed the **12-step programme** model for recovery (Box 17.6), which is based on the philosophy that total abstinence is essential and that alcoholics need the help and support of others to maintain sobriety. Key slogans reflect the ideas in the 12 steps, such as 'one day at a time' (approach sobriety one day at a time), 'easy does it' (don't get in a frenzy about

daily life and problems), and 'let go and let God' (turn your life over to a higher power). People who are early in recovery are encouraged to have a sponsor to help them progress through the 12 steps of AA. Once sober, a member can be a sponsor for another person.

Similar approaches are used by Narcotics Anonymous and other groups working with people who misuse drugs and with other 'addictive' problems such as gambling, overeating and sex.

Regular attendance at meetings is emphasized. Meetings are available daily in large cities and towns and at least weekly in smaller towns or rural areas. AA (or other 12-step-type) meetings may be 'closed' (only those who are pursuing recovery can attend) or 'open' (anyone can attend). Meetings may be educational with a featured speaker; other meetings focus on a reading, daily meditation or a theme, and then offer the opportunity for members to relate their battles with alcohol and to ask the others for help staying sober.

Many other treatment programmes – particularly in the independent sector – use the 12-step approach and emphasize participation in AA or the equivalent. They also include individual counselling and a wide variety of groups. Group experiences involve education about substances and their use, problem-solving techniques and cognitive techniques to identify and to modify faulty ways of thinking. An overall theme is coping with life, stress and other people without the use of substances.

Although traditional treatment programmes and AA have been successful for many people, they are not effective for everyone. Some object to the emphasis on God and spirituality; others do not respond well to the confrontational approach sometimes used in treatment or to identifying himself or herself as an alcoholic or an addict. Women and minorities have reported feeling overlooked or ignored by an essentially 'white, male, middle-class' organization.

Al-Anon is a support group for spouses, partners and friends of alcoholics; and AlaTeen, a group for children (aged 12 to 17 inclusive) whose parents have substance misuse problems (see Internet Resources).

MOTIVATIONAL, COGNITIVE AND OTHER THERAPEUTIC APPROACHES

Gibbins and Kipping (2006) identify three overlapping psychotherapeutic approaches to working with people with dual diagnosis problems, which can be applied equally to specific substance misuse problems. These are:

1. Prochaska and DiClemente's (1986) transtheoretical model of change, which incorporates a four-stage model in which the practitioner works alongside the client to move from '*precontemplation*' (not yet recognizing a problem and not ready to begin an active process of change), through to '*contemplation*' (an embryonic conscious awareness of the problem and first consideration of the possibilities of change), through to '*determination and action*' (preparing for and actually making changes) and, finally, through to the '*maintenance*' stage – ensuring changes are embedded and strategies are in place to prevent relapse (Table 17.1).
2. A framework that parallels Prochaska and DiClemente's is that of Osher and Kofoed (1989) whose 'staged-treatment' model moves from '*engagement*' (absolutely vital with substance-misusing and dual diagnosis clients), through to '*persuasion*' (employing a collaborative therapeutic alliance built on the trust and honesty of the engagement stage), through to '*active treatment*' (psycho-educational, pharmacological, practical and psychotherapeutic interventions) and, finally, to '**relapse prevention**' – the consolidation of skills and changes and the identification of danger signs and prophylactic measures to tackle 'risky' events.
3. Miller and Rollnick's '**motivational interviewing**' model (Miller & Rollnick, 1991) draws on CBT and other approaches to explicitly explore issues of ambivalence: people who take substances do so for a reason and get something out of it – they are, by definition, ambivalent about losing something that has, at least in the short term, sig-

nificant apparent benefits. Validation and gentle, empathic exploration of the beliefs, negative automatic thinking, affect, behaviour and environmental factors motivating and maintaining people's use of substances is undertaken in a structured, respectful, planned way. Autonomy is vital to the process, alongside genuine acceptance that change – and resistance to change – are natural and normal.

These three overlapping psychotherapeutic approaches to substance misuse and the treatment of dual diagnosis can be drawn on to offer effective individual and group help to people. CBT, DBT, psychodynamic and solution-focused approaches are used also, although the evidence base for all – particularly in dual diagnosis work – remains in a relatively early stage of development.

HARM REDUCTION/MINIMIZATION

There is an increasing emphasis in both private and NHS settings on the concept of **harm minimization** or **harm reduction**. The philosophy here is one that assumes – as Philips (2006, p. 130) points out – that 'therapeutic work with service users with substance misuse problems should initially be focused on reducing substance-related harms for their family, friends and community'. It should only then start looking at the actual reduction and elimination of the substance misuse. This approach is, as Philips remarks, contextualized, 'pragmatic, user-focused and meets users "as they are" with no hard and fast rules'.

Pharmacological Treatment

Pharmacological treatment in substance abuse has two main purposes: to permit safe withdrawal from alcohol, sedative-hypnotics and benzodiazepines, and to prevent relapse. Table 17.2 summarizes drugs used in substance misuse treatment. For clients whose primary substance is alcohol, vitamin B$_1$ (thiamine) is often prescribed to prevent or to treat Wernicke's syndrome and Korsakoff's syndrome, which are neurological conditions that can result from heavy alcohol use. Cyanocobalamin (vitamin B$_{12}$) and folic acid are often prescribed for clients with nutritional deficiencies.

Alcohol withdrawal is usually managed with a benzodiazepine, which is used to suppress the symptoms of abstinence. The most commonly used benzodiazepines are lorazepam, chlordiazepoxide and diazepam. These medications can be administered on a fixed schedule around the clock during withdrawal. Giving these medications on an as-needed basis according to symptom parameters, however, is just as effective and often results in a speedier withdrawal (Lehne, 2006).

Disulfiram (Antabuse) is occasionally prescribed to help deter clients from drinking. If a client taking disulfiram drinks alcohol, a severe adverse reaction occurs, with flushing, a throbbing headache, sweating, nausea and vomiting. In severe cases, severe hypotension, confusion, coma and even death may result (see Chapter 3). The client must also

Table 17.1   THE STAGES OF TREATMENT–INTERVENTION MATRIX

Stage of Change	Stage of Treatment	Intervention
Pre-contemplation: no recognition of problem	Engagement	Relationship building
		Information gathering
		Screening and assessment
		Eliciting change talk
		Practical assistance
		Appropriate response to resistance
		Stabilizing symptoms
		Carers' needs evaluation
Contemplation: recognition and exploration of the problem areas	Persuasion	Cost benefit analysis of change
		Specialized assessment
		Relationship building
		Information exchange
		Healthy social sampling
		Reframing events
		Negotiating appropriate goals
Action: planning, rehearsing and refining strategies for change to reduce and stabilize symptoms and substance use	Active treatment	Detoxification or reduction strategies
		Review medication
		Coping skills training
		Lifestyle modification
		Psycho-educational work
		Group work for SUD (substance use disorder) and/or SMI (serious mental illness)
		Engagement into self-help groups
		Relapse prevention, exploration and planning
Maintenance: ongoing review and practice of strategies to maintain changes in the long term	Relapse prevention	Relapse prevention planning
		Healthy social sampling
		Therapeutic occupational roles
		Lapse analysis
		Consolidation of skills learned

From Gibbins, J. & Kipping, C. (2006). Coexistent substance use and psychiatric disorders. In C. Gamble & G. Brennan (Eds.), *Working with serious mental illness* (p. 260). London: Elsevier. Copyright © Elsevier.

avoid a wide variety of products that contain alcohol, such as cough syrup, lotions, mouthwash, perfume, aftershave, vinegar and vanilla and other extracts. The client must read product labels carefully because any product containing alcohol can produce symptoms. Ingestion of alcohol may cause unpleasant symptoms for 1 to 2 weeks after the last dose of disulfiram.

Acamprosate may be prescribed for clients recovering from alcohol abuse or dependence, to help reduce cravings for alcohol and decrease the physical and emotional discomfort that occurs especially in the first few months of recovery. These include sweating, anxiety and sleep disturbances. People with renal impairment cannot take this drug.

Side-effects are reported as mild, and include diarrhoea, nausea, flatulence and pruritus.

Drugs used in opioid dependence are discussed in Boxes 17.4 and 17.7 and Table 17.2.

APPLICATION OF THE NURSING PROCESS: SUBSTANCE MISUSE

Identifying people with substance-use problems can be difficult. From a psychodynamic perspective, substance use typically includes the use of defence mechanisms, especially **denial**. Clients may deny directly having any problems or may minimize the extent of problems or actual substance use.

Table 17.2	DRUGS USED IN TREATMENT OF SUBSTANCE MISUSE		
Drug	**Use**	**Dosage**	**Indicative Nursing Considerations**
Chlordiazepoxide (Librium)	Alcohol withdrawal	10–50 mg 4 times daily, gradually reducing over 7–14 days	Monitor vital signs and global assessments for effectiveness; may cause dizziness or drowsiness. Avoid if likelihood of continued alcohol use
Disulfiram (Antabuse)	Maintain abstinence from alcohol	800 mg as a single dose on first day, reducing over 5 days to 100–200 mg daily	Focus on comprehensive education and monitoring: teach client to read labels to avoid products with alcohol
Chlomethiazole (Heminevrin)	Alcohol withdrawal	Initially 2–4 capsules, if necessary repeated after some hours; day 1 (first 24 hours), 9–12 capsules in 3–4 divided doses; day 2, 6–8 capsules in 3–4 divided doses; day 3, 4–6 capsules in 3–4 divided doses; then gradually reduced over days 4–6; total treatment for not more than 9 days	Inpatient setting only; risk of dependence
Acamprosate calcium (Campral)	Maintain abstinence from alcohol	18–65 years, body weight 60 kg and over, 666 mg 3 times daily; body weight less than 60 kg, 666 mg at breakfast, 333 mg at mid-day and 333 mg at night	Maintain even if patient relapses: 1 year treatment period
Methadone	Maintain abstinence from opiates	Single daily dose 1mg/ml	Itself addictive: only use where physical dependence on opioid exists
Buprenorphine (Subutex)	Maintenance therapy adjunct	0.8–4 mg as a single daily dose, adjusted according to response; max. 32 mg daily	Withdraw gradually
Naltrexone hydrochloride (Nalorex/ Opizone)	Prevention of relapse in opioid dependence	25 mg initially then 50 mg daily; total weekly dose (350 mg) may be divided and given on 3 days of the week for improved compliance (e.g. 100 mg on Monday and Wednesday, and 150 mg on Friday)	For prevention of relapse. Client may not respond to narcotics used to treat cough, diarrhoea or pain; take with food or milk; may cause headache, restlessness or irritability

Adapted from British National Formulary Online. (2008). http://www.bnf.org/bnf/bnf/55/

For all, pharmacological treatments should be an adjunct to full psychotherapeutic input. Social, psychological and other factors must be taken into account and appropriate care and treatment offered. Both effective educational programmes and high levels of physical health care are vital. Medical supervision is essential.

The Alcohol Use Disorders Identification Test (AUDIT) is a screening device to detect hazardous drinking patterns that may be precursors to full-blown substance use disorders (Bohn et al., 1995). This tool (Box 17.8) promotes recognition of problem drinking in the early stage, when resolution without formal treatment is more likely. Early detection and treatment are associated with more positive outcomes. According to Heather et al. (2006), 'The AUDIT (Alcohol Use Disorders Identification Test) is a screening instrument of good sensitivity and specificity for detecting hazardous and harmful drinking among people not seeking treatment for alcohol problems', and 'should be considered as the screening instrument of first choice in community settings'.

Assessment

HISTORY

People may report a chaotic family life, although this is not always the case. They generally describe some crisis

| | |

Box 17.7 — NICE GUIDANCE FOR DRUG USE IN OPIOID DEPENDENCE

METHADONE AND BUPRENORPHINE FOR THE MANAGEMENT OF OPIOID DEPENDENCE (JANUARY 2007)

Oral methadone and buprenorphine are recommended for maintenance therapy in the management of opioid dependence. Patients should be committed to a supportive care programme including a flexible dosing regimen administered under supervision for at least 3 months, until compliance is assured. Selection of methadone or buprenorphine should be made on a case-by-case basis, but methadone should be prescribed if both drugs are equally suitable.

NALTREXONE FOR THE MANAGEMENT OF OPIOID DEPENDENCE (JANUARY 2007)

Naltrexone is recommended for the prevention of relapse in detoxified, formerly opioid-dependent patients who are motivated to remain in a supportive care abstinence programme. Naltrexone should be administered under supervision and its effectiveness in preventing opioid misuse reviewed regularly.

From British National Formulary Online. (2008). http://www.bnf.org/bnf/bnf/55/

that precipitated contact with the services, such as contact with the police, physical problems or development of withdrawal symptoms while being treated for another condition. Usually, other people, such as an employer threatening loss of a job or a spouse or partner threatening loss of a relationship, are involved in a client's decision to seek treatment. It seems to be relatively rare for clients to decide to seek treatment independently with no outside influence.

GENERAL APPEARANCE AND MOTOR BEHAVIOUR

Assessment of general appearance and behaviour usually reveals appearance and speech to be normal. Clients may appear anxious, tired and dishevelled if they have just completed a difficult course of detoxification. Depending on their overall health status and any health problems resulting from substance use, clients may appear physically ill. Most clients are somewhat apprehensive about treatment, resent being in treatment or feel pressured by others to be there. This may be the first time in a long time that clients have had to deal with any difficulty without the help of a psychoactive substance.

MOOD AND AFFECT

Wide ranges of mood and affect are possible. Some clients are sad and tearful, expressing guilt and remorse for their behaviour and circumstances. Others may be angry and sarcastic, or quiet and sullen, unwilling to talk to the nurse. Irritability is common because clients are newly free of substances. Clients may be pleasant and seemingly happy, appearing unaffected by the situation, especially if they are still in denial about the substance use.

THOUGHT PROCESS AND CONTENT

During assessment of thought process and content, clients are likely to minimize their substance use, blame others for their problems and rationalize their behaviour. They may believe they cannot survive without the substance or may express no desire to do so. They may focus their attention on finances, legal issues or employment problems as the main source of difficulty, rather than their substance use. They may believe that they could quit 'on their own' if they wanted to, and they continue to deny or minimize the extent of the problem.

SENSORY AND INTELLECTUAL PROCESSES

Clients generally are orientated and alert unless they are experiencing lingering effects of withdrawal. Intellectual abilities are intact unless clients have experienced neurological deficits from long-term alcohol or inhalant use.

JUDGEMENT AND INSIGHT

Clients are likely to have exercised poor judgement, especially while under the influence of the substance. Judgement may still be affected: clients may behave impulsively, such as leaving treatment to obtain the substance of choice. Insight is usually limited regarding substance use. Clients may have difficulty acknowledging their behaviour while using, or may not see loss of jobs or relationships as connected to the substance use. They may still believe they can control the substance use.

SELF-CONCEPT

Clients generally have low self-esteem, which they may express directly or cover with grandiose behaviour. They do not feel adequate to cope with life and stress without the substance and are often uncomfortable around others when not using. They often have difficulty identifying and expressing true feelings; in the past, they have preferred to escape feelings and to avoid any personal pain or difficulty with the help of the substance.

Box 17.8 ALCOHOL USE DISORDER IDENTIFICATION TEST (AUDIT)

The following questionnaire will give you an indication of the level of risk associated with your current drinking pattern. To accurately assess your situation, you will need to be honest in your answers. This questionnaire was developed by the World Health Organization and is used in many countries to assist people to better understand their current level of risk in relation to alcohol consumption.

1. How often do you have a drink containing alcohol? (0) Never, (1) Monthly or less, (2) 2 to 4 times a month, (3) 2 to 3 times a week, (4) 4 or more times a week.
2. How many standard drinks do you have on a typical day when you are drinking? (0) 1 or 2, (1) 3 or 4, (2) 5 or 6, (3) 7 to 9, (4) 10 or more.
3. How often do you have six or more drinks on one occasion? (0) Never, (1) Less than monthly, (2) Monthly, (3) Weekly, (4) Daily or almost daily.
4. How often during the last year have you found that you were not able to stop drinking once you had started? (0) Never, (1) Less than monthly, (2) Monthly, (3) Weekly, (4) Daily or almost daily.
5. How often during the past year have you failed to do what was normally expected of you because of drinking?

(0) Never, (1) Less than monthly, (2) Monthly, (3) Weekly, (4) Daily or almost daily.
6. How often during the last year have you needed a drink in the morning to get yourself going after a heavy drinking session? (0) Never, (1) Less than monthly, (2) Monthly, (3) Weekly, (4) Daily or almost daily.
7. How often during the last year have you had a feeling of guilt or remorse after drinking? (0) Never, (1) Less than monthly, (2) Monthly, (3) Weekly, (4) Daily or almost daily.
8. How often during the last year have you been unable to remember what happened the night before because you had been drinking? (0) Never, (1) Less than monthly, (2) Monthly, (3) Weekly, (4) Daily or almost daily.
9. Have you or someone else been injured as a result of your drinking? (0) Never, (1) Less than monthly, (2) Monthly, (3) Weekly, (4) Daily or almost daily.
10. Has a relative, a doctor or other health worker been concerned about your drinking or suggested that you cut down? (0) No, (2) Yes, but not in the last year, (4) Yes, during the last year.

Adapted from Babor, T., de la Fuente, J. R., Saunders, J., *et al*. (1992). Alcohol Use Disorders Identification Test (AUDIT): Guidelines for use in primary health care. World Health Organization, Geneva. Used with permission. Bohn, Babor, & Kranzler (1995).

ROLES AND RELATIONSHIPS

Clients usually have experienced many difficulties with social, family and occupational roles. Absenteeism and poor work performance are common. Often, family members have told these clients that the substance use was a concern, and it may have been the subject of family arguments. Relationships in the family are often strained. Clients may be angry with family members who were instrumental in bringing them to treatment or who threatened loss of a significant relationship.

PHYSIOLOGICAL CONSIDERATIONS

Many clients have a history of poor nutrition – often using rather than eating – and sleep disturbances that persist beyond detoxification. They may have liver damage from drinking alcohol, hepatitis or HIV infection from intravenous drug use or lung or neurological damage from using inhalants.

Data Analysis

Each client has nursing diagnoses specific to his or her physical health status. These may include the following:

- Imbalanced nutrition: less than body requirements
- Risk of infection
- Risk of injury
- Diarrhoea
- Excess fluid volume
- Activity intolerance
- Self-care deficits.

Nursing formulations commonly used when working with clients with substance use include the following:

- Ineffective denial of impact of substance use
- Ineffective role performance
- Dysfunctional family processes: alcoholism
- Ineffective coping.

Outcome Identification

Treatment outcomes for clients with substance use may include the following:

- The client will abstain from (or reduce the harm from) alcohol and drug use.
- The client will express feelings openly and directly.

CLINICAL VIGNETTE: ALCOHOLISM

Sam, age 38, is married with two children. Sam's father was an alcoholic, and his childhood was chaotic. His father was seldom around for Sam's school activities or family events, and when he was there, his drunken behaviour often spoiled the occasion. Sam both hated and loved his father and felt he had to protect his mother as he was growing up; when he left school, he vowed he would never be like his father. He had had many hopes and dreams: he wanted to become an architect and bring up a family with love and affection.

But he'd had some bad luck. He got into trouble after drinking too much one night at college, and his grades slipped because he missed classes after celebrating with his friends. He dropped out of college after that and found himself moving from one job to another, rarely really happy but always seen as sociable and outgoing. He married when he was 19; they'd had a few problems (they had a 'fiery marriage' and

he'd been attacked a couple of times on a Friday night in town after he'd had a few: the police had blamed him for starting it), but he pictured himself still as a devoted and loving spouse.

Sam believes life has treated him unfairly – after all, he only has a few beers with friends to relax. Sometimes he overdoes it and he drinks a bit more than he intended – but doesn't everybody? He knows all those big plans for the future are on hold – but it's just temporary.

This morning, Sam's boss told him he'd be fired if he was late or absent from work even once in the next month. Sam tells himself that the boss is being unreasonable; after all, Sam is an excellent worker, when he's there. The last straw is when Sam's wife tells him she's tired of his drinking and irresponsible behaviour. She threatens to leave if Sam doesn't stop drinking. Her parting words are, 'You're just like your father!'

- The client will verbalize acceptance of responsibility for his or her own behaviour.
- The client will practise non-chemical alternatives to deal with stress or difficult situations.
- The client will establish an effective long-term plan.

DSM-IV-TR DIAGNOSTIC CRITERIA: SYMPTOMS OF SUBSTANCE ABUSE

- Low self-esteem
- Denial of problems
- Minimizes use of substance
- Rationalization
- Blaming others for problems
- Anxiety
- Irritability
- Impulsivity
- Feelings of guilt and sadness, or anger and resentment
- Poor judgement
- Limited insight
- Ineffective coping strategies
- Difficulty expressing genuine feelings
- Impaired role performance
- Strained interpersonal relationships
- Physical problems such as sleep disturbances and inadequate nutrition

Adapted from American Psychiatric Association. (2000). Diagnostic and Statistical Manual of Mental Disorders (4th edn, text revision). Washington, DC: American Psychiatric Association.

Intervention

PROVIDING HEALTH TEACHING FOR CLIENT AND FAMILY

Clients and family members need facts about the substance, its effects, and recovery. The nurse must dispel the following myths and misconceptions:

- 'It's a matter of will power.'
- 'I can't be an alcoholic if I only drink beer or if I only drink on weekends.'
- 'I can learn to use drugs socially.'
- 'I'm okay now; I could handle using once in a while.'

Education about relapse is important. Family members and friends should be aware that clients who begin to revert to old behaviours, return to substance-using acquaintances, or believe they can 'handle myself now' are at high risk for relapse, and loved ones need to take action. Whether a client plans to attend a self-help group or has other resources, a specific plan for continued support and involvement after treatment increases the client's chances of recovery.

ADDRESSING FAMILY ISSUES

Alcoholism (and other substance abuse) has been called 'a family illness'. All those who have a close relationship with a person who abuses substances suffer emotional, social and sometimes physical anguish.

Co-dependence is a concept meaning a maladaptive coping pattern on the part of family members or others that results from a prolonged relationship with the person who uses substances. Characteristics of co-dependence are poor relationship skills, excessive anxiety and worry, compulsive behaviours and resistance to change. Family members learn these dysfunctional behaviour patterns as they try to adjust to the behaviour of the substance user. One type of co-dependent behaviour is called enabling, which is a behaviour that seems helpful on the surface but actually perpetuates the substance use. For example, a wife who continually calls in to report that her husband is sick when he is really drunk or hung-over prevents the husband from having to face the true implications and repercussions of his behaviour. What appears to be a helpful action really just assists the husband to avoid the consequences of his behaviour and to continue abusing the substance.

Roles may shift dramatically, such as when a child actually looks out for or takes care of a parent. Co-dependent behaviours have also been identified in health-care professionals when they make excuses for a client's behaviour or do things for clients that clients can do for themselves.

An adult child of an alcoholic is someone who was raised in a family in which one or both parents were addicted to alcohol and who has been subjected to the many dysfunctional aspects associated with parental alcoholism. In addition to being at high risk of alcoholism and eating disorders, children of alcoholics often develop an inability to trust, an extreme need to control, an excessive sense of responsibility and denial of feelings; these characteristics persist into adulthood. Many people growing up in homes with parental alcoholism believe their problems will be solved when they are old enough to leave and escape the situation. They may begin to have problems in relationships, low self-esteem, and excessive fears of abandonment or insecurity as adults (Kelley et al., 2005). Never having experienced a healthy family life, they may find that they do not know what might make them healthy and happy.

Without support and help to understand and cope, many family members may develop substance abuse problems of their own, thus perpetuating the dysfunctional cycle. Treatment and support groups are available to address the issues of family members. Clients and family also need information about support groups, their purpose and their locations in the community.

PROMOTING COPING SKILLS

Nurses can encourage clients to identify problem areas in their lives and to explore the ways that substance use may have intensified those problems. Clients should not believe that all life's problems will disappear with sobriety; rather, sobriety will assist them to think about the problems clearly. The nurse may need to redirect a client's attention to his or her behaviour and how it influenced his or her problems. The nurse should not allow clients to focus exclusively on external events or other people without discussing their role in the problem.

It may be helpful to role-play situations that clients have found difficult. This is also an opportunity to help clients learn to solve problems or to discuss situations with others calmly and more effectively. In the group setting in treatment, it is helpful to encourage clients to give and to receive feedback about how others perceive their interaction or ability to listen.

The nurse can also help clients to find ways to relieve stress or anxiety that do not involve substance use. Relaxing, exercising, listening to music or engaging in activities may be effective. Clients may also need to develop new social activities or leisure pursuits if most of their friends or habits of socializing involved the use of substances.

The nurse can help clients to focus on the present, not the past. It is not necessarily helpful for clients to dwell on past problems and regrets: while validating past distress, the nurse needs to be exploring with the client strengths, competencies and exceptions to the problem. There will need to be a focus on what can now be done in terms of changing behaviour and improving relationships. Clients may need support from the nurse to view life and sobriety in feasible terms – 'taking it one day at a time'. The nurse can encourage clients to set attainable goals such as, 'What can I do today to stay sober?' instead of feeling overwhelmed by thinking 'How can I avoid substances for the rest of my life?' Clients need to believe that they can succeed – so do the people caring for them.

Evaluation

The effectiveness of substance abuse treatment is based heavily on the client's abstinence or ability to minimize the harm from substances. In addition, successful treatment should result in more stable role performance, improved interpersonal relationships and increased satisfaction with quality of life.

CONSIDERATIONS WHEN NURSING OLDER PEOPLE

According to Mehta et al. (2006), and many others, 'alcohol misuse in older people is underestimated and often goes undetected'. The problem seems to be increasing. Some older people with alcohol use problems are those who had a drinking problem early in life, had a significant period of abstinence and then resumed drinking again in later life. Others may have been heavy or reactive consumers of alcohol early in life. However, estimates are that 30% to 60% of older people in treatment programmes began drinking abusively after age 60.

Risk factors for late-onset substance abuse in elders include chronic illness that causes pain, long-term use of prescription medication (sedative-hypnotics, anxiolytics), life stress, loss, social isolation, grief, depression and an

CLIENT-FAMILY EDUCATION FOR SUBSTANCE ABUSE

- Substance abuse is distressing for the client and for others.
- Dispel myths about substance abuse.
- Abstinence from substances is not simply a matter of willpower.
- Any alcohol, whether beer, wine or spirits, can be an abused substance.
- Prescribed medication can be an abused substance.
- Feedback from family about relapse signs, e.g. a return to previous maladaptive coping mechanisms, is vital.
- Continued participation in therapeutic or support programmes is important.

abundance of discretionary time and money (Atkinson, 2004). Older people may experience physical problems associated with substance abuse rather quickly, especially if their overall medical health is compromised by other illnesses.

MENTAL HEALTH PROMOTION

In whatever role or service setting, it is the responsibility of mental health nurses to encourage a healthy approach to substances: to provide information, challenge misconceptions, support people through the process of motivation and change – from pre-contemplation to contemplation, to action, to maintenance.

NURSING INTERVENTIONS FOR SUBSTANCE ABUSE

- Health promotion for the client and family.
- Dispel myths surrounding substance abuse.
- Decrease co-dependent behaviours among family members.
- Make appropriate referrals for family members.
- Establish CBT, motivational interviewing and/or harm minimization approaches.
- Promote coping skills.
- Role-play potentially difficult situations.
- Offer validation of past distress while focusing on goal-setting and the here-and-now.
- Set realistic goals such as staying sober today.

SUBSTANCE ABUSE IN HEALTH PROFESSIONALS

Nurses, doctors and dentists have far higher rates of dependence on **controlled substances** such as opioids, stimulants and sedatives than other professionals of comparable educational. One reason is thought to be the ease of obtaining controlled substances (Jaffe & Anthony, 2005). Health-care professionals also have higher rates of alcoholism than the general population.

The issue of reporting colleagues with suspected substance misuse problems is an important and extremely sensitive one. It is difficult for colleagues and supervisors to report their peers for suspected abuse. Nurses may hesitate to report suspected problems for several reasons: they have difficulty believing that a trained health-care professional would do something like this; they may feel guilty or fear falsely accusing someone; or they may simply want to avoid conflict. Substance abuse by health professionals is very serious, however, because it can endanger the lives of clients. Nurses have an ethical and professional responsibility to report any behaviour they feel is detrimental (or potentially detrimental) to clients to a line-manager. Nurses should not try to handle such situations alone by merely warning the co-worker; this often just allows the co-worker to continue to abuse the substance without suffering any repercussions.

General warning signs of misuse of substances include poor work performance, frequent absenteeism, unusual behaviour, slurred speech and isolation from peers. More specific behaviours and signs that might indicate substance abuse include the following:

- Drug errors
- Excessive controlled substances listed as wasted or contaminated
- Reports by clients of ineffective pain relief from medications, especially if relief had been adequate previously
- Damaged or torn packaging on controlled substances
- Consistent offers to obtain controlled substances from pharmacy
- Unexplained absences from the unit
- Trips to the bathroom after contact with controlled substances
- Consistent early arrivals at or late departures from work for no apparent reason.

Nurses can become involved in substance misuse just as any other person might. Nurses with misuse problems deserve the opportunity for treatment and recovery as well. Reporting suspected substance abuse could be the crucial first step toward a nurse getting the help he or she needs.

Dual Diagnosis

Increasingly, and belatedly, a large proportion of resources (time, money and personnel) in mental health care is becoming focused on people with a 'dual diagnosis'. It is probable that between 33% and 50% of inpatient admissions in the UK involve people who have a severe mental disorder *and* misuse substances, whether alcohol, prescribed or illicit drugs. Somewhere between 33% and 75% of people who come into contact with specialist substance misuse services have a diagnosable mental disorder (Department of Health, 2002; MIND, 2007).

RETHINK (2008) cites research by the Royal College of Psychiatrists (2002) that suggests that people with a diagnosis of schizophrenia are more likely to misuse alcohol; according to Chrome (cited by RETHINK, 2008), they are also six times more likely to use street drugs.

The client with both substance abuse and another diagnosed mental health disorder is said to have a **dual diagnosis**. According to the *Dual Diagnosis Practice Guide* (Department of Health, 2002): 'The term 'dual diagnosis' covers a broad spectrum of mental health and substance misuse problems that an individual might experience concurrently. The nature of the relationship between these two conditions is complex. Possible mechanisms include:

- Primary psychiatric illness precipitating or leading to substance misuse
- Substance misuse worsening or altering the course of a psychiatric illness
- Intoxication and/or substance dependence leading to psychological symptoms
- Substance misuse and/or withdrawal leading to psychiatric symptoms or illnesses.'

Traditional methods of care and treatment for 'dual diagnosis' clients have often had little success, for the following reasons:

- Clients with a major mental disorder may have impaired abilities to process abstract concepts or work in sophisticated psychotherapeutic ways; this has been a major barrier in some substance abuse programmes.
- Much substance misuse treatment emphasizes avoidance of all psychoactive drugs. This may not be possible for the client who needs psychotropic drugs to treat his or her mental health problems.
- The notion of lifelong abstinence, which is central to some substance-use treatment approaches, may seem overwhelming and impossible to the client who lives 'day-to-day' with a chronic mental health problem.
- The use of alcohol and other drugs can precipitate psychotic behaviour; this makes it difficult for professionals to identify whether symptoms are the result of active mental disorder or substance abuse.
- The use of illicit drugs may – at least in the short term – significantly reduce the distress caused by psychotic symptoms, by anxiety symptoms or by low mood.
- There has been, and remains, despite national policy guidance (e.g. Department of Health, 2002), often poor communication between specialist services and generic

services, whereby each claims the other is best suited to cope with someone's needs. Attempts to understand which came first – mental health problem or substance misuse – can fatally distract from timely and effective interventions.

Clients with a dual diagnosis present challenges that traditional settings cannot meet. Studies of successful treatment and relapse prevention strategies for this population have, though, found several key elements that need to be addressed. These include healthy, nurturing, supportive living environments; assistance with fundamental life changes, such as finding a job; abstinent friends; connections with other recovering people; and treatment of their co-morbid conditions (Drake *et al*., 2005). Clients themselves have identified the need for stable housing, positive social support, using prayer or relying on a higher power, participation in meaningful activity, eating regularly, getting sufficient sleep and looking presentable as important components of relapse prevention (Davis & O'Neill, 2005). In addition, the policy of 'mainstreaming' first advocated by the *Dual Diagnosis Good Practice Guide* (2002) (that is, caring for and treating dual diagnosis clients in general mental health settings, with substance misuse services acting in a consultancy capacity) promises more coherent and person-centred (rather than service-centred) care.

APPLICATION OF THE NURSING PROCESS: DUAL DIAGNOSIS

Assessing, formulating, intervening and evaluating as part of the nursing process for people who have – or may have – the dual problems of a mental disorder and substance misuse is a complex one. In many ways, though, the skills, attitudes and knowledge necessary are those needed in all other spheres of nursing: **respect**, openness to evidence, curiosity and a genuine desire to work collaboratively. Nurses need to be optimistic, genuine and willing to see people as complex, ever-changing and full of resources – experiences, support and strengths – they can use to help tackle their problems and find the solutions they need.

In a specialist substance-misuse setting, nurses need always to approach people with the assumption they may well have other mental health problems (and assess, plan, intervene and evaluate care appropriately). In other mental health settings, nurses must always be aware of – and assess for – the possible (maybe even probable) coexistence of substance misuse alongside mental disorder – and, again, offer appropriate care.

Both motivational interviewing and harm reduction approaches have a growing evidence-base, although the need for far greater integration of generic mental health and substance misuse services seems to be key to ensuring that clients receive high-quality care (Heather *et al*., 2006; Laker, 2007).

The measurement of alcohol-related problems can be undertaken using the Alcohol Problems Questionnaire (APQ) (Williams & Drummond, 1994). The Readiness to Change Questionnaire (RCQ) (can be viewed online at http://www.ncbi.nlm.nih.gov/books/bv.fcgi?rid=hstat5.table.62295) is

Nursing Care Plan

Dual Diagnosis

Nursing Formulation

Ineffective Coping With Substance Misuse In The Context Of A Mental Health Problem: *Inability to form a valid appraisal of the stressors, inadequate choices of practised responses and/or inability to use available resources.*

ASSESSMENT DATA

- Poor impulse control
- Low self-esteem
- Lack of social skills
- Dissatisfaction with life circumstances
- Lack of purposeful daily activity

EXPECTED OUTCOMES (FOCUSED ON SUBSTANCE MISUSE)

Immediate
The client will
- Take only prescribed medication
- Interact appropriately with professionals and others
- Express feelings openly
- Develop plans to manage unstructured time

Medium-term
The client will
- Demonstrate appropriate or social skills
- Identify social activities in drug- and alcohol-free environments
- Assess own strengths and weaknesses realistically

Ongoing
The client will
- Maintain contacts with a professional in the community
- Verbalize plans to join a community support group that meets the needs of clients with a dual diagnosis, if available
- Participate in drug- and alcohol-free programmes and activities

IMPLEMENTATION

Nursing Interventions *denotes collaborative interventions	**Rationale**
Encourage open expression of feelings.	Verbalizing feelings is an initial step toward dealing constructively with those feelings.
Validate the client's frustration or anger in dealing with dual problems (e.g. 'I know this must be really difficult.').	Expressing feelings outwardly, especially negative ones, may relieve some of the client's stress and anxiety.
Consider alcohol or substance use as a factor that influences the client's ability to live in the community, similar to such factors as attending for CBT, taking medications, keeping appointments and so forth.	Substance use is not necessarily the major problem the client with a dual diagnosis experiences, only one of several problems. Overemphasis on any single factor does not guarantee success.
Maintain frequent contact with the client, even if it is only brief telephone calls.	Frequent contact decreases the length of time the client feels 'stranded' or left alone to deal with problems.
Give positive feedback for abstinence on a day-to-day basis.	Positive feedback reinforces abstinent behaviour.
If drinking or substance use occurs, discuss the events that led to the incident with the client in a non-judgemental manner.	The client may be able to see the relatedness of the events or a pattern of behaviour while discussing the situation.

continued ⋯⟩

Nursing Care Plan: Dual Diagnosis, cont.

Discuss ways to avoid similar circumstances in the future.	Anticipatory planning may prepare the client to avoid similar circumstances in the future.
Assess the amount of unstructured time with which the client must cope.	The client is more likely to experience frustration or dissatisfaction, which can lead to substance use, when he or she has excessive amounts of unstructured time.
Assist the client to plan daily or weekly schedules of purposeful activities: errands, appointments, taking walks and so forth.	Scheduled events provide the client with something to anticipate or look forward to doing.
Writing the schedule on a calendar may be beneficial.	Visualization of the schedule provides a concrete reference for the client.
Encourage the client to record activities, feelings and thoughts in a journal.	A journal can provide a focus for the client and yield information that is useful in future planning but may otherwise be forgotten or overlooked.
Teach the client social skills. Describe and demonstrate specific skills, such as eye contact, attentive listening, nodding and so forth. Discuss the kind of topics that are appropriate for social conversation, such as the weather, news, local events and so forth.	The client may have little or no knowledge of social interaction skills. Modelling the skills provides a concrete example of the desired skills.
Give positive support to the client for appropriate use of social skills.	Positive feedback will encourage the client to continue attempts at socialization and enhance self-esteem.
*Refer the client to volunteer or vocational services if indicated.	Purposeful activity makes better use of the client's unstructured time and can enhance the client's feelings of worth and self-esteem.
*Refer the client to community support services that address mental health and substance dependence-related needs.	Clients with dual diagnoses have complicated and long-term problems that require ongoing, extended assistance.

Adapted from Schultz, J. M. & Videbeck, S. L. (2005). *Lippincott's manual of psychiatric nursing care plans* (7th edn). Philadelphia: Lippincott Williams & Wilkins.

another useful tool for assessing and engaging with people who may or may not be ready to tackle their alcohol use (Heather *et al.*, 2006).

SELF-AWARENESS ISSUES

We live in a culture in which legal, socially condoned use and misuse of substances is endemic. The nurse must examine his or her beliefs and attitudes about both alcohol (and other legal drugs) and the use of illicit substances. A history of substance use in the nurse's family can strongly influence his or her interaction with clients. The nurse may be overly harsh and critical, telling the client that he or she should 'realize how you're hurting your family'. Conversely, the nurse may unknowingly act out old family roles and engage in enabling behaviour, such as sympathizing with the client's reasons for using substances. Examining one's own substance use, or the use by close friends and family, may be difficult and unpleasant but is necessary if the nurse is to have therapeutic relationships with clients.

The nurse might also have different attitudes about various substances of abuse. For example, a nurse may have genuine empathy for clients who are addicted to prescription medication but be disgusted by clients who use heroin or other illegal substances. It is important to remember that the treatment process and underlying issues of substance abuse, remission and relapse are quite similar regardless of the substance, and that nurses have an obligation to engage compassionately and effectively with everyone.

Many clients experience periodic relapses. For some, being sober is a lifelong struggle. The nurse may become cynical or pessimistic when clients return for multiple attempts at substance use treatment. Such thoughts as 'he deserves health problems if he keeps drinking' or 'she should expect to get hepatitis or HIV infection if she keeps doing intravenous drugs' are signs that the nurse has some personal attitudinal problems that prevent him or her from working effectively with clients and their families.

Laker (2006) identified three areas of difficulty for nurses working with people with substance misuse and dual diagnoses:

1. Difficulties in understanding the concept of dual diagnosis

2. Feeling deskilled when working with people who have a dual diagnosis
3. Struggling to work in a system that seeks to avoid people with dual diagnosis.

All nurses have an obligation to do what they can to address each of these issues.

Points to Consider When Working With Clients and Families With Substance Abuse Problems

• Remember that substance abuse feels like – and appears to be like – a chronic, recurring disease for many people, just like diabetes or heart disease. Even though clients look like they should be able to control their substance abuse easily, they cannot without assistance and understanding.

• Examine substance abuse problems in your own family and friends, even though it may be painful. Recognizing your own background, beliefs and attitudes is the first step toward managing those feelings effectively so that they do not interfere with the care of clients and families.

Critical Thinking Questions

1. You discover that another nurse on your ward has taken Valium from the trolley. You confront the nurse, and she replies, 'I'm under a lot of stress at home. I've never done anything like this before, and I promise it will never happen again.' What should you do, and why?
2. A client of yours – diagnosed with paranoid schizophrenia – tells you he's just started taking cannabis and that it really helps reduce the voices. How should you respond?

KEY POINTS

• Substance use and substance-related disorders can involve alcohol, stimulants, cannabis, opioids, hallucinogens, inhalants, sedatives, hypnotics, anxiolytics, caffeine and nicotine.

• A large proportion of people with diagnosed mental health problems misuse substances – perhaps as many as 75%. A significant proportion of people with an identified substance misuse problem have a concomitant mental health problem, often undiagnosed.

• Clients who are dually diagnosed with substance use problems and major mental health problems do poorly in traditional treatment settings and need specialized attention.

• Substance use and dependence include major impairment in the user's social and occupational functioning, and behavioural and psychological changes.

• Psychotherapeutic approaches include CBT, harm minimization approaches and motivational interviewing.

• After caffeine, alcohol is the substance used most often in the UK; tobacco is next, followed by cannabis.

• Intoxication is the use of a substance that results in maladaptive behaviour.

• Withdrawal syndrome is defined as negative psychological and physical reactions when use of a substance ceases or dramatically decreases.

• Detoxification is the process of safely withdrawing from a substance. Detoxification from alcohol and barbiturates can be life-threatening and requires medical supervision.

• The most significant risk factors for alcoholism seem to be having an alcoholic parent, genetic vulnerability and growing up in 'an alcoholic home'.

• Approach each treatment experience with an open and objective attitude. The client may be successful in maintaining abstinence after his or her second or third (or more) treatment experience.

INTERNET RESOURCES

RESOURCES
• Al-Anon/Alateen
• Alcoholics Anonymous
• Alcohol Concern
• Drugscope
• London Drug and Alcohol Network
• National Treatment Agency
• Tackling Drugs Changing Lives
• FRANK

INTERNET ADDRESS
http://www.al-anonuk.org.uk
http://www.alcoholics-anonymous.org
www.alcoholconcern.org.uk
www.drugscope.org.uk
http://www.ldan.org.uk/
www.nta.nhs.uk
http://drugs.homeoffice.gov.uk/
www.talktofrank.com

- Routine screening with tools such as the AUDIT in a wide variety of settings (GP surgeries, CMHTs, crisis and home treatment teams) can be used to help detect substance misuse problems.
- After any detoxification, treatment of substance use continues in various outpatient and inpatient settings. Approaches are often based on the 12-step philosophy of abstinence, altered lifestyles and peer support.
- Substance misuse can be seen as a family disorder, meaning that it affects all members in some way. Family members and close friends need education and support to cope with their feelings toward the misuser. Many support groups are available to family members and close friends.
- Nursing interventions for clients being treated for substance misuse include teaching clients and families about substance abuse, dealing with family issues and helping clients to learn more effective coping skills.
- Health-care professionals have increased rates of substance use problems, particularly involving opioids, stimulants and sedatives. Reporting suspected substance abuse in colleagues is an ethical (and sometimes legal) responsibility of all health-care professionals.

REFERENCES

Action on Smoking and Health (ASH). (2008a). *Essential information on smoking statistics.* Available: http://www.ash.org.uk/files/documents/ASH_107.pdf

Action on Smoking and Health (ASH). (2008b). *Essential information on smoking and mental health.* Available: http://www.ash.org.uk/files/documents/ASH_120.pdf

American Psychiatric Association. (2000). *Diagnostic and statistical manual of mental disorders* (4th edn, text revision). Washington, DC: American Psychiatric Association.

Atkinson, R. M. (2004). Substance abuse. In J. Sadavoy, L. F. Jarvik, G. T. Greenberg, *et al.* (Eds.), *Comprehensive textbook of geriatric psychiatry* (3rd edn, pp. 723–761). New York: W. W. Norton and Company.

Bayard, M., McIntyre, J., Hill, K. R., & Woodside, J. Jr. (2004). Alcohol withdrawal syndrome. *American Family Physician,* 69(6), 1443–1450.

Bischof, G., Rumpf, H. J., Meyer, C., *et al.* (2005). Influence of psychiatric comorbidity in alcohol-dependent subjects in a representative population survey on treatment utilization and natural recovery. *Addiction,* 100(3), 405–413.

Bohn, M. J., Babor, T. F., & Kranzler, H. R. (1995). The alcohol use disorder identification test (AUDIT): validation of a screening instrument for use in medical settings. *Journal of Studies on Alcohol,* 56(4), 423–432.

Brown University Digest. (2001). Integrated services for dually diagnosed can be effective, but rarely offered. DATA. *The Brown University Digest of Addiction Theory & Application,* 20(12), 1, 6.

Cabinet Office. (2003). Alcohol misuse: How much does it cost? Available: http://www.cabinetoffice.gov.uk/media/cabinetoffice/strategy/assets/econ.pdf

Ciraulo, D. A. & Sarid-Segal, O. (2005). Sedative-, hypnotic- or anxiolytic-related abuse. In B. J. Sadock & V. A. Sadock (Eds.), *Comprehensive textbook of psychiatry, Vol. 1* (8th edn, pp. 1300–1318). Philadelphia: Lippincott Williams & Wilkins.

Crowley, T. J. & Sakai, J. (2005). Inhalant-related disorders. In B. J. Sadock & V. A. Sadock (Eds.), *Comprehensive textbook of psychiatry, Vol. 1* (8th edn, pp. 1247–1257). Philadelphia: Lippincott Williams & Wilkins.

Davis, K. E. & O'Neill, S. J. (2005). A focus group analysis of relapse prevention strategies for persons with substance use and mental disorders. *Psychiatric Services,* 56(10), 1288–1291.

Department of Health. (2002). *Mental health policy implementation guide: Dual diagnosis good practice guide.* Available: http://www.dh.gov.uk/en/Publicationsandstatistics/Publications/PublicationsPolicyAndGuidance/DH_4009058

Dick, D. M. & Bierut, L. J. (2006). The genetics of alcohol dependence. *Current Psychiatry Reports,* 8(2), 151–157.

Drake, R. E., Wallach, M. A., & McGovern, M. P. (2005). Future directions in preventing relapse to substance abuse among clients with severe mental illness. *Psychiatric Services,* 56(10), 1297–1302.

Drugscope. (2008). *How many people die from drugs?* Available: http://www.drugscope.org.uk/resources/faqs/faqpages/how-many-people-die-from-drugs.htm

Foster, T. (2001). Dying for a drink. Global suicide prevention should focus more on alcohol use disorders. *British Medical Journal,* 323(7317), 817–818.

Gibbins, J. & Kipping, C. (2006). Coexistent substance use and psychiatric disorders. In C. Gamble & G. Brennan (Eds.), *Working with serious mental illness.* London: Elsevier.

Grogan, L. (2006). Alcoholism, tobacco and drug use in the countries of central and eastern Europe and the former Soviet Union. *Substance Use & Misuse,* 41(4), 567–571.

Hall, W. & Degenhardt, L. (2005). Cannabis-related disorders. In B. J. Sadock & V. A. Sadock (Eds.), *Comprehensive textbook of psychiatry, Vol. 1* (8th edn, pp. 1211–1220). Philadelphia: Lippincott Williams & Wilkins.

Heather, N., Raistrik, D., & Godfrey, C. (2006). *A summary of the Review of the Effectiveness of Treatment for Alcohol Problems.* National Treatment Agency For Substance Misuse. Available: http://www.nta.nhs.uk/publications/documents/nta_review_of_the_effectiveness_of_treatment_for_alcohol_problems_summary_2006_alcohol3.pdf

International Centre for Drug Policy. (2008). *National programme on Substance Abuse Deaths (np-SAD). 20th Surveillance Report: January–June 2007.* Available: http://www.sgul.ac.uk/dms/CB928511C0A2A2CE54046F74F4AA8DE8.pdf

Jaffe, J. H. & Anthony, J. C. (2005). Substance-related disorders: Introduction and overview. In B. J. Sadock & V. A. Sadock (Eds.), *Comprehensive textbook of psychiatry, Vol. 1* (8th edn, pp. 1137–1168). Philadelphia: Lippincott Williams & Wilkins.

Jaffe, J. H. & Strain, E. C. (2005). Opioid-related disorders. In B. J. Sadock & V. A. Sadock (Eds.), *Comprehensive textbook of psychiatry, Vol. 1* (8th edn, pp. 1265–1291). Philadelphia: Lippincott Williams & Wilkins.

Jaffe, J. H., Ling, W., & Rawson, R. A. (2005). Amphetamine (or amphetamine-like) related disorders. In B. J. Sadock & V. A. Sadock (Eds.), *Comprehensive textbook of psychiatry, Vol. 1* (8th edn, pp. 1188–1201). Philadelphia: Lippincott Williams & Wilkins.

Jones, R. T. (2005). Hallucinogen-related disorders. In B. J. Sadock & V. A. Sadock (Eds.), *Comprehensive textbook of psychiatry, Vol. 1* (8th edn, pp. 1238–1247). Philadelphia: Lippincott Williams & Wilkins.

Kelley, M. L., Nair, V., Rawlings, T., *et al.* (2005). Retrospective reports of parenting received in their families of origin: Relationships to adult attachment in adult children of alcoholics. *Addictive Behaviours,* 30(8), 1479–1495.

Laker, C. (2006). How successful is the Dual Diagnosis Good Practice Guide? *British Journal of Nursing,* 15(14), 787–790.

Laker, C. (2007). How reliable is the current evidence looking at the efficacy of harm reduction and motivational interviewing interventions in the treatment of patients with a dual diagnosis? *Journal of Psychiatric and Mental Health Nursing,* 14(8), 720–726.

Lehne, R. A. (2006). *Pharmacology for nursing care* (6th edn). Philadelphia: W. B. Saunders.

Mehta, M., Moriarty, K., Proctor, D., Bird, M., & Darling, W. (2006). Alcohol misuse in older people: heavy consumption and protean presentations. *Journal of Epidemiology and Community Health,* 60, 1048–1052.

Miller, W. R. & Rollnick, S. (1991). *Motivational interviewing: preparing people to change addictive behaviour.* New York: Guilford Press.

Milne, D. (2002). Alcohol consumption in Japan. *Canadian Medical Association Journal,* 167(4), 388.

MIND. (2007). *Understanding dual diagnosis*. Available: http://www.mind.org.uk/Information/Booklets/Understanding/Understanding+dual+diagnosis.htm

National Institute on Alcohol Abuse and Alcoholism. (2007). *A family history of alcoholism*. Available: http://www.pubs.niaaa.nih.gov/publications/FamilyHistory/famhist.htm

National Institute For Mental Health In England. (2008). *National Suicide Prevention Strategy for England Annual Report*. Available: http://www.nimhe.csip.org.uk/silo/files/suicide-prevention-strategy-report-2007.pdf

Osher, F. C. & Kofoed, I. (1989). Treatment of patients with psychiatric and psychoactive substance buse disorders. *Hospital and Community Psychiatry, 40*, 1025–1030.

Philips, P. (2006). Principles of working with service users with substance misuse problems. In P.Callaghan & H.Waldock (Eds.), *Oxford handbook of mental health nursing*. Oxford: Oxford University Press.

Prochaska, J. & DiClemente, C. (1986). Towards a comprehensive model of change. In W. Miller, & N. Heather (Eds.), *Treating addictive behaviours: processes of change*. New York: Plenum Press.

RETHINK. (2008). *Dual diagnosis*. Available: http://www.rethink.org/about_mental_illness/dual_diagnosis/index.html

Royal College of Physicians Working Party Report. (2001). *Alcohol – can the NHS afford it?* Available: http://www.rcplondon.ac.uk/pubs/contents/ea90ff6a-fcd3-4112-b958-d98f0cc2246a.pdf

Schuckit, M. A. (2005). Alcohol-related disorders. In B. J. Sadock & V. A. Sadock (Eds.), *Comprehensive textbook of psychiatry, Vol. 1* (8th edn, pp. 1168–1188). Philadelphia: Lippincott Williams & Wilkins.

Wakabayashi, I. & Masuda, H. (2006). Influence of drinking alcohol on atherosclerotic risk in alcohol flushers and non-flushers of Oriental patients with type 2 diabetes mellitus. *Alcohol and Alcoholism, 41*(6), 672–677.

Williams, B. T. & Drummond, D. C. (1994). The Alcohol Problems Questionnaire: reliability and validity. *Drug and Alcohol Dependence, 35*(3), 239–243.

ADDITIONAL READING

Menninger, J. A. (2002). Assessment and treatment of alcoholism and substance-related disorders in the elderly. *Bulletin of the Menninger Clinic, 66*(2), 166–183.

National Institute on Alcohol Abuse and Alcoholism. (2005a). *Alcohol and minorities*. Available: http://www.niaaa.nih.gov/

National Institute on Alcohol Abuse and Alcoholism. (2005b). *A snapshot of high-risk college drinking consequences*. Available: http://www.collegedrinkingprevention.gov

O'Brien, C. P. (2005). Anticraving medications for relapse prevention: a possible new class of psychoactive medications. *American Journal of Psychiatry, 162*(8), 1423–1431.

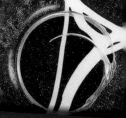

Chapter Study Guide

MULTIPLE CHOICE QUESTIONS

Select the best answer for each of the following questions.

1. Which of the following statements would indicate that teaching about naltrexone has been effective?
   a. 'I'll get sick if I use heroin while taking this medication.'
   b. 'This medication will block the effects of any opioid substance I take.'
   c. 'If I use opioids while taking naltrexone, I'll become extremely ill.'
   d. 'Using naltrexone may make me dizzy.'

2. Which of the following would the nurse recognize as signs of alcohol withdrawal?
   a. Coma, disorientation and hypervigilance
   b. Tremulousness, sweating and elevated blood pressure
   c. Increased temperature, lethargy and hypothermia
   d. Talkativeness, hyperactivity and blackouts

3. Which of the following behaviours would indicate stimulant intoxication?
   a. Slurred speech, unsteady gait, impaired concentration
   b. Hyperactivity, talkativeness, euphoria
   c. Relaxed inhibitions, increased appetite, distorted perceptions
   d. Depersonalization, dilated pupils, visual hallucinations

4. The 12 steps of AA teach that
   a. Acceptance of being an alcoholic will help prevent urges to drink.
   b. A Higher Power will protect individuals if they feel like drinking.
   c. Once a person has learned to be sober, he or she can graduate and leave AA.
   d. Once a person is sober, he or she remains at risk to drink.

5. The nurse consultant has provided an in-service training programme on helping professionals with substance misuse problems. She knows that teaching has been effective when staff identify the following as the greatest risk for substance abuse among professionals:
   a. Nurses tend to come from dysfunctional families.
   b. Nurses tend to be weak and passive-aggressive in their behaviour.
   c. Nurses are exposed to stressful work, to a culture that minimizes the impact of addiction and to a system that often seems to insist on a rigid separation between 'them' (clients) and 'us' (professionals).
   b. Nurses tend to socialize a lot.

6. A client comes to day treatment intoxicated, but says he is not. The nurse identifies that the client may be exhibiting signs of
   a. Denial
   b. Reaction formation
   c. Projection
   d. Transference

7. The client tells the nurse that she takes a drink every morning to calm her nerves and stop her tremors. The nurse realizes the client is at risk of
   a. An anxiety disorder
   b. A neurological disorder
   c. Physical dependence
   d. Psychological addiction

FILL-IN-THE-BLANK QUESTIONS

Give two examples of drugs for each of the following categories.

_____ Stimulants

_____ Opioids

_____ Hallucinogens

_____ Inhalants

GROUP DISCUSSION TOPICS

How much does your own substance use (or abstinence) affect you when you meet someone who misuses drugs or alcohol?

Should all mental health facilities be free of drugs such as tobacco or caffeine?

CLINICAL EXAMPLE

Sharon, 43 years of age, is attending a CMHT-based group for help with alcohol abuse. She is divorced, and her two children live with their father. Sharon broke up with her boyfriend of 3 years just last week. She was recently arrested for the second time for driving while intoxicated, which is why she is in this treatment programme. Sharon tells anyone who will listen that she is 'not an alcoholic' but is in this programme only to avoid serving time in prison.

1. Identify two nursing formulations for Sharon.

2. Write an expected outcome for each identified formulation.

3. List three interventions for each of the formulations.

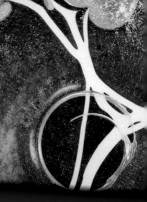

Chapter

18

Eating Disorders

Key Terms

- alexithymia
- anorexia nervosa
- autonomy
- binge eating
- body image
- body image disturbance
- bulimia nervosa
- enmeshment
- family therapy
- identity
- invalidating environment
- purging
- satiety
- self-image
- self-monitoring

Learning Objectives

After reading this chapter, you should be able to:

1. Understand some of the emotional, cognitive and behavioural aspects of eating disorders.

2. Compare and contrast the symptoms of anorexia nervosa and bulimia nervosa.

3. Discuss various aetiological theories of eating disorders.

4. Identify effective treatment for clients with eating disorders.

5. Apply the nursing process to the care of clients with eating disorders.

6. Provide teaching to clients, families and community members to increase knowledge and understanding of eating disorders.

7. Evaluate your feelings, beliefs and attitudes about clients with eating disorders.

Eating is part of everyday life. It is necessary for survival but it is also a social activity and part of many happy – and important – occasions. People go out for dinner, invite friends and family for meals in their homes and celebrate special events such as marriages, holidays and birthdays with food. Yet, for all sorts of people, eating is a source of worry and anxiety. Are they eating too much? Do they look fat? Is some new weight-loss fad going to be the answer? Food, eating and weight are inexorably tied-up with our sense of ourselves and with our interactions with others. For some people they become all-encompassing – and even fatal.

Hundreds of thousands of women – and men – are either starving themselves or engaging in chaotic eating patterns that can lead to death. This chapter focuses on anorexia nervosa and bulimia nervosa, the two most common eating disorders found in the mental health setting. It discusses strategies for early identification and prevention of these disorders and approaches to ensure compassionate and effective care.

OVERVIEW OF EATING DISORDERS

Although many believe that eating disorders are relatively new, in the Middle Ages, for example, women sometimes fasted to the point of starvation in order to achieve 'purity'. In the late 1800s, doctors in England and France described young women who apparently used self-starvation to avoid obesity. It was not until the 1960s, however, that anorexia nervosa became established as a recognized mental disorder. Bulimia nervosa was first described as a distinct syndrome in 1979 (Andersen & Yager, 2005).

Eating disorders can be viewed on a continuum, with clients with anorexia eating too little or starving themselves, clients with bulimia eating chaotically, and clients with obesity eating too much. The distinguishing features of anorexia include an earlier age at onset and below-normal body weight; the person usually fails to recognize the eating behaviour as a problem. Clients with bulimia tend to have a later age at onset and near-normal body weight. The majority are ashamed and embarrassed by the eating behaviour but find it impossible to control without outside help.

There is much overlap among the eating disorders: 30% to 35% of normal-weight people with bulimia have a history of anorexia nervosa and low body weight, and about 50% of people with anorexia nervosa exhibit bulimic behaviour. There are significant overlaps between people with eating disorders and people diagnosed with a personality disorder, people who have substance misuse problems and people who are depressed or anxious: rarely do any of these appear in a 'pure', textbook form.

Anorexia nervosa most commonly starts in the mid-teens. About 1% of 16- to 18-year-olds has the disorder, around 0.5% of young women overall (Fletcher, 2003). It is much more common in girls than in boys – somewhere between 70% and 95% of cases are reported in girls (Callaghan, 2006).

Bulimia nervosa usually starts when people are a bit older; again it is far more common in girls. Bulimia seems to be more common than anorexia (around 2% of young women) (Fletcher, 2003), although people with anorexia, and young men in particular, don't always ask for treatment and this may distort the statistics.

About 40% of people with diagnosed anorexia make a full recovery, and many others improve. About 30% continue to have major long-term difficulties. Untreated, about 15% of all sufferers will die from the disorder within 20 years of its onset (Royal College of Psychiatrists, 2008).

Anorexia Nervosa

Anorexia nervosa is a life-threatening eating disorder characterized by a person's refusal or inability to maintain a minimally normal body weight, intense fear of gaining weight or becoming fat, significantly disturbed perception of the shape or size of the body and steadfast inability or refusal to acknowledge the seriousness of the problem or even that one exists (American Psychiatric Association, 2000). Clients with anorexia have a body weight that is 85% or less of that expected for their age and height, have experienced amenorrhoea for at least three consecutive cycles, and have a preoccupation with food and food-related activities.

For *DSM-IV-TR* diagnostic criteria for anorexia nervosa (American Psychiatric Association, 2000), please refer to the box below.

People with anorexia nervosa can be classified into two sub-groups depending on how they control their weight. Clients with the *restricting* sub-type lose weight primarily through dieting, fasting or excessively exercising. Those with the *binge-eating and purging* sub-type engage regularly in binge-eating followed by purging. **Binge eating** means consuming a large amount of food (far greater than most people eat at one time) in a discrete period of usually 2 hours or less. **Purging** means the compensatory behaviours designed to eliminate food by means of self-induced vomiting or misuse of laxatives, enemas and diuretics. Some clients with anorexia do not binge but still engage in purging behaviours after ingesting small amounts of food.

Clients with anorexia nervosa become totally absorbed in their quest for weight loss and thinness. The term *anorexia* is actually a misnomer: these clients do not lose their appetites. They still experience hunger but ignore it, deny it and suppress both it and signs of physical weakness and fatigue; they often believe that if they eat anything, they will not be able to stop eating and will become fat. Clients with anorexia nervosa are often preoccupied with food-related activities such as grocery shopping, collecting recipes or cookbooks, counting calories, creating fat-free meals and cooking family meals. They may also engage in unusual or ritualistic food behaviours such as refusing to eat around others, cutting food into minute pieces or not allowing the food they eat to touch their lips. These behaviours increase

---

DSM-IV-TR DIAGNOSTIC CRITERIA: SYMPTOMS OF ANOREXIA NERVOSA

Fear of gaining weight or becoming fat even when severely underweight

Body image disturbance

Amenorrhoea

Depressive symptoms such as depressed mood, social withdrawal, irritability and insomnia Preoccupation with thoughts of food

Feelings of ineffectiveness

Inflexible thinking

Strong need to control environment

Limited spontaneity and overly restrained emotional expression

Complaints of constipation and abdominal pain

Cold intolerance

Lethargy

Emaciation

Hypotension, hypothermia and bradycardia

Hypertrophy of salivary glands

Elevated blood urea nitrogen (BUN)

Electrolyte imbalances

Leucopenia and mild anaemia

Elevated liver function studies

Adapted from American Psychiatric Association. (2000). *Diagnostic and Statistical Manual of Mental Disorders* (4th edn, text revision). Washington, DC: American Psychiatric Association.

---

their sense of control. Excessive exercise is common; it may occupy several hours a day.

Anorexia nervosa typically begins between 14 and 18 years of age. In the early stages, clients often deny they have a negative body image or anxiety regarding their appearance. They are very pleased with their ability to control their weight and may express this. When they initially come for treatment, they may be unable to identify or to explain their emotions about life events such as school or relationships with family or friends. A profound sense of emptiness is common.

As the illness progresses, depression and lability in mood become more apparent. As dieting and compulsive behaviours increase, clients isolate themselves. This social isolation can lead to a basic mistrust of others and even paranoia. Clients may believe their peers are jealous of their weight loss and may believe that family and health-care professionals are trying to make them 'fat and ugly'.

In long-term studies of clients with anorexia nervosa, Andersen and Yager (2005) reported that clients with the lowest body weights and longest durations of illness tended to relapse most often and have the poorest outcomes. Clients who abuse laxatives are at a greater risk for medical complications. Table 18.1 lists common medical complications of eating disorders.

Bulimia Nervosa

Bulimia nervosa, often simply called bulimia, is an eating disorder characterized by recurrent episodes (at least twice a week for 3 months) of binge-eating followed by inappropriate compensatory behaviours to avoid weight gain, such as purging (self-induced vomiting or use of laxatives, diuretics, enemas or emetics), fasting or excessively exercising

(American Psychiatric Association, 2000). The amount of food consumed during a binge episode is much larger than a person would normally eat. The client often engages in binge eating secretly. Between binges, the client may eat low-calorie foods or fast. Bingeing or purging episodes are often precipitated by strong emotions and followed by guilt, remorse, shame or self-contempt.

The weight of clients with bulimia is usually in the normal range, although some clients are overweight or underweight. Recurrent vomiting destroys tooth enamel, and incidence of dental caries and ragged or chipped teeth increases in these clients. Dentists are often the first health-care professionals to identify people with bulimia.

Bulimia nervosa usually begins in late adolescence or early adulthood; 18 or 19 years old is the typical age at onset. Binge eating frequently begins during or after dieting. Between bingeing and purging episodes, clients may eat restrictively, choosing salads and other low-calorie foods. This restrictive eating effectively sets them up for the next episode of bingeing and purging, and the cycle continues.

Clients with bulimia are usually aware that their eating behaviour is pathological and go to great lengths to hide it from others. They may store food in their cars, desks or secret locations around the house. They may drive from one fast-food restaurant to another, ordering a normal amount of food at each but stopping at half a dozen places in a couple of hours. Some people order food from the internet in an attempt to keep it secret. Such patterns may exist for years until family or friends discover the client's behaviour or medical complications develop for which the person seeks treatment.

Follow-up studies in the USA with people with bulimia show that 10 years after treatment, 30% continued to engage

Table 18.1   MEDICAL COMPLICATIONS OF EATING DISORDERS

Body System	Symptoms
Related to weight loss	
Musculoskeletal	Loss of muscle mass, loss of fat, osteoporosis and pathological fractures
Metabolic	Hypothyroidism (symptoms include lack of energy, weakness, intolerance to cold and bradycardia), hypoglycaemia and decreased insulin sensitivity
Cardiac	Bradycardia, hypotension, loss of cardiac muscle, small heart, cardiac arrhythmias (including atrial and ventricular premature contractions, prolonged QT interval, ventricular tachycardia) and sudden death
Gastrointestinal	Delayed gastric emptying, bloating, constipation, abdominal pain, gas and diarrhoea
Reproductive	Amenorrhoea and low levels of luteinizing and follicle-stimulating hormones
Dermatological	Dry, cracking skin due to dehydration, lanugo (i.e. fine, baby-like hair over body), oedema and acrocyanosis (i.e. blue hands and feet)
Haematological	Leucopenia, anaemia, thrombocytopenia, hypercholesterolaemia and hypercarotenaemia
Neuropsychiatric	Abnormal taste sensation, apathetic depression, mild organic mental symptoms and sleep disturbances
Related to purging (vomiting and laxative abuse)	
Metabolic	Electrolyte abnormalities, particularly hypokalaemia, hypochloraemic alkalosis, hypomagnesaemia and elevated BUN
Gastrointestinal	Salivary gland and pancreas inflammation and enlargement with an increase in serum amylase, oesophageal and gastric erosion or rupture, dysfunctional bowel and superior mesenteric artery syndrome
Dental	Erosion of dental enamel (perimyolysis), particularly front teeth
Neuropsychiatric	Seizures (related to large fluid shifts and electrolyte disturbances), mild neuropathies, fatigue, weakness and mild organic mental symptoms

Adapted from Andersen, A. E. & Yager, J. (2005). Eating disorders. In B. J. Sadock & V. A. Sadock (Eds.), *Comprehensive textbook of psychiatry, Vol. 2* (8th edn, pp. 2002–2021). Philadelphia: Lippincott Williams & Wilkins.

in recurrent binge-eating and purging behaviours, whereas 38% to 47% had fully recovered (Andersen & Yager, 2005). One-third of fully recovered clients relapse. Clients with a co-morbid personality disorder tend to have poorer outcomes than those without. The death rate from bulimia is estimated at 3% or less.

For *DSM-IV-TR* diagnostic criteria for bulimia nervosa, please refer to the box below.

Related Disorders

Eating disorders usually first diagnosed in infancy and childhood include *rumination disorder, pica* and *feeding disorder* (see Chapter 20). Common elements in clients with these disorders are family dysfunction and parent–child conflicts.

Binge eating disorder is listed as a research category in *DSM-IV-TR* (American Psychiatric Association, 2000); it is

CLINICAL VIGNETTE: ANOREXIA NERVOSA

Maggie, 15 years old, is 5 feet 7 inches tall and weighs 6 stone exactly. Though it is August, she is wearing baggy trousers and three layers of shirts. Her hair is dry, brittle and uncombed, and she wears no make-up. Maggie's GP has referred her to the eating disorders team because she has lost 20 pounds in the last 4 months and her menstrual periods have ceased. She is also lethargic and weak, yet has trouble sleeping. Maggie is an avid ballet student and believes she still needs to lose more weight to achieve the figure she wants. Her ballet instructor has expressed concern to Maggie's parents about her appearance and fatigue.

Maggie's family reports that she has gone from being an excellent student academically to barely scraping by in school. She spends much of her time isolated in her room and is often exercising for long hours, even in the middle of the night. Maggie seldom goes out with friends, and they have stopped calling her. The nurse interviews Maggie but gains little information, as Maggie is reluctant to discuss her eating. Maggie does say she is too fat and has no interest in gaining weight. She does not understand why her parents are forcing her to come to see people who 'just want to fatten you up and keep you ugly.'

DSM-IV-TR DIAGNOSTIC CRITERIA:
SYMPTOMS OF BULIMIA NERVOSA

Recurrent episodes of binge eating

Compensatory behaviour such as self-induced vomiting, misuse of laxatives, diuretics, enema or other medications or excessive exercise

Self-evaluation overly influenced by body shape and weight

Usually within normal weight range, possible underweight or overweight

Restriction of total calorie consumption between binges, selecting low-calorie foods while avoiding foods perceived to be fattening or likely to trigger a binge

Depressive and anxiety symptoms

Possible substance use involving alcohol or stimulants

Loss of dental enamel

Chipped, ragged or moth-eaten appearance of teeth

Increased dental caries

Menstrual irregularities

Dependence on laxatives

Oesophageal tears

Fluid and electrolyte abnormalities

Metabolic alkalosis (from vomiting) or metabolic acidosis (from diarrhoea)

Mildly elevated serum amylase levels

Adapted from American Psychiatric Association. (2000). *Diagnostic and Statistical Manual of Mental Disorders* (4th edn, text revision). Washington, DC: American Psychiatric Association

being investigated to determine its classification as a mental disorder but is increasingly recognized as such in the UK. The essential features are recurrent episodes of binge eating; no regular use of inappropriate compensatory behaviours, such as purging or excessive exercise or abuse of laxatives; guilt, shame and disgust about eating behaviours; and marked psychological distress. Binge eating disorder frequently affects people over age 35, and it often occurs in men (Pope *et al.*, 2006). Individuals are more likely to be overweight or obese, overweight as children and teased about their weight at an early age. Thirty-five per cent reported that binge eating preceded dieting; 65% reported dieting before binge eating.

Night eating syndrome is characterized by morning anorexia, evening hyperphagia (consuming 50% of daily calories after the last evening meal), and night-time awakening (at least once a night) to consume snacks. It is associated with life stress, low self-esteem, anxiety, depression and adverse reactions to weight loss. Most people with night eating syndrome are obese (O'Reardon *et al.*, 2005). Treatment with SSRI antidepressants has shown positive effects.

As mentioned before, co-morbid mental disorders are common in clients with anorexia nervosa and bulimia nervosa. Mood disorders, anxiety disorders and substance abuse/dependence are frequently seen in clients with eating disorders. Of those, depression and OCD are most common (Andersen & Yager, 2005). Anorexia and bulimia are both characterized by perfectionism, obsessive-compulsiveness, neuroticism, negative emotionality, harm avoidance, low self-directedness, low co-operativeness and traits associated with avoidant and borderline personality disorders. In addition, clients with bulimia may also exhibit high impulsivity, sensation seeking, novelty seeking and traits associated with borderline personality disorder (Cassin & von Ranson, 2005).

Eating disorders are often linked to a history of sexual abuse, especially if the abuse occurred before puberty (Preti *et al.*, 2006). Such a history may be a factor contributing to problems with intimacy, sexual attractiveness and low interest in sexual activity. Clients with eating disorders and a history of sexual abuse also have higher levels of depression and anxiety, lower self-esteem, more interpersonal problems and more severe obsessive-compulsive symptoms (Carter *et al.*, 2006). Whether or not sexual abuse has a direct cause-and-effect relationship with the development of eating disorders, however, remains unclear.

CLINICAL VIGNETTE: BULIMIA NERVOSA

Susan is driving home from the supermarket and eating from the bags as she drives. In the 15-minute trip, she has already eaten a packet of biscuits, a large bag of crisps and a pound of cheese from the deli counter. She thinks 'I have to hurry, I'll be home soon. No one can see me like this!' She knew when she bought these food items that she would never get home with them.

Susan hurriedly drops the groceries on the kitchen counter and races for the bathroom. Tears are streaming down her face as she vomits to get rid of what she has just eaten. She feels guilty and ashamed and does not understand why she cannot stop what she's doing. If only she didn't eat those things. She thinks, 'I'm 30 years old, married with two beautiful daughters and a successful design consultant. What would my clients say if they could see me now? If my husband and daughters saw me, they would be disgusted.' As Susan leaves the bathroom to put away the remainder of the groceries, she promises herself to stay away from all those bad foods. If she just does not eat them, this won't happen. This is a promise she has made many times before.

AETIOLOGY

A specific cause for eating disorders is unknown. Initially, dieting may be the stimulus that leads to their development. Biological vulnerability, developmental problems and family and social influences can turn dieting into an eating disorder as they interact with the development of core beliefs about the self, the world and other people (Table 18.2). Psychological and physiological reinforcement of maladaptive eating behaviour sustains the cycle (Andersen & Yager, 2005).

Biological Factors

Studies of anorexia nervosa and bulimia nervosa have shown that these disorders tend to run in families. Genetic vulnerability might also result from a particular personality type or a general susceptibility to mental health disorders. It may directly involve a dysfunction of the hypothalamus. A family history of mood or anxiety disorders (e.g. OCD) places a person at risk for an eating disorder (Andersen & Yager, 2005).

Disruptions of the nuclei of the hypothalamus may produce many of the symptoms of eating disorders. Two sets of nuclei are particularly important in many aspects of hunger and **satiety** (satisfaction of appetite): the lateral hypothalamus and the ventromedial hypothalamus. Deficits in the lateral hypothalamus result in decreased eating and decreased responses to sensory stimuli that are important to eating. Disruption of the ventromedial hypothalamus leads to excessive eating, weight gain and decreased responsiveness to the satiety effects of glucose, which are seen in bulimia.

Many neurochemical changes accompany eating disorders, but it is difficult to tell whether they cause or result from eating disorders and the characteristic symptoms of starvation, bingeing and purging. For example, noradrenaline levels normally rise in response to eating, allowing the body to metabolize and to use nutrients. Noradrenaline levels do not rise during starvation, however, because few nutrients are available to metabolize. Therefore, low noradrenaline levels are seen in clients during periods of restricted food intake. Also, low adrenaline levels are related to the decreased heart rate and blood pressure seen in clients with anorexia.

Increased levels of the neurotransmitter serotonin and its precursor tryptophan have been linked with increased satiety. Low levels of serotonin as well as low platelet levels of monoamine oxidase have been found in clients with bulimia and the binge and purge sub-type of anorexia nervosa (Andersen & Yager, 2005); this may explain bingeing behaviour. The positive response of some clients with bulimia to treatment with SSRI antidepressants supports the idea that serotonin levels at the synapse may be low in these clients.

Developmental Factors

ANOREXIA NERVOSA

Onset of anorexia nervosa usually occurs during adolescence or young adulthood. Some researchers believe its causes are directly related to developmental issues.

Two essential tasks of adolescence are the struggle to develop *autonomy* and the establishment of a unique *identity*. Autonomy, or exerting control over oneself and the environment, may be difficult in families that are overprotective or in which **enmeshment** (lack of clear role boundaries) exists. Such families do not support members' efforts to gain independence, and teenagers may feel as though they have little or no control over their lives. They begin to control their eating through severe dieting and thus gain control over their weight. Losing weight becomes reinforcing: by

Table 18.2	RISK FACTORS FOR EATING DISORDERS			
Disorder	**Biological Risk Factors**	**Developmental Risk Factors**	**Family Risk Factors**	**Sociocultural Risk Factors**
Anorexia nervosa	Obesity; dieting at an early age	Issues of developing autonomy and having control over self and environment; developing a unique identity; dissatisfaction with body image	Family lacks emotional support; parental maltreatment; cannot deal with conflict	Cultural ideal of being thin; media focus on beauty, thinness, fitness; preoccupation with achieving the ideal body
Bulimia nervosa	Obesity; early dieting; possible serotonin and noradrenaline disturbances; chromosome 1 susceptibility	Self-perceptions of being overweight, fat, unattractive and undesirable; dissatisfaction with body image	Chaotic family with loose boundaries; parental maltreatment including possible physical or sexual abuse	Same as above; weight-related teasing

continuing the weight loss, these clients exert control over one aspect of their lives.

It is important to identify potential risk factors for developing eating disorders so that prevention programmes can target those at greatest risk. Johnson and Wardle (2005) found that adolescent girls who expressed body dissatisfaction were most likely to experience adverse outcomes, such as emotional eating, binge eating, abnormal attitudes about eating and weight, low self-esteem, stress and depression. In a US study of almost 3000 dieters, 104 developed an eating disorder within 2 years of screening and characteristics of those who developed an eating disorder included disturbed eating habits; disturbed attitudes toward food; eating in secret; preoccupation with food, eating, shape or weight; fear of losing control overeating; and wanting to have a completely empty stomach (Fairburn *et al.*, 2005).

The need to develop a unique identity, or a sense of who one is as a person, is another essential task of adolescence. It coincides with the onset of puberty, which initiates many emotional and physiological changes. Self-doubt and confusion can result if the adolescent does not measure up to the person she or he wants to be.

Adverts, magazines and films that feature thin women reinforce the cultural belief that slimness is attractive. The obsession with celebrity and the looks of celebrities has become pandemic in our culture; excessive dieting and weight loss may be the way an adolescent chooses to achieve the ideal of becoming like these empty heroes and heroines.

Body image is how a person perceives his or her body, that is, a mental **self-image**. For most people, body image is relatively consistent with how others view them. For people with anorexia nervosa, however, their body image differs greatly from the perception of others. They perceive themselves as fat, unattractive and undesirable even when they are severely underweight and malnourished. **Body image disturbance** occurs when there is an extreme discrepancy between one's body image and the perceptions of others, and extreme dissatisfaction with one's body image.

BULIMIA NERVOSA

Self-perceptions of the body can influence the development of identity in adolescence greatly, and often persist into adulthood. Self-perceptions that include being overweight lead to the belief that dieting is necessary before one can be happy or satisfied. Clients with bulimia nervosa report dissatisfaction with their bodies as well as the belief that they are fat, unattractive and undesirable. The bingeing and purging cycle of bulimia can begin at any time – after dieting has been unsuccessful, before the severe dieting begins or at the same time as part of a 'weight loss plan'.

Family Influences

Girls growing up amid family problems and abuse are at higher risk for both anorexia and bulimia. Disordered eating seems to

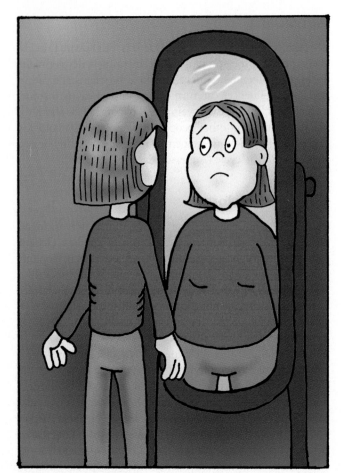

Body image disturbance

be a common response to family discord. Girls growing up in families without emotional support often try to escape their negative emotions. They place an intense focus outward on something concrete: physical appearance. Disordered eating becomes a distraction from emotions.

'Childhood adversity' has been identified as a significant risk factor in the development of problems with eating or weight in adolescence or early adulthood. Adversity can be defined as physical neglect, sexual abuse or parental maltreatment that included little care, affection and empathy, as well as excessive paternal control, unfriendliness or overprotectiveness: similar in many ways to the '**invalidating environment**' first identified by Linehan (1993) in her work with people with borderline personality disorder.

Sociocultural Factors

In the UK and other Western countries, the media fuels the image of the 'ideal woman' as thin. The culture equates beauty, desirability and, ultimately, happiness with being very thin, perfectly toned and physically fit. Adolescents often idealize actresses and models as having the perfect 'look' or body, even though many of these celebrities are underweight or use special effects to appear thinner than they are. Books, magazines, dietary supplements, exercise equipment, plastic surgery advertisements and weight loss programmes abound; the dieting industry is a billion-pound business. Western culture considers being overweight a sign of laziness, lack of self-control or indifference; it equates pursuit of the 'perfect' body with beauty, desirability, success and willpower. Thus, many women speak of being 'good' when they stick to their diet and 'bad' when they eat desserts or snacks.

Pressure from others may also contribute to eating disorders. Pressure from coaches, parents and peers, and the emphasis placed on body form in sports such as gymnastics, ballet and wrestling, can promote eating disorders in athletes (Waldrop, 2005; Eating Disorders Association, 2008a, b). Parental concern over a girl's weight and teasing from parents or peers reinforces a girl's body dissatisfaction and her need to diet or control eating in some way.

CULTURAL CONSIDERATIONS

Both anorexia nervosa and bulimia nervosa are far more prevalent in industrialized societies, where food is abundant and beauty is linked with thinness. Eating disorders are most common in the United States, Canada, Europe, Australia, Japan, New Zealand and South Africa. Immigrants from cultures in which eating disorders are rare may develop eating disorders as they assimilate the thin-body ideal (American Psychiatric Association, 2000). In the UK, anorexia nervosa seems at present to be less frequent among people from ethnic minorities but this appears to be shifting and minority women who are younger, better educated and more closely identified with white, middle-class values are at increased risk for developing an eating disorder. The influence of culture seems undeniable: for example, before 1995, there was little television on the island of Fiji. Eating disorders were almost non-existent, and being 'plump' was considered the ideal shape for girls and women. In the 5 years following the widespread introduction of television, the number of eating disorders in Fiji skyrocketed.

During the past few years, eating disorders have shown an increase among all UK social classes and ethnic groups. With today's technology, the entire world is exposed to the Western ideal, which equates thinness with beauty and desirability. As this ideal becomes widespread to non-Western cultures, anorexia and bulimia will almost certainly increase there as well.

CARE AND TREATMENT

Anorexia Nervosa

Clients with anorexia nervosa can be very difficult to treat because they are often actively resistant to change, appear uninterested and deny their problems. Treatment settings include specialist inpatient eating disorder units, partial hospitalization or day treatment programmes and community-based therapy (often CBT or DBT). Rigid inpatient behaviour modification programmes should not be used in the management of anorexia nervosa (NICE, 2004). The choice of setting depends on the severity of the illness, such as weight loss, physical symptoms, duration of bingeing and purging, drive for thinness, body dissatisfaction and co-morbid mental disorders. Major life-threatening complications that indicate the need for hospital admission include severe fluid, electrolyte and metabolic imbalances; cardiovascular complications; severe weight loss and its consequences (Andreasen & Black, 2006); and risk of suicide. Short hospital stays are most effective for people who are amenable to weight gain, and gain weight rapidly while hospitalized. Longer inpatient stays are required for those who gain weight more slowly and are more resistant to gaining additional weight (Willer et al., 2005). Focused community-based therapy has the best success with clients who have been ill for less than 6 months, are not bingeing and purging and have parents likely to participate effectively in **family therapy**.

Extra care needs to be taken when a person with anorexia is being looked after on a 'generic' acute inpatient ward or in a general hospital setting: this group of people (like those diagnosed with borderline personality disorder) are – because of the likelihood of their own previous experiences of abuse (sexual, emotional and physical) – both exceptionally vulnerable to abuse by others and at risk of being re-traumatized if approached by either staff or other clients in a way that can be seen as potentially threatening or abusive. Careful, considered, compassionate nursing care is essential.

PSYCHOLOGICAL TREATMENTS

'There is insufficient evidence to suggest that any particular psychological treatment (including CAT, CBT, interpersonal therapy (IPT), family therapy, focal psychodynamic therapy) is superior to any other in the treatment of adult patients with anorexia nervosa' (National Collaborating Centre For Mental Health, 2004).

Family therapy – focused on the client's disorder and mobilizing family resources rather than on family dysfunction *per se* – may be beneficial, particularly for families of clients younger than 18 years (NICE, 2004). Families who demonstrate enmeshment, unclear boundaries among members and difficulty handling emotions and conflict can begin to resolve these issues and improve communication. Family therapy is also useful to help members to be effective participants in the client's treatment, though significant improvements in family functioning may take 2 years or more.

Individual therapy – CBT, DBT, motivational-based work, CAT, supportive psychotherapy, for example – that is focused on the client's particular issues and circumstances, including coping skills, self-esteem, self-acceptance, interpersonal relationships and assertiveness, can both help during acute crises and improve overall functioning and life satisfaction in the longer term (Marcus & Levine, 2004; Middleton, 2007; Waller et al., 2007).

Bulimia Nervosa

'Psychological treatment should be provided which has a focus both on eating behaviour and attitudes to weight and shape, and on wider psychosocial issues with the expectation of weight gain' (NICE, 2004).

CBT for bulimia nervosa (CBT-BN) has been found to be the most effective treatment for bulimia, normally involving 16 to 20 sessions over 4 or 5 months (NICE, 2004). The approach involves strategies designed to change the client's thinking and feelings about, and actions around, food, focusing on interrupting the cycle of dieting, bingeing and purging and altering dysfunctional thoughts and beliefs about food, weight, body image and overall self-concept.

CAT and IPTs can be effective in preventing relapse and improving overall outcomes; DBT has recently begun to be used with some success. Focal psychodynamic therapy and family interventions focused explicitly on eating disorders can also be helpful (NICE, 2004). Integrative therapeutic group work has shown promising results (Seamoore et al., 2006).

MEDICAL MANAGEMENT

Medical management focuses, in the first instance, on saving life: weight restoration, nutritional rehabilitation, rehydration and correction of electrolyte imbalances. Clients receive nutritionally balanced meals and snacks that gradually increase caloric intake to a normal level for size, age and activity. Severely malnourished clients may require total parenteral nutrition, tube feedings or hyperalimentation to receive adequate nutritional intake. Generally, access to a bathroom is supervised to prevent purging as clients begin to eat more food. Weight gain and adequate food intake are most often the criteria for determining the effectiveness of treatment.

PSYCHOPHARMACOLOGY

Several classes of drugs have been studied, but few have shown clinical success. Pharmacological interventions may be helpful in managing co-morbid disorders – for example, antidepressants may be helpful. Drugs with cardiac side-effects – antipsychotics, tricyclic antidepressants and some antibiotics and antihistamines – may prove dangerous to people with anorexia. If absolutely necessary, electrocardiogram (ECG) monitoring is essential.

At present in the UK, only antidepressants are recommended for the treatment of bulimia nervosa. Since the 1980s, several controlled studies have been conducted to evaluate the effectiveness of antidepressants to treat bulimia. Drugs such as amitriptyline, phenelzine (Nardil) and fluoxetine (Prozac) were prescribed in the same dosages used to treat depression (see Chapter 3). In all the studies, the antidepressants were more effective than were the placebos in reducing binge eating. They also improved mood and reduced preoccupation with shape and weight. Most of the positive results, however, were short term, with about one-third relapsing within a 2-year period (Agras, 2006).

SSRIs are now recommended as the drug of first choice in the UK, due to the fact that in terms of their acceptability to clients, their tolerability and their effectiveness, they appear to offer a better alternative than other antidepressants.

APPLICATION OF THE NURSING PROCESS

Although anorexia and bulimia have several differences, many similarities are found in assessing, planning, implementing and evaluating nursing care for clients with these disorders. Thus, this section addresses both eating disorders but highlights differences where they exist.

Assessment

Several specialized tests have been developed for eating disorders. An assessment tool such as the Eating Attitudes Test (see Box 18.1) is often used in studies of anorexia and bulimia. This test can also be used at the end of treatment to evaluate outcomes because it is sensitive to clinical changes.

NICE guidelines (2004) suggest two very straightforward questions that can help identify the need for further assessment:

- 'Do you think you have an eating problem?'
- 'Do you worry excessively about your weight?'

HISTORY

Family members often describe clients with anorexia nervosa as perfectionists with above-average intelligence, achievement oriented, dependable, eager to please and seeking approval before their condition began. Parents describe clients as being 'good, causing us no trouble' until the onset of anorexia. Likewise, clients with bulimia often are focused on pleasing others and avoiding conflict. Clients with bulimia, however, often have a history of impulsive behaviour, such as substance abuse and shoplifting, as well as anxiety, depression and personality disorders (Schultz & Videbeck, 2005).

GENERAL APPEARANCE AND MOTOR BEHAVIOUR

Clients with anorexia can appear slow, lethargic and fatigued; they may be emaciated, depending on the amount of weight loss. They may be slow to respond in conversation and have difficulty deciding what to say. They are often reluctant to answer questions fully because they do not want to acknowledge any problem. They often wear loose-fitting clothes in layers, regardless of the weather, both to hide weight loss and to keep warm (clients with anorexia are generally cold). Eye contact may be limited. Clients may turn away from the nurse, indicating their unwillingness to discuss problems or to enter treatment.

Clients with bulimia may be underweight or overweight but are generally close to expected body weight for age and size. General appearance is not unusual, and they appear open and willing to talk.

MOOD AND AFFECT

Clients with eating disorders have labile moods that usually correspond to their eating or dieting behaviours. Avoiding 'bad' or fattening foods gives them a sense of power and control over their bodies, whereas eating, bingeing or purging leads to anxiety, depression and feeling out of control. People with eating disorders often seem sad, anxious and worried. Those with anorexia seldom smile, laugh or enjoy any attempts at humour; they are sombre and serious most of the time. In contrast, clients with bulimia are initially pleasant and cheerful as though nothing is wrong. The pleasant façade usually disappears when they begin describing binge eating and purging; they may express intense guilt, shame and embarrassment.

It is important to ask clients with eating disorders about thoughts of self-harm or suicide. It is not uncommon for these clients to engage in self-mutilating behaviours such as cutting. Concern about self-harm and suicidal behaviour should increase even more when clients have a history of sexual abuse (see Chapters 11 and 15).

THOUGHT PROCESSES AND CONTENT

Clients with eating disorders spend most of the time thinking about dieting, food and food-related behaviour. They are preoccupied with their attempts to avoid eating or eating 'bad' or 'wrong' foods. Clients cannot think about themselves without thinking about weight and food. The body image disturbance can seem delusional; even if clients are severely underweight, they can point to areas on their buttocks or thighs that are 'still fat', thereby fuelling their need to continue dieting. Clients with anorexia who are severely underweight may have paranoid ideas about their family and health-care professionals, believing they are their 'enemies' who are trying to make them fat by forcing them to eat.

SENSORY AND INTELLECTUAL PROCESSES

Generally, clients with eating disorders are alert and oriented; their intellectual functions are intact. The exception is clients with anorexia who are severely malnourished and showing signs of starvation such as mild confusion, slowed mental processes and difficulty with concentration and attention.

JUDGEMENT AND INSIGHT

Clients with anorexia have very limited insight and poor judgement about their health status. They do not believe they have a problem; rather, they believe others are trying to interfere with their ability to lose weight and to achieve the desired body image. Facts about failing health status are not enough to convince these clients of their true problems. Clients with anorexia continue to restrict food intake or to engage in purging despite the negative effect on health.

In contrast, clients with bulimia are ashamed of the binge eating and purging. They recognize these behaviours as abnormal and go to great lengths to hide them. They feel out of control and unable to change even though they recognize their behaviours as pathological. Box 18.1 shows an Eating Attitudes Test.

SELF-CONCEPT

Low self-esteem is prominent in clients with eating disorders. They see themselves only in terms of their ability to control their food intake and weight. They tend to judge themselves harshly and see themselves as 'bad' if they eat certain foods or fail to lose weight. They overlook or ignore other personal characteristics or achievements as less important than thinness. Clients often perceive themselves as helpless, powerless and ineffective. This feeling of lack of control over themselves and their environment only strengthens their desire to control their weight.

ROLES AND RELATIONSHIPS

Eating disorders interfere with the ability to fulfil roles and to have satisfying relationships. Clients with anorexia may begin to fail at school, which is in sharp contrast to previously successful academic performance. They withdraw from peers and pay little attention to friendships. They believe that others will not understand, or fear they will begin out-of-control eating with others.

Clients with bulimia feel great shame about their binge eating and purging behaviours. As a result, they tend to lead secret lives that include sneaking behind the backs of friends and family to binge and purge in privacy. The time spent buying and eating food and then purging can interfere with role performance both at home and at work.

PHYSIOLOGICAL AND SELF-CARE CONSIDERATIONS

The health status of clients with eating disorders relates directly to the severity of self-starvation, purging behaviours or both (see Table 18.1). In addition, clients may exercise excessively, almost to the point of exhaustion, in an effort to control weight. Many clients have sleep disturbances such as insomnia, reduced sleep time and early-morning wakening. Those who frequently vomit have many dental problems such as loss of tooth enamel, chipped and ragged teeth and dental caries. Frequent vomiting also may result in sores in the mouth. Complete medical and dental examinations are essential.

Data Analysis

Nursing formulations for clients with eating disorders include the following:

- Imbalanced nutrition: less than/more than body requirements
- Ineffective coping
- Disturbed body image.

Box 18.1 EATING ATTITUDES TEST

Please place an (X) under the column that applies best to each of the numbered statements. All the results will be strictly confidential. Most of the questions relate to food or eating, although other types of questions have been included. Please answer each question carefully. Thank you.

	Always	Very Often	Often	Sometimes	Rarely	Never
1. Like eating with other people.						X
2. Prepare foods for others but do not eat what I cook.	X					
3. Become anxious prior to eating.	X					
4. Am terrified about being overweight.	X					
5. Avoid eating when I am hungry.	X					
6. Find myself preoccupied with food.	X					
7. Have gone on eating binges where I feel that I may not be able to stop.	X					
8. Cut food into small pieces.	X					
9. Aware of the calorie content of foods that I eat.	X					
10. Particularly avoid foods with a high carbohydrate content (e.g. bread, potatoes, rice, etc.).	X					
11. Feel bloated after meals.	X					
12. Feel that others would prefer I ate more.	X					
13. Vomit after I have eaten.	X					
14. Feel extremely guilty after eating.	X					
15. Am preoccupied with a desire to be thinner.	X					
16. Exercise strenuously to burn off calories.	X					
17. Weigh myself several times a day.	X					
18. Like my clothes to fit tightly.						X
19. Enjoy eating meat.						X
20. Wake up early in the morning.	X					
21. Eat the same foods day after day.	X					
22. Think about burning up calories when I exercise.	X					
23. Have regular menstrual periods.						X
24. Other people think I am too thin.	X					
25. Am preoccupied with the thought of having fat on my body.	X					
26. Take longer than others to eat.	X					
27. Enjoy eating at restaurants.						X
28. Take laxatives.	X					
29. Avoid foods with sugar in them.	X					
30. Eat diet foods.	X					
31. Feel that food controls my life.	X					
32. Display self-control around food.	X					
33. Feel that others pressure me to eat.	X					
34. Give too much time and thought to food.	X					
35. Suffer from constipation.		X				
36. Feel uncomfortable after eating sweets.	X					
37. Engage in dieting behaviour.	X					
38. Like my stomach to be empty.	X					
39. Enjoy trying new rich foods.						X
40. Have impulse to vomit after meals.	X					

Scoring: The patient is given the questionnaire without the Xs, just blank. Three points are assigned to endorsements that coincide with the Xs; the adjacent alternatives are weighted as 2 points and 1 point, respectively. A total score of over 30 indicates significant concerns with eating behaviour.

Other nursing formulations may be pertinent, such as deficient fluid volume, constipation, fatigue and activity intolerance.

Outcome Identification

For severely malnourished clients, their medical condition must be stabilized before formal psychological treatment can begin. Medical stabilization may include parenteral fluids, total parenteral nutrition and cardiac monitoring.

Examples of expected outcomes for clients with eating disorders include the following:

- The client will establish adequate nutritional eating patterns.
- The client will eliminate use of compensatory behaviours such as excessive exercise and use of laxatives and diuretics.
- The client will demonstrate coping mechanisms not related to food.
- The client will verbalize feelings of guilt, anger, anxiety or an excessive need for control.
- The client will verbalize acceptance of body image with stable body weight.

Interventions

ESTABLISHING NUTRITIONAL EATING PATTERNS

Typically, inpatient treatment is for clients with anorexia nervosa who are severely malnourished, and clients with bulimia whose binge eating and purging behaviours are out of control. Primary nursing roles are to implement and to supervise the regimen for nutritional rehabilitation. Total parenteral nutrition or enteral feedings may be prescribed initially when a client's health status is severely compromised.

Avoiding distressing 'battles' with clients requires high levels of empathy and engagement, good team-work and open, transparent approaches to care. Adult–adult relationships are essential, though there may be times where nurses have to adopt a nurturing parental role in order to intervene to save someone's life.

When clients can eat, a diet of 1200 to 1500 calories per day is often ordered, with gradual increases in calories until clients are ingesting adequate amounts for height, activity level and growth needs. Allotted calories may be divided into three meals and three snacks. A liquid protein supplement can be given to replace any food not eaten, to ensure consumption of the total number of prescribed calories. The nurse is responsible for monitoring meals and snacks and often, initially, will sit with a client during eating at a table away from other clients. Depending on the treatment programme, diet beverages and food substitutions may be prohibited, and a specified time may be set for consuming each meal or snack. Clients may also be discouraged from performing food rituals such as cutting food into tiny pieces or mixing food in unusual combinations. The nurse must be alert for any attempts by clients to hide or to discard food.

After each meal or snack, clients may be required to remain in view of staff for 1 to 2 hours to ensure they do not empty the stomach by vomiting. Some treatment programmes limit client access to bathrooms without supervision, particularly after meals, to discourage vomiting. As clients begin to gain weight and to become more independent in eating behaviour, these restrictions are lessened gradually.

In most treatment programmes, clients are weighed only once daily, usually on awakening and after they have emptied the bladder. Clients should wear minimal clothing - the same as worn when previously weighed and ideally without pockets- each time they are weighed. They may attempt to place objects in their clothing to give the appearance of weight gain.

Clients with bulimia are nearly always treated in the community. The nurse must work closely with clients to establish normal eating patterns and to interrupt the binge and purge cycle. He or she encourages clients to eat meals with their families or, if they live alone, with friends. Clients should always sit at a table in a designated eating area such as a kitchen or dining room. It is easier for clients to follow a nutritious eating plan if it is written in advance and groceries are purchased for the planned menus. Clients must avoid buying foods frequently consumed during binges, such as biscuits, sweets, fizzy drinks and crisps. They should discard, or move to the kitchen, food that was kept at work, in the car or in the bedroom.

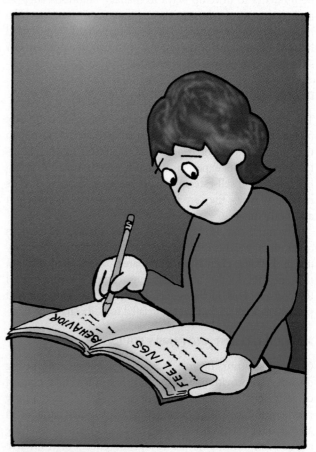

Keeping a feelings diary

IDENTIFYING EMOTIONS AND DEVELOPING COPING STRATEGIES

Because clients with anorexia frequently have problems with self-awareness, they often have difficulty identifying and expressing feelings (**alexithymia**). They may often, therefore, express these feelings in terms of somatic complaints such as feeling fat or bloated. The nurse can help clients begin to recognize emotions such as anxiety or guilt by asking them to describe how they are feeling and allowing adequate time for response. The nurse should not ask, 'Are you sad?' or 'Are you anxious?' because a client may quickly agree rather than struggle for an answer. The nurse encourages the client to describe his or her feelings. This approach can eventually help clients to recognize their emotions and to connect them to their eating behaviours.

Self-monitoring is a cognitive-behavioural technique designed to help clients with bulimia. It may help clients to identify behaviour patterns and then implement techniques to avoid or to replace them (Carter *et al.*, 2003). Self-monitoring techniques raise client awareness about behaviour and help them to regain a sense of control. The nurse encourages clients to keep a diary of all food eaten throughout the day, including binges, and to record moods, emotions, thoughts, circumstances and interactions surrounding eating and bingeing or purging episodes. In this way, clients begin to see connections between emotions and situations and eating behaviours. The nurse can then help clients to develop ways to manage emotions such as anxiety by using relaxation techniques or distraction with music or another activity. This is an important step toward helping clients find ways to cope with people, emotions or situations that do not involve food.

DEALING WITH BODY IMAGE ISSUES

The nurse can help clients to accept a more normal body image. This may involve clients agreeing to weigh more than they would like, to be healthy and to stay out of the hospital. When clients experience relief from emotional distress, have increased self-esteem and are meeting emotional needs in healthy ways, they are more likely to accept their weight and body image.

The nurse can also help clients to view themselves in terms other than weight, size, shape and satisfaction with body image. Helping clients to identify areas of personal strength that are not food-related broadens clients' perceptions of themselves. This includes identifying talents, interests and positive aspects of character unrelated to body shape or size.

PROVIDING CLIENT AND FAMILY EDUCATION

One primary nursing role in caring for clients with eating disorders is providing education to help them take control of nutritional requirements independently. This teaching can be done in an inpatient setting prior to discharge or in an outpatient setting. The nurse provides extensive teaching about basic nutritional needs and the effects of restrictive eating, dieting and the binge and purge cycle. Clients need encouragement to set realistic goals for eating throughout the day (Muscari, 2002). Eating only salads and vegetables during the day may set up clients for later binges as a result of too little fat and carbohydrates.

For clients who purge, the most important goal is – simply – to stop. Teaching should include information about the harmful effects of purging by vomiting and laxative abuse. The nurse should explain – sensitively and respectfully – that purging is an ineffective means of weight control and only disrupts the neuroendocrine system. In addition, purging promotes binge-eating by decreasing the anxiety that follows the binge. The nurse should explain that if clients can avoid purging, they may be less likely to engage in binge-eating. The nurse also teaches the techniques of distraction and delay because they are useful against both bingeing and purging. The longer clients can delay either bingeing or purging, the less likely they are to carry out the behaviour.

The nurse explains to family and friends that they can be most helpful by providing emotional support, love and attention. They can express concern about the client's health, but it is rarely helpful to focus on food intake, calories and weight.

NURSING INTERVENTIONS FOR EATING DISORDERS

- **Establishing nutritional eating patterns**
  Sit with the client during meals and snacks. Avoid confrontation and belittling. Offer liquid protein supplement if client is unable to complete meal.
  Adhere to treatment programme guidelines regarding restrictions.
  Observe client following meals and snacks for 1 to 2 hours.
  Weigh client daily in similar clothing.
  Be alert for attempts to hide or discard food or inflate weight.
- **Helping the client identify emotions and develop non-food-related coping strategies**
  Ask the client to identify thoughts and feelings.
  Self-monitoring using a journal
  Relaxation techniques
  Distraction
  Assist client to change stereotypical beliefs.
- **Helping the client deal with body image issues**
  Recognize benefits of a more near-normal weight.
  Assist to view self in ways not related to body image.
  Identify personal strengths, interests, talents.
- **Providing client and family education** (see Client/ Family Education for Eating Disorders)

CLIENT/FAMILY INTERVENTION FOR EATING DISORDERS

Client
- Basic nutritional needs
- Harmful effects of restrictive eating, dieting, purging
- Realistic goals for eating
- Acceptance of healthy body image

Family and Friends
- Provide emotional support.
- Express concern about client's health.
- Encourage client to seek professional help.
- Avoid talking only about weight, food intake, calories.
- Become informed about eating disorders.
- It is not possible for family and friends to force the client to eat. The client needs professional help.

Evaluation

The nurse can use assessment tools such as the Eating Attitudes Test to detect improvement for clients with eating disorders. Both anorexia and bulimia are chronic for many clients. Residual symptoms such as dieting, compulsive exercising and experiencing discomfort when eating in a social setting are common. Treatment could be considered successful if the client maintains a body weight within 5% to 10% of normal with no medical complications from starvation or purging.

MENTAL HEALTH PROMOTION

Nurses can educate parents, children and young people about strategies to prevent eating disorders. Important aspects include realizing that the 'ideal' figures portrayed in advertisements and magazines are unrealistic, developing realistic ideas about body size and shape, resisting peer pressure to diet, improving self-esteem and learning coping strategies for dealing with emotions and life issues.

The Atlanta Center for Eating Disorders (2006) offers the following advice:

- Read the research about fad diets: they don't work. No-fat diets are unhealthy, and claims about diets that use special combinations of food are unfounded.
- Send the right message to children about food and body image issues. Parents who are constantly worrying about, or talking about, weight, or are always 'on a diet', powerfully influence their children. Give up dieting and eat well-balanced meals.

- Listen to your conversations. Weight, dieting and appearance are among the most common topics for women. Make a pact with friends to stop talking about your bodies negatively.
- Focus on the positive aspects of yourself and others that have nothing to do with physical appearance.
- Encourage healthy expression of emotions. Learn positive ways to communicate.
- Give up wanting to be thin before doing anything, and get on with enjoying your life.
- Increase physical activity by focusing on the enjoyment of movement, not on how many calories you'll burn.

School nurses, CAMHS nurses, CMHNs in primary care and early intervention teams and many others may encounter clients in various settings who are at risk of developing, or who already have, an eating disorder. In these settings, early identification and appropriate referral are primary responsibilities of the nurse. Routine screening of all young women in these settings would help identify those at risk for an eating disorder. Box 18.2 contains a sample of questions that can be used for such screening. Such early identification could result in early intervention and prevention of a full-blown eating disorder.

SELF-AWARENESS ISSUES

Many health professionals themselves have problematic relationships with food, eating and weight: they need to develop awareness of these and address them honestly wherever possible.

An emaciated, starving client with anorexia can be a shocking sight, and the nurse may want to 'take care of this person' and nurse her back to health. When the client rejects this help and resists the nurse's caring actions, the nurse can become angry and frustrated and feel incompetent to handle the situation.

Box 18.2 SAMPLE SCREENING QUESTIONS

- How often do you feel dissatisfied with your body shape or size?
- Do you think you are fat or need to lose weight, even when others say you are thin?
- Do thoughts about food, weight, dieting and eating dominate your life?
- Do you eat to make yourself feel better emotionally, and then feel guilty about it?

Nursing Care Plan *Bulimia*

Nursing Formulation

Ineffective Coping: *Inability to form a valid appraisal of the stressors, inadequate choices of practised responses and/or inability to use available resources.*

ASSESSMENT DATA

- Inability to meet basic needs
- Inability to ask for help
- Inability to problem solve
- Inability to change behaviours
- Self-destructive behaviour
- Suicidal thoughts or behaviour
- Inability to delay gratification
- Poor impulse control
- Stealing or shoplifting behaviour
- Desire for perfection
- Feelings of worthlessness
- Feelings of inadequacy or guilt
- Unsatisfactory interpersonal relationships
- Self-deprecatory verbalization
- Denial of feelings, illness or problems
- Anxiety
- Sleep disturbances
- Low self-esteem
- Excessive need to control
- Feelings of being out of control
- Preoccupation with weight, food or diets
- Distortions of body image
- Overuse of laxatives, diet pills or diuretics
- Secrecy regarding eating habits or amounts eaten
- Fear of being fat
- Recurrent vomiting
- Binge eating
- Compulsive eating
- Substance use

EXPECTED OUTCOMES

Immediate
The client will
- Be free from self-inflicted harm
- Identify methods not related to food of dealing with stress or crises
- Verbalize feelings of guilt, anxiety, anger or an excessive need for control

Medium-term
The client will
- Demonstrate more satisfying interpersonal relationships
- Demonstrate alternative methods of dealing with stress or crises
- Eliminate shoplifting or stealing behaviours
- Express feelings in ways not related to food
- Verbalize understanding of disease process and safe use of medications, if any

Ongoing
The client will
- Verbalize more realistic body image
- Follow through with discharge planning, including support groups or therapy as indicated
- Verbalize increased self-esteem and self-confidence

IMPLEMENTATION

Nursing Interventions *denotes collaborative interventions	**Rationale**
Set limits with the client about eating habits, e.g. food will be eaten in a dining room setting, at a table, only at conventional mealtimes.	Limits will discourage binge behaviour, such as hiding, sneaking and gulping food, and help the client return to normal eating patterns. Eating three meals a day will prevent starvation and subsequent overeating in the evening.
Encourage the client to eat with other clients, when tolerated.	Eating with other people will discourage secrecy about eating, though initially the client's anxiety may be too high to join others at mealtime.
Encourage the client to express feelings, such as anxiety and guilt about having eaten.	Expressing feelings can help decrease the client's anxiety and the urge to engage in purging behaviours.

Nursing Care Plan: Bulimia, cont.

IMPLEMENTATION

Nursing Interventions *denotes collaborative interventions	Rationale
Ask the client directly about thoughts of suicide or self-harm.	The client's safety is a priority. You will NOT 'give the client ideas' about suicide by addressing the issue directly.
Encourage the client to use a diary to write types and amounts of foods eaten and feelings that occur before, during and after eating, especially related to urges to engage in binge or purge behaviour.	A diary can help the client explore food intake, feelings and relationships among these feelings and behaviours. Initially, the client may be able to write about these feelings and behaviours more easily than talk about them.
Encourage the client to describe and discuss feelings verbally. Begin to separate dealing with feelings from eating or purging behaviours. Maintain a non-judgemental approach.	Being non-judgemental gives the client permission to discuss feelings that may be negative or unacceptable to him or her without fear of rejection or reprisal.
Discuss the types of foods that are soothing to the client and that relieve anxiety.	You may be able to help the client see how he or she has used food to deal with feelings.
Help the client explore ways to relieve anxiety, express feelings and experience pleasure that are not related to food or eating.	It is important to help the client separate emotional issues from food and eating behaviours.
Give positive feedback for the client's efforts to discuss feelings.	Your sincere praise can promote the client's attempts to deal openly and honestly with anxiety, anger and other feelings.
*Teach the client and significant others about bulimic behaviours, physical complications, nutrition and so forth. Refer the client to a dietitian if indicated.	The client and significant others may have little knowledge of the disorder, food and nutrition. Factual information can be useful in dispelling incorrect beliefs and in separating food from emotional issues.
*Teach the client and significant others about the purpose, action, timing and possible adverse effects of medications, if any.	Antidepressants and other medications may be prescribed for bulimia. Remember, some antidepressant medications may take several weeks to achieve a therapeutic effect.
Teach the client about the use of the problem-solving process.	Successful use of the problem-solving process can help increase the client's self-esteem and confidence.
Explore with the client his or her personal strengths. Making a written list is sometimes helpful.	You can help the client discover his or her strengths; he or she needs to identify them, so it will not be useful for you to make a list for the client.
Discuss with the client the idea of accepting a less than 'ideal' body weight.	The client's previous expectations or perception of an ideal weight may have been unrealistic, and even unhealthy.
Encourage the client to incorporate fattening (or 'bad') foods into the diet as he or she tolerates.	This will enhance the client's sense of control of overeating.
Encourage the client to express his or her feelings about family members and significant others, their roles and relationships.	Expressing feelings can help the client to identify, accept and work through feelings in a direct manner.
*Refer the client to assertiveness training books or classes if indicated.	Many bulimic clients are passive in interpersonal relationships. Assertiveness training may foster a sense of increased confidence and healthier relationship dynamics.
*Refer the client to long-term therapy if indicated. Contracting with the client may be helpful to promote follow through with continuing therapy.	Treatment for eating disorders is often a long-term process. The client may be more likely to engage in ongoing therapy if he or she has contracted to do this.

continued ···>

Nursing Care Plan: Bulimia, cont.

IMPLEMENTATION

Nursing Interventions *denotes collaborative interventions	Rationale
*Ongoing therapy may need to include significant others to sustain the client's non-food-related coping skills. *Refer the client and family and significant others to support groups in the community or via the Internet (e.g. BEAT at http://www.b-eat.co.uk/Home). *Refer the client to a substance misuse treatment programme or support group (e.g. AA), if appropriate.	Dysfunctional relationships with significant others are often a primary issue for clients with eating disorders. These groups can offer support, education and resources to clients and their families or significant others. Substance use is common among clients with bulimia.

Adapted from Schultz, J. M. & Videbeck, S. L. (2005). *Lippincott's manual of psychiatric nursing care plans* (7th edn). Philadelphia: Lippincott Williams & Wilkins.

The client may initially view the nurse, who is responsible for making the client eat, as the enemy. The client may hide or throw away food or become overtly hostile as anxiety about eating increases. The nurse must remember that the person's behaviour is a symptom of anxiety and fear about gaining weight and not personally directed toward the nurse. Taking the client's behaviour personally may cause the nurse to feel angry and behave in a rejecting manner – thus compounding the person's view of themselves and others.

Because eating is such a basic part of everyday life, the nurse may wonder why the client cannot just eat 'like everyone else'. The nurse may also find it difficult to understand how a four and a half stone client sees herself as fat when she looks in the mirror. Likewise, when working with a client who binges and purges, the nurse may wonder why the client cannot exert the willpower to stop. The nurse must remember that the client's eating behaviour has become out of control. Eating disorders are mental disorders, just like schizophrenia and bipolar affective disorder.

Points to Consider When Working With Clients With Eating Disorders

- Remain empathic and non-judgemental, even though this is not easy. Remember the client's perspective and fears about weight and eating. Ensure that ongoing formal clinical supervision is available.
- Avoid being parental when talking about nutrition or why laxative use is harmful. Presenting information factually without chiding the client will obtain more positive results.
- Do not label clients as 'good' when they avoid purging or eat an entire meal. Otherwise, clients may believe they are 'bad' on days when they purge or fail to eat enough food.

Critical Thinking Questions

1. You notice a friend or family member has been losing weight, has strange eating rituals and constantly talks about dieting. You suspect an eating disorder. How would you approach this person?
2. A client has the right to refuse treatment. How might a CMHN address this right when working with a client with anorexia who is losing weight rapidly and who doesn't want treatment?

 ## KEY POINTS

- Anorexia nervosa is a life-threatening eating disorder characterized by body weight less than 85% of normal, an intense fear of being fat, a severely distorted body image and refusal to eat, or binge eating and purging.
- Bulimia nervosa is an eating disorder that involves recurrent episodes of binge eating and compensatory behaviours such as purging, using laxatives and diuretics or exercising excessively.
- Ninety per cent of clients with eating disorders are female. Anorexia usually begins between the ages of 14 and 18, and bulimia usually begins around age 18 or 19.
- Many neurochemical changes are present in individuals with eating disorders, but it is uncertain whether these changes cause or are a result of the eating disorders.
- Persons with eating disorders feel unattractive and ineffective and may be poorly equipped to deal with the challenges of maturity.
- Societal attitudes regarding thinness, beauty, desirability and physical fitness may influence the development of eating disorders.

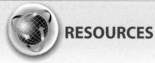

INTERNET RESOURCES

RESOURCES	INTERNET ADDRESS
• Anorexia and Bulimia Care (a Christian organization)	http://www.anorexiabulimiacare.co.uk/
• BEAT: Eating Disorders Association	http://www.b-eat.co.uk/Home
• BMJ Clinical Evidence	http://clinicalevidence.bmj.com/ceweb/conditions/meh/1011/1011.jsp
• Bodywhys – The Eating Disorders Association of Ireland	www.bodywhys.ie

- Severely malnourished clients with anorexia nervosa may require intensive medical treatment and nursing care to restore homeostasis before any psychiatric treatment can begin.
- CBT, DBT and family therapies seem to be effective for clients with anorexia; CBT seems to be most effective for clients with bulimia.
- Interventions for clients with eating disorders include establishing nutritional eating patterns, helping the client to identify emotions and to develop coping strategies not related to food, helping the client to deal with body image issues and providing client and family education.
- Focus on healthy eating and pleasurable physical exercise; avoid fad or stringent dieting.
- Parents must become aware of their own behaviour and attitudes and the way they influence children.

REFERENCES

Agras, W. S. (2006). Treatment of eating disorders. In A. F. Schatzberg & C. B. Nemeroff (Eds.), *Essentials of clinical psychopharmacology* (2nd edn, pp. 669–687). Washington DC: American Psychiatric Publishing.

American Psychiatric Association. (2000). *Diagnostic and statistical manual of mental disorders* (4th edn, text revision). Washington, DC: American Psychiatric Association.

Andersen, A. E. & Yager, J. (2005). Eating disorders. In B. J. Sadock & V. A. Sadock (Eds.), *Comprehensive textbook of psychiatry, Vol. 1* (8th edn, pp. 2002–2021). Philadelphia: Lippincott Williams & Wilkins.

Andreasen, N. C. & Black, D. W. (2006). *Introductory textbook of psychiatry* (4th edn). Washington DC: American Psychiatric Publishing.

Atlanta Center for Eating Disorders. (2006). How can you help prevent eating disorders? Available: http://eatingdisorders.home.mindspring.com/causes2.htm.

Callaghan, P. (2006). Working with a person with anorexia nervosa. In P. Callaghan & H. Waldock (Eds.), *Oxford handbook of mental health nursing*. Oxford: Oxford University Press.

Carter, J. C., Olmsed, M. P., Kaplan, A. S., et al. (2003). Self-help for bulimia nervosa: A randomized controlled trial. *American Journal of Psychiatry, 160*(5), 973–978.

Carter, J. C., Bewell, C., Blackmore, E., & Woodside, D. B. (2006). The impact of childhood sexual abuse in anorexia nervosa. *Child Abuse & Neglect, 30*(3), 257–269.

Cassin, S. E. & von Ranson, K. M. (2005). Personality and eating disorders: A decade in review. *Clinical Psychology Review, 25*(7), 895–916.

Eating Disorders Association. (2008a). *Eating disorders . . . an athlete's guide.* Available: http://www.b-eat.co.uk/Publications/InformationSheets/main_content/Eatingdisorders-Anathletesguide.pdf

Eating Disorders Association. (2008b). *Eating disorders . . . a coach's guide.* Available: http://www.b-eat.co.uk/Publications/InformationSheets/main_content/Eatingdisorders-Ancoachsguide.pdf

Fairburn, C. G., Cooper, Z., Doll, H. A., & Davies, B. A. (2005). Identifying dieters who will develop an eating disorder: A prospective, population-based study. *American Journal of Psychiatry, 162*(12), 2249–2255.

Fletcher, E. (2003). The person with an eating disorder. In P. Barker (Ed.), *Psychiatric and mental health nursing: the craft of caring*. London: Arnold.

Johnson, F. & Wardle, J. (2005). Dietary restraint, body dissatisfaction, and psychological distress: A prospective analysis. *Journal of Abnormal Psychology, 114*(1), 119–125.

Linehan, M. (1993). *Cognitive behavioural treatment of borderline personality disorder.* New York: Guilford.

Marcus, M. & Levine, M. (2004). Use of dialectical behaviour therapy in the eating disorders. In T. Brewerton (Ed.) *Clinical handbook of eating disorders: an integrated approach*. New York: Marcel Dekker.

Middleton, K. (2007). *Eating disorders: the path to recovery*. Oxford: Lion Hudson.

Muscari, M. (2002). Effective management of adolescents with anorexia and bulimia. *Journal of Psychosocial Nursing, 40*(2), 23–31.

National Collaborating Centre For Mental Health. (2004). *Eating disorders: Core interventions in the treatment and management of anorexia nervosa, bulimia nervosa and related eating disorders*. Available: http://www.nice.org.uk/guidance/index.jsp?action=byID&r=true&o=10932

NICE. (2004). Eating disorders: Core interventions in the treatment and management of anorexia nervosa, bulimia nervosa and related eating disorders. Available: http://www.nice.org.uk/guidance/index.jsp?action=byID&r=true&o=10932

O'Reardon, J. P., Peshek, A., & Allison K. C. (2005). Night eating syndrome: diagnosis, epidemiology, and management. *CNS Drugs, 19*(12), 997–1008.

Pope, H. G. Jr, Lalonde, J. K., Pindyck, L. J., et al. (2006). Binge eating disorder: A stable syndrome. *American Journal of Psychiatry, 163*(12), 2181–2183.

Preti, A., Incani, E., Camboni, M. V., et al. (2006). Sexual abuse and eating disorder symptoms: The mediator role of bodily dissatisfaction. *Comprehensive Psychiatry, 47*(6), 475–481.

Royal College of Psychiatrists. (2008). Changing minds: anorexia and bulimia. Available: http://www.rcpsych.ac.uk/default.aspx?page=1428

Schultz, J. M. & Videbeck, S. L. (2005). *Lippincott's manual of psychiatric nursing care plans* (7th edn). Philadelphia: Lippincott Williams & Wilkins.

Seamoore, D., Buckroyd, J., & Stott, D. (2006). Changes in eating behaviour following group therapy for women who binge eat: a pilot study. *Journal of Psychiatric and Mental Health Nursing, 13*(3), 337–346.

Waldrop, J. (2005). Early identification and interventions for female athlete triad. *Journal of Pediatric Health Care, 19*(4), 213–220.

Waller, G., Cordery, H., Corstophine, E., *et al.* (2007). *Cognitive behavioural therapy for eating disorders: A comprehensive treatment guide.* Cambridge: Cambridge University Press

Willer, M. G., Thuras, P., & Crow, S. J. (2005). Implications of the changing use of hospitalization to treat anorexia nervosa. *American Journal of Psychiatry, 162*(12), 2374–2376.

ADDITIONAL READING

Shiina, A., Nakazato, M., Mitsumori, M., *et al.* (2005). An open trial of outpatient group therapy for bulimic disorders: Combination program of cognitive behavioural therapy with assertive training and self-esteem enhancement. *Psychiatry and Clinical Neurosciences, 59*(6), 690–696.

Wiser, S. & Telch, C. F. (1999). Dialectic behaviour therapy for binge eating disorder. *Journal of Clinical Psychology, 55*(6), 755–768.

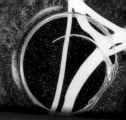

Chapter Study Guide

MULTIPLE-CHOICE QUESTIONS

Select the best answer for each of the following questions.

1. Treating clients with anorexia nervosa with a SSRI antidepressant such as fluoxetine (Prozac) may present which of the following problems?
   a. Clients object to the side-effect of weight gain.
   b. Fluoxetine can cause appetite suppression and weight loss.
   c. Fluoxetine can cause clients to become giddy and silly.
   d. Clients with anorexia get no benefit from fluoxetine.

2. Which of the following is an example of a specifically cognitive-behavioural technique?
   a. Distraction
   b. Relaxation
   c. Self-monitoring
   d. Verbalization of emotions

3. The nurse is working with a client with anorexia nervosa. Even though the client has been eating all her meals and snacks, her weight has remained unchanged for a week. Which of the following interventions is indicated?
   a. Supervise the client closely for 2 hours after meals and snacks.
   b. Increase the daily caloric intake from 1500 to 2000 calories.
   c. Increase the client's fluid intake.
   d. Request a prescription for fluoxetine.

4. Which of the following statements is true?
   a. Anorexia nervosa was not recognized as an 'illness' until the 1960s.
   b. Cultures where beauty is linked to thinness have an increased risk of eating disorders.
   c. Eating disorders are a major health problem only in Europe and North America.
   d. People with anorexia nervosa are popular with their peers as a result of their thinness.

5. All but which of the following are initial goals for treating the severely malnourished client with anorexia nervosa?
   a. Correction of body image disturbance
   b. Correction of electrolyte imbalances
   c. Nutritional rehabilitation
   d. Weight restoration

6. The nurse is evaluating the progress of a client with bulimia. Which of the following behaviours would indicate that the client is making positive progress?
   a. The client can identify calorie content for each meal.
   b. The client identifies healthy ways of coping with anxiety.
   c. The client spends time resting in her room after meals.
   d. The client verbalizes knowledge of former eating patterns as unhealthy.

7. A teenage girl is being evaluated for an eating disorder. Which of the following might suggest anorexia nervosa?
   a. Guilt and shame about eating patterns
   b. Lack of knowledge about food and nutrition
   c. Refusal to talk about food-related topics
   d. Unrealistic perception of body size

8. A client with bulimia is learning to use the technique of self-monitoring. Which of the following interventions by the nurse would be most beneficial for this client?
   a. Ask the client to write about all feelings and experiences related to food.
   b. Assist the client to make out daily meal plans for 1 week.
   c. Encourage the client to ignore feelings and impulses related to food.
   d. Teach the client about nutrition content and calories of various foods.

FILL-IN-THE-BLANK QUESTIONS

Identify each of the following characteristics as being typical of anorexia nervosa, bulimia nervosa or both.

_____ Person puts on a pleasant and cheerful face for others.

_____ Person spends the majority of time thinking about food and food-related activities.

_____ Person believes if she starts eating, she will not be able to stop.

_____ Person believes there is no problem with her dieting behaviour.

_____ Person is guilty and ashamed about her eating behaviour.

GROUP DISCUSSION TOPICS

1. How much do you think the culture you grew up in has put pressure on you to be a certain weight?

2. Why are there different cultural expectations for men and women regarding weight?

3. Should a nurse who is overweight work with people with anorexia?

CLINICAL EXAMPLE

Judy is a 17-year-old sixth-former who is active in gymnastics. She is 5 feet, 7 inches tall, weighs six and a half stone and has not had a period for 5 months. The GP referred her to the eating disorders team with a diagnosis of anorexia nervosa. During the admission interview, Judy is defensive about her weight loss, stating she needs to be thin to be competitive in her sport. Judy points to areas on her buttocks and thighs, saying, 'See this? I still have plenty of fat. Why can't everyone just leave me alone?'

1. Identify two nursing formulations that might be helpful for Judy.

2. Write an expected outcome for each identified nursing formulation.

3. List three nursing interventions for each nursing formulation.

Somatoform Disorders and the Mind–Body Relationship

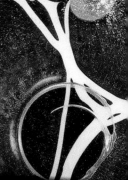

Key Terms

- **body dysmorphic disorder**
- **conversion disorder**
- **disease conviction**
- **disease phobia**
- **emotion-focused coping strategies**
- **factitious disorders**
- **hypochondriasis**
- **hysteria**
- **internalization**
- ***la belle indifférence***
- **malingering**
- **Munchausen syndrome**
- **Munchausen syndrome by proxy**
- **pain disorder**
- **primary gain**
- **problem-focused coping strategies**
- **psychosomatic**
- **secondary gain**
- **somatization**
- **somatization disorder**
- **somatoform disorders**

Learning Objectives

After reading this chapter, you should be able to:

1. Examine and begin to explain the interrelationship between physical health and mental health.

2. Understand what is meant by 'psychosomatic' or 'psychogenic' illness.

3. Describe somatoform disorders and identify their three central features.

4. Discuss the aetiological theories related to somatoform disorders.

5. Discuss the characteristics and dynamics of specific somatoform disorders.

6. Distinguish somatoform disorders from factitious disorders and malingering.

7. Apply the nursing process to the care of clients with somatoform disorders.

8. Provide education to clients, families and the community to increase knowledge and understanding of somatoform disorders.

9. Evaluate your feelings, beliefs and attitudes regarding clients with somatoform disorders.

There is much debate in scientific circles and within mental health nursing and other allied professions about the relative influences of environmental (both physical and political/social), physical (genetics, biology, chemistry) and psychological (meaning and purpose, cognitions, beliefs, emotions, feelings) factors on people's well-being, on mental health and on mental disorder. What we even mean by 'mental' or 'psychological' is, of course, debatable: are thoughts and beliefs and emotions not, in themselves, ultimately functions of the brain and nervous system and, therefore, physical?

That a whole host of factors – social, psychological, political, economic, genetic, biological, chemical – have significant roles to play in health and illness (and in helping us try to understand people and work with them effectively) is indisputable. Yet services and related professions have, traditionally, separated themselves (and their clients) into the 'social', the 'physical' and the 'psychological', often with the result of fragmenting care and fragmenting people: mental health services are notoriously poor at assessing and treating physical health problems, physical health services may be poor at assessing and intervening when someone has a mental health problem. 'Holistic' care is much talked about, but rarely delivered.

The influence of physical factors on the psychological and the social – and vice versa – is, of course, exceptionally difficult to define and it may well be that we all experience a cyclical process (rather than the 'dualistic' one we tend to adopt as a culture) in which each impacts endlessly on the other. This complexity is brought into relief by so-called 'psychosomatic' or 'somatoform' disorders.

In the early 1800s, medicine began to consider the various social and psychological factors that influence physical illness. The term '**psychosomatic**' began to be used to convey the connection between the mind (*psyche*) and the body (*soma*) in states of health and illness. Essentially, the argument was that the 'mind' can cause the body to create physical symptoms or to worsen physical illnesses. Real symptoms can begin, continue or be worsened as a result of emotional factors. Examples include diabetes, hypertension and colitis, all of which are medical illnesses undoubtedly influenced by people's environment and by their cognitions, emotions and behaviour. When a person is under a lot of stress or is not coping well with stress, symptoms of these medical illnesses may well worsen. In addition, stress can cause physical symptoms unrelated to a diagnosable medical illness. After a stressful day at work, many of us experience 'tension headaches' that can be very real and very uncomfortable. These headaches are a manifestation of stress rather than a symptom of an underlying medical problem.

Though rarely used in contemporary UK mental health care, due to its pejorative, often sexist connotations, the term '**hysteria**' refers – in psychiatry – to physical complaints with no organic basis; these complaints are often described dramatically. The concept probably originated in Egypt around 4000 years old; in the Middle Ages, hysteria was associated with witchcraft, demons and sorcerers. People with 'hysteria' – usually women (the term derives from the same Greek root as 'hysterectomy') – were considered evil or possessed by evil spirits.

At the end of the 19th century, Paul Briquet and Jean Martin Charcot, both (male!) French physicians, identified 'hysteria' as a disorder of the nervous system. Sigmund Freud, working with Charcot, observed that his patients (usually women!) with hysteria seemed to improve with hypnosis and experienced relief from their physical symptoms when they recalled memories and expressed emotions. This development led Freud to propose that people can *convert* unexpressed emotions into physical symptoms (Hollifield, 2005), a process now referred to as *conversion* or *somatization*. This chapter discusses **somatoform disorders**, which are based on this concept of somatization.

OVERVIEW OF SOMATOFORM DISORDERS

Somatization can be defined, then, as the transference of mental experiences and states into bodily symptoms. Somatoform disorders can be characterized as the presence of physical symptoms that suggest a medical condition without a demonstrable organic basis to account fully for them. The three central features of somatoform disorders are as follows:

- Physical complaints that suggest major medical illness but have no demonstrable organic basis.
- Psychological factors and conflicts seem important in initiating, exacerbating and maintaining the symptoms.
- Symptoms or magnified health concerns are not under the client's conscious control (Hollifield, 2005).

Clients are convinced that they harbour serious physical problems despite negative results during diagnostic testing. They actually experience these physical symptoms as well as the accompanying pain, distress and functional limitations such symptoms induce. Clients do not wilfully control the physical symptoms. Although their symptoms are psychological in nature and driven by anxiety, many clients do not seek help from mental health professionals. Unfortunately, many professionals who do not understand the nature of somatoform disorders are not sympathetic to these clients' complaints (Andreasen & Black, 2006). Nurses must remember that these clients really experience the symptoms they describe and cannot control them voluntarily.

The five specific somatoform disorders are as follows (American Psychiatric Association, 2000):

- **Somatization disorder** is characterized by multiple physical symptoms. It begins by 30 years of age, extends over several years, and includes a combination of pain and gastrointestinal, sexual and pseudoneurological symptoms.
- **Conversion disorder**, sometimes called conversion reaction, involves unexplained, usually sudden deficits

DSM-IV-TR DIAGNOSTIC CRITERIA: SYMPTOMS OF SOMATIZATION DISORDER

Pain symptoms: complaints of headache; pain in the abdomen, head, joints, back, chest, rectum; pain during urination, menstruation or sexual intercourse

Gastrointestinal symptoms: nausea, bloating, vomiting (other than during pregnancy), diarrhoea or intolerance of several foods

Sexual symptoms: sexual indifference, erectile or ejaculatory dysfunction, irregular menses, excessive menstrual bleeding, vomiting throughout pregnancy

Pseudoneurological symptoms: conversion symptoms such as impaired co-ordination or balance, paralysis or localized weakness, difficulty swallowing or lump in throat, aphonia, urinary retention, hallucinations, loss of touch or pain sensation, double vision, blindness, deafness, seizures; dissociative symptoms such as amnesia; or loss of consciousness other than fainting

Adapted from American Psychiatric Association. (2000). *Diagnostic and Statistical Manual of Mental Disorders* (4th edn, text revision). Washington, DC: APA.

in sensory or motor function (e.g. blindness, paralysis). These deficits suggest a neurological disorder but are associated with psychological factors. An attitude of *la belle indifférence*, a seeming lack of concern or distress, is a key feature.

- **Pain disorder** has the primary physical symptom of pain, which generally is unrelieved by analgesics and greatly affected by psychological factors in terms of onset, severity, exacerbation and maintenance.
- **Hypochondriasis** is preoccupation with the fear that one has a serious disease (**disease conviction**) or will get a serious disease (**disease phobia**). It is thought that clients with this disorder misinterpret bodily sensations or functions.
- **Body dysmorphic disorder** is preoccupation with an imagined or exaggerated defect in physical appearance, such as thinking one's nose is too large or teeth are crooked and unattractive.

Somatization disorder, conversion disorder and pain disorder seem to be more common in women than in men; hypochondriasis and body dysmorphic disorder (BDD) seem to be distributed equally by gender, though UK statistics are hard to find (the work of Philips & Castle (2001) and Lucas (2002) suggests there has been an increase in men with BDD over the past few years and that it may be associated with increased risk of suicide and – in rare instances – be a trigger for aggression and violence). In the US, somatization disorder occurs in 0.2% to 2% of the gen-

eral population, conversion disorder in less than 1% of the population. Hypochondriasis is estimated to occur in 4% to 9% of people seen in general practice. No clear statistics of the incidence of body dysmorphic disorder or of pain disorder are available (American Psychiatric Association, 2000).

ONSET AND CLINICAL COURSE

Clients with somatization disorder and body dysmorphic disorder often experience symptoms in adolescence, although these diagnoses may not be made until early adulthood (about 25 years of age). Conversion disorder usually occurs between 10 and 35 years of age. Pain disorder and hypochondriasis can occur at any age (American Psychiatric Association, 2000).

All the somatoform disorders are usually either chronic or recurrent, lasting for decades for many people. Clients with somatization disorder and conversion disorder will most likely seek help from mental health professionals after they have exhausted efforts at finding a diagnosed medical condition. Clients with hypochondriasis, pain disorder and body dysmorphic disorder are unlikely to receive treatment in mental health settings unless they have a co-morbid condition. Clients with somatoform disorders tend to go from one GP or clinic to another, or they may see multiple professionals at once in an effort to obtain relief of symptoms. They tend to be pessimistic about the medical establishment and often believe

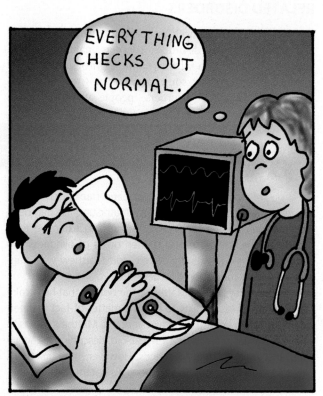

Somatoform disorders

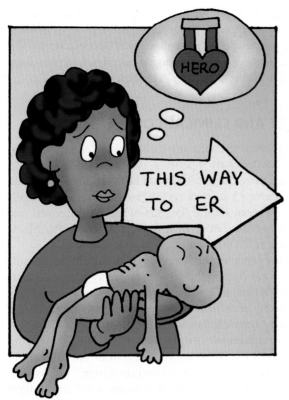

Munchausen syndrome by proxy

their disease could be diagnosed if clinicians were more competent.

RELATED DISORDERS

Somatoform disorders need to be distinguished from other body-related mental disorders, such as malingering and factitious disorders, in which people feign or intentionally produce symptoms for some purpose or gain. In malingering and factitious disorders, people wilfully control

the symptoms. In somatoform disorders, clients *do not* voluntarily control their physical symptoms.

Malingering is the intentional production of false or grossly exaggerated physical or psychological symptoms; it is motivated by external incentives such as avoiding work, evading criminal prosecution, obtaining financial compensation or obtaining drugs. People who malinger have no real physical symptoms or grossly exaggerate relatively minor symptoms. Their purpose is some external incentive or outcome that they view as important and results directly from the illness. People who malinger can stop the physical symptoms as soon as they have gained what they wanted (Wang *et al.*, 2005). Though there is no doubt there are people who 'malinger', it is a sad reflection on attitudes within the mental health services that many people with genuine psychological difficulties – particularly those who meet the criteria for personality disorders – are dismissed as 'malingering'.

Factitious disorder occurs when a person intentionally produces or feigns physical or psychological symptoms solely to gain attention. People with factitious disorder may even inflict injury on themselves to receive attention. The common term for factitious disorder is **Munchausen syndrome**. A variation of factitious disorder, **Munchausen syndrome by proxy**, occurs when a person inflicts illness or injury on someone else to gain the attention of emergency medical personnel or to be a 'hero' for saving the victim. An example would be a nurse who gives excess intravenous potassium to a client and then 'saves his life' by performing cardiopulmonary resuscitation. Although factitious disorders are uncommon, they seem to occur most often in people who are in, or familiar with, medical professions, such as nurses, physicians, medical technicians or hospital volunteers. People who injure or kill clients or their children through 'Munchausen syndrome by proxy' are generally arrested and prosecuted through the legal system (Ragaisis, 2004), though recent expert opinion (especially in the UK and Australia) has

---

CLINICAL VIGNETTE: CONVERSION DISORDER

Matthew, 13, has just been transferred from a medical ward to the adolescent psychiatric unit. He had been on the medical unit for 3 days, undergoing extensive tests to determine the cause of a sudden onset of blindness. No organic pathology was discovered, and Matthew was diagnosed with a conversion disorder.

As the nurse talks to Matthew, she notices that he is calm and speaks of his inability to see in a matter-of-fact manner, demonstrating no distress at his blindness. Matthew seems to have the usual interests of a 13-year-old, describing his activities at school and with his friends. However, the nurse finds that Matthew has little to say about his parents, his younger brother or activities at home.

Later, the nurse has a chance to talk to Matthew's mother when she comes to the unit after work. Soon, Matthew's mother is crying, telling the nurse that her husband has a drinking problem and has been increasingly violent at home. She admitted that 2 days before Matthew's symptoms developed, Matthew witnessed one of his father's rages, which included breaking furniture and hitting her. When Matthew tried to help his mother, his father called him spineless and worthless and told him to go to his bedroom and stay there. The nurse wonders if the violence Matthew has witnessed and his inability to change the situation may be the triggering event for his conversion disorder.

thrown doubt on the existence of the syndrome as a separate clinical entity, rather than merely as a set of behaviours.

AETIOLOGY

Psychosocial Theories

Many psychosocial theorists believe that people with somatoform disorders keep stress, anxiety or frustration inside rather than expressing them outwardly. This is called **internalization**. Clients express these internalized feelings and stress through physical symptoms (somatization). Both internalization and somatization are unconscious defence mechanisms. Clients are not consciously aware of the process, and they do not voluntarily control it.

People with somatoform disorders do not readily and directly express their feelings and emotions verbally. They have tremendous difficulty dealing with interpersonal conflict. When placed in situations involving conflict or emotional stress, their physical symptoms appear to worsen. The worsening of physical symptoms helps them to meet psychological needs for security, attention and affection through primary and secondary gain (Hollifield, 2005). **Primary gains** are the direct external benefits that being sick provides, such as relief of anxiety, conflict or distress. **Secondary gains** are the internal or personal benefits received from others because one is sick, such as attention from family members and comfort measures (e.g. being brought tea, receiving a back rub). The person soon learns that he or she 'needs to be sick' to have their emotional needs met.

Somatization is associated most often with women, as evidenced by the old term *hysteria* (Greek for 'wandering uterus'). Ancient theorists believed that unexplained female pains resulted from migration of the uterus throughout the woman's body. Psychosocial theorists posit that increased incidence of somatization in women may be related to various factors:

- Boys in the UK are still taught to be stoical and to 'act like a man', causing them to offer fewer physical complaints as adults.
- Women seek medical treatment more often than men, and it is more socially acceptable for them to do so.
- Childhood sexual abuse, which is related to somatization, happens more frequently to girls.
- Women more often receive treatment for psychiatric disorders with strong somatic components, such as depression.

Biological Theories

Research has shown differences in the way that clients with somatoform disorders regulate and interpret stimuli. These clients cannot sort relevant from irrelevant stimuli, and respond equally to both types. In other words, they may experience a normal body sensation such as peristalsis

and attach a pathological rather than a normal meaning to it (Hollifield, 2005). Too little inhibition of sensory input amplifies awareness of physical symptoms and exaggerates response to bodily sensations. For example, minor discomfort such as muscle tightness becomes amplified because of the client's concern and attention to the tightness. This amplified sensory awareness causes the person to experience somatic sensations as more intense, noxious and disturbing (Andreasen & Black, 2006).

Somatization disorder is found in 10% to 20% of female first-degree relatives of people with this disorder. Conversion symptoms are found more often in relatives of people with conversion disorder. First-degree relatives of those with pain disorder are more likely to have depressive disorders, alcohol dependence and chronic pain (American Psychiatric Association, 2000).

CULTURAL CONSIDERATIONS

The type and frequency of somatic symptoms and their meaning may vary across cultures. Pseudoneurological symptoms of somatization disorder in Africa and South Asia include burning hands and feet and the non-delusional sensation of worms in the head or ants under the skin. Symptoms related to male reproduction are more common in some countries or cultures – for example, men in India often have *dhat*, which is a hypochondriacal concern about loss of semen. Somatization disorder is rare in men in the UK or US but more common in Greece and Puerto Rico.

Many culture-bound syndromes have corresponding somatic symptoms not explained by a medical condition (Table 19.1). *Koro* occurs in South-East Asia and may be related to body dysmorphic disorder. It is characterized by the belief that the penis is shrinking and will disappear into the abdomen, causing the man to die. Falling-out episodes, found in the southern US and the Caribbean islands, are characterized by a sudden collapse during which the person cannot see or move. *Hwa-byung* is a Korean folk syndrome attributed to the suppression of anger and includes insomnia, fatigue, panic, indigestion and generalized aches and pains. *Sangue dormido* ('sleeping blood') occurs among Portuguese Cape Verde Islanders who report pain, numbness, tremors, paralysis, seizures, blindness, heart attacks and miscarriages. *Shenjing shuariuo* occurs in China and includes physical and mental fatigue, dizziness, headache, pain, sleep disturbance, memory loss, gastrointestinal problems and sexual dysfunction (Mojtabai, 2005).

TREATMENT

Treatment focuses on managing symptoms and improving quality of life. The nurse must show empathy and sensitivity to the client's physical complaints (Karvonen *et al.*, 2004). A trusting relationship helps to ensure that clients stay with and receive care from one provider instead of 'doctor-shopping'.

Table 19.1 CULTURE-BOUND SYNDROMES

Syndrome	Culture	Characteristics
Dhat	India	Hypochondriacal concern about semen loss
Koro	South-East Asia	Belief that penis is shrinking and will disappear into abdomen, resulting in death
Falling-out episodes	Southern United States, Caribbean islands	Sudden collapse; person cannot see or move
Hwa-byung	Korea	Suppressed anger causes insomnia, fatigue, panic, indigestion and generalized aches and pains
Sangue dormido ('sleeping blood')	Portuguese Cape Verde Islands	Pain, numbness, tremors, paralysis, seizures, blindness, heart attack, miscarriage
Shenjing shuariuo	China	Physical and mental fatigue, dizziness, headache, pain, sleep disturbance, memory loss, gastrointestinal problems, sexual dysfunction

Adapted from Mojtabai, R. (2005). Culture-bound syndromes with psychotic features. In B. J. Sadock & V. A. Sadock (Eds.) *Comprehensive textbook of psychiatry, Vol. 1* (8th edn, pp. 1538–1542). Philadelphia: Lippincott Williams & Wilkins. © American Psychiatric Association. Reprinted with permission

For many clients, depression may accompany or result from somatoform disorders. Thus, antidepressants help in some cases. SSRIs such as fluoxetine (Prozac), sertraline (Lustral) and paroxetine (Seroxat) are used most commonly (Table 19.2).

For clients with pain disorder, referral to a chronic pain clinic may be useful. Clients learn cognitive-behavioural methods of pain management and techniques such as visual imaging and relaxation. Services such as physical therapy to maintain and build muscle tone help to improve functional abilities. Providers should avoid prescribing and administering narcotic analgesics to these clients because of the risk for dependence or abuse. Clients can use non-steroidal anti-inflammatory agents to help reduce pain.

Involvement in therapy groups is beneficial for some people with somatoform disorders. Studies of clients with somatization disorder who participated in a structured cognitive-behavioural group showed evidence of improved physical and emotional health 1 year later (Hollifield, 2005). The overall goals of the group were offering peer support, sharing methods of coping and perceiving and expressing emotions. Abramowitz and Braddock (2006) found that clients with hypochondriasis who were willing to participate in CBT and take medications were able to alter their erroneous perceptions of threat (of illness) and improve. CBT also produced significant improvement in clients with somatization disorder (Allen *et al.*, 2006).

In terms of prognosis, somatoform disorders tend to be chronic or recurrent. With treatment, conversion disorder often remits in a few weeks but recurs in 25% of clients. Somatization disorder, hypochondriasis and pain disorder often last for many years, and clients report being in poor health. People with body dysmorphic disorder may be preoccupied with the same or a different perceived body flaw throughout their lives (American Psychiatric Association, 2000).

Table 19.2 ANTIDEPRESSANTS USED TO TREAT SOMATOFORM DISORDERS

Drug	Usual Dose (mg/day)	Nursing Considerations
Fluoxetine (Prozac)	20–60	Monitor for rash, hives, insomnia, headache, anxiety, drowsiness, nausea, loss of appetite; avoid alcohol
Paroxetine (Seroxat)	20–60	Monitor for nausea, loss of appetite, dizziness, dry mouth, somnolence or insomnia, sweating, sexual dysfunction; avoid alcohol
Sertraline (Lustral)	50–200	Monitor for nausea, loss of appetite, diarrhoea, headache, insomnia, sexual dysfunction; avoid alcohol

Adapted from British National Formulary Online (2008) http://www.bnf.org/bnf/bnf/55/

APPLICATION OF THE NURSING PROCESS

The underlying mechanism of somatization is consistent for clients with somatoform disorders of all types. This section discusses application of the nursing process for clients with somatization; differences among the disorders are highlighted in the appropriate places.

Assessment

The nurse must investigate physical health status thoroughly to ensure there is no underlying pathology requiring treatment. Box 19.1 contains a useful screening test for symptoms of somatization disorder. When a client has been diagnosed with a somatoform disorder, it is important not to dismiss all future complaints because, at any time, the client could develop a physical condition that would require medical attention.

HISTORY

Clients usually provide a lengthy and detailed account of previous physical problems, numerous diagnostic tests and perhaps even a number of surgical procedures. It is likely that they have seen many professionals over several years. They may express dismay or anger at the medical community with comments such as 'They just can't find out what's wrong with me' or 'They're all incompetent, and they're trying to tell me I'm crazy!' The exception may be clients with conversion disorder, who show little emotion when describing physical limitations or lack of a medical diagnosis (*la belle indifférence*).

GENERAL APPEARANCE AND MOTOR BEHAVIOUR

Overall appearance is usually not remarkable. Often, clients walk slowly or with an unusual gait because of the pain or disability caused by the symptoms. They may exhibit a facial expression of discomfort or physical distress. In many cases, they brighten and look much better as the assessment interview begins because they have the nurse's undivided attention. Clients with somatization disorder usually describe their complaints in colourful, exaggerated terms, but often lack specific information.

MOOD AND AFFECT

Mood is often labile, shifting from seeming depressed and sad when describing physical problems to looking bright and excited when talking about how they had to go to the hospital in the middle of the night by ambulance. Emotions are often exaggerated, as are reports of physical symptoms. Clients describing a series of personal crises related to their physical health may appear pleased rather than distressed about these situations. Clients with conversion disorder display an unexpected lack of distress.

THOUGHT PROCESS AND CONTENT

Clients who somatize do not experience disordered thought processes. The content of their thinking is primarily about often exaggerated physical concerns: for example, when they have a simple cold, they may be convinced it is pneumonia. They may even talk about dying and what music they want played at their funeral.

Clients are unlikely to be able to think about or to respond to questions about emotional feelings. They will answer questions about how they feel in terms of physical health or sensations. For example, the nurse may ask, 'How did you feel about having to quit your job?' The client might respond, 'Well, I thought I'd feel better with the extra rest, but my back pain was just as bad as ever.'

Clients with hypochondriasis focus on the fear of serious illness rather than the existence of illness, as seen in clients

---

Box 19.1 ASSESSMENT QUESTIONS FOR SYMPTOMS IN SCREENING TEST FOR SOMATIZATION DISORDER

1. Have you ever had trouble breathing?
2. Have you ever had trouble with menstrual cramps?
3. Have you ever had burning sensations in your sexual organs, mouth or rectum?
4. Have you ever had difficulties swallowing or had an uncomfortable lump in your throat that stayed for at least an hour?
5. Have you ever found that you could not remember what you had been doing for hours or days at a time? If yes, did this happen even though you had not been drinking or using drugs?
6. Have you ever had trouble with frequent vomiting?
7. Have you ever had frequent pain in your fingers or toes?

Adapted from Othmer, E. & DeSouza, C. (1983). A screening test for somatization disorder (hysteria). *American Journal of Psychiatry, 142*(10), 1146–1149. © American Psychiatric Association. Reprinted with permission.

with other somatoform disorders. However, they are just as preoccupied with physical concerns as other somatizing clients and are likewise very limited in their abilities to identify emotional feelings or interpersonal issues. Fink and colleagues (2004) found that clients with hypochondriasis were preoccupied with bodily functions ruminated about illness, were fascinated about medical information and had unrealistic fears about potential infection and prescription medications.

SENSORY AND INTELLECTUAL PROCESSES

Clients are alert and oriented. Intellectual functions are unimpaired.

JUDGEMENT AND INSIGHT

Exaggerated responses to their physical health may affect clients' judgement. They have little or no insight into their behaviour. They are firmly convinced that their problem is entirely physical and often believe that others don't understand.

SELF-CONCEPT

Clients focus almost exclusively on the physical part of themselves. They are unlikely to think about personal characteristics or strengths and are uncomfortable when asked to do so. Clients who somatize have low self-esteem and seem to deal with it by totally focusing on physical concerns. They lack confidence, have little success in work situations and have difficulty managing daily life issues, which they relate solely to their physical status.

ROLES AND RELATIONSHIPS

Clients may have employment difficulties. They often lose jobs because of excessive absenteeism or inability to perform work; clients may have given up working voluntarily because of poor physical health. Consumed with seeking medical care, they often have difficulty fulfilling family roles. It is likely that these clients have few friends and spend little time in social activities. They may decline to see friends or to go out socially for fear that they would become desperately ill away from home. Most socialization takes place with members of the health-care community.

Clients may report a lack of family support and understanding. Family members may tire of the ceaseless complaints and the client's refusal to accept the absence of a medical diagnosis. The illnesses and physical conditions often interfere with planned family events such going on vacations or attending family gatherings. Home life is often chaotic and unpredictable.

PHYSIOLOGICAL AND SELF-CARE CONCERNS

In addition to the multitude of physical complaints, these clients often have legitimate needs in terms of their health practices (Box 19.2). Clients who somatize often have sleep

Box 19.2   CLINICAL NURSE ALERT

Just because a client has been diagnosed with a somatoform disorder, do not automatically dismiss all future complaints. They should be completely assessed because the client could, at any time, develop a physical condition that would require medical attention.

pattern disturbances, lack basic nutrition and get no exercise. In addition, they may be taking multiple prescriptions for pain or other complaints. If a client has been using anxiolytics or analgesics, the nurse must consider the possibility of dependence (see Chapter 17).

Data Analysis

Nursing formulations commonly used when working with clients who somatize include the following:

- Ineffective coping
- Ineffective denial
- Impaired social interaction
- Anxiety
- Disturbed sleep pattern
- Fatigue
- Pain.

Clients with conversion disorder may be at risk for 'disuse syndrome' from having pseudo-neurological paralysis symptoms. In other words, if clients do not use a limb for a long time, the muscles may weaken or atrophy from lack of use.

Outcome Identification

Treatment outcomes for clients with a somatoform disorder may include the following:

- The client will identify the relationship between stress and physical symptoms.
- The client will verbally express thoughts and feelings.
- The client will follow an established daily routine.
- The client will demonstrate alternative ways to deal with stress, anxiety and other feelings.
- The client will demonstrate healthier behaviours regarding rest, activity and nutritional intake.

Intervention

HEALTH PROMOTION

The nurse must help the client to establish a daily routine that includes improved health behaviours. Adequate nutritional intake, improved sleep patterns and a realistic balance of activity and rest are all areas with which the client may need assistance. The nurse should expect resistance, including protests from the client that he or she does not feel well enough to do these things. The challenge for the nurse is to validate the client's feelings while encouraging him or her to participate in activities.

Nurse: *'Let's take a walk outside for some fresh air.'* (encouraging collaboration)

Client: *'I wish I could, but I feel so terrible, I just can't do it.'*

Nurse: *'I know this is difficult, but some exercise is really important. Let's make it just a short walk.'* (validation; encouraging collaboration)

The nurse can use a similar approach to gain client participation in eating more nutritious foods, getting up and dressed at a certain time every morning and setting a regular bedtime. The nurse also can explain that inactivity and poor eating habits perpetuate discomfort and that often it is necessary to engage in behaviours even when one doesn't feel like it.

Client: *'I just can't eat anything. I have no appetite.'*

Nurse: *'I know you don't feel well, but it's important to begin eating.'* (validation; encouraging collaboration)

Client: *'I promise I'll eat just as soon as I'm hungry.'*

Nurse: *'Actually, if you begin to eat a few bites, you'll begin to feel better, and your appetite may improve.'* (encouraging collaboration)

The nurse should not attempt to strip clients of their somatizing defences until he or she has collected adequate assessment data and clients have learned other coping mechanisms. The nurse should not attempt to confront clients about somatic symptoms or attempt to tell them that these symptoms are not 'real'. They are very real to clients, who actually experience the symptoms and associated distress.

ASSISTING THE CLIENT TO EXPRESS EMOTIONS

Teaching about the relationship between stress and physical symptoms is a useful way to help clients begin to see the mind–body relationship. Clients may keep a detailed journal of their physical symptoms. The nurse might ask them to describe the situation at the time, such as whether they were alone or with others, whether any disagreements were occurring and so forth. The journal may help clients to see when physical symptoms seemed worse or better and what other factors may have affected that perception.

Limiting the time that clients can focus on physical complaints alone may be necessary. Encouraging them to focus on emotional feelings is important, although this can

---

CLIENT/FAMILY EDUCATION FOR SOMATOFORM DISORDERS

- Establish daily health routine, including adequate rest, exercise and nutrition.
- Teach about relationship of stress and physical symptoms and mind–body relationship.
- Educate about proper nutrition, rest and exercise.
- Educate client in relaxation techniques: progressive relaxation, deep breathing, guided imagery and distraction such as music or other activities.
- Educate client by role-playing social situations and interactions.
- Encourage family to provide attention and encouragement when client has fewer complaints.
- Encourage family to decrease special attention when client is in 'sick' role.

---

be difficult for clients. The nurse should provide attention and positive feedback for efforts to identify and discuss feelings.

It may help for the nurse to explain to the family about primary and secondary gains. For example, if the family can provide attention to clients when they are feeling better or fulfilling responsibilities, clients are more likely to continue doing so. If family members have lavished attention on clients when they have physical complaints, the nurse can encourage the relatives to stop reinforcing the sick role.

TEACHING COPING STRATEGIES

Two categories of coping strategies are important for clients to learn and to practise: **emotion-focused coping strategies**, which help clients relax and reduce feelings of stress, and **problem-focused coping strategies**, which help to resolve or change a client's behaviour or situation or manage life stressors. Emotion-focused strategies include progressive relaxation, deep breathing, guided imagery and distractions such as music or other activities. Many approaches to stress relief are available for clients to try. The nurse should help clients to learn and practise these techniques, emphasizing that their effectiveness usually improves with routine use. Clients must not expect such techniques to eliminate their pain or physical symptoms; rather, the focus is helping them to manage or diminish the intensity of the symptoms.

Problem-focused coping strategies include learning problem-solving methods, applying the process to identified problems and role-playing interactions with others. For example, a client may complain that no one comes to visit or that she has no friends. The nurse can help the

NURSING INTERVENTIONS FOR SOMATOFORM DISORDERS

- Health education
  Establish a daily routine.
  Promote adequate nutrition and sleep.
- Expression of emotional feelings
  Recognize relationship between stress/coping and physical symptoms.
  Keep a journal.
  Limit time spent on physical complaints.
  Limit primary and secondary gains.
- Coping strategies
  Emotion-focused coping strategies such as relaxation techniques, deep breathing, guided imagery and distraction
  Problem- and skills-focused coping strategies such as CBT and DBT approaches and role-play.

client to plan social contact with others, can role-play what to talk about (other than the client's complaints) and can improve the client's confidence in making relationships. The nurse also can help clients to identify stressful life situations and plan strategies to deal with them. For example, if a client finds it difficult to accomplish daily household tasks, the nurse can help him to plan a schedule with difficult tasks followed by something the client may enjoy.

Evaluation

Somatoform disorders are usually chronic or recurrent, so changes are likely to occur slowly. If treatment is effective, the client should make fewer visits to GPs as a result of physical complaints, use less medication and more positive coping techniques and increase functional abilities. Improved family and social relationships are also a positive outcome that may follow improvements in the client's coping abilities.

MHNs sometimes encounter clients with somatoform disorders in health centres, clinics, CMHTs or in settings other than those related to mental health. Building a trusting relationship with the client, providing empathy and support and being sensitive to, rather than dismissive of, complaints are skills that the nurse can use in any setting where clients are seeking assistance. Making appropriate referrals such as to a pain clinic for clients with pain disorder or providing information about support groups in the community may be helpful. Encouraging clients to find pleasurable activities or hobbies may help to meet their needs for attention and

security, thus diminishing the psychological needs for somatic symptoms.

MENTAL HEALTH PROMOTION

A common theme in somatoform disorders is their occurrence in people who do not express conflicts, stress and emotions verbally. They express themselves through physical symptoms; the resulting attention and focus on their physical ailments somewhat meet their needs. As these clients are better able to express their emotions and needs directly, physical symptoms subside. Thus, assisting them to deal with emotional issues directly is a strategy for mental health promotion.

Micale (2000) suggests that 'hysteria' and 'neuroses' (now called somatization disorder) have decreased in the US since 1900 (as they appear to have done in the UK). He cites the following reasons for this decline:

- People now have more 'psychological self-knowledge'.
- The sexual confinement, emotional oppression and social suffocation of the Victorian era have dissipated.
- The interaction of mind and body now has a scientific foundation.

As people continue to gain knowledge about themselves and to express their emotional needs and desires directly, the incidence of coping through physical symptoms may continue to decline.

SELF-AWARENESS ISSUES

Clients who cope through physical symptoms can be frustrating for the nurse. Initially, they may well be unwilling to consider that anything other than major physical illness is the root of all their problems. When health professionals tell clients there is no physical illness and refer them to mental health professionals, the response, often, is anger: clients may express anger directly or passively at the medical community and be highly critical of the inadequate care they believe they have received. The nurse must not respond in kind with anger to such outbursts or criticism.

The client's progress is usually slow and painstaking, if any happens at all. Clients coping with somatization have been doing so for years. Changes are rarely rapid or drastic. The nurse may feel frustrated because, after giving the client his or her best efforts, the client returns time after time with the same focus on physical symptoms. The nurse should be realistic about the small successes that can be achieved in any given period. To enhance the ongoing relationship, the nurse must be able to accept the client and his or her continued complaints and criticisms while remaining non-judgemental.

Nursing Care Plan   *Hypochondriasis*

Nursing Formulation

Ineffective Coping: *Inability to form a valid appraisal of the stressors, inadequate choices of practised responses and/or inability to use available resources.*

ASSESSMENT DATA

- Denial of emotional problems
- Difficulty identifying and expressing feelings
- Apparent lack of insight
- Self-preoccupation, especially with physical functioning
- Fears of or rumination on disease
- Numerous somatic complaints (may involve many different organs or systems)
- Sensory complaints (pain, loss of taste sensation, olfactory complaints)
- Reluctance or refusal to participate in psychiatric treatment programme or activities
- Reliance on medications or physical treatments (such as laxative dependence)
- Extensive use of over-the-counter medications, home remedies, enemas and so forth
- Ritualistic behaviours (such as exaggerated bowel routines)
- Tremors
- Limited gratification from interpersonal relationships
- Lack of emotional support system
- Anxiety
- Secondary gains received for physical problems
- History of repeated visits to physicians or hospital admissions
- History of repeated medical evaluations with no findings of abnormalities

EXPECTED OUTCOMES

Immediate
The client will
- Participate in the treatment programme
- Decrease the number and frequency of physical complaints
- Demonstrate concordance with medical therapy and medications
- Demonstrate adequate energy, food and fluid intake
- Identify life stresses and anxieties
- Identify the relationship between stress and physical symptoms
- Express feelings verbally
- Identify alternative ways to deal with stress, anxiety or other feelings

Medium-term
The client will
- Decrease ritualistic behaviours
- Decrease physical attention-seeking complaints
- Verbalize increased insight into the dynamics of hypochondriacal behaviour, including secondary gains
- Verbalize an understanding of therapeutic regimens and medications, if any

Ongoing
The client will
- Eliminate overuse of medications or physical treatments
- Demonstrate alternative ways to deal with stress, anxiety or other feelings

IMPLEMENTATION

Nursing Interventions *denotes collaborative interventions

The initial nursing assessment should include a complete physical assessment, a history of previous complaints and treatment and a consideration of each current complaint.

*The nursing staff should note the medical assessment of each complaint on the client's admission.

Rationale

The nursing assessment provides a baseline from which to begin planning care.

Real physical problems must be noted and treated.

continued ···⫸

Nursing Care Plan: Hypochondriasis, cont.

IMPLEMENTATION

Nursing Interventions *denotes collaborative interventions	Rationale
*Each time the client voices a new complaint, the client should be referred to the medical staff for assessment (and treatment if appropriate).	It is unsafe to assume that all physical complaints are hypochondriacal – the client could really be ill or injured. The client may attempt to establish the legitimacy of complaints by being genuinely injured or ill.
*Minimize the amount of time and attention given to complaints. When the client makes a complaint, refer him or her to the medical staff (if it is a new complaint) or follow the team treatment plan; then tell the client you will discuss something else but not bodily complaints. Tell the client that you are interested in the client as a person, not just in his or her physical complaints. If the complaint is not acute, ask the client to discuss the complaint during a regular appointment with the medical staff.	If physical complaints are unsuccessful in gaining attention, they should decrease in frequency over time.
Respectfully withdraw your attention if the client insists on making complaints the sole topic of conversation. Tell the client your reason for withdrawal and that you will return later to discuss other topics.	It is important to make clear to the client that attention is withdrawn from physical complaints, not from the client as a person.
Allow the client a specific time limit (like 5 minutes per hour) to discuss physical complaints with one person. The remaining staff will discuss only other issues with the client.	Because physical complaints have been the client's primary coping strategy, it is less threatening to the client if you limit this behaviour initially rather than forbid it. If the client is denied this coping mechanism before new skills can be developed, hypochondriacal behaviour may increase.
Acknowledge the complaint as the client's perception and then follow the previous approaches; do not argue about the somatic complaints.	Arguing gives the client's complaints attention, albeit negative, and the client is able to avoid discussing feelings.
Use minimal objective reassurance in conjunction with questions to explore the client's feelings. ('Your tests have shown that you have no lesions. Do you still feel that you do? What are your feelings about this?')	This approach helps the client make the transition to discussing feelings.
Encourage the client to discuss his or her feelings about the fears rather than the fears themselves.	The focus is on feelings of fear, not fear of physical problems.
Explore the client's feelings of lack of control over stress and life events.	The client may have helpless feelings but may not recognize this independently.
Initially, carefully assess the client's self-image, social patterns and ways of dealing with anger, stress and so forth.	This assessment provides a knowledge base regarding hypochondriacal behaviours.
Talk with the client about sources of satisfaction and dissatisfaction, relationships, employment and so forth.	Open-ended discussion is usually non-threatening and helps the client begin self-assessment.
After some discussion of the above and developing a trust relationship, talk more directly with the client and encourage him or her to identify specific stresses, recent and ongoing.	The client's perception of stressors forms the basis of his or her behaviour and usually is more significant than others' perception of those stressors.
If the client is using denial as a defence mechanism, point out apparent or possible stresses (in a non-threatening way) and ask the client for feedback.	If the client is in denial, more direct approaches may produce anger or hostility and threaten the trust relationship.

Nursing Care Plan: Hypochondriasis, cont.

IMPLEMENTATION

Nursing Interventions *denotes collaborative interventions	Rationale
Gradually, help the client identify possible connections between anxiety and the occurrence of physical symptoms, such as: What makes the client more or less comfortable? What is the client doing, or what is going on around the client, when he or she experiences symptoms?	The client can begin to see the relatedness of stress and physical problems at his or her own pace. Self-realization will be more acceptable to the client than the nurse telling the client the problem.
Encourage the client to keep a diary of situations, stresses and occurrence of symptoms, and use it to identify relationships between stresses and symptoms.	Reflecting on written items may be more accurate and less threatening to the client.
Talk with the client at least once per shift, focusing on the client's identifying and expressing feelings	Demonstrating consistent interest in the client facilitates the relationship and can desensitize the discussion of emotional issues.
Encourage the client to ventilate feelings by talking or crying, through physical activities and so forth.	The client may have difficulty expressing feelings directly. Your support may help him or her develop these skills.
*Teach the client and his or her family or significant others about the dynamics of hypochondriacal behaviour and the treatment plan, including plans after discharge.	The client and his or her family or significant others may have little or no knowledge of these areas. Knowledge of the treatment plan will promote long-term behaviour change.
*Talk with the client and significant others about secondary gains and together develop a plan to reduce those gains. Identify the needs the client is attempting to meet with secondary gains (such as attention or escape from responsibilities).	Maintaining limits to reduce secondary gain requires everyone's participation to be successful. The client's family and significant others must be aware of the client's needs if they want to be effective in helping to meet those needs.
Help the client plan to meet his or her needs in more direct ways. Show the client that he or she can gain attention when he or she does not exhibit symptoms, deals with responsibilities directly or asserts himself or herself in the face of stress.	Positive feedback and support for healthier behaviour tend to make that behaviour recur more frequently. The client's family and significant others also must use positive reinforcement.
Compassionately and transparently reduce the 'benefits' of illness as much as possible. Do not allow the client to avoid responsibilities or allow special privileges, such as staying in bed by voicing somatic discomfort.	If physical problems do not get the client what he or she wants, the client is less likely to cope in that manner.
*Work with the medical staff to limit the number, variety, strength and frequency of medications, enemas and so forth, which are made available to the client.	A team effort helps to prevent the client's manipulation of staff members to obtain additional medication.
When the client requests a medication or treatment, encourage the client to identify what precipitated his or her complaint and to deal with it in other ways.	If the client can obtain stress relief in a non-chemical, non-medical way, he or she is less likely to use the medication or treatment.
Observe and record the circumstances related to complaints; talk about your observations with the client.	Alerting the client to situations surrounding the complaint helps him or her see the relatedness of stress and physical symptoms.
Help the client identify and use non-chemical methods of pain relief, such as relaxation techniques.	Using non-chemical pain relief shifts the focus of coping away from medications and increases the client's sense of control.
Teach the client more healthful daily living habits, including diet, stress management techniques, daily exercise, rest, possible connection between caffeine and anxiety symptoms and so forth.	Optimal physical wellness is especially important with clients using physical symptoms as a coping strategy.

continued ⋯⫶

Nursing Care Plan: Hypochondriasis, cont.

IMPLEMENTATION

Nursing Interventions *denotes collaborative interventions	Rationale
Encourage the client to ventilate feelings by talking or crying, through physical activities and so forth.	The client may have difficulty expressing feelings. Your support may help the client develop these skills.
Encourage the client to express feelings directly, especially feelings with which the client is uncomfortable (such as anger or resentment).	Direct expression of feelings will minimize the need to use physical symptoms to express them.
Notice the client's interactions with others and give positive feedback for self-assertion and expressing feelings, especially anger, resentment and other so-called negative emotions.	The client needs to know that appropriate expressions of anger or other negative emotions are acceptable and that he or she can feel better physically as a result of these expressions.

Adapted from Schultz, J. M. & Videbeck, S. L. (2005). *Lippincott's manual of psychiatric nursing care plans* (7th edn). Philadelphia: Lippincott Williams & Wilkins.

Points to Consider When Working With Clients With Somatoform Disorders

- Carefully assess the client's physical complaints. Even when a client has a history of a somatoform disorder, the nurse must not dismiss physical complaints or assume they are psychological. The client may actually have a medical condition.
- Validate the client's feelings while trying to engage him or her in treatment; for example, use a reflective yet engaging comment such as 'I know you're not feeling well, but it is important to get some exercise each day.'
- Remember that the somatic complaints are not under the client's voluntary control. The client will have fewer somatic complaints when he or she improves coping skills and interpersonal relationships.

Critical Thinking Questions

1. What do you think the relationship is between environmental, physiological and psychological factors in the causation of mental health problems generally?
2. Why do you think somatoform disorders are more common in women than in men?
3. When a client has somatoform pain disorder, powerful analgesics such as narcotics are generally contraindicated, even though the client is suffering unremitting pain. How might the nurse feel when working with this client? How should the nurse respond when the client says, 'You know I'm in pain! Why won't you do anything? Why do you let me suffer?'
4. Should there be limits on expensive medical tests and procedures for clients with somatoform disorder? Who should decide when health-care benefits are limited?

5. A mother is found to have caused a medical crisis by giving her 6-year-old child a medication to which the child has a known severe allergy. The mother is diagnosed as having Munchausen syndrome by proxy. Should she be treated in the mental health setting? Charged with a criminal act? Why?

 KEY POINTS

- Somatization means transforming mental experiences and states into bodily symptoms.
- The three central features of somatoform disorders are physical complaints that suggest major medical illness but have no demonstrable organic basis, psychological factors and conflicts that seem important in initiating, exacerbating and maintaining the symptoms and symptoms or magnified health concerns that are not under the client's conscious control.
- Somatoform disorders include somatization disorder, conversion disorder, hypochondriasis, pain disorder and body dysmorphic disorder.
- Malingering means feigning physical symptoms for some external gain such as avoiding work.
- Factitious disorders are characterized by physical symptoms that are feigned or inflicted for the sole purpose of drawing attention to oneself and gaining the emotional benefits of assuming the sick role.
- Internalization and somatization are the chief defence mechanisms seen in somatoform disorders.
- Clients with somatization disorder and conversion reactions may eventually be treated in mental health settings. Clients with other somatoform disorders are seen typically in medical settings.

- Clients who cope with stress through somatizing are reluctant or unable to identify emotional feelings and interpersonal issues and have few coping abilities unrelated to physical symptoms.
- Nursing interventions that may be effective with clients who somatize involve providing health teaching, identifying emotional feelings and stress and using alternative coping strategies.
- Coping strategies that are helpful to clients with somatoform disorders include CBT, relaxation techniques such as guided imagery and deep breathing, distractions such as music and problem-solving strategies such as identifying stressful situations, learning new methods of managing them and role-playing social interactions.
- Clients with somatization disorder actually experience symptoms and the associated discomfort and pain. The nurse should never try to confront the client about the origin of these symptoms until the client has learned other coping strategies.
- Somatoform disorders are chronic or recurrent, so progress toward treatment outcomes can be slow and difficult.
- Nurses caring for clients with somatoform disorders must show patience and understanding toward them as they struggle through years of recurrent somatic complaints and attempts to learn new emotion- and problem-focused coping strategies.

REFERENCES

Abramowitz, J. S. & Braddock, A. E. (2006). Hypochondriasis: Conceptualization, treatment, and relationship to obsessive-compulsive disorder. *Psychiatric Clinics of North America, 29*(2), 503–519.

Allen, L. A., Woolfolk, R. L., Escobar, J. I., Gara, M. A., & Hamer, R. M. (2006). Cognitive-behavioural therapy for somatization disorder: A randomized controlled trial. *Archives of Internal Medicine, 166*(14), 1512–1518.

American Psychiatric Association. (2000). *Diagnostic and statistical manual of mental disorders* (4th edn, text revision). Washington, DC: American Psychiatric Association.

Andreasen, N. C. & Black, D. W. (2006). *Introductory textbook of psychiatry* (2nd edn). Washington DC: American Psychiatric Publishing.

Fink, P., Ornbol, E., Toft, T., et al. (2004). A new empirically established hypochondriasis diagnosis. *American Journal of Psychiatry, 161*(9), 1680–1691.

Hollifield, M. A. (2005). Somatoform disorders. In B. J. Sadock & V. A. Sadock (Eds.), *Comprehensive textbook of psychiatry, Vol. 1* (8th edn, pp. 1800–1828). Philadelphia: Lippincott Williams & Wilkins.

Karvonen, J. T., Veijola, J., Jokelainen, J., et al. (2004). Somatisation disorder in young adult population. *General Hospital Psychiatry, 26*(1), 9–12.

Lucas, P. (2002). Body dysmorphic disorder and violence. *Journal of Forensic Psychiatry, 13*(1), 145–156.

Micale, M. S. (2000). The decline of hysteria. *Harvard Mental Health Letter, 17*(1), 4–6.

Mojtabai, R. (2005). Culture-bound syndromes with psychotic features. In B. J. Sadock & V. A. Sadock (Eds.), *Comprehensive textbook of psychiatry, Vol. 1* (8th edn, pp. 1538–1541). Philadelphia: Lippincott Williams & Wilkins.

Philips, K. & Castle, D. (2001). Body dysmorphic disorder in men. *British Medical Journal, 323*, 1015–1016.

Ragaisis, K. (2004). When the system works: Rescuing a child from Munchausen's syndrome by proxy. *Journal of Child and Adolescent Psychiatric Nursing, 17*(4), 173–176.

Wang, D., Nadiga, D. N., & Jenson, J. J. (2005). Factitious disorders. In B. J. Sadock & V. A. Sadock (Eds.), *Comprehensive textbook of psychiatry, Vol. 1* (8th edn, pp. 1829–1843). Philadelphia: Lippincott Williams & Wilkins.

ADDITIONAL READING

Bahtia, M. S. & Sapra, S. (2005). Pseudoseizures in children: A profile of 50 cases. *Clinical Pediatrics, 44*(7), 617–621.

Creed, F. (2006). Should general psychiatry ignore somatization and hypochondriasis? *World Psychiatry, 5*(3), 146–150.

Gregory, R. J. & Jindal, S. (2006). Factitious disorder on an inpatient psychiatry ward. *American Journal of Orthopsychiatry, 76*(1), 31–36.

Szepietowski, J.C., Salomon, J., Pacan, P., Hrehorów, E., & Zalewska, A. (2008). Body dysmorphic disorder and dermatologists. *Journal of the European Academy of Dermatology and Venereology, 22*(7), 795–799.

Weardon, A., Perryman, K., & Ward, V. (2006). Adult attachment, reassurance seeking, and hypochondriacal concerns in college students. *Journal of Health Psychology, 11*(6), 877–886.

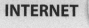 **INTERNET** **RESOURCES**

RESOURCES

- OCD Action: Body Dysmorphic Disorder
- Munchausen Syndrome by Proxy Resources

INTERNET ADDRESS

http://www.ocdaction.org.uk/ocdaction/index.asp?id=37
http://www.vachss.com/help_text/msp.html

Chapter Study Guide

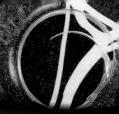

MULTIPLE CHOICE QUESTIONS

Select the best answer for each of the following questions.

1. The nurse is caring for a client with a conversion disorder. Which of the following assessments will the nurse expect to see?
   a. Extreme distress over the physical symptom
   b. Indifference about the physical symptom
   c. Labile mood
   d. Multiple physical complaints

2. Which of the following statements would indicate that teaching about somatization disorder has been effective?
   a. 'The doctor believes I am faking my symptoms.'
   b. 'If I try harder to control my symptoms, I will feel better.'
   c. 'I will feel better when I begin handling stress more effectively.'
   d. 'Nothing will help me feel better physically.'

3. Paroxetine (Seroxat) has been prescribed for a client with a somatoform disorder. The nurse instructs the client to watch for which of the following side-effects?
   a. Constipation
   b. Increased appetite
   c. Increased flatulence
   d. Nausea

4. Emotion-focused coping strategies are designed to accomplish which of the following outcomes?
   a. Helping the client manage difficult situations more effectively
   b. Helping the client manage the intensity of symptoms
   c. Teaching the client the relationship between stress and physical symptoms
   d. Relieving the client's physical symptoms

5. Which of the following is true about clients with hypochondriasis?
   a. They may interpret normal body sensations as signs of disease.
   b. They often exaggerate or fabricate physical symptoms for attention.
   c. They do not show signs of distress about their physical symptoms.
   d. All the above are true statements.

6. The client's family asks the nurse, 'What is hypochondriasis?' The best response by the nurse is, 'Hypochondriasis is
   a. A persistent preoccupation with getting a serious disease.'
   b. An illness not fully explained by a diagnosed medical condition.'
   c. Characterized by a variety of symptoms over a number of years.'
   d. The eventual result of excessive worrying about diseases.'

7. A client with somatization disorder has been attending group therapy. Which of the following statements indicates that therapy is having a positive outcome for this client?
   a. 'I feel better physically just from getting a chance to talk.'
   b. 'I haven't said much, but I get a lot from listening to others.'
   c. 'I shouldn't complain too much; my problems aren't as bad as others.'
   d. 'The other people in this group have emotional problems.'

8. A client who developed numbness in the right hand could not play the piano at a scheduled recital. The consequence of the symptom, not having to perform, is best described as
   a. Emotion-focused coping
   b. Phobia
   c. Primary gain
   d. Secondary gain

FILL-IN-THE-BLANK QUESTIONS

Identify the type of somatoform disorder that is described by each of the following statements.

_____ Preoccupation with an imagined or exaggerated body defect

_____ Multiple physical symptoms including pain and gastrointestinal, sexual and pseudoneurological symptoms

_____ Sudden, unexplained deficits in sensory or motor function

_____ Pain that is unrelieved by analgesics and greatly affected by psychological factors

_____ Preoccupation with the fear of having or acquiring a serious illness

GROUP DISCUSSION TOPICS

Why do you think somatoform disorders are rarely talked about in contemporary mental health care?:

CLINICAL EXAMPLE

Mary Jones, 34 years old, was referred to a chronic pain clinic with a diagnosis of pain disorder. She has been unable to work for 7 months because of back pain. Mary has seen several doctors, has had an MRI, and has tried various anti-inflammatory medications. She tells the CMHN that she is at the CMHT as a last resort because none of her doctors will 'do anything' for her. Mary's gait is slow, her posture is stiff, and she grimaces frequently while trying to sit in a chair. She reports being unable to drive a car, play with her children, do housework or enjoy any of her previous leisure activities.

1. Identify three nursing formulations that would be pertinent for Mary's plan of care.

2. Identify two expected outcomes for Mary's plan of care.

3. Describe five interventions that the nurse might implement to achieve the outcomes.

4. What other disciplines might make a contribution to Mary's care at the clinic?

5. Identify any appropriate referrals the nurse might make for Mary.

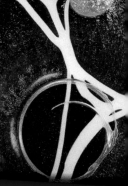

20

Child and Adolescent Mental Health

Key Terms

- Asperger syndrome
- attention deficit hyperactivity disorder (ADHD)
- autistic disorder
- autistic spectrum disorders
- conduct disorder
- encopresis
- enuresis
- learning disability
- limit-setting
- pica
- stereotypic movements
- therapeutic play
- tic
- time-out
- Tourette syndrome

Learning Objectives

After reading this chapter, you should be able to:

1. Discuss the characteristics, risk factors and family dynamics of mental health problems in childhood and adolescence.

2. Apply the nursing process to the care of children and adolescents with mental health problems and their families.

3. Provide education to clients, families, teachers, carers and members of the public about mental health problems in young people.

4. Discuss the nurse's role as an advocate for children and adolescents.

5. Evaluate your feelings, beliefs and attitudes about young people with mental health problems and their parents and other carers.

Mental health problems are usually harder to recognize or diagnose in children than in adults. Children often lack the abstract cognitive abilities and verbal skills to describe what is happening. Because they are constantly changing and developing, children have a limited sense of a stable, normal self to allow them to discriminate unusual or unwanted symptoms from normal feelings and sensations. Additionally, behaviours that are normal in a child of one age may indicate problems in a child of another age. For example, an infant who cries and wails when separated from her mother is normal. However, if the same child at 5 years of age cries and shows extreme anxiety when separated only briefly from her or his mother, this behaviour might suggest a problem and warrant investigation.

Children and adolescents experience many of the same mental health problems as adults, particularly mood and anxiety disorders, and are diagnosed with these disorders using the same criteria as for adults. Eating disorders, especially anorexia, usually begin in adolescence and continue into adulthood. Discussions of mood, anxiety and eating disorders are presented in separate chapters of this book.

This chapter focuses on those mental health problems usually first diagnosed in infancy, childhood or adolescence (Box 20.1); many of these can persist into adulthood. Mental health nurses working with child and adolescent teams, **learning disability** teams, CMHTs, crisis/home treatment teams and in acute inpatient settings may come across people – children and adults – with a disorder or disability first diagnosed in childhood. They may also be in an excellent position to recognize possible signs of childhood disorder in the families of adult clients.

Box 20.1 DISORDERS FIRST DIAGNOSED IN INFANCY, CHILDHOOD AND ADOLESCENCE

MENTAL RETARDATION

- Mild
- Moderate
- Severe
- Profound

LEARNING DISORDERS

- Reading disorder
- Mathematics disorder
- Disorder of written expression

MOTOR SKILLS DISORDER

- Developmental co-ordination disorder

COMMUNICATION DISORDERS

- Expressive language disorder
- Mixed receptive and expressive language disorder
- Phonologic disorder
- Stuttering

PERVASIVE DEVELOPMENTAL DISORDERS

- Autistic disorder
- Rett's disorder
- Childhood disintegrative disorder
- Asperger syndrome

ATTENTION DEFICIT AND DISRUPTIVE BEHAVIOUR DISORDERS

- ADHD
- Conduct disorder
- Oppositional defiant disorder

FEEDING AND EATING DISORDERS

- Pica
- Rumination disorder
- Feeding disorder of infancy or early childhood

TIC DISORDERS

- Tourette syndrome
- Chronic motor or tic syndrome
- Transient tic disorder

ELIMINATION DISORDERS

- Encopresis
- Enuresis

OTHER DISORDERS OF INFANCY, CHILDHOOD OR ADOLESCENCE

- Separation anxiety disorder
- Selective mutism
- Reactive attachment disorder
- Stereotypic movement disorder

Each category except feeding and eating disorders has an additional diagnosis 'Not Otherwise Specified' (NOS) for similar problems that do not meet the criteria for other diagnoses in the category (*DSM-IV-TR*, 2000).

Adapted from American Psychiatric Association. (2000). *Diagnostic and Statistical Manual of Mental Disorders* (4th edn, text revision). Washington, DC: American Psychiatric Association.

The childhood disorders most common in mental health settings include mild learning disabilities, pervasive developmental disorders, ADHD and disruptive behaviour disorders. For this reason, the chapter presents an in-depth discussion of ADHD and conduct disorder (the most prevalent disruptive behaviour disorder) with appropriate nursing formulations and interventions as well as sample nursing care plans. It discusses less common disorders briefly; generally, most of these disorders are not treated in the mental health system unless they coexist with other disorders. Learning disabilities are explored in Appendix A.

It is important to note again that effective, compassionate nursing care involves far more than awareness of a diagnosis. Diagnoses are notoriously changeable over time, frequently debatable and restrictive: they can be helpful in targeting effective care and treatment, but openness and flexibility, and a readiness to be taught by the experts – the child and his or her carers – are absolutely crucial.

Specific Educational Problems/'Learning Disorders'

Sometimes a child doesn't have a **learning disability** *per se* (see Appendix A) but his or her achievement in reading, mathematics or written expression is below that expected for his or her age, formal education and intelligence. These 'learning problems' interfere with academic achievement and life activities requiring reading, maths or writing (American Psychiatric Association, 2000).

Low self-esteem and poor social skills are common in children with these problems. As adults, some have difficulties with employment or social adjustment; others have minimal difficulties. Early identification of the specific 'learning disorder', effective intervention and no coexisting problems seem to be associated with better outcomes. Children with specific 'learning disorders' are often assisted with academic achievement through special education classes or individual help in mainstream schools.

Developmental Co-ordination Disorder

The essential feature of *developmental co-ordination disorder* is impaired co-ordination severe enough to interfere with academic achievement or activities of daily living (American Psychiatric Association, 2000). This diagnosis is not made if the problem with motor co-ordination is part of a general medical condition, such as cerebral palsy or muscular dystrophy. This disorder becomes evident as a child attempts to crawl or walk, or as an older child tries to dress independently or manipulate toys such as building blocks. Developmental co-ordination disorder often coexists with a communication disorder. Its course is variable; sometimes lack of co-ordination persists into adulthood (American

Psychiatric Association, 2000). Schools provide adaptive physical education and sensory integration programmes to treat motor skills disorder. Adaptive physical education programmes emphasize inclusion of movement games such as kicking a football. Sensory integration programmes are specific physical therapies prescribed to target improvement in areas where the child has difficulties. For example, a child with tactile defensiveness (discomfort at being touched by another person) might be involved in touching and rubbing skin surfaces (Pataki & Spence, 2005). Mental health disorders may result from or coexist with developmental co-ordination disorder (as with many other disorders).

Communication Disorders

A communication disorder is diagnosed when a communication deficit is severe enough to hinder development, academic achievement or activities of daily living, including socialization. *Expressive language disorder* involves an impaired ability to communicate through verbal and sign language. The child has difficulty learning new words and speaking in complete and correct sentences; his or her speech is limited. *Mixed receptive-expressive language disorder* includes the problems of expressive language disorder along with difficulty understanding (receiving) and determining the meaning of words and sentences. Both disorders can be present at birth (developmental) or may be acquired as a result of neurological injury or insult to the brain. *Phonological disorder* involves problems with articulation (forming sounds that are part of speech). *Stuttering* is a disturbance of the normal fluency and time patterning of speech. Phonologic disorder and stuttering run in families and occur more frequently in boys than in girls.

Communication disorders may be mild-to-severe. Difficulties that persist into adulthood are related most closely to the severity of the disorder. Speech and language therapists work with children who have communication disorders to improve their communication skills and to teach parents to continue speech therapy activities at home (Johnson & Beitchman, 2005).

Autistic Spectrum Disorders/ Pervasive Developmental Disorders

Autistic spectrum disorders (known as pervasive developmental disorders in the US) are characterized by pervasive and usually severe impairment of reciprocal social interaction skills, communication deviance and restricted stereotypical behavioural patterns (Volkmar *et al.*, 2005). This category of disorders is an umbrella term and includes autistic disorder (classic autism), Rett's disorder, childhood disintegrative disorder and Asperger's disorder (National Autistic Society, 2008b). Approximately 75% of children with pervasive developmental disorders also have a learning disability (American Psychiatric Association, 2000).

The National Autistic Society in the UK suggests there may be around half a million people (1%) with an autism spectrum disorder, although figures on the prevalence of autism *per se* in adults are unreliable (National Autistic Society, 2008a), and a recent study cited by the National Autistic Society suggests a total of 116 in 10,000 for all autism spectrum disorders in children (National Autistic Society, 2008a).

AUTISTIC DISORDER (AUTISM)

Autistic disorder (autism), the best known of the autistic spectrum disorders, seems to be more prevalent in boys than in girls and is usually identified by 18 months – and no later than 3 years of age. Children with autism usually display little eye contact with and make few facial expressions toward others; they may use limited gestures to communicate. They have limited capacity to relate to peers or parents. They lack spontaneous enjoyment, express no moods or emotional affect and cannot engage in play or make-believe with toys. There is frequently little intelligible speech. Children may engage in stereotyped motor behaviours such as hand flapping, body twisting or head banging.

Eighty per cent of cases of autism are 'early onset', with developmental delays starting in infancy. The other 20% of children with autism have seemingly normal growth and development until 2 or 3 years of age, when developmental regression or loss of abilities begins. They stop talking and relating to parents and peers and begin to demonstrate the behaviours described previously (Volkmar *et al.*, 2005). In the UK, estimates are 38.9 in 10,000 for childhood autism (National Autistic Society, 2008a).

The causes are unknown. Autism does seem to have a genetic link; many children with autism have a relative with autism or autistic traits. Despite seemingly convincing evidence, controversy continues about whether measles, mumps and rubella (MMR) vaccinations contribute to the development of late-onset autism. The general medical view is that there is no proven link (backed up by recent research, such as that of Baird *et al.*, 2008), but the lack of clear reasons why some children develop autism remains worrying, particularly for parents and carers.

Autism tends to improve, in some cases substantially, as children start to acquire and to use language to communicate with others. If behaviour deteriorates in adolescence, it may reflect the effects of hormonal changes or the difficulty meeting increasingly complex social demands. Autistic traits persist into adulthood, and most people with autism remain dependent to some degree on others. Manifestations vary from little speech and poor daily living skills throughout life to adequate social skills that allow relatively independent functioning. Social skills rarely improve enough to permit marriage and child rearing. Adults with autism may be viewed as merely odd or reclusive, or they may be given a diagnosis of OCD, schizoid personality disorder or learning disability.

Typical goals of care and treatment of children with autism are to reduce behavioural symptoms (e.g. stereotyped motor behaviours) and to promote learning and development, particularly the acquisition of language skills (Cashin, 2005). Comprehensive and individualized treatment, including special education and language therapy, is associated with more favourable outcomes. Music and art therapies, diet and the use of vitamins and a whole host of communication-based therapies are also used (National Autistic Society, 2008a).

Pharmacological treatment with antipsychotics such as haloperidol (Haldol) or risperidone (Risperdal) may be effective for specific target symptoms such as temper tantrums, aggressiveness, self-injury, hyperactivity and stereotyped behaviours. Other medications such as anticonvulsants, naltrexone (Nalorex), SSRIs and tricyclics, and stimulants, to diminish self-injury and hyperactive and obsessive behaviours, have had varied but unremarkable results (Volkmar *et al.*, 2005; Research Autism, 2008).

RETT'S DISORDER

Rett's disorder is an autistic spectrum disorder characterized by the development of multiple deficits after a period of normal functioning. It occurs almost exclusively in girls, is rare (affecting around 1 in 10,000 girls), and persists throughout life. Developmentally normal from around 6 months to around 18 months, the child loses motor skills and begins showing stereotyped movements instead. She loses interest in the social environment (although this can improve again by school age) and severe impairment of expressive and receptive language becomes evident as she grows older. Movement disorders are common. Care and treatment are similar to that of autism.

CHILDHOOD DISINTEGRATIVE DISORDER

Childhood *disintegrative disorder* is characterized by marked regression in multiple areas of functioning after at least 2 years of apparently normal growth and development (American Psychiatric Association, 2000). Typical age at onset is between 3 and 4 years. Children with childhood disintegrative disorder have the same social and communication deficits and behavioural patterns seen with autistic disorder. This rare disorder occurs slightly more often in boys than in girls.

ASPERGER SYNDROME

Asperger syndrome – more common in males than females – is an autistic spectrum disorder characterized by the same impairments of social interaction and restricted stereotyped behaviours seen in autistic disorder, but there are no language or cognitive delays, and people with Asperger's tend to be of average or above-average intelligence and less likely to have a learning disability, although they may have specific learning difficulties such as dyslexia or dyspraxia, and conditions such as ADHD (see below) and epilepsy.

According to the National Autistic Society (2008b), people with Asperger's have difficulties in three main areas:

- Social communication (not understanding nuance, tone, non-verbal cues, for example)
- Social interaction (appearing aloof, struggling to understand social rules and others' motivation and behaviour)
- Social imagination (finding it hard to predict outcome, empathizing and fantasizing).

Asperger syndrome remains something of a mystery in terms of cause; various behavioural, psychological and nutritional approaches are being tried to help affected people and their carers.

Attention Deficit and Disruptive Behaviour Disorders

ATTENTION DEFICIT HYPERACTIVITY DISORDER (ATTENTION DEFICIT DISORDER (ADD)/HYPERKINETIC DISORDER)

Attention deficit hyperactivity disorder (ADHD) (sometimes referred to as hyperkinetic disorder) is characterized by inattentiveness, overactivity and impulsiveness. ADHD is the most common childhood disorder, affecting an estimated 3% to 9% of all school-aged children (and around 2% to 4% of adults). The ratio of boys to girls ranges from 3:1 in non-clinical settings to 9:1 in clinical settings (Hechtman, 2005). Despite growing awareness, many feel that too many children still remain undiagnosed or are not receiving the most appropriate care and treatment (NICE, 2008); equally, there is controversy about possible over-diagnosis of ADHD: there is a belief that 'different', mentally disordered, unhappy or challenging children are misdiagnosed and labelled because of their behaviour and without adequate contextualization of that behaviour (and, potentially, are prescribed drugs unnecessarily). In addition, there is contested evidence for a neurobiological (rather than a psychosocial) cause for ADHD and the context of children's behaviour and distress must always be addressed (Southall, 2007). These controversies need to be taken into account by all clinicians; nevertheless, regardless of the 'truth' of the diagnosis, there is no doubt that the nursing role can be vital in helping a group of unhappy, underachieving children live more satisfying and productive lives.

The two essential groupings of ADHD features are:

1. Inattention and
2. Hyperactivity and impulsivity

with three subtypes:

- ADHD mainly inattentive
- ADHD mainly hyperactive-impulsive or
- ADHD combined.

CLINICAL VIGNETTE: ATTENTION DEFICIT HYPERACTIVITY DISORDER

Scott is 8 years old. At 7 AM, his mother looks into Scott's bedroom and sees him playing. 'Scott, you know the rules: no playing before you're ready for school. Get dressed and come and have your breakfast.' Although these rules for a school day have been set for the past 7 months, Scott always tests them. In about 10 minutes, he is still not in the kitchen. His mother checks his room and finds Scott on the floor, still in his pyjamas, playing with miniature cars. Once he gets started doing or talking about something, it is often difficult for Scott to stop.

'Scott, you need to get dressed first. Your jeans and shirt are over here on the chair.' 'Mum, after school today, can we go shopping? There is the coolest new car game that anyone can play. I'd love to try it out.' As he is talking, Scott walks over to the chair and begins to pull his shirt over his head. 'Scott, you're putting your shirt over your pyjamas. You need to take your pyjamas off first,' his mother reminds him.

Ten minutes later, Scott bounds into the kitchen, still without socks and shoes, and hair in a mess. 'You forgot your socks, and your hair isn't combed,' his mother reminds him. 'Oh yeah. What's for breakfast?' he says. 'Scott, finish dressing first.' 'Well, where are my shoes?' 'By the back door where you left them.' This is the special designated place where Scott is supposed to leave his shoes so he doesn't forget.

Scott starts toward his shoes but spots his younger sister playing with blocks on the floor. He hurries to her. 'Wow, Amy, watch this—I can make these blocks into a huge tower, all the way to the ceiling.' He grabs the blocks and begins to stack them higher and higher. 'Scott makes a better tower than Amy,' he chants. Amy shrieks at this intrusion, but she is used to Scott grabbing things from her. The shriek brings their mother into the room. She notices Scott's feet still do not have socks and shoes.

'Scott, get your socks and shoes on now and leave Amy alone!' 'Where are my socks?' he asks. 'Go to your room and get a clean pair of socks and brush your teeth and hair. Then come eat your breakfast or you'll miss the bus.'

'I will in just a minute, Mum.' 'No! Now! Go get your socks.' Scott continues stacking blocks.

Wearily, his mother directs him toward his room. As he is looking for the socks, he is still chattering away. He finds a pair of socks and bolts in the direction of the kitchen, grabbing Amy and pinching her cheek as he swirls by her. Amy shrieks again and he begins to chant, 'Amy's just a baby! Amy's just a baby!' 'Scott, stop it right now and come eat something! You've got just 10 minutes until the bus comes.'

Typical warning signs for ADHD are:

- Poor concentration
- A tendency to be easily distracted
- Restless, fidgety behaviour
- Difficulty in sitting down or remaining still when told to
- Difficulty following instructions
- Finding it hard to wait their turn in a group situation
- Interrupting others
- Difficulty in playing quietly
- Often shifting from one incomplete activity to another and
- Little or no sense of danger, taking part in potentially dangerous activities seemingly without thinking about the consequences.

However, these broad problems need – for diagnosis – to be more common than generally observed in children of the same age, and children who are very active or hard to handle in the classroom can be diagnosed and treated mistakenly for ADHD. Some of these overly active children may suffer from psychosocial stressors at home, inadequate parenting or other mental health problems. Distinguishing bipolar disorder from ADHD can be difficult but is crucial in order to prescribe the most effective treatment (Faedda & Teicher, 2005). Girls may be less frequently diagnosed because they are less likely to come to adults' attention.

Onset and Clinical Course

ADHD is usually identified and diagnosed when the child begins nursery or school, although many parents report problems from a much younger age. As infants, children with ADHD are often fussy and temperamental and have poor sleeping patterns. Toddlers may be described as 'always on the go' and 'into everything', at times dismantling toys and cribs. They dart back and forth, jump and climb on furniture, run through the house, and cannot tolerate sedentary activities such as listening to stories. At this point in a child's development, it can be difficult for parents to distinguish normal active behaviour from excessive hyperactive behaviour.

By the time the child starts school, symptoms of ADHD begin to interfere significantly with behaviour and performance (Raggi & Chronis, 2006). The child fidgets constantly, is in and out of assigned seats and makes excessive noise by tapping or playing with pencils or other objects.

Normal environmental noises, such as someone coughing, distract the child. He or she cannot listen to directions or complete tasks. The child interrupts and blurts out answers before questions are completed. Academic performance suffers because the child makes hurried, careless mistakes in schoolwork, often loses or forgets homework assignments and fails to follow directions.

Socially, peers may ostracize or even ridicule the child for his or her behaviour. Forming positive peer relationships is difficult because the child cannot play co-operatively or take turns, and constantly interrupts others (American

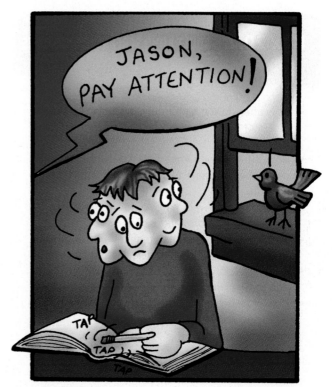

Attention deficit

Psychiatric Association, 2000). Studies have shown that both teachers and peers perceive children with ADHD as more aggressive, more bossy and less likeable (Hechtman, 2005). This perception results from the child's impulsivity, inability to share or take turns, tendency to interrupt, and failure to listen to and follow directions. Thus, peers and teachers may exclude the child from activities and play, may refuse to socialize with the child or may respond to the child in a harsh, punitive or rejecting manner.

About two-thirds of children diagnosed with ADHD continue to have problems in adolescence. Typical impulsive behaviours include truanting, getting speeding tickets, failing to maintain interpersonal relationships and adopting risk-taking behaviours such as using drugs or alcohol, engaging in sexual promiscuity, fighting and staying out late. Many adolescents with ADHD have discipline problems serious enough to warrant suspension or expulsion from school (Hechtman, 2005). The secondary complications of ADHD, such as low self-esteem and peer rejection, continue to pose serious problems.

Previously, it was believed that children outgrew ADHD, but it is now known that ADHD can persist into adulthood (McGough, 2005; Royal College of Psychiatrists 2008). Some estimates are that 30% to 50% of children with ADHD have symptoms that continue into adulthood (ADDISS ADHD Information Service, 2008). In one study, adults who had been treated for hyperactivity 25 years earlier were three to four times more likely than their brothers to experience nervousness, restlessness, depression, lack of friends and low frustration tolerance (McGough, 2005). Adults in

Box 20.2 ADULT ADHD SCREENING QUESTIONS

- How often do you have trouble wrapping up the final details of a project once the challenging parts have been done?
- How often do you have difficulty getting things in order when you have to do a task that requires organization?
- How often do you have problems remembering appointments or obligations?
- When you have a task that requires a lot of thought, how often do you avoid or delay getting started?
- How often do you fidget or squirm with your hands or feet when you have to sit down for a long time?
- How often do you feel overly active and compelled to do things, like you were driven by a motor?

Adapted from *World Health Organization Composite Diagnostic Interview* (2003).

whom ADHD was diagnosed in childhood also have higher rates of impulsivity, alcohol and drug use, legal troubles and personality disorders. Box 20.2 contains a screening questionnaire for ADHD in adults.

Aetiology

Although much research is taking place, the definitive causes of ADHD remain unknown. There may be cortical-arousal, information-processing or maturational abnormalities in the brain (Rowe & Hermens, 2006). A combination of factors such as environmental toxins, prenatal influences, heredity and damage to brain structure and functions may be at least partially responsible (Hechtman, 2005). Prenatal exposure to alcohol, tobacco and lead, and severe malnutrition in early childhood increase the likelihood of ADHD. Although the relation between ADHD and dietary sugar and vitamins has been studied, results have been inconclusive (Hechtman, 2005).

Brain images of people with ADHD have suggested decreased metabolism in the frontal lobes, which are essential for attention, impulse control, organization and sustained goal-directed activity. Studies have also shown decreased blood perfusion of the frontal cortex in children with ADHD, and frontal cortical atrophy in young adults with a history of childhood ADHD. Another study showed decreased glucose use in the frontal lobes of parents of children with ADHD, who had ADHD themselves (Hechtman, 2005). Evidence is not conclusive, but research in these areas seems promising.

There seems to be a genetic link for ADHD that is most likely associated with abnormalities in catecholamine and possibly serotonin metabolism. Despite the strong evidence supporting a genetic contribution, there are also cases of ADHD with no family history of ADHD; this furthers the theory of multiple contributing factors.

Risk factors for ADHD include family history of ADHD; male relatives with antisocial personality disorder or alcoholism; female relatives with somatization disorder; lower socioeconomic status; male gender; marital or family discord, including divorce, neglect, abuse or parental deprivation; low birth weight; and various kinds of brain insult (Hechtman, 2005).

DSM-IV-TR DIAGNOSTIC CRITERIA: SYMPTOMS OF ADHD

Inattentive Behaviours	Hyperactive/Impulsive Behaviours
Misses details	Fidgets
Makes careless mistakes	Often leaves seat (e.g. during a meal)
Has difficulty sustaining attention	Runs or climbs excessively
Doesn't seem to listen	Can't play quietly
Does not follow-through on chores or homework	Is always on the go; driven
Has difficulty with organization	Talks excessively
Avoids tasks requiring mental effort	Blurts out answers
Often loses necessary things	Interrupts
Is easily distracted by other stimuli	Can't wait for turn
Is often forgetful in daily activities	Is intrusive with siblings/playmates

Adapted from American Psychiatric Association. (2000). *Diagnostic and Statistical Manual of Mental Disorders* (4th edn, text revision). Washington, DC: APA.

Cultural Considerations

ADHD is known to occur in various cultures. It is more prevalent in Western cultures, but that may be the result of different diagnostic practices rather than actual differences in existence (American Psychiatric Association, 2000). Pierce and Reid (2004) found that, in the US, increasing numbers of children from culturally diverse groups were being diagnosed with ADHD. They believe this increase may represent over-identification of ADHD in culturally diverse children and urge practitioners to consider cultural context before making the diagnosis.

Care and Treatment

No one treatment has been found to be effective for all children with ADHD; this gives rise to many different approaches, including sugar-controlled diets and megavitamin therapy. Parents need to know that any treatment heralded as the 'cure' for ADHD is probably too good to be true (Hechtman, 2005). Goals of treatment involve managing symptoms, reducing hyperactivity and impulsivity and increasing the child's attention so that he or she can grow and develop normally: a large proportion of children (probably around 50%) simply 'grow out of it'. Effective treatments can include CBT or other psychotherapies, pharmacotherapy, psychosocial and educational interventions (Raggi & Chronis, 2006; NICE, 2008).

The Strengths and Difficulties Questionnaire (Youth in Mind, 2008) is a rating scale frequently used to determine problem areas and competencies. It and other scales are often part of a comprehensive assessment of ADHD in children.

PSYCHOPHARMACOLOGY

Medications are often effective in decreasing hyperactivity and impulsiveness and improving attention; this enables the child to participate in school and family life. The most common medications are methylphenidate (Ritalin), atomoxetine (Strattera) and dexamfetamine (Dexedrine)

Though possibly over-prescribed and used on occasion as a way of avoiding more complex and resource-intensive psychological and social packages of care, methylphenidate seems to be effective for some children with ADHD; it can reduce hyperactivity, impulsivity and mood lability and helps the child to pay attention. According to NICE guidelines, however,

> Drug treatment is not indicated as the first-line treatment for all school-age children and young people with ADHD. It should be reserved for those with severe symptoms and impairment or for those with moderate levels of impairment who have refused non-drug interventions, or whose symptoms have not responded sufficiently to parent-training/ education programmes or group psychological treatment.
>
> (NICE, 2008)

The most common side-effects of these drugs are insomnia, loss of appetite and weight loss or failure to gain weight.

Giving stimulants during daytime hours usually effectively combats insomnia. Eating a good breakfast with the morning dose and substantial nutritious snacks late in the day and at bedtime helps the child to maintain an adequate dietary intake. When stimulant medications are not effective, or their side-effects are intolerable, antidepressants are the second choice for treatment (see Chapter 3).

Atomoxetine (Strattera) is an antidepressant, specifically a selective noradrenaline reuptake inhibitor. The most common side-effects in children during clinical trials were decreased appetite, nausea, vomiting, tiredness and upset stomach. In adults, side-effects were similar to those of other antidepressants, including insomnia, dry mouth, urinary retention, decreased appetite, nausea, vomiting, dizziness and sexual side-effects. In addition, atomoxetine can cause liver damage, so individuals taking the drug need to have liver function tests. Table 20.1 lists, drugs, dosages and nursing considerations for clients with ADHD.

STRATEGIES FOR HOME AND SCHOOL

Medications do not automatically improve the child's academic performance or ensure that he or she makes friends: in many cases they may not be an answer at all. Cognitive-behavioural and other psychotherapeutic strategies, such as solution-focused and systemic therapy (individual and group), are necessary to help validate the child's experiences, thoughts and feelings, to help them understand others and to assist the child to master appropriate behaviours. Environmental strategies at school and home can help the child to succeed in those settings. Educating parents and helping them with parenting strategies are crucial components of effective treatment of ADHD. Effective approaches include validation and respectful listening strategies, providing consistent rewards and consequences for behaviour, offering consistent praise, using time-out and giving verbal reprimands.

In **therapeutic play**, play techniques are used to understand the child's thoughts and feelings, and to promote communication. Dramatic play is acting out an anxiety-producing situation, such as allowing the child to be a doctor or use a stethoscope or other equipment to take care of a patient (a doll). Play techniques to release energy could include pounding pegs, running or working with modelling clay. Creative play techniques can help children to express themselves, for example, by drawing pictures of themselves, their family and peers. These techniques are especially useful when children are unable or unwilling to express themselves verbally.

APPLICATION OF THE NURSING PROCESS: ATTENTION DEFICIT HYPERACTIVITY DISORDER

Assessment

During assessment, the nurse may gather information from the child, through direct observation and from the child's parents, other professionals and teachers. Assessing the

Table 20.1   DRUGS USED TO TREAT ADHD

Generic (Trade) Name	Dosage (mg/day)	Nursing Considerations
Stimulants		
Methylphenidate (Ritalin)	Child over 6: 5 mg 1–2 times daily, increased if necessary at weekly intervals by 5–10 mg daily to maximum of 60 mg in divided doses	Discontinue if no response after a month Avoid abrupt withdrawal Monitor for appetite suppression or growth delays Suspend every 1 to 2 years to assess child's condition Monitor blood pressure (BP) and full blood count
Modified release (Equasym XL, Concerta XL, Medikinet XL)	60 mg maximum (Concerta 54 mg maximum)	In morning with breakfast Alert client that full drug effect takes 2 days
Dexamfetamine sulphate (Dexedrine)	Child over 6: 5–40 (5–10 mg daily, increased if necessary by 5 mg daily at intervals of 1 week; usual max. 20 mg daily in 2–3 divided doses)	Monitor for insomnia Monitor height, weight, BP
Antidepressant (SNRI)		
Atomoxetine (Strattera)	Maximum 1.2 mg/kg/day in 1 or 2 divided doses (children <70 kg) 40–80 mg in 1 or 2 divided doses (children >70 kg and adults)	Monitor for suicidal ideation Give with food Monitor for appetite suppression Use calorie-free drinks to relieve dry mouth Monitor for elevated liver function tests

Adapted from *Lexi-comp's Psychotrophic Drug Information Handbook* (2005) and British National Formulary Online (2008) http://www.bnf.org/bnf/bnf/55/

child in a group of peers is likely to yield useful information because the child's behaviour may be subdued or different in a focused one-to-one interaction with the nurse. It is often helpful to use a checklist when talking with parents to help focus their input on the target symptoms or behaviours their child exhibits.

HISTORY

Parents may report that the child was fussy and had problems as an infant, or they may not have noticed the hyperactive behaviour until the child was a toddler or entered day care or school. The child probably has difficulties in all major life areas such as school or play, and he or she may well display overactive or even dangerous behaviour at home. Often, parents say the child is 'out of control', and they feel unable to deal with the behaviour. Parents may report many, largely unsuccessful, attempts to discipline the child or to change the behaviour.

GENERAL APPEARANCE AND MOTOR BEHAVIOUR

The child may be unable to sit still in a chair and squirms and wriggles while trying to do so. He or she may dart around the room with little or no apparent purpose. Speech may be unimpaired, but the child cannot carry on a conversation: he or she interrupts, blurts out answers before the question is finished and fails to pay attention to what has been said. Conversation topics may jump

abruptly. The child may appear immature or lag behind in developmental milestones.

MOOD AND AFFECT

Mood may be labile, even to the point of verbal outbursts or temper tantrums. Anxiety, frustration and agitation are common. The child appears to be driven to keep moving or talking and appears to have little control over movement or speech. Attempts to focus the child's attention or redirect the child to a topic may evoke resistance and anger.

THOUGHT PROCESS AND CONTENT

There are generally no impairments in this area, although assessment can be difficult, depending on the child's activity level and age or developmental stage.

SENSORY AND INTELLECTUAL PROCESSES

The child is alert and oriented with no sensory or perceptual alterations such as hallucinations. Ability to pay attention or to concentrate is markedly impaired. The child's attention span may be as little as 2 or 3 seconds with severe ADHD, or 2 or 3 minutes in milder forms of the disorder. Assessing the child's memory may be difficult; he or she may frequently answer, 'I don't know,' because he or she cannot pay attention to the question or stop the mind from racing. The child with ADHD is very distractible and rarely able to complete tasks.

JUDGEMENT AND INSIGHT

Children with ADHD usually exhibit poor judgement and often do not think before acting. They may fail to perceive harm or danger and engage in impulsive acts such as running into the street or jumping off high objects. Although assessing judgement and insight in young children is difficult, children with ADHD display more lack of judgement when compared with others of the same age. Most young children with ADHD are totally unaware that their behaviour is different from that of others, and cannot perceive how it harms others. Older children might report, 'No one at school likes me,' but they cannot relate the lack of friends to their own behaviour.

SELF-CONCEPT

Again, this may be difficult to assess in a very young child, but generally the self-esteem of children with ADHD is low. Because they are not successful at school, may not develop many friends, and have trouble getting along at home, they generally feel out of place and bad about themselves. The negative reactions their behaviour evokes from others often cause them to see themselves as bad or stupid.

ROLES AND RELATIONSHIPS

The child is often unsuccessful academically and socially at school. He or she frequently is disruptive and intrusive at home, which causes friction with siblings and parents. Until the child is diagnosed and treated, parents often believe that the child is wilful, stubborn and purposefully misbehaving. Generally, measures to discipline have limited success; in some cases, the child becomes physically out of control, even hitting parents or destroying family possessions. Parents find themselves chronically exhausted mentally and physically. Teachers often feel the same frustration as parents, and day-care providers or baby-sitters may refuse to care for the child with ADHD, which adds to the child's rejection.

PHYSIOLOGICAL AND SELF-CARE CONSIDERATIONS

Children with ADHD may be thin if they do not take time to eat properly or cannot sit through meals. Trouble settling down and difficulty sleeping are problems as well. If the child engages in reckless or risk-taking behaviours, there also may be a history of physical injuries.

Data Analysis and Planning

Nursing formulations commonly used when working with children with ADHD include the following:

- Risk of injury
- Ineffective role performance
- Impaired social interaction
- Compromised family coping.

Outcome Identification

Treatment outcomes for clients with ADHD may include the following:

- The child will feel comfortable with self and others.
- The client will be free of injury.
- The client will not violate the boundaries of others.
- The client will demonstrate age-appropriate social skills.
- The client will complete tasks.
- The client will follow directions.

Intervention

Interventions described in this section can be adapted to various settings and used by nurses and other health professionals, teachers and parents or carers.

ENSURING SAFETY

Safety of the child and others is always a priority. If the child is engaged in a potentially dangerous activity, the first step is to stop the behaviour. This may require physical intervention if the child is running into the street or attempting to jump from a high place. Attempting to talk to or reason with a child engaged in a dangerous activity is unlikely to succeed because his or her ability to pay attention and to listen is limited. When the incident is over and the child is safe, the adult should talk to the child directly about the expectations for safe behaviour. Close supervision may be required for a time to ensure compliance and to avoid injury.

> **NURSING INTERVENTIONS FOR ADHD**
>
> - Ensure the child's safety and that of others
>   Stop unsafe behaviour.
>   Provide close supervision.
>   Give clear directions about acceptable and unacceptable behaviour.
> - Improved role performance
>   Give positive feedback for meeting expectations.
>   Manage the environment (e.g. provide a quiet place free of distractions for task completion).
> - Simplifying instructions/directions
>   Get child's full attention.
>   Break complex tasks into small steps.
>   Allow breaks.
> - Structured daily routine
>   Establish a daily schedule.
>   Minimize changes.
> - Child/family education and support
>   Listen to parent's feelings and frustrations.

Explanations should be short and clear, and the adult should not use a punitive or belittling tone of voice. The adult should not assume that the child knows acceptable behaviour but instead should state expectations clearly. For example, if the child was jumping down a flight of stairs, the adult might say,

'It is unsafe to jump down stairs. From now on, you are to walk down the stairs, one at a time.'

If the child pushes ahead of others, the adult should walk the child back to the proper place in line and say, gently but firmly,

'It's not okay to push ahead of others. Take your place please at the end of the line.'

To prevent physically intrusive behaviour, it also may be necessary to supervise the child closely while he or she is playing. Again, it is often necessary to act first to stop the harmful behaviour by separating the child from the friend, such as stepping between them or physically removing the child. Afterward, the adult should clearly explain expected and unacceptable behaviour. For example, the adult might say,

'It's not okay to grab other people. When you're playing with others, you must ask for the toy.'

IMPROVING ROLE PERFORMANCE

It is extremely important to give the child specific positive feedback when he or she meets stated expectations. Doing so reinforces desired behaviours and gives the child a sense of accomplishment. For example, the adult might say,

'You walked down the stairs safely' or *'You did a good job of asking to play with the guitar and waited until it was your turn.'*

Managing the environment helps the child to improve his or her ability to listen, pay attention and complete tasks. A quiet place with minimal noise and distraction is desirable. At school, this may be a seat directly facing the teacher at the front of the room and away from the distraction of a window or door. At home, the child should have a quiet area for homework away from the television or radio.

SIMPLIFYING INSTRUCTIONS

Before beginning any tasks, adults must gain the child's full attention. It is helpful to face the child on his or her level and use good eye contact. The adult should tell the child what needs to be done and break the task into smaller steps if necessary. For example, if the child has 25 maths problems,

it may help to give him or her five problems at a time, then five more when those are completed and so on. This approach prevents overwhelming the child and provides the opportunity for feedback about each set of problems he or she completes. With sedentary tasks, it is also important to allow the child to have breaks or opportunities to move around.

Adults can use the same approach for tasks such as cleaning or picking up toys. Initially, the child needs the supervision or at least the presence of the adult. The adult can direct the child to do one portion of the task at a time; when the child shows progress, the adult can give only occasional reminders and then allow the child to complete the task independently. It helps to provide specific, step-by-step directions rather than give a general direction such as 'Please clean your room.' The adult could say,

'Put your dirty clothes in the basket please.'

After this step is completed, the adult gives another direction:

'Now make the bed, please.'

The adult assigns specific tasks until the child has completed the overall chore.

PROMOTING A STRUCTURED DAILY ROUTINE

A structured daily routine is helpful. The child will accomplish getting up, dressing, doing homework, playing, going to bed and so forth much more readily if there is a routine time for these daily activities. Children with ADHD do not adjust to changes readily and are less likely to meet expectations if times for activities are arbitrary or differ from day to day.

PROVIDING CLIENT AND FAMILY EDUCATION AND SUPPORT

It is important to include parents in planning and providing care for the child with ADHD. The nurse can teach parents the approaches described previously for use at home. Parents feel empowered and relieved to have specific strategies that can help both them and their child be more successful.

The nurse must listen to parents' feelings. They may feel frustrated, angry or guilty, and blame themselves or the school system for their child's problems. Parents need to hear that neither they nor their child are at fault and that techniques and therapeutic programmes are available to help.

Because raising a child with ADHD can be frustrating and exhausting, it often helps parents to attend support groups that can provide information and encouragement from other parents with the same problems. Parents must learn

CLIENT/FAMILY EDUCATION FOR ADHD

- Include parents in planning and providing care.
- Refer parents to support groups.
- Focus on child's strengths as well as problems.
- Teach accurate administration of medication and possible side-effects.
- Assist parents to identify behavioural approaches to be used at home.
- Help parents achieve a balance of praising child and correcting child's behaviour.
- Emphasize the need for structure and consistency in child's daily routine and behavioural expectations.

strategies to help their child improve his or her social and academic abilities, but they also must understand how to help rebuild their child's self-esteem. Most of these children have low self-esteem because they have been labelled as having 'behaviour problems' and have been corrected continually by parents and teachers for not listening, not paying attention and misbehaving. Parents should give positive comments as much as possible to encourage the child and acknowledge his or her strengths. One technique to help parents to achieve a good balance is to ask them to count the numbers of times they praise or criticize their child each day or for several days.

Although medication can help reduce hyperactivity and inattention and allow the child to focus during school, it is by no means a cure-all. The child needs strategies and practice to improve social skills and academic performance. Because these children often are not diagnosed until they are 7 or 8 years old, they may have missed much basic learning for reading and maths. Parents should know that it takes time for them to catch up to other children of the same age.

Evaluation

Parents and teachers are likely to notice positive outcomes of treatment before the child does. Medications are often effective in decreasing hyperactivity and impulsivity and improving attention relatively quickly, if the child responds to them. Improved sociability, peer relationships and academic achievement happen more slowly and gradually, but are possible with effective treatment.

CONDUCT DISORDERS

'Conduct disorder' is characterized by persistent antisocial behaviour in children and adolescents that significantly impairs their ability to function in social, academic or occupational areas. Symptoms are clustered in four areas: aggression

to people and animals, destruction of property, deceitfulness and theft and serious violation of rules (Thomas, 2005). People diagnosed with conduct disorder have little empathy for others; they have low self-esteem, poor frustration tolerance and temper outbursts. Conduct disorder is frequently associated with early onset of sexual behaviour, drinking, smoking, use of illegal substances and other reckless or risky behaviours. It occurs three times more often in boys than in girls.

Children diagnosed with conduct disorders are more likely to experience a range of related health and social problems in adulthood. As many as 30% to 50% of children with conduct disorders will be diagnosed with antisocial personality disorders as adults, and others will receive diagnoses including substance misuse, schizophrenia and depressive disorders. They are also at a high risk of experiencing future disadvantage through poor school achievement and long-term unemployment (NICE, 2006).

Onset and Clinical Course

Two subtypes of 'conduct disorder' are based on age at onset. The childhood-onset type involves symptoms before 10 years of age, including physical aggression toward others and disturbed peer relationships. These children are more likely to have persistent conduct disorder and to develop antisocial personality disorder as adults. Adolescent-onset type is defined by no behaviours of conduct disorder until after 10 years of age. These adolescents are less likely to be aggressive, and they have more normal peer relationships. They are less likely to have persistent conduct disorder or antisocial personality disorder as adults (American Psychiatric Association, 2000).

Box 20.3 CONDUCT DISORDERS AND OPPOSITIONAL DEFIANT DISORDERS

Be very wary of these diagnoses:

- Conduct disorder
- Oppositional defiant disorder.

These labels are most unhelpful. They simply name the behaviour without any indication of the underlying cause.

It is possible for a child or adult with an autistic spectrum disorder to be given one of these diagnoses if a proper history is not taken and the proper psychological investigations are not carried out.

If this happens the needs of the child or adult concerned and their family are likely to be misjudged, with disastrous results.

From National Autistic Society. (2008). http://www.nas.org.uk/nas/jsp/polopoly.jsp?d=364&a=9120. Reproduced with permission.

Nursing Care Plan *Children with Attention Deficit Hyperactivity Disorder*

Nursing Diagnosis

Impaired Social Interaction: *Insufficient or excessive quantity or ineffective quality of social exchange.*

ASSESSMENT DATA

- Short attention span
- High level of distractibility
- Labile moods
- Low frustration tolerance
- Inability to complete tasks
- Inability to sit still or fidgeting
- Excessive talking
- Inability to follow directions

EXPECTED OUTCOMES

Immediate
The child will
- Successfully complete tasks or assignments with assistance
- Demonstrate effective social skills while interacting with staff or family members

Stabilization
The child will
- Participate successfully in educational, occupational and social settings
- Demonstrate the ability to complete tasks with reminders
- Demonstrate successful interactions with family members

Ongoing
The child will
- Verbalize positive statements about himself or herself
- Complete tasks independently

IMPLEMENTATION

Nursing Interventions *denotes collaborative interventions

Identify the factors that aggravate and alleviate the child's performance.

Provide an environment as free from distractions as possible. Institute interventions on a one-to-one basis. Gradually increase the amount of environmental stimuli.

Engage the child's attention before giving instructions (i.e. call the child's name and establish eye contact).

Give instructions slowly, using simple language and concrete directions.

Ask the child to repeat instructions before beginning tasks.

Separate complex tasks into small steps.

Provide positive feedback for completion of each step.

Rationale

The external stimuli that exacerbate the child's problems can be identified and minimized. Likewise, ones that positively influence the child can be effectively used.

The child's ability to deal with external stimulation is impaired.

The child must hear instructions as a first step toward carrying them out.

The child's ability to comprehend instructions (especially if they are complex or abstract) is impaired.

Repetition demonstrates that the child has accurately received the information.

The likelihood of success is enhanced with less complicated components of a task.

The child's opportunity for successful experiences is increased by treating each step as an opportunity for success.

Nursing Care Plan: Children with Attention Deficit Hyperactivity Disorder, cont.

IMPLEMENTATION

Nursing Interventions *denotes collaborative interventions	Rationale
Allow breaks, during which the child can move around.	The child's restless energy can be given an acceptable outlet, so he or she can attend to future tasks more effectively.
State expectations for task completion clearly.	The child must understand the request before he or she can attempt task completion.
Initially, assist the child to complete tasks.	If the child is unable to complete a task independently, having assistance will allow success and will demonstrate how to complete the task.
Progress to prompting or reminding the child to perform tasks or assignments.	The amount of intervention gradually is decreased to increase child independence as his or her abilities increase.
Give the child positive feedback for performing behaviours that come close to task achievement.	This approach, called *shaping*, is a behavioural procedure in which successive approximations of a desired behaviour are positively reinforced. It allows rewards to occur as the child gradually masters the actual expectation.
Gradually decrease reminders.	Child independence is promoted as staff participation is decreased.
Assist the child to verbalize by asking sequencing questions to keep on the topic ('Then what happens?' and 'What happens next?').	Sequencing questions provide a structure for discussions to increase logical thought and decrease tangentiality.
*Teach the child's family or caregivers to use the same procedures for his or her tasks and interactions at home.	Successful interventions can be instituted by the child's family or caregivers by using this process. This will promote consistency and enhance the child's chances for success.
*Explain and demonstrate 'positive parenting' techniques to family or carers, such as *time-in* for good behaviour or being vigilant in identifying and responding positively to the child's first bid for attention; *special time*, or guaranteed time spent daily with the child with no interruptions and no discussion of problem-related topics; *ignoring minor transgressions* by immediate withdrawal of eye contact or physical contact and cessation of discussion with the child to avoid secondary gains.	It is important for parents or caregivers to engage in techniques that will maintain their loving relationship with the child while promoting, or at least not interfering with, therapeutic goals. Children need to have a sense of being lovable to their significant others that is not crucial to the nurse–child therapeutic relationship.

Adapted from Schultz, J. M. & Videbeck, S. L. (2005). *Lippincott's manual of psychiatric nursing care plans* (7th edn). Philadelphia: Lippincott Williams & Wilkins.

Conduct disorders can be classified as mild, moderate or severe (American Psychiatric Association, 2000):

- Mild: The person has some conduct problems that cause relatively minor harm to others. Examples include lying, truancy and staying out late without permission.
- Moderate: The number of conduct problems increases, as does the amount of harm to others. Examples include vandalism and theft.
- Severe: The person has many conduct problems that cause considerable harm to others. Examples include forced sex, cruelty to animals, use of a weapon, burglary and robbery.

The course of conduct disorder is variable. People with the adolescent-onset type or mild problems can achieve adequate social relationships and academic or occupational success as adults. Those with the childhood-onset type or more severe problem behaviours are more likely to develop antisocial personality disorder as adults. Even those who do not have antisocial personality disorder may lead troubled lives with difficult interpersonal relationships, unhealthy lifestyles and an inability to support themselves (Thomas, 2005).

Aetiology

Researchers generally accept that genetic vulnerability, environmental adversity and factors such as poor coping interact to cause the disorder. Risk factors include poor parenting, low academic achievement, poor peer relationships and low self-esteem; protective factors include resilience, family support, positive peer relationships and good health (Thomas, 2005).

There is a genetic risk for conduct disorder, although no specific gene marker has been identified (Thomas, 2005). The disorder is more common in children who have a sibling with conduct disorder or a parent with antisocial personality disorder, substance abuse, mood disorder, schizophrenia or ADHD (American Psychiatric Association, 2000).

A lack of reactivity of the autonomic nervous system has been found in children with conduct disorder; this non-responsiveness is similar to that of adults with antisocial

personality disorder. The abnormality may cause more aggression in social relationships as a result of decreased normal avoidance or social inhibitions. Research into the role of neurotransmitters is promising (Thomas, 2005).

Poor family functioning, marital discord, poor parenting and a family history of substance abuse and psychiatric problems are all associated with the development of conduct disorder. Child abuse is an especially significant risk factor. The specific parenting patterns considered ineffective are inconsistent parental responses to the child's demands and giving in to demands as the child's behaviour escalates. Many childhood, adolescent and, indeed, adult mental health problems have their roots in abuse by carers- often, depressingly, by those professionals working in children's homes and wider children's services. Exposure to violence in the media and community is a contributing factor for the child at risk in other areas. Socioeconomic disadvantages such as inadequate housing, crowded conditions and poverty also increase the likelihood of conduct disorder in at-risk children (McGuinness, 2006).

Academic underachievement, learning disabilities, hyperactivity and problems with attention span are all associated with conduct disorder. Children with conduct disorder have difficulty functioning in social situations. They lack the abilities to respond appropriately to others and to negotiate conflict, and they lose the ability to restrain themselves when emotionally stressed. They are often accepted only by peers with similar problems (Thomas, 2005).

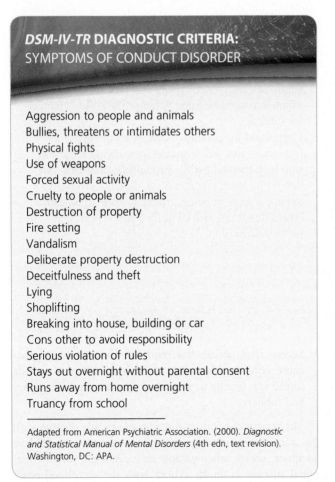

DSM-IV-TR DIAGNOSTIC CRITERIA:
SYMPTOMS OF CONDUCT DISORDER

Aggression to people and animals
Bullies, threatens or intimidates others
Physical fights
Use of weapons
Forced sexual activity
Cruelty to people or animals
Destruction of property
Fire setting
Vandalism
Deliberate property destruction
Deceitfulness and theft
Lying
Shoplifting
Breaking into house, building or car
Cons other to avoid responsibility
Serious violation of rules
Stays out overnight without parental consent
Runs away from home overnight
Truancy from school

Adapted from American Psychiatric Association. (2000). *Diagnostic and Statistical Manual of Mental Disorders* (4th edn, text revision). Washington, DC: APA.

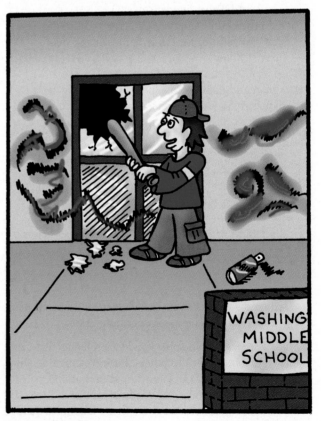

Conduct disorder

Cultural Considerations

As is the case with ADHD, concerns have been raised that 'difficult' children may be mistakenly labelled as having conduct disorder. Knowing the client's history and circumstances is essential for accurate diagnosis. In high-crime areas, aggressive behaviour may be protective and not necessarily indicative of conduct disorder. In immigrants from war-ravaged countries, aggressive behaviour may have been necessary for survival, so these individuals should not be diagnosed with conduct disorder (American Psychiatric Association, 2000).

Treatment

Many treatments have been used for conduct disorder with only modest effectiveness. Early intervention is more effective, and prevention is more effective than treatment. Dramatic interventions such as 'boot camp' or incarceration have not proved effective and may even worsen the situation (Thomas, 2005). Care and treatment must be sensitive, respectful, curious and collaborative, and geared toward the client's developmental age; no one treatment is suitable for all ages. Preschool programmes such as Sure Start result in lower rates of delinquent behaviour and conduct disorder through use of parental education about normal growth and development, stimulation for the child and parental support during crises.

For school-aged children with conduct disorder, the child, family and school environment are the focus of treatment. Techniques include parenting education, social skills training to improve peer relationships and attempts to improve academic performance and increase the child's ability to comply with demands from authority figures. Family therapy is considered to be essential for children in this age group (Thomas, 2005).

Adolescents rely less on their parents and more on peers, so treatment for this age group includes individual therapy. Many adolescent clients have some involvement with the legal system as a result of criminal behaviour, and they may have restrictions on their freedom as a result. Use of alcohol and other drugs plays a more significant role for this age group; any treatment plan must address this issue. The most promising treatment approach includes keeping the client in his or her environment with family and individual therapies. The plan usually includes conflict resolution, anger management and teaching social skills.

Medications alone have little effect but may be used in conjunction with treatment for specific symptoms. For example, the client who presents a clear danger to others may be prescribed an antipsychotic medication, or a client with a labile mood may benefit from lithium or another mood stabilizer such as carbamazepine (Tegretol) or valproic acid (Depakote) (Thomas, 2005).

APPLICATION OF THE NURSING PROCESS: 'CONDUCT DISORDER'

Assessment

HISTORY

Children diagnosed with conduct disorder have a history of disturbed relationships with peers, aggression toward people or animals, destruction of property, deceitfulness or theft and serious violation of rules (e.g. truancy, running away from home, staying out all night without permission). The behaviours and problems may be mild-to-severe.

GENERAL APPEARANCE AND MOTOR BEHAVIOUR

Appearance, speech and motor behaviour are typically normal for the age group but may be somewhat extreme (e.g. body piercings, tattoos, hairstyle, clothing). These clients

CLINICAL VIGNETTE: 'CONDUCT DISORDER'

Tom, 14 years of age, leaves the headmaster's office after being involved in a physical fight in the dining room. He knows his parents will be furious because he is suspended for one week. 'It wasn't my fault,' he thinks to himself, 'What am I supposed to do when someone calls me names?' Tom is angry that he even came to school today; he'd much rather spend time hanging out with his friends and having a few drinks or smoking weed.

On his way home, Tom sees a car parked next to the newsagents; it is unlocked and running. Tom jumps in, thinking, 'This is my lucky day!' He speeds away, but soon he can hear police sirens as a patrol car closes in on him. He is eventually stopped and arrested. As he waits for his parents at the station, he's not sure what to do next. He tells the police officer that the car belongs to a friend and he just borrowed it. He promises never to get into trouble again if the officer will let him go. But the officer has Tom's record, which includes truancy, underage drinking, suspicion in the disappearance of a neighbour's pet cat and shoplifting.

When Tom's father arrives, he smacks Tom across the face and says, 'You stupid kid! I told you the last time you'd better straighten up. And look at you now! What a sorry excuse for a son!' Tom slumps in his chair with a sullen, defiant look on his face. 'Go ahead and hit me! Who cares? I'm not gonna do what you say, so you might as well give up!'

often slouch and are sullen and unwilling to be interviewed. They may use excessive obscenities, call the nurse names and make disparaging remarks about parents, teachers, police and other authority figures (even more than 'normal' adolescents!).

MOOD AND AFFECT

Clients may be quiet and reluctant to talk or openly hostile and angry. Their attitude is likely to be disrespectful toward parents, the nurse or anyone in a position of authority. Irritability, frustration and temper outbursts are common. Clients may be unwilling to answer questions or to co-operate with the interview; they believe they do not need help or treatment. If a client has legal problems, he or she may express superficial guilt or remorse, but it is unlikely that these emotions are sincere.

THOUGHT PROCESS AND CONTENT

Thought processes are usually intact – that is, clients are capable of logical, rational thinking. Nevertheless, they perceive the world to be aggressive and threatening, and they respond in the same manner. Clients may be preoccupied with looking out for themselves and behave as though everyone is 'out to get me'. Thoughts or fantasies about death or violence are common.

SENSORY AND INTELLECTUAL PROCESSES

Clients are alert and oriented with intact memory and no sensory-perceptual alterations. Intellectual capacity is not impaired, but typically these clients have poor results because of academic underachievement, behavioural problems in school, or failure to attend class and to complete assignments.

JUDGEMENT AND INSIGHT

Judgement and insight are limited for developmental stage. Clients consistently break rules with no regard for the consequences. Thrill-seeking or risky behaviour is common, such as use of drugs or alcohol, reckless driving, sexual activity and illegal activities such as theft. Clients lack insight and usually blame others or society for their problems; they rarely believe their behaviour is the cause of difficulties.

SELF-CONCEPT

Although these clients generally try to appear tough, their self-esteem is low. They do not value themselves any more than they value others. Their identity is related to their behaviours, such as being cool if they have had many sexual encounters or feeling important if they have stolen expensive merchandise or been expelled from school.

ROLES AND RELATIONSHIPS

Relationships with others, especially those in authority, are disruptive and may be violent. This includes parents, teachers, police and most other adults. Verbal and physical aggression is common. Siblings may be a target for ridicule or aggression. Relationships with peers are limited to others who display similar behaviours; these clients see peers who follow rules as dumb or afraid. Clients usually have poor grades, have been expelled or have dropped out. It is unlikely that they have a job (if old enough) because they would prefer to steal. Their idea of fulfilling roles is being tough, breaking rules and taking advantage of others.

PHYSIOLOGICAL AND SELF-CARE CONSIDERATIONS

Clients are often at risk of unplanned pregnancy and sexually transmitted diseases because of their early and frequent sexual behaviour. Use of drugs and alcohol is an additional risk to health. Clients with conduct disorders are involved in physical aggression and violence including weapons; this results in more injuries and deaths than compared with others of the same age.

Data Analysis and Planning

Nursing formulations commonly used for clients with conduct disorders include the following:

- Risk of violence towards others
- Non-collaboration
- Ineffective coping
- Impaired social interaction
- Chronic low self-esteem.

Outcome Identification

Treatment outcomes for clients with conduct disorders may include the following:

- The client will not hurt others or damage property.
- The client will participate in treatment.
- The client will learn effective problem-solving and coping skills.
- The client will use age-appropriate and acceptable behaviours when interacting with others.
- The client will verbalize positive, age-appropriate statements about self.

Intervention

DECREASING VIOLENCE AND INCREASING COLLABORATIVE APPROACH TO TREATMENT

The nurse must protect others from the manipulative or aggressive behaviours common with these clients. He or she must set limits on unacceptable behaviour at the beginning of treatment. **Limit-setting** involves three steps:

1. Inform clients of the rule or limit.
2. Explain the consequences if clients exceed the limit.
3. State expected behaviour.

Providing consistent limit-enforcement with no exceptions by all members of the health team, including parents, is essential. For example, the nurse might say,

'It's not OK to hit another person. If you're angry, tell a staff member about your anger. If you hit someone, you'll be restricted from recreation time for 24 hours.'

For limit setting to be effective, the consequences must have meaning for clients – that is, they must value or desire recreation time (in this example). If a client wanted to be alone in his or her room, then this consequence would not be effective.

The nurse can negotiate with a client a behavioural contract outlining expected behaviours, limits and rewards to increase treatment compliance. The client can refer to the written agreement to remember expectations, and staff can refer to the agreement if the client tries to change any terms. A contract can help staff to avoid power struggles over requests for special favours or attempts to alter treatment goals or behavioural expectations.

Whether there is a written contract or treatment plan, staff must be consistent with these clients. They will attempt to bend or break rules, blame others for non-compliance or make excuses for behaviour. Consistency in following the treatment plan is essential to decrease manipulation; equally, staff themselves must earn trust, carry out promises and maintain their own boundaries.

Time-out is retreat to a neutral place so clients can regain self-control. It is not a punishment. When a client's behaviour begins to escalate, such as when he or she yells at or threatens someone, a time-out may prevent aggression or acting out. Staff may need to institute a time-out for clients if they are unwilling or unable to do so. Eventually, the goal is for clients to recognize signs of increasing agitation and take a self-instituted time-out to control emotions and outbursts. After the time-out, the nurse should discuss the events with the client. Doing so can help clients to recognize situations that trigger emotional responses and to learn more effective ways of dealing with similar situations in the future. Providing positive feedback for successful efforts at avoiding aggression helps to reinforce new behaviours for clients.

It helps for clients to have a schedule of daily activities, including personal hygiene, school, homework and leisure time. Clients are more likely to establish positive habits if they have routine expectations about tasks and responsibilities. They are more likely to follow a daily routine if they have input concerning the schedule.

IMPROVING COPING SKILLS AND SELF-ESTEEM

The nurse must show acceptance of clients as worthwhile persons even if their behaviour is unacceptable. This means that the nurse must be matter-of-fact about setting limits and must not make judgemental statements about clients. He or she must focus only on the behaviour. For example, if a client broke a chair during an angry outburst, the nurse would say,

'John, breaking chairs is unacceptable. You need to let staff know you're upset so you can talk about it instead of breaking things and upsetting people.'

The nurse must avoid saying things like,

'What's the matter with you? Don't you know any better?'

Comments such as these are subjective and judgemental and do not focus on the specific behaviour; they reinforce the client's self-image as a 'bad person' and maintain a non-therapeutic distance between nurse and client.

Clients diagnosed with a conduct disorder often have a tough exterior and are unable or reluctant to discuss feelings and emotions. Keeping a diary may help them to identify and express their feelings. The nurse can discuss these feelings with clients and explore better, safer expressions than through aggression or acting out.

Clients may also need to learn how to solve problems effectively. Problem solving involves identifying the problem, exploring all possible solutions, choosing and implementing one of the alternatives and evaluating the results (see Chapter 16). The nurse can help clients to work on actual problems using this process. Problem-solving skills are likely to improve with practice.

PROMOTING SOCIAL INTERACTION

Clients diagnosed with conduct disorder may not have age-appropriate social skills, so teaching social skills is important. The nurse can role model these skills and help clients to practise appropriate social interaction. The nurse identifies what is not appropriate, such as profanity and name calling, and also what is appropriate. Clients may have little experience discussing the news, current events, sports or other topics. As they begin to develop social skills, the nurse can include other peers in these discussions. Positive feedback is essential to let clients know they are meeting expectations.

PROVIDING CLIENT AND FAMILY EDUCATION

Parents may also need help in learning social skills, solving problems and behaving appropriately. Often, parents have their own problems, and they have had difficulties with the client for a long time before treatment was instituted. Parents need to replace old patterns such as yelling, hitting or simply ignoring behaviour with more effective strategies. The nurse can teach parents age-appropriate activities and expectations for clients, such as reasonable curfews, household responsibilities and acceptable behaviour at home. The parents may need to learn effective limit setting with appropriate consequences. Parents often need to learn to communicate their feelings and expectations clearly and directly to these clients. Some parents may need to let clients experience the consequences of their behaviour rather than rescuing them. For example, if a client gets a speeding ticket, the parents should not pay the fine for him or her. If a client causes a disturbance in school and receives detention, the parents can support the teacher's actions instead of blaming the teacher or school.

Evaluation

Treatment is considered effective if the client stops behaving in an aggressive or illegal way, attends school and follows reasonable rules and expectations at home. The client will not become a model child in a short period; instead, he or she may make modest progress with some setbacks over time.

Clients with 'conduct disorder' are seen in acute care settings only when their behaviour is severe and only for short periods of stabilization. Much long-term work takes place at school and home or another community setting. Some clients are placed outside their parents' home for short or long periods. Group homes, halfway houses, and residential treatment settings are designed to provide safe, structured environments and adequate supervision if that cannot be provided at home. Younger clients with legal issues may be placed in young offender institutions or prison. Chapter 4 discusses treatment settings and programmes.

NURSING INTERVENTIONS FOR 'CONDUCT DISORDER'

- Decreasing violence and increasing concordance with treatment
  Protect others from client's aggression and manipulation.
  Set limits for unacceptable behaviour.
  Provide consistency with client's treatment plan.
  Use behavioural contracts.
  Institute time-out.
  Provide a routine schedule of daily activities.
- Improving coping skills and self-esteem
  Show acceptance of the person, not necessarily the behaviour.
  Encourage the client to keep a diary.
  Teach and practise problem-solving skills.
- Promoting social interaction
  Teach age-appropriate social skills.
  Role model and practise social skills.
  Provide positive feedback for acceptable behaviour.
- Providing client and family education

Nursing Care Plan *'Conduct Disorder'*

Nursing Diagnosis

Ineffective Coping: *Inability to form a valid appraisal of the stressors, inadequate choices of practised responses and/or inability to use available resources.*

ASSESSMENT DATA

- Few or no meaningful peer relationships
- Inability to empathize with others
- Inability to give and receive affection
- Low self-esteem, masked by 'tough' act

EXPECTED OUTCOMES

Immediate
The client will

- Engage in social interaction
- Verbalize feelings
- Learn problem-solving skills

Medium-term
The client will

- Demonstrate effective problem-solving and coping skills
- Assess own strengths and weaknesses realistically

Longer-term
The client will

- Demonstrate development of relationships with peers
- Verbalize real feelings of self-worth that are age appropriate
- Perform at a satisfactory academic level

Nursing Care Plan: Conduct Disorder, cont.

IMPLEMENTATION

Nursing Interventions *denotes collaborative interventions	**Rationale**
Encourage the client to discuss his or her thoughts and feelings.	Verbalizing feelings is an initial step toward dealing with them in an appropriate manner.
Give positive feedback for appropriate discussions.	Positive feedback increases the likelihood of continued performance.
Tell the client that he or she is accepted as a person, although a particular behaviour may not be acceptable.	Clients with conduct disorders frequently experience rejection. The client needs support to increase self-esteem, while understanding that behavioural changes are necessary.
Give the client positive attention when behaviour is not problematic.	The client may have been receiving the majority of attention from others when he or she was engaged in problematic behaviour, a pattern that needs to change.
Teach the client about limit setting and the need for limits. Include time for discussion.	This allows the client to hear about the relationship between harmful behaviour and consequences when behaviour is not problematic. The client may have no knowledge of the concept of limits and how limits can be beneficial.
Teach the client the problem-solving process as an alternative to acting out (identify the problem, consider alternatives, select and implement an alternative, evaluate the effectiveness of the solution).	The client may not know how to solve problems constructively or may not have seen this behaviour modelled in the home.
Help the client practise the problem-solving process with situations (for example) on an inpatient unit, then situations the client may face at home, school and so forth.	The client's ability and skill will increase with practice. He or she will experience success with practice.
Role-model appropriate conversation and social skills for the client.	This allows the client to see what is expected in a non-threatening situation.
Specify and describe the skills you are demonstrating.	Clarification of expectations decreases the chance for misinterpretation.
Practise social skills with the client on a one-to-one basis.	As the client gains comfort with the skills through practice, he or she will increase their use.
Gradually introduce other clients into the interactions and discussions.	Success with others is more likely to occur once the client has been successful with the staff.
Assist the client to focus on age- and situation-appropriate topics.	Peer relationships are enhanced when the client is able to interact as other adolescents do.
Encourage the client to give and receive feedback with others in his or her age group.	Peer feedback can be influential in shaping the behaviour of an adolescent.
Facilitate expression of feelings among clients in supervised group situations.	Adolescents are reluctant to be vulnerable to peers and may need encouragement to share feelings.
Teach the client about transmission of HIV infection and other sexually transmitted diseases (STDs).	Because these clients may act out sexually or use intravenous drugs, it is especially important that they be educated about preventing transmission of HIV and STDs.
*Assess the client's use of alcohol or other substances, and provide referrals as indicated.	Often adolescents with conduct disorders also have substance abuse issues.

Adapted from Schultz, J. M. and Videbeck, S. L. (2005). *Lippincott's manual of psychiatric nursing care plans* (7th edn). Philadelphia: Lippincott Williams & Wilkins.

MENTAL HEALTH PROMOTION

- Teach parents social and problem-solving skills when needed.
- Encourage parents to seek treatment for their own problems.
- Help parents to identify age-appropriate activities and expectations.
- Assist parents with direct, clear communication.
- Help parents to avoid 'rescuing' the client.
- Teach parents effective **limit-setting** techniques.
- Help parents identify appropriate discipline strategies.

Parental behaviour profoundly influences children's behaviour. Parents who engage in risky behaviours, such as smoking, drinking and ignoring their health, are more likely to have children who also engage in risky behaviours, including early unprotected sex. Group-based parenting classes are effective to deal with problem behaviours in children and to prevent later development of conduct disorders (Zubrick *et al.*, 2005; Turner & Sanders, 2006).

The SNAP-IV Teacher and Parent Rating Scale (Swanson, 2000) is an assessment tool that can be used for initial evaluation in many areas of concern such as ADHD, oppositional defiant disorder, conduct disorder and depression (Box 20.4). Such tools can identify problems or potential problems that signal a need for further evaluation and follow-up. Early detection and successful intervention are often the key to mental health promotion.

OPPOSITIONAL DEFIANT DISORDER (ODD)

Oppositional defiant disorder consists of an enduring pattern of unco-operative, defiant and hostile behaviour toward authority figures without major antisocial violations. It is another controversial diagnosis. *DSM-IV* suggests that children must have behaved in this way for at least 6 months and meet at least four of the following criteria:

- Often loses temper
- Often argues with adults
- Often actively defies or refuses to comply with adults' requests or rules
- Often deliberately annoys people
- Often blames others for his or her mistakes or misbehaviour
- Is often touchy or easily annoyed by others
- Is often angry and resentful
- Is often spiteful or vindictive.

The reason for the controversy may seem obvious from this description: it appears vague – and most parents of adolescents may well recognize their own children

---

Box 20.4 **THE SNAP-IV TEACHER AND PATIENT RATING SCALE**

Name: _____ Gender: _____ Age: _____ Grade: _____

Ethnicity (circle one which best applies):   African–American   Asian   Caucasian   Hispanic   Other _____

Completed by: _____ Type of Class: _____ Class size: _____

For each item, check the column which best describes this child:	Not at All	Just a Little	Quite a Bit	Very Much
1. Often fails to give close attention to details or makes careless mistakes in schoolwork or tasks	_____	_____	_____	_____
2. Often has difficulty sustaining attention in task or play activities	_____	_____	_____	_____
3. Often does not seem to listen when spoken to directly	_____	_____	_____	_____
4. Often does not follow through on instructions and fails to finish schoolwork, chores or duties	_____	_____	_____	_____
5. Often has difficulty organizing tasks and activities	_____	_____	_____	_____
6. Often avoids, dislikes or reluctantly engages in tasks requiring sustained mental effort	_____	_____	_____	_____
7. Often loses things necessary for activities (e.g. toys, school assignments, pencils or books	_____	_____	_____	_____
8. Often is distracted by extraneous stimuli	_____	_____	_____	_____
9. Often is forgetful in daily activities	_____	_____	_____	_____
10. Often has difficulty maintaining alertness, orienting to requests or executing directions	_____	_____	_____	_____

Box 20.4: The Snap-IV Teacher and Patient Rating scale, cont.

For each item, check the column which best describes this child:	Not at All	Just a Little	Quite a Bit	Very Much
11. Often fidgets with hands or feet or squirms in seat	_____	_____	_____	_____
12. Often leaves seat in classroom or in other situations in which remaining seated is expected	_____	_____	_____	_____
13. Often runs about or climbs excessively in situations in which it is inappropriate	_____	_____	_____	_____
14. Often has difficulty playing or engaging in leisure activities quietly	_____	_____	_____	_____
15. Often is 'no the go' or often acts as if 'driven by a motor'	_____	_____	_____	_____
16. Often talks excessively	_____	_____	_____	_____
17. Often blurts out answers before questions have been completed	_____	_____	_____	_____
18. Often has difficulty awaiting turn	_____	_____	_____	_____
19. Often interrupts or intrudes on others (e.g. butts into conversations/games)	_____	_____	_____	_____
20. Often has difficulty sitting still, being quiet or inhibiting impulses in the classroom or at home	_____	_____	_____	_____
21. Often loses temper	_____	_____	_____	_____
22. Often argues with adults	_____	_____	_____	_____
23. Often actively defies or refuses adult requests or rules	_____	_____	_____	_____
24. Often does things that annoy other people	_____	_____	_____	_____
25. Often blames others for his or her mistakes or misbehaviour	_____	_____	_____	_____
26. Often is touchy or easily annoyed by others	_____	_____	_____	_____
27. Often is angry and resentful	_____	_____	_____	_____
28. Often is spiteful or vindictive	_____	_____	_____	_____
29. Often is quarrelsome	_____	_____	_____	_____
30. Often is negative defiant, disobedient or hostile towards authority figures	_____	_____	_____	_____
31. Often makes noises (e.g. humming or odd sounds)	_____	_____	_____	_____
32. Often is excitable, impulsive	_____	_____	_____	_____
33. Often cries easily	_____	_____	_____	_____
34. Often is uncooperative	_____	_____	_____	_____
35. Often acts 'smart'	_____	_____	_____	_____
36. Often is restless or overactive	_____	_____	_____	_____
37. Often disturbs other overactive children	_____	_____	_____	_____
38. Often changes mood quickly and drastically	_____	_____	_____	_____
39. Often easily frustrated if demands are not met immediately	_____	_____	_____	_____
40. Often teases other children and interferes with their activities	_____	_____	_____	_____
41. Often is aggressive to other children (e.g. picks fights or bullies)	_____	_____	_____	_____
42. Often is destructive with property of others (e.g. vandalism)	_____	_____	_____	_____
43. Often is deceitful (e.g. steals, lies, forges, copies the work of others or 'cons' others)	_____	_____	_____	_____
44. Often and seriously violates rules (e.g. is truant, runs away or completely ignores class rules)	_____	_____	_____	_____
45. Has persistent pattern of violating the basic rights of others or major societal norms	_____	_____	_____	_____

continued ⋯⟶

Box 20.4: The Snap-IV Teacher and Patient Rating scale, cont.

For each item, check the column which best describes this child:	Not at All	Just a Little	Quite a Bit	Very Much
46. Has episodes of failure to resist aggressive impulses (to assault others or to destroy property	_____	_____	_____	_____
47. Has motor or verbal tics (sudden, rapid, recurrent, nonrhythmic motor or verbal activity	_____	_____	_____	_____
48. Has repetitive motor behaviour (e.g. hand waving, body rocking or picking at skin)	_____	_____	_____	_____
49. Has obsessions (persistent and intrusive inappropriate ideas, thoughts or impulses	_____	_____	_____	_____
50. Has compulsions (repetitive behaviour or mental acts to reduce anxiety or distress	_____	_____	_____	_____
51. Often is restless or seems keyed up on edge	_____	_____	_____	_____
52. Often is easily fatigued	_____	_____	_____	_____
53. Often has difficulty concentrating (mind goes blank)	_____	_____	_____	_____
54. Often is irritable	_____	_____	_____	_____
55. Often has muscle tension	_____	_____	_____	_____
56. Often has excessive anxiety and worry (e.g. apprehensive expectation)	_____	_____	_____	_____
57. Often has daytime sleepiness (unintended sleeping in inappropriate situations)	_____	_____	_____	_____
58. Often has excessive emotionality and attention-seeking behaviour	_____	_____	_____	_____
59. Often has need for undue admiration, grandiose behaviour or lack of empathy	_____	_____	_____	_____
60. Often has instability in relationships with others, reactive mood and impulsivity	_____	_____	_____	_____
61. Sometimes for at least a week has inflated self-esteem or grandiosity	_____	_____	_____	_____
62. Sometimes for at least a week is more talkative than usual or seems pressured to keep talking	_____	_____	_____	_____
63. Sometimes for at least a weak has flight of ideas or says that thoughts are racing	_____	_____	_____	_____
64. Sometimes for at least a week has elevated, expansive or euphoric mood	_____	_____	_____	_____
65. Sometime for at least a week is excessively involved by pleasurable but risky activities	_____	_____	_____	_____
66. Sometimes for at least 2 weeks has depressed mood (sad, hopeless, discouraged)	_____	_____	_____	_____
67. Sometimes for at least 2 weeks has irritable or cranky mood (not just when frustrated)	_____	_____	_____	_____
68. Sometimes for at least 2 weeks has markedly diminished interest or pleasure in most activities	_____	_____	_____	_____
69. Sometimes for at least 2 weeks has psychomotor agitation (even more active than usual)	_____	_____	_____	_____
70. Sometimes for at least 2 weeks has psyshomotor retardation (slowed down in most activities)	_____	_____	_____	_____
71. Sometimes for at least 2 weeks is fatigued or has loss of energy	_____	_____	_____	_____

Box 20.4: The Snap-IV Teacher and Patient Rating scale, cont.

For each item, check the column which best describes this child:	Not at All	Just a Little	Quite a Bit	Very Much
72. Sometimes for at least 2 weeks has feelings of worthlessness or excessive, inappropriate guilt				
73. Sometimes for at least 2 weeks has diminished ability to think or concentrate				
74. Chronic low self-esteem most of the time for at least a year				
75. Chronic poor concentration or difficulty making decisions most of the time for at least a year				
76. Chronic feelings of hopelessness most of the time for at least a year				
77. Currently is hypervigilant (overly watchful or alert) or has exaggerated startle response				
78. Currently is irritable, has anger outbursts, or has difficulty concentrating				
79. Currently has an emotional (e.g. nervous, worried, hopeless, tearful) response to stress				
80. Currently has a behavioural (e.g. fighting, vandalism, truancy) response to stress				
81. Has difficulty getting started on classroom assignments				
82. Has difficulty staying on task for an entire classroom period				
83. Has problems in completion of work on classroom assignments				
84. Has problems in accuracy or neatness of written work in the classroom				
85. Has difficulty attending to a group classroom activity or discussion				
86. Has difficulty making transitions to the next topic or classroom period				
87. Has problems in interactions with peers in the classroom				
88. Has problems in interactions with staff (teacher or aide)				
89. Has difficulty remaining quiet according to classroom rules				
90. Has difficulty staying seated according to classroom rules				

Developed by James M. Swanson, Ph. D., University of California, Irvaine.

in the criteria, children who may in fact be 'normal'! A certain level of oppositional behaviour is, of course, common in children and adolescents; indeed, it is almost expected at some phases, such as 2 to 3 years of age and in early adolescence. Oppositional defiant disorder should be diagnosed only when behaviours are more frequent and intense than in unaffected peers and cause dysfunction in social, academic or work situations. The disorder is diagnosed in about 5% of the population and occurs equally among male and female adolescents. Most authorities believe that genes, temperament and adverse social conditions interact to create oppositional defiant disorder. Twenty-five per cent of people with this disorder develop conduct disorder; 10% are diagnosed with antisocial personality disorder as adults (Thomas, 2005). Treatment approaches are similar to those used for conduct disorder. ODD is often found in combination with ADHD. Table 20.2 contrasts acceptable characteristics with abnormal behaviour in adolescents.

Feeding and Eating Disorders of Infancy and Early Childhood

The disorders of feeding and eating included in this category are persistent in nature and are not explained by underlying medical conditions. They include pica, rumination disorder and feeding disorder.

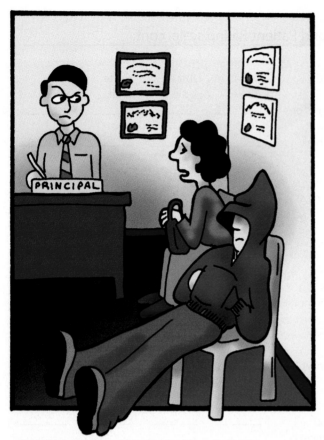

Oppositional defiant disorder

PICA

Pica is persistent ingestion of non-nutritive substances such as paint, hair, cloth, leaves, sand, clay or soil. Pica is commonly seen in children with learning disabilities; it occasionally occurs in pregnant women. It tends to come to the clinician's attention only if a medical complication develops

such as a bowel obstruction or an infection, or if a toxic condition develops such as lead poisoning. In most instances, the behaviour lasts for several months and then remits.

RUMINATION DISORDER

Rumination disorder is the repeated regurgitation and rechewing of food. The child brings partially digested food up into the mouth and usually rechews and reswallows the food. The regurgitation does not involve nausea, vomiting or any medical condition (American Psychiatric Association, 2000). This disorder is relatively uncommon and occurs more often in boys than in girls; it results in malnutrition, weight loss and even death in about 25% of affected infants. In infants, the disorder frequently remits spontaneously, but it may continue in severe cases.

FEEDING DISORDER

Feeding disorder of infancy or early childhood is characterized by persistent failure to eat adequately, which results in significant weight loss or failure to gain weight. Feeding disorder is equally common in boys and in girls and occurs most often during the first year of life. Estimates are that 5% of all paediatric hospital admissions are for failure to gain weight, and up to 50% of those admissions reflect a feeding disorder with no predisposing medical condition. In severe cases, malnutrition and death can result, but most children have improved growth after some time (American Psychiatric Association, 2000).

Tic Disorders

A **tic** is a sudden, rapid, recurrent, non-rhythmic, stereotyped motor movement or vocalization (American Psychiatric Association, 2000). Tics can be suppressed but

Table 20.2	'ACCEPTABLE' CHARACTERISTICS AND POSSIBLE 'ABNORMAL' BEHAVIOURS IN ADOLESCENCE
'Acceptable'	**Potentially 'Abnormal'**
Occasional psychosomatic complaints	Frequent or prolonged hypochondriacal complaints
Inconsistent and unpredictable behaviour	Frequent or prolonged and distressing defiant, negative or depressed behaviour
Eagerness for peer approval	Consistently poor personal relationships with peers
Competitive in play	Learning problematic, irregular and deficient
Erratic work–leisure patterns	Complete or major inability to work or socialize
Critical of self and others	Frequent or prolonged and distressing fears, anxiety and guilt about sex, health, education
Highly ambivalent toward parents	Frequent or major acts of delinquency, ritualism, obsessions
Anxiety about lost parental nurturing	Absolute unwillingness to assume greater autonomy
Verbal aggression to parents	Sexual aberrations
Strong moral and ethical perceptions	Inability to postpone gratification

Adapted from Pataki, C. (2005). Normal adolescence. In B. J. Sadock & V. A. Sadock (Eds.), *Comprehensive textbook of psychiatry* (8th edn, pp. 3035–3043). Philadelphia: Lippincott Williams & Wilkins.

not indefinitely. Stress exacerbates tics, which diminish during sleep and when the person is engaged in an absorbing activity. Common simple motor tics include blinking, jerking the neck, shrugging the shoulders, grimacing and coughing. Common simple vocal tics include clearing the throat, grunting, sniffing, snorting and barking. Complex vocal tics include repeating words or phrases out of context, coprolalia (use of socially unacceptable words, frequently obscene), palilalia (repeating one's own sounds or words), and echolalia (repeating the last-heard sound, word or phrase) (American Psychiatric Association, 2000). Complex motor tics include facial gestures, jumping or touching or smelling an object.

Tic disorders tend to run in families. Abnormal transmission of the neurotransmitter dopamine is thought to play a part in tic disorders (Scahill & Leckman, 2005). Tic disorders usually are treated with risperidone (Risperdal) or olanzapine (Zyprexa), which are atypical antipsychotics. It is important for clients with tic disorders to get plenty of rest and to manage stress because fatigue and stress increase symptoms.

TOURETTE SYNDROME

Tourette syndrome involves multiple motor tics and one or more vocal tics, which occur many times a day for more than 1 year. The complexity and severity of the tics change over time, and the person experiences almost all the possible tics described previously during his or her lifetime. The person has significant impairment in academic, social or occupational areas and feels ashamed and self-conscious. This rare disorder (4 or 5 in 10,000) is more common in boys and is usually identified by 7 years of age. Some people have lifelong problems; others have no symptoms after early adulthood (American Psychiatric Association, 2000).

CHRONIC MOTOR OR TIC DISORDER

Chronic motor or vocal tic differs from Tourette syndrome in that either the motor or the vocal tic is seen, but not both. Transient tic disorder may involve single or multiple vocal or motor tics, but the occurrences last no longer than 12 months.

Elimination Disorders

Encopresis is the repeated passage of faeces into inappropriate places, such as clothing or the floor, by a child who is at least 4 years of age either chronologically or developmentally. It is often involuntary, but it can be intentional. Involuntary encopresis usually is associated with constipation that occurs for psychological, not medical, reasons. Intentional encopresis is often associated with oppositional defiant disorder or conduct disorder.

Enuresis is the repeated voiding of urine during the day or at night into clothing or bed by a child at least 5 years of age either chronologically or developmentally. Most often enuresis is involuntary; when intentional, it is associated with a disruptive behaviour disorder. Seventy-five per cent of children with enuresis have a first-degree relative who had the disorder. Most children with enuresis do not have a coexisting mental disorder.

Both encopresis and enuresis are more common in boys than in girls; 1% of all 5 year olds have encopresis, and 5% of all 5 year olds have enuresis. Encopresis can persist with intermittent exacerbations for years; it is rarely chronic. Most children with enuresis are continent by adolescence; only 1% of all cases persist into adulthood.

Impairment associated with elimination disorders depends on the limitations on the child's social activities, effects on self-esteem, degree of social ostracism by peers and anger, punishment and rejection on the part of parents or carers (American Psychiatric Association, 2000).

Enuresis can be treated effectively with imipramine (Tofranil), an antidepressant with a side-effect of urinary retention. Both elimination disorders respond to behavioural approaches such as a pad with a warning bell and to positive reinforcement for continence. For children with a disruptive behaviour disorder, psychological treatment of that disorder may improve the elimination disorder (Mikkelsen, 2005).

Other Disorders of Infancy, Childhood or Adolescence

SEPARATION ANXIETY DISORDER

Separation anxiety disorder is characterized by anxiety exceeding that expected for developmental level, related to separation from the home or those to whom the child is attached (American Psychiatric Association, 2000). When apart from attachment figures, the child insists on knowing their whereabouts and may need frequent contact with them, such as phone calls. These children are miserable away from home and may fear never seeing their homes or loved ones again. They often follow parents like a shadow, cannot be in a room alone and have trouble going to bed at night unless someone stays with them. Fear of separation may lead to avoidance behaviours such as refusal to attend school or go on errands. Separation anxiety disorder often is accompanied by nightmares and multiple physical complaints such as headaches, nausea, vomiting and dizziness.

Separation anxiety disorders are thought to result from an interaction between temperament and parenting behaviours. Inherited temperament traits such as passivity, avoidance, fearfulness or shyness in novel situations coupled with parenting behaviours that encourage avoidance as a way to deal with strange or unknown situations are thought to cause anxiety in the child (Bernstein & Layne, 2005).

Depending on the severity of the disorder, children may have academic difficulties and social withdrawal if their avoidance behaviour keeps them from school or relationships with others. Children may be described as demanding, intrusive and in need of constant attention or they may be compliant and eager to please. As adults, they may be slow to leave the family home or overly concerned about, and protective of, their own spouses and children. They may continue to have marked discomfort when separated from home or family. Parent education and family therapy are essential components of treatment; 80% of children experience remission at 4-year follow-up (Bernstein & Layne, 2005).

SELECTIVE MUTISM

Selective mutism is characterized by persistent failure to speak in social situations where speaking is expected, such as school (American Psychiatric Association, 2000). Children may communicate by gestures, nodding or shaking the head or occasionally one-syllable vocalizations in a voice different from their natural voice. These children are often excessively shy, socially withdrawn or isolated and clinging; they may have temper tantrums. Selective mutism is rare and slightly more common in girls than in boys. It usually lasts only a few months but may persist for years.

REACTIVE ATTACHMENT DISORDER

Reactive attachment disorder involves a markedly disturbed and developmentally inappropriate social relatedness in most situations. This disorder usually begins before 5 years of age and is associated with grossly pathogenic care such as parental neglect, abuse or failure to meet the child's basic physical or emotional needs. Repeated changes in primary carers, such as multiple foster care placements, also can prevent the formation of stable attachments (American Psychiatric Association, 2000). The disturbed social relatedness may be evidenced by the child's failure to initiate or respond to social interaction (inhibited type) or indiscriminate sociability or lack of selectivity in choice of attachment figures (disinhibited type). In the first type, the child will not cuddle or desire to be close to anyone. In the second type, the child's response is the same to a stranger or to a parent.

Initially, treatment focuses on the child's safety, including removal of the child from the home if neglect or abuse is found. Individual and family therapy (either with parents or foster carers) is most effective. With early identification and effective intervention, remission or considerable improvements can be attained. Otherwise, the disorder follows a continuous course, with relationship problems persisting into adulthood.

STEREOTYPIC MOVEMENT DISORDER

Stereotypic movement disorder is associated with many genetic, metabolic and neurological disorders and often accompanies learning disabilities. The precise cause is unknown. It involves repetitive motor behaviour that is non-functional and either interferes with normal activities or results in self-injury requiring medical treatment (American Psychiatric Association, 2000). **Stereotypic movements** may include waving, rocking, twirling objects, biting fingernails, banging the head, biting or hitting oneself or picking at the skin or body orifices. Generally speaking, the more severe the learning disabiliy, the higher the risk for self-injury behaviours. Stereotypic movement behaviours are relatively stable over time but may diminish with age (Shah, 2005).

No specific treatment has been shown to be effective. Clomipramine (Anafranil) is effective in treating severe nail biting; haloperidol (Haldol) and chlorpromazine (Largactil) have been effective for stereotypic movement disorder associated with learning disability and autistic disorder.

SELF-AWARENESS ISSUES

Working with children and adolescents can be both incredibly rewarding and incredibly difficult. Many disorders of childhood, such as severe developmental disorders, severely limit the child's abilities. It may be difficult for the nurse to remain positive with the child and parents when the prognosis for improvement seems to be poor. Even in overwhelming and depressing situations, the nurse has an opportunity to influence positively children and adolescents, who are still in crucial phases of development. The nurse can often help these clients to develop coping mechanisms they'll use throughout adulthood.

Working with parents is a crucial aspect of dealing with children with these disorders. Parents often have the most influence on how these children learn to cope with their disorders. The nurse's beliefs and values about raising children affect how he or she deals with children and parents. The nurse must not be overly critical about how parents handle their children's problems until the situation is fully understood: caring for a child as a nurse is very different from being responsible around the clock. Given their own skills and problems, parents often give their best efforts. Given the opportunity, resources, support and education, many parents can improve their parenting.

Critical Thinking Questions

1. What values or beliefs about child rearing and families do you have as a result of your own experiences growing up? Have these values and beliefs changed over time? If so, how?

INTERNET RESOURCES

RESOURCES	INTERNET ADDRESS
• Every Child Matters	http://www.everychildmatters.gov.uk
• CSIP Children, Young People and Families Programme	http://www.camhs.org.uk
• Choosing What's Best For You	http://www.annafreudcentre.org/ebpu/choosingjv.pdf
• National Autistic Society	www.nas.org.uk

Points to Consider When Working With Children and Adolescents and Their Parents

- Remember to focus on the client's and parents' strengths and assets, not just their problems.
- Support parents' efforts to remain hopeful while dealing with the reality of their child's situation.
- Ask parents how they are doing. Offer to answer questions, and provide support or make referrals to meet their needs as well as those of the client.

KEY POINTS

- Diagnostic categories in children are controversial and problematic.
- Mental disorders are more difficult to diagnose in children than in adults because their basic development is incomplete and children may lack the ability to recognize or to describe what they are experiencing.
- Children and adolescents can experience some of the same mental health problems as adults, and can be diagnosed with depression, bipolar disorder and anxiety.
- The disorders of childhood and adolescence most often encountered in mental health settings include autistic spectrum disorders, ADHD and disruptive behaviour disorders. Many, though by no means all, mental health problems in childhood and adolescence are the direct or indirect result of inadequate nurturing—within families, within the education system and/or within the health and social care systems.
- Learning disorders include categories for substandard achievement in reading, mathematics and written expression. They tend to be treated through special education in schools.
- Communication disorders may be expressive or receptive and expressive. They primarily involve articulation or stuttering and are treated by speech and language therapists.
- Autistic spectrum disorders are characterized by severe impairment of reciprocal social interaction skills, communication difficulties and restricted stereotyped behavioural patterns.
- Children with autism, the best known of the autistic spectrum disorders, seem detached and usually make little eye contact with and few facial expressions toward others. They do not relate to peers or parents, lack spontaneous enjoyment and cannot engage in play or make-believe with toys. Autism is often treated with cognitive-behavioural approaches. Months or years of treatment may be needed before positive outcomes appear.
- The essential feature of ADHD (also known as ADD or hyperkinetic disorder) is a persistent pattern of inattention and/or hyperactivity and impulsivity. ADHD, the most common disorder in childhood, can result in poor academic performance, strained family relations and rejection by peers.
- Interventions for ADHD include a combination of individual and group psychotherapeutic approaches, medication, behavioural interventions and parental education. Often, special educational assistance is needed to help with academic achievement.
- Conduct disorder, seen by some as the most common disruptive behaviour disorder, is characterized by aggression to people and animals, destruction of property, deceitfulness and theft and serious violation of rules. Its diagnosis is problematic.
- Interventions for conduct disorder include decreasing violent behaviour, increasing concordance and effective therapeutic alliances, improving coping skills and self-esteem, promoting social interaction and educating and supporting parents.
- Feeding and eating disorders of infancy and childhood include pica, rumination and feeding disorders. Pica and rumination often improve with time, and most cases of feeding disorders can be treated successfully.
- Tic disorders involve various combinations of involuntary vocal and/or motor tics. Tourette syndrome is most common. Tic disorders are usually treated successfully with atypical antipsychotic medications.
- Elimination disorders cause impairment for the child based on the response of parents, the level of self-esteem and the degree of ostracism by peers.

REFERENCES

ADDISS ADHD Information Service. (2008). http://www.addiss.co.uk/adhd.htm

American Psychiatric Association. (2000). *Diagnostic and statistical manual of mental disorders* (4th edn, text revision). Washington, DC: American Psychiatric Association.

Baird, G., Pickles, A., Simonoff, E., *et al.* (2008) Measles vaccination and antibody response in autism spectrum disorders. *Archives of Disease in Childhood*, 93, 832–837.

Bernstein, G. A. & Layne, A. E. (2005). Separation anxiety disorder and other anxiety disorders. In B. J. Sadock & V. A. Sadock (Eds.), *Comprehensive textbook of psychiatry* (8th edn, pp. 3292–3302). Philadelphia: Lippincott Williams & Wilkins.

Cashin, A. J. (2005). Autism: understanding conceptual processing deficits. *Journal of Psychosocial Nursing*, 43(4), 22–30.

Faedda, G. L. & Teicher, M. H. (2005). Objective measures of activity and attention in the differential diagnosis of psychiatric disorders of childhood. *Essential Psychopharmacology*, 6(5), 239–249.

Hechtman, L. (2005). Attention deficit disorders. In B. J. Sadock & V. A. Sadock (Eds.), *Comprehensive textbook of psychiatry* (8th edn, pp. 3183–3198). Philadelphia: Lippincott Williams & Wilkins.

Johnson, C. J. & Beitchman, J. H. (2005). Communication disorders. In B. J. Sadock & V. A. Sadock (Eds.), *Comprehensive textbook of psychiatry* (8th edn, pp. 3136–3154). Philadelphia: Lippincott Williams & Wilkins.

McGough, J. J. (2005). Adult manifestations of attention deficit/hyperactivity disorder. In B. J. Sadock & V. A. Sadock (Eds.), *Comprehensive textbook of psychiatry* (8th edn, pp. 3198–3204). Philadelphia: Lippincott Williams & Wilkins.

McGuinness, T. M. (2006). Update on conduct disorder. *Journal of Psychosocial Nursing*, 44(12), 21–25.

Mikkelsen, E. J. (2005). Elimination disorders. In B. J. Sadock & V. A. Sadock (Eds.), *Comprehensive textbook of psychiatry* (8th edn, pp. 3237–3246). Philadelphia: Lippincott Williams & Wilkins.

National Autistic Society. (2008a). Statistics: how many people have autistic spectrum disorders? http://www.nas.org.uk/nas/jsp/polopoly.jsp?d=235&a=3527

National Autistic Society. (2008b). Asperger syndrome: what is it? http://www.nas.org.uk/nas/jsp/polopoly.jsp?d=212

NICE. (2006). *Conduct disorders in children – new guidance to help parents.* Available: http://www.nice.org.uk/newsevents/infocus/infocusarchive/conduct_disorders_in_children_new_guidance_to_help_parents.jsp

NICE. (2008). *Attention deficit hyperactivity disorder. Diagnosis and management of ADHD in children, young people and adults.* Available: http://www.nice.org.uk/nicemedia/pdf/CG072NiceGuidelinev4.pdf

Pataki, C. S. & Spence, S. J. (2005). Motor skills disorder: Developmental coordination disorder. In B. J. Sadock & V. A. Sadock (Eds.), *Comprehensive textbook of psychiatry* (8th edn, pp. 3130–3135). Philadelphia: Lippincott Williams & Wilkins.

Pierce, C. D. & Reid, R. (2004). Attention deficit hyperactivity disorder: Assessment and treatment of children from culturally different groups. *Seminars in Speech and Language*, 25(3), 233–240.

Raggi, V. L. & Chronis, A. M. (2006). Interventions to address the academic impairment of children and adolescents with ADHD. *Clinical Child and Family Psychology Review*, 9(2), 85–111.

Research Autism. (2008). Available: http://www.researchautism.net/pages/welcome/home.ikml

Rowe, D. L. & Hermens, D. F. (2006). Attention-deficit/hyperactivity disorder: Neurophysiology, information processing, arousal, and drug development. *Expert Review of Neurotherapeutics*, 6(11), 1721–1734.

Royal College of Psychiatrists. (2008). Attention-deficit hyperactivity disorder and hyperkinetic disorder: for parents and teachers. Available: http://www.rcpsych.ac.uk/mentalhealthinformation/mentalhealthandgrowingup/5adhdhyperkineticdisorder.aspx

Scahill, L. & Leckman, J. F. (2005). Tic disorders. In B. J. Sadock & V. A. Sadock (Eds.), *Comprehensive textbook of psychiatry* (8th edn, pp. 3228–3236). Philadelphia: Lippincott Williams & Wilkins.

Shah, B. G. (2005). Stereotypic movement disorder of infancy. In B. J. Sadock & V. A. Sadock (Eds.), *Comprehensive textbook of psychiatry* (8th edn, pp. 3254–3257). Philadelphia: Lippincott Williams & Wilkins.

Southall, A. (2007). *The other side of ADHD*. Oxford: Radcliffe.

Swanson, J. M. (2000). The SNAP-IV Teacher and Parent Rating Scale. Available: http://www.adhd.net/snap-iv-form.pdf.

Thomas, C. R. (2005). Disruptive behaviour disorders. In B. J. Sadock & V. A. Sadock (Eds.), *Comprehensive textbook of psychiatry* (8th edn, pp. 3205–3216). Philadelphia: Lippincott Williams & Wilkins.

Turner, K. M. & Sanders, M. R. (2006). Help when it's needed first: A controlled evaluations of brief, preventive behavioural family intervention in a primary care setting. *Behaviour Therapy*, 37(2), 131–142.

Volkmar, F. R., Klin, A., & Schultz, R. T. (2005). Pervasive developmental disorders. In B. J. Sadock & V. A. Sadock (Eds.), *Comprehensive textbook of psychiatry* (8th edn, pp. 3164–3182). Philadelphia: Lippincott Williams & Wilkins.

Youth In Mind. (2008). *Strengths and Difficulties Questionnaire*. Available: http://www.sdqinfo.com/

Zubrick, S. R., Ward, K. A., Silburn, S. A., *et al.* (2005). Prevention of child behaviour problems through implementation of a group behavioural family intervention. *Prevention Science*, 6(4), 287–304.

ADDITIONAL READING

Cooper, M., Hooper, C. & Thompson, M. (Eds.). (2005). Child and adolescent mental health: theory and practice. London: Hodder Arnold.

NICE. (2006). Attention deficit hyperactivity disorder (ADHD) – methylphenidate, atomoxetine and dexamfetamine (review). Available: http://www.nice.org.uk/guidance/index.jsp?action=byID&o=11572

Oward, P., Grant, G., Ramcharan, P., Richardson, M. (2005). *Learning disability: A life cycle*. Milton Keynes: Open University Press.

Pataki, C. S. (2005). Normal adolescence. In B. J. Sadock & V. A. Sadock (Eds.), *Comprehensive textbook of psychiatry* (8th edn, pp. 3035–3043). Philadelphia: Lippincott Williams & Wilkins.

Yeh, M., Hough, R. L., McCabe, K., *et al.* (2004). Parental beliefs about the causes of child problems: Exploring racial/ethnic patterns. *Journal of the American Academy of Child and Adolescent Psychiatry*, 43(5), 605–612.

Young Minds/CSIP. (2006). Looking after the health of looked-after children. Available: http://www.csip.org.uk/silo/files/looked-after-children-exemplar.pdf

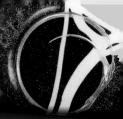

MULTIPLE-CHOICE QUESTIONS

Select the best answer for each of the following questions.

1. Teaching about methylphenidate (Ritalin) should include which of the following?
   a. Give the medication after meals.
   b. Give the medication when the child becomes overactive.
   c. Increase the child's fluid intake when he or she is taking the medication.
   d. Take the child's temperature daily.

2. The nurse might expect to see all the following symptoms in a child with ADHD, except
   a. Easily distracted and forgetful
   b. Excessive running, climbing and fidgeting
   c. Moody, sullen and pouting behaviour
   d. Interrupts others and can't take turns

3. Which of the following is 'normal' adolescent behaviour?
   a. Critical of self and others
   b. Defiant, negative and depressed behaviour
   c. Frequent hypochondriacal complaints
   d. Unwillingness to assume greater autonomy

4. Which of the following is used to treat enuresis?
   a. Imipramine (Tofranil)
   b. Methylphenidate (Ritalin)
   c. Olanzapine (Zyprexa)
   d. Risperidone (Risperdal)

5. An effective nursing intervention for the impulsive and aggressive behaviours that accompany conduct disorder is
   a. Assertiveness training
   b. Respectful, consistent limit setting
   c. Negotiation of rules
   d. Open expression of feelings

6. The nurse recognizes which of the following as a common behavioural sign of autism?
   a. Clinging behaviour toward parents
   b. Creative imaginative play with peers
   c. Early language development
   d. Indifference to being hugged or held

FILL-IN-THE-BLANK QUESTIONS

Identify the disorder associated with the following behaviours.

_____ Ingestion of paint, clay, sand or soil

_____ Repeated regurgitation and rechewing of food

_____ Disturbed and developmentally inappropriate social functioning

_____ Persistent failure to speak in specific social situations

GROUP DISCUSSION TOPICS

1. Why are diagnoses controversial in childhood mental health problems?

2. Who should be the main focus of service input – the child, parents or society as a whole?

3. How has your childhood affected your attitude to mental health nursing?

CLINICAL EXAMPLE

Lucy, 7 years of age, has been brought by her parents to the GP because she has been very rough with her 18-month-old brother. She cannot sit still at school or at meals and is beginning to fall behind academically in Year 3. Her parents report that they have 'tried everything', but Lucy will not listen to them. She doesn't seem to be able to follow directions, pick up toys or get ready for school on time.

   After a thorough examination of Lucy and a lengthy interview with the parents, the psychiatrist diagnoses ADHD and prescribes methylphenidate (Ritalin), 10 mg in the morning, 5 mg at noon and 5 mg in the afternoon. The nurse meets with the parents to provide teaching and to answer questions before they go home.

1. What information should the nurse offer about methylphenidate?

2. What information might the nurse provide about ADHD?

3. What suggestions for managing the home environment might be helpful for the parents?

4. What other psychological interventions can the nurse make for Lucy and her parents?

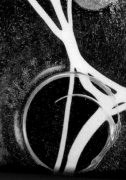

Chapter 21

Dementia and Other Cognitive Disorders

Key Terms

- agnosia
- Alzheimer's disease
- amnestic disorder
- aphasia
- apraxia
- confabulation
- Creutzfeldt–Jakob disease
- delirium
- dementia
- distraction
- echolalia
- executive functioning
- going along
- Huntington's disease
- Korsakoff's syndrome
- palilalia
- Parkinson's disease
- Pick's disease
- reframing
- reminiscence therapy
- supportive touch
- time away
- validation therapy
- vascular dementia

Learning Objectives

After reading this chapter, you should be able to:

1. Describe the characteristics of and risk factors for cognitive disorders.

2. Distinguish between delirium and dementia in terms of symptoms, course, treatment and prognosis.

3. Apply the nursing process to the care of people with a range of cognitive disorders.

4. Identify methods for meeting the needs of people who provide care to people with dementia.

5. Provide education to clients, families, carers and community members to increase knowledge and understanding of cognitive disorders.

6. Evaluate your feelings, beliefs and attitudes regarding people with cognitive disorders.

Cognition is the brain's ability to process, retain and use information. Cognitive abilities include reasoning, judgement, perception, attention, comprehension and memory. These cognitive abilities are essential for many important tasks, including making decisions, solving problems, interpreting the environment and learning new information.

A 'cognitive disorder' is a disruption or impairment in these higher-level functions of the brain. Cognitive disorders can have devastating effects on the ability to function in daily life. They can cause people to forget the names of immediate family members, to be unable to perform daily household tasks and to neglect personal hygiene (Davis, 2005). The primary categories of cognitive disorders are delirium, dementia and amnestic disorders. All involve impairment of cognition, but they vary with respect to cause, treatment, prognosis and effect on people and family members or carers. This chapter focuses on delirium and dementia. It emphasizes not only the care of people with cognitive disorders but also the needs of their carers.

Despite the presence very often of a much clearer organic basis to their development, cognitive disorders are – like all other mental disorders – indivisible from their context: as Adams (2008, p. 10) says, 'people's experience of dementia arises out of an interrelationship between physical/biomedical and social/psychological phenomena.' Nurses – whether generic mental health clinicians or dementia care specialists, and whether in working-age or older adult services – are at the very forefront of helping people make sense of – and live satisfying lives within – this interrelationship.

DEMENTIA

In the UK, there were, in 2007, an estimated 683,597 people with dementia; this will gradually increase, it is estimated, to nearly a million in 2021 and to around 1.7 million by 2051 (Alzheimer's Society, 2007) as the numbers of older people – particularly those over 85 – rise.

Dementia is a mental disorder that involves multiple cognitive deficits, primarily memory impairment and at least one of the following cognitive disturbances (American Psychiatric Association, 2000):

- **Aphasia**, which is deterioration of language function
- **Apraxia**, which is impaired ability to execute motor functions despite intact motor abilities
- **Agnosia**, which is inability to recognize or name objects despite intact sensory abilities
- Disturbance in **executive functioning**, which is the ability to think abstractly and to plan, initiate, sequence, monitor and stop complex behaviour

These cognitive deficits must be sufficiently severe to impair social or occupational functioning and must represent a decline from previous functioning.

Dementia must be distinguished from delirium; if the two diagnoses coexist, the symptoms of dementia remain even when the delirium has cleared. Table 21.1 compares delirium and dementia and the second half of this chapter addresses issues in the nursing care of people with delirium.

Memory impairment is the prominent early sign of dementia. People have difficulty learning new material and forget previously learned material. Initially, recent memory is impaired – for example, forgetting where certain objects were placed or that food is cooking on the stove. In later stages, dementia affects remote memory; people forget the names of adult children, their lifelong occupations and even their own names.

Aphasia usually begins with the inability to name familiar objects or people and then progresses to speech that becomes vague or empty with excessive use of terms such as *it* or *thing*. People may exhibit **echolalia** (echoing what

Table 21.1	COMPARISON OF DELIRIUM AND DEMENTIA	
Indicator	**Delirium**	**Dementia**
Onset	Rapid	Gradual and insidious
Duration	Brief (hours to days)	Progressive deterioration
Level of consciousness	Impaired, fluctuates	Not affected
Memory	Short-term memory impaired	Short- then long-term memory impaired, eventually destroyed
Speech	May be slurred, rambling, pressured, irrelevant	Normal in early stage, progressive aphasia in later stage
Thought processes	Temporarily disorganized	Impaired thinking, eventual loss of thinking abilities
Perception	Visual or tactile hallucinations, delusions	Often absent, but can have paranoia, hallucinations, illusions
Mood	Anxious, fearful if hallucinating; weeping, irritable	Depressed and anxious in early stage, labile mood, restless pacing, angry outbursts in later stages

Adapted from American Psychiatric Association. (2000). *Diagnostic and Statistical Manual of Mental Disorders* (4th edn, text revision). Washington, DC: APA; and Ribby, K. J. & Cox, K. R. (1996). Development, implementation, and evaluation of a confusion protocol. *Clinical Nurse Specialist, 10*(5), 241–247.

is heard) or **palilalia** (repeating words or sounds over and over) (American Psychiatric Association, 2000). *Apraxia* may cause people to lose the ability to perform routine self-care activities such as dressing or cooking. Agnosia is frustrating for people: they may look at a table and chairs but are unable to name them. Disturbances in executive functioning are evident as people lose the ability to learn new material, solve problems or carry out daily activities such as meal planning or budgeting.

People with dementia also may underestimate the risks associated with activities or overestimate their ability to function in certain situations. For example, while driving, people may cut in front of other drivers, sideswipe parked cars or fail to slow down when they should.

Onset and Clinical Course

When an underlying, treatable cause is not present, the course of dementia is usually progressive. Dementia is often described in stages:

- *Mild*: Forgetfulness is the hallmark of early, mild dementia. It exceeds the normal, occasional forgetfulness experienced as part of the aging process. The person has difficulty finding words, frequently loses objects, and begins to experience anxiety about these losses. Occupational and social settings are less enjoyable, and the person may avoid them. Most people remain in the community during this stage.
- *Moderate*: Confusion is apparent, along with progressive memory loss. The person can no longer perform complex tasks but remains oriented to person and place. He or she still recognizes familiar people. Toward the end of this stage, the person loses the ability to live independently and requires assistance because of disorientation to time and loss of information such as his or her address and telephone number. The person may remain in the community if adequate support is available, but some people move to supervised living situations.
- *Severe*: Personality and emotional changes occur. The person may be delusional, wander at night, forget the names of his or her spouse and children and require assistance in activities of daily living (ADLs). Most people still have to live in facilities with intensive nursing support when they reach this stage unless an exceptional degree of community support is available.

Aetiology

Causes vary, although the clinical picture is similar for most dementias. Often, no definitive diagnosis can be made until completion of a postmortem examination. Metabolic activity is decreased in the brains of people with dementia; it is not known whether dementia causes decreased metabolic activity or if decreased metabolic activity results in dementia. A genetic component has been identified for some dementias

> ### *DSM-IV-TR* DIAGNOSTIC CRITERIA:
> SYMPTOMS OF DEMENTIA
>
> - Loss of memory (initial stages, recent memory loss such as forgetting food cooking on the stove; later stages, remote memory loss such as forgetting names of children, occupation)
> - Deterioration of language function (forgetting names of common objects such as chair or table, palilalia (echoing sounds), and echoing words that are heard (echolalia))
> - Loss of ability to think abstractly and to plan, initiate, sequence, monitor or stop complex behaviours (loss of executive function): the client loses the ability to perform self-care activities
>
> Adapted from American Psychiatric Association. (2000). *Diagnostic and Statistical Manual of Mental Disorders* (4th edn, text revision). Washington, DC: APA.

such as Huntington's disease. An abnormal *APOE* gene is known to be linked with Alzheimer's disease. Other causes of dementia are related to infections such as HIV infection or Creutzfeldt–Jakob disease.

There are over 100 dementias. Around 700,000 people in the UK have dementia and this is increasing. By 2025 there will be over a million people with dementia. Sixty

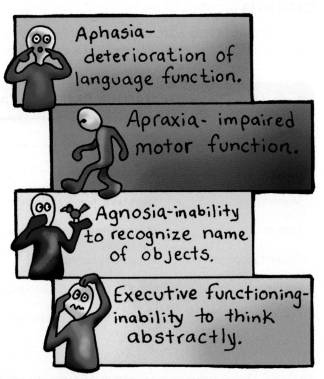

Multiple cognitive deficits of dementia

thousand deaths a year are directly attributable to dementia. Approximately two-thirds of people with dementia live in the community, a third in care homes. Carers who are family members – historically a highly pressured, frequently ignored or sidelined group of people – save the taxpayer over £6 billion a year (Alzheimer's Society, 2008a). Standards of care in state and private homes remains mixed: people living with dementias are only now beginning to be given a voice in their own care and in the services that provide that care.

The most common types and their known or hypothesized causes are as follows (American Psychiatric Association, 2000; Neugroschl et al., 2005; Adams, 2008).

Alzheimer's disease is a progressive brain disorder that has a gradual onset but causes an increasing decline in functioning, including loss of speech, loss of motor function and profound personality and behavioural changes, such as paranoia, delusions, hallucinations, inattention to hygiene and irritability and aggression. An estimated 417,000 people in the UK had Alzheimer's disease in 2007, around 62% of all dementias.

In Alzheimer's a person's level of consciousness remains intact. It is evidenced by atrophy of cerebral neurons, senile plaque deposits and enlargement of the third and fourth ventricles of the brain. Risk for Alzheimer's disease increases with age (it is characterized by an onset over the age of 40), and average duration from onset of symptoms to death is 8 to 10 years. Dementia of the Alzheimer's type, especially with late onset (after 65 years of age), may have a genetic component. There are two forms of Alzheimer's disease – an 'early-onset' familial Alzheimer's disease (EOFAD) and a 'sporadic late-onset' Alzheimer's disease (LOAD) (American Psychiatric Association, 2000; Adams, 2008).

Recent studies have suggested that Alzheimer's disease may be connected to depression: Alzheimer's was found to be 2.5 times more likely in those with a history of depression (Geerlings et al., 2008)). Much research still needs to be done to determine what the relationship between the two actually is.

Vascular dementia has symptoms similar to those of Alzheimer's disease, but onset is typically abrupt, followed by rapid changes in functioning; a plateau, or levelling-off period; more abrupt changes; another levelling-off period; and so on. Computed tomography or magnetic resonance imaging usually shows multiple vascular lesions of the cerebral cortex and subcortical structures, resulting from the decreased blood supply to the brain (caused by stroke or small vessel disease). When a single stroke causes vascular dementia, it is termed a 'single-infarct dementia' (Adams, 2008).

Pick's disease is a degenerative brain disease that particularly affects the frontal and temporal lobes and results in a clinical picture similar to that of Alzheimer's disease. Early signs include personality changes, loss of social skills and inhibitions, emotional blunting and language abnormalities. Onset is most commonly 50 to 60 years of age; death occurs in 2 to 5 years. It is one of a number of conditions – including frontal lobe degeneration and dementia associated with motor neuron disease – which are classed under the term 'fronto-temporal dementia' (Adams, 2008).

Creutzfeldt–Jakob disease is a central nervous system disorder that typically develops in adults between 40 and 60 years of age. It involves altered vision, loss of co-ordination or abnormal movements, and dementia that usually progresses rapidly (a few months). The cause of the encephalopathy is an infectious particle resistant to boiling, some disinfectants (e.g. formalin, alcohol) and ultraviolet radiation. Pressured autoclaving or bleach can inactivate the particle.

Dementia with Lewy bodies (DLB) is another progressive condition – accounting for something between 10% and 15% of all cases of dementia (Adams, 2008) – that leads to people developing some symptoms of Alzheimer's disease (e.g. memory loss, impaired communication) and some symptoms of Parkinson's disease (e.g. movement difficulties and the typical mask-like expression). DLB may also involve fluctuating abilities throughout the day, feeling faint, experiencing vivid visual hallucinations and sleep disturbance (Adams, 2008, p. 5).

Dementias related to other conditions:

- **HIV infection** can lead to dementia and other neurological problems; these may result directly from invasion of nervous tissue by HIV or from other acquired immunodeficiency syndrome-related illnesses, such as toxoplasmosis and cytomegalovirus. This type of dementia can result in a wide variety of symptoms ranging from mild sensory impairment to gross memory and cognitive deficits to severe muscle dysfunction.

- **Parkinson's disease** is a slowly progressive neurological condition characterized by tremor, rigidity, bradykinesia and postural instability. It results from loss of neurons of the basal ganglia. Dementia has been reported in approximately 20% to 60% of people with Parkinson's disease and is characterized by cognitive and motor slowing, impaired memory and impaired executive functioning.

- **Huntington's disease** is an inherited, dominant gene disease that primarily involves cerebral atrophy, demyelination and enlargement of the brain ventricles. Initially, there are choreiform movements that are continuous during waking hours and involve facial contortions, twisting, turning and tongue movements. Personality changes are the initial psychosocial manifestations, followed by memory loss, decreased intellectual functioning and other signs of dementia. The disease begins in the late thirties or early forties and may last 10 to 20 years or more before death.

- Dementia can be a direct pathophysiological consequence of head trauma. The degree and type of cognitive impairment and behavioural disturbance depend on the location and extent of the brain injury. When it occurs as a single injury, the dementia is usually stable rather than progressive. Repeated head injury (e.g. from boxing) may lead to progressive dementia.

CLINICAL VIGNETTE: DEMENTIA

Jack Smith, 74, and his wife, Marion, 69, have been living in their home and managing fairly well until recently. The Smiths have two grown-up children who both live an hour or so away but visit every 2 months or so and at holidays and birthdays. Jack recently had a stroke and entered a rehabilitation centre to try to help him learn to walk and talk again. Marion wanted to stay at home and wait for his return, but whenever the children called to check on her, she would often be crying and confused or frightened. On one visit, they found her looking very tired, dressed in a wrinkled dress that looked soiled. She looked as if she had lost weight, and she couldn't remember what she had eaten for breakfast or lunch.

Marion's daughter remembered that before her father had the stroke, she noticed that Jack had taken over several routine tasks her mother had always done, such as making the shopping list and planning and helping to cook their meals. Her mother seemed more forgetful and would ask the same questions over and over and often related the same story several times during their visit.

A few weeks after Jack entered the rehab centre and Marion was living at home alone, the neighbours found Marion wandering around the streets one morning, lost and confused. It was now clear to her children that their mother could not remain in her home alone and take care of herself. It was uncertain how long Jack would need to remain at the rehabilitation centre, and they were not sure what his physical capabilities would be when he did return.

Her daughter decided that Marion (and eventually Jack) would come to live with her family. They moved her in with them, but even after getting settled at her daughter's home, Marion continued to be confused and often did not know where she was. She kept asking where Jack was and forgot her grandchildren's names. At times, she grew agitated and would accuse them of stealing her purse or other possessions (later, she would always find them). Marion would sometimes forget to go to the bathroom and would soil her clothes. She would forget to brush her hair and teeth and take a bath and often needed help with these activities. When her daughter came home from work in the evening, the sandwich she had made for her mother was often left untouched in the fridge. Marion spent much of her time packing her bags to go home and 'see Jack'.

Prevalence of dementia rises with age: estimated prevalence of moderate to severe dementia in people older than 65 years is about 5%; dementia is found in 20% to 40% of the general population older than 85 years. Dementia of the Alzheimer's type is the most common type in the UK, US (60% of all dementias), Scandinavia and Europe; vascular dementia is more prevalent in Russia and Japan. Dementia of the Alzheimer's type is more common in women; vascular dementia is more common in men.

Cultural Considerations

There are at least 12,000 people with dementia from black and ethnic minority groups in the UK, with numbers increasing sharply. People from other cultures may find the questions used in many traditional assessment tools for dementia difficult or impossible to answer: examples include the names of former Prime Ministers. To avoid drawing erroneous conclusions, the nurse *must* be aware of differences in the person's knowledge base.

The nurse also must be aware of different culturally influenced perspectives and beliefs about elderly family members. In many Eastern countries, older people hold a position of authority, respect, power and decision making for the family; this may not change despite memory loss or confusion. Direct client involvement and partnership is essential with people in all cultures, although, on occasion – and especially in advanced stages of some dementias – decisions may need to be made by others. For fear of seeming disrespectful, other family members may be reluctant to make decisions or plans for older people with dementia. The nurse must work with family members to accomplish goals without making them feel they have betrayed the revered older person.

Dementia Care Mapping

Dementia care mapping, originally developed by Kitwood and Bredin in the late 1980s and early 1990s and subsequently by Goldsmith (1996) and Brooker (2004; 2007; 2008) among others, is a process whereby formal and informal processes and structures are put in place in an attempt to ensure the client's voice and perspective are at the centre of evaluations of care treatment. Observations are made, recorded and analysed and findings – and their interpretations – are fed back to staff. Renewed person-centred plans for care and engagement are then drawn up and put into place (Brooker et al., 2004; 2007).

Medical Treatment and Prognosis

Whenever possible, the underlying cause of dementia is identified so that treatment can be instituted. For example, the progress of vascular dementia, the second most common type, may be halted with appropriate treatment of the underlying vascular condition (e.g. changes in diet, exercise, control of hypertension or diabetes). Improvement of cerebral blood flow may arrest the progress of vascular dementia in some people (Neugroschl et al., 2005).

Table 21.2	DRUGS USED IN ADJUNCTIVE TREATMENT OF MODERATE ALZHEIMER'S DISEASE (FOR THOSE WHO SCORE 10–20 ON MMSE)	
Name	**Dosage Range and Route**	**Nursing Considerations**
Memantine (Ebixa)	5–20 mg in divided doses	Monitor for nausea, vomiting, abdominal pain and loss of appetite
Donepezil (Aricept)	5–10 mg orally per day	Monitor for nausea, diarrhoea and insomnia. Test stools periodically for GI bleeding
Rivastigmine (Exelon)	3–12 mg orally per day divided into 2 doses	Monitor for nausea, vomiting, abdominal pain and loss of appetite
Galantamine (Reminyl)	8–16 mg orally per day divided into 2 doses	Monitor for nausea, vomiting, loss of appetite, dizziness and syncope

GI, gastrointestinal; MMSE, mini mental-state examination. Adapted from *Drug facts and comparisons*. (2007). 61st edn. St. Louis: Wolters Kluwer; and British National Formulary Online (2008) http://www.bnf.org/bnf/bnf/55/

The prognosis for the progressive types of dementia may vary as described earlier, but all prognoses involve progressive deterioration of physical and mental abilities until death. Typically, in the later stages, people have minimal cognitive and motor function, are totally dependent on carers and are unaware of their surroundings or people in the environment. They may be totally uncommunicative or make unintelligible sounds or attempts to verbalize.

For degenerative dementias, no direct therapies have been found to reverse or retard the fundamental pathophysiological processes. Levels of numerous neurotransmitters such as acetylcholine, dopamine, noradrenaline and serotonin are decreased in dementia. This has led to attempts at replenishment therapy with acetylcholine precursors, cholinergic agonists and cholinesterase inhibitors. Donepezil (Aricept), rivastigmine (Exelon) and galantamine (Reminyl) are cholinesterase inhibitors and have shown modest therapeutic effects and temporarily slow the progress of dementia. They have no effect, however, on the overall course of the disease. Memantine (Ebixa) is used in moderate-to-severe dementia in Alzheimer's disease (Table 21.2, Box 21.1).

People with dementia demonstrate a broad range of cognitions, emotions and behaviours that can be treated symptomatically. Doses of medications are usually one-half to two-thirds lower than usually prescribed. Antidepressants are effective for significant depressive symptoms. Antipsychotics such as haloperidol (Haldol), olanzapine (Zyprexa), risperidone (Risperdal) and quetiapine (Seroquel) may be used to manage psychotic symptoms of delusions, hallucinations or paranoia. However, there has undoubtedly been over-prescription of antipsychotics as an

Box 21.1	NICE GUIDANCE: DONEPEZIL, GALANTAMINE, RIVASTIGMINE, AND MEMANTINE FOR ALZHEIMER'S DISEASE (SEPTEMBER 2007)

Donepezil, galantamine and rivastigmine are recommended for the adjunctive treatment of moderate Alzheimer's disease in those whose mini mental-state examination (MMSE) score is 10–20 points, under the following conditions:

- Alzheimer's disease must be diagnosed in a specialist clinic; the clinic should also assess cognitive, global and behavioural functioning, activities of daily living and the likelihood of compliance with treatment.
- Treatment should be initiated by specialists but can be continued by GPs under a shared-care protocol.
- The carers' views of the condition should be sought before and during drug treatment.
- The patient should be assessed every 6 months and drug treatment should normally continue only if the MMSE score remains at or above 10 points and if treatment is

considered to have a worthwhile effect on the global, functional and behavioural condition.

- Patients receiving acetylcholinesterase inhibitors for mild Alzheimer's disease can continue treatment until they, their carers or their specialist consider it appropriate to stop.

Healthcare professionals should not rely solely on the MMSE score to assess the severity of Alzheimer's disease when the patient has learning or other disabilities, or other communication difficulties.

NICE does not recommend memantine for moderately severe-to-severe Alzheimer's disease except as part of well-designed clinical studies; patients already receiving memantine can continue treatment until they, their carers or their specialist consider it appropriate to stop.

From British National Formulary Online (2008) http://www.bnf.org/bnf/bnf/55/

attempt to control people rather than engage with people and help them be active. Human emotions – sadness, fear, anger – can be dismissed as 'symptomatic' and then treated pharmacologically rather than with compassionate interaction (Alzheimer's Society, 2008c).

Lithium carbonate, carbamazepine (Tegretol) and valproic acid (Depakote) can help to stabilize affective lability and to diminish aggressive outbursts, though similar concerns arise. Benzodiazepines are used cautiously because they may cause delirium and can worsen already compromised cognitive abilities (Neugroschl *et al.*, 2005). These medications are discussed in Chapter 3.

APPLICATION OF THE NURSING PROCESS: DEMENTIA

This section focuses on caring for people with progressive dementia, in particular Alzheimer's, which is the most common type. The nurse can use these guidelines as indicated for people with dementia that is not progressive.

The emphasis here is on person-centred care (Box 21.2) and draws on Brooker's use of the equation (cited in Adams, 2008, p. 45):

$$\text{Person-centred care} = V + I + P + S$$

in which:

V = a value base that asserts the absolute value of all human lives regardless of age or cognitive ability

I = an individualized approach, recognizing uniqueness

P = understanding the world from the perspective of the service user

S = providing a social environment that supports psychological needs.

Relevant to the nursing care of people with any mental health difficulty, these components of the 'person-centred equation' are absolutely essential as a foundation for good care for people with dementia.

Assessment

The assessment process itself – potentially baffling and confusing for anyone – may seem particularly so for people with dementia. They may not know or may forget the purpose of the interview. The nurse needs to provide simple explanations as often as people need them, such as 'I'm asking these questions so we can see how your health is.' People

---

Box 21.2 KEY MESSAGES: STRENGTHENING THE INVOLVEMENT OF PEOPLE WITH DEMENTIA

FOR PEOPLE WITH DEMENTIA

As a person using a service you have a right to be involved:

- You have a personal perspective about dementia that no one else can provide.
- Involvement can increase confidence and self-esteem.
- It can provide a role and occupation and contribute to a better quality of life.
- You can provide positive examples of living with dementia, encouraging others to get involved.
- You will contribute to removing the stigma associated with dementia, as with mental health in general.

FOR COMMISSIONERS

Involving people who use a service is a policy requirement:

- It can evidence where services are no longer required and how new services should be shaped, optimizing the value of available resources.
- Feedback through involvement gathers data for audit and evaluation purposes and feeds into performance assessment frameworks.

- It ensures fair access to public services and benefits.
- It ensures equality of treatment and protection.
- Involvement improves standards and responsiveness.
- Involvement generates new ideas.

FOR PRACTITIONERS

People who are involved, whether practitioners or those receiving services, feel empowered:

- Information gathered and acted upon ensures that the most relevant services are provided.
- It meets the personal and social needs of people using services.
- It can assist people with dementia and practitioners to develop their potential.
- It illustrates respect for individuals and their communities.
- It promotes dignity, individuality, rights, responsibilities, identity and personal preferences.
- Involvement promotes trust in services and may guard against abuse.

From CSIP. (2007). *Strengthening the involvement of people with dementia: a resource for implementation*. Available: http://www.olderpeoplesmentalhealth. csip.org.uk/silo/files/strengthening-the-involvement-of-people-with-dementia.pdf

may become confused or tire easily, so frequent breaks in the interview may be needed. It helps to ask simple rather than compound questions and to allow people ample time to answer (Box 21.3).

Box 21.3 WHAT SKILLS ARE REQUIRED TO COMMUNICATE?

Ten tips to improve communication:

- Always believe that communication is possible.
- Try to focus on the non-verbal signs as well as verbal.
- Avoid making assumptions: check things out with the person.
- Make your communication a two-way process that engages the person.
- Avoid the use of jargon or complicated explanations. Keep your conversation as simple as possible without being patronizing or sounding childish.
- Try to avoid questions that have 'why' in them. The reasoning involved in giving an answer may be too difficult. This in turn could make them annoyed or upset.
- Be a good listener. Give the person your full attention and resist the temptation to finish their sentences or talk at them.
- Talk at a slower pace so that the person has an opportunity to grasp what is being said.
- Maintain a calm and unhurried approach.
- Above all, don't be afraid to try or say 'I don't understand'.

From CSIP. (2007). Strengthening the involvement of people with dementia: a resource for implementation. Available: http://www.olderpeoplesmentalhealth.csip.org.uk/silo/files/strengthening-the-involvement-of-people-with-dementia.pdf

---

A mental status examination such as the MMSE (available: http://www3.parinc.com/products/product.aspx?Productid=MMSE) can provide information about the client's cognitive abilities such as memory, concentration and abstract information processing. Typically, the client is asked to interpret the meaning of a proverb, perform subtraction of figures without paper and pencil, recall the names of objects, make a complete sentence and copy two intersecting pentagons. Although this does not replace a thorough assessment, it gives a cursory evaluation of the client's cognitive abilities. It is important to remember that people with severe depression or psychosis may also be unable to perform some of these cognitive tasks correctly.

HISTORY

Considering the impairment of recent memory, people may be unable to provide an accurate and thorough history of the onset of problems. Interviews with family, friends, or carers may be necessary to obtain information.

GENERAL APPEARANCE AND MOTOR BEHAVIOUR

Dementia progressively impairs the ability to carry on meaningful conversation. People display aphasia when they cannot name familiar objects or people. Conversation becomes repetitive because people often perseverate on one idea. Eventually, speech may become slurred, followed by a total loss of language function.

The initial finding with regard to motor behaviour is the loss of ability to perform familiar tasks (*apraxia*) such as dressing or combing one's hair, although actual motor abilities are intact. People cannot imitate the task when others demonstrate it for them. In the severe stage, people may experience a gait disturbance that makes unassisted ambulation unsafe, if not impossible.

Some people with dementia show uninhibited behaviour, including making inappropriate jokes, neglecting personal hygiene, showing undue familiarity with strangers or disregarding social conventions for acceptable behaviour. This can include swearing excessively or making disparaging remarks about others when people have never displayed these behaviours before.

MOOD AND AFFECT

Initially, people with dementia usually experience anxiety and fear over the losses of memory and cognitive functions. They may nevertheless not express these feelings to anyone. Mood often becomes more labile over time and may shift rapidly and drastically for no apparent reason. Emotional outbursts are common but usually pass quickly. People may display anger and hostility, sometimes toward other people. They begin to demonstrate catastrophic emotional reactions in response to environmental changes that people may not perceive or understand accurately or when they cannot respond adaptively. These catastrophic reactions may include verbal or physical aggression, wandering at night, agitation or other behaviours that seem to indicate a loss of personal control.

People may display a pattern of withdrawal from the world they no longer understand. They can be lethargic, look apathetic and pay little attention to the environment or the people in it. They appear to lose all emotional affect and seem dazed and listless.

THOUGHT PROCESS AND CONTENT

Initially, the ability to think abstractly is impaired, resulting in loss of the ability to plan, sequence, monitor, initiate or stop complex behaviour (American Psychiatric Association, 2000). The client loses the ability to solve problems or to take action in new situations because he or she cannot think about what to do. The ability to generalize knowledge from one situation to another is lost because the client cannot recognize similarities or differences in situations. These problems with cognition almost certainly make it impossible for the employed person to continue working. The client's ability to perform tasks such as planning activities, budgeting or planning meals is lost.

As the dementia progresses, delusions of persecution are common. The client may accuse others of stealing objects he or she has lost or may believe he or she is being cheated or pursued.

SENSORY AND INTELLECTUAL PROCESSES

People lose intellectual function, which eventually involves the almost complete loss of their abilities. Memory deficits are the initial and essential feature of dementia. Dementia first affects recent and immediate memory and then eventually impairs the ability to recognize close family members and even oneself. In mild and moderate dementia, people may make up answers to fill in memory gaps (**confabulation**). Agnosia is another hallmark of dementia. People lose visual spatial relations, which is often evidenced by deterioration of the ability to write or draw simple objects.

Attention span and ability to concentrate are increasingly impaired until people lose the ability to do either. People are chronically confused about the environment, other people and eventually themselves. Initially, they may be disoriented to time in mild dementia, time and place in moderate dementia and finally to self in the severe stage.

Hallucinations are a frequent problem. Visual hallucinations are most common and generally unpleasant. People are likely to believe the hallucination is reality.

JUDGEMENT AND INSIGHT

People with dementia have poor judgement in the light of the cognitive impairment. They underestimate risks and unrealistically appraise their abilities, which result in a high risk for injury. People cannot evaluate situations for risks or danger. For example, they may wander outside in the winter wearing only thin nightclothes and not consider this to be a risk.

Insight is limited. Initially, the client may be aware of problems with memory and cognition and may worry that he or she is 'losing my mind'. Quite quickly, these concerns about the ability to function diminish, and people have little or no awareness of the more serious deficits that have developed. In this context, people may accuse others of stealing possessions that the people themselves have actually lost or forgotten.

SELF-CONCEPT

Initially, people may be angry or frustrated with themselves for losing objects or forgetting important things. Some people express sadness at their bodies for getting old and at the loss of functioning. Soon, though, they lose that awareness of self, which gradually deteriorates until they can look in a mirror and fail to recognize their own reflection.

ROLES AND RELATIONSHIPS

Dementia profoundly affects the person's roles and relationships. If he or she is still employed, work performance

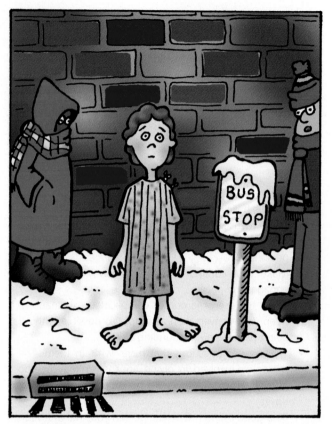

Judgement

suffers, even in the mild stage of dementia, to the point that work is no longer possible given the memory and cognitive deficits. Roles as spouse, partner or parent deteriorate as people lose the ability to perform even routine tasks or recognize familiar people. Eventually, people cannot meet even the most basic needs.

Inability to participate in meaningful conversation or social events severely limits relationships. People quickly become confined to the house or apartment because they are unable to venture outside unassisted. Close family members often begin to assume carer roles; this can change previously established relationships. Grown children of people with dementia experience role reversal; that is, they care for parents who once cared for them. Spouses or partners may feel as if they have lost the previous relationship and now are in the role of custodian.

PHYSIOLOGICAL AND SELF-CARE CONSIDERATIONS

People with dementia often experience disturbed sleep–wake cycles; they nap during the day and wander at night. Some people ignore internal cues such as hunger or thirst; others have little difficulty with eating and drinking until dementia is severe. People may experience bladder and even bowel incontinence or have difficulty cleaning themselves after elimination. They frequently neglect bathing and grooming. Eventually, people are likely to require complete care from someone else to meet these basic physiological needs.

Data Analysis

Many nursing formulations can be appropriate because the effects of dementia on people are profound; the disease touches virtually every part of their lives. Commonly used formulations include the following:

- Risk of injury
- Disturbed sleep pattern
- Risk of deficient fluid balance
- Risk of imbalanced nutrition: less than body requirements
- Chronic confusion
- Impaired environmental interpretation syndrome
- Impaired memory
- Impaired social interaction
- Impaired verbal communication
- Ineffective role performance.

In addition, the nursing formulations of Disturbed Thought Processes and Disturbed Sensory Perception would be appropriate for a client with psychotic symptoms. Multiple nursing formulations related to physiological status also may be indicated based on the nurse's assessment, such as alterations in nutrition, hydration, elimination, physical mobility and activity tolerance.

Outcome Identification

Care and treatment outcomes for people with progressive dementia do not involve regaining or maintaining abilities to function. In fact, the nurse must reassess overall health status and revise treatment outcomes periodically as the client's condition changes. Outcomes and nursing care that focus on the client's medical condition or deficits have, traditionally, been common. Current literature proposes a re-focusing on genuinely holistic psychosocial care that maximizes the client's strengths and abilities for as long as possible (Adams, 2008). Psychosocial care involves maintaining the client's independence as long as possible, validating the client's feelings, keeping the client involved in the environment and in care-planning and evaluation, adopting a whole systems approach and dealing with behavioural challenges respectfully (Hendry & Douglas, 2003; Mittelman *et al.*, 2004; Yuhas *et al.*, 2006; Adams, 2008). Treatment outcomes for a client with dementia may include the following:

- The person will be safe and remain free of injury.
- The person will maintain an adequate balance of activity and rest, nutrition, hydration and elimination.
- The person will function as independently and satisfyingly as possible, given his or her cogntitive limitations.
- The person will feel respected and supported.
- The person will remain involved in his or her surroundings.
- The person will interact with others in the environment.

Intervention

Psychosocial models for care of people with dementia are based on the approach that each client is a unique person and remains so, even as the disease's progression blocks the client's ability to demonstrate those unique characteristics. Interventions are rooted in the belief that people with dementia have personal strengths. They focus on demonstrating caring, keeping people involved by relating to the environment and other people and validating feelings and dignity of people by being responsive to them, offering choices and reframing (offering alternative points of view to explain events; Hendry & Douglas, 2003). This is in contrast to medical models of care that focus on progressive loss of function and identity.

Nurses can use the following interventions in any setting for people with dementia. Education for family members caring for people at home and for professional carers in residential or skilled facilities is an essential component of providing safe and supportive care. The discussion provides examples that apply to various settings.

PROMOTING THE CLIENT'S SAFETY

Safety considerations involve protecting against injury, meeting physiological needs and managing risks posed by the environment, including internal stimuli such as delusions and hallucinations. People cannot accurately appraise the environment and their abilities; therefore, they do not exercise normal caution in daily life. For example, the client living at home may forget food cooking on the stove; the client living in a residential care setting may leave for a walk in cold weather without a coat and gloves. Assistance or supervision that is as unobtrusive as possible protects people from injury while preserving their dignity. A family member might say,

'I'll sit in the kitchen and talk to you while you make lunch' (suggesting collaboration) rather than, 'You can't cook by yourself because you might set the house on fire.'

In this way, the nurse or carer supports the client's desire and ability to engage in certain tasks while providing protection from injury.

People with dementia may believe that their physical safety is jeopardized; they may feel threatened or suspicious and paranoid. These feelings can lead to agitated or erratic behaviour that compromises safety. Avoiding direct confrontation of the client's fears is important. People with dementia may struggle with fears and suspicion throughout their illness. Triggers of suspicion include strangers, changes in the daily routine or impaired memory. The nurse must discover and address these environmental triggers rather than confront the paranoid ideas.

For example, a client reports that his belongings have been stolen. The nurse might say,

NURSING INTERVENTIONS FOR PEOPLE WITH DEMENTIA

- Promoting client's safety and protecting from injury
  Offer unobtrusive assistance with or supervision of cooking, bathing or self-care activities.
  Identify environmental triggers to help client avoid them.
- Promoting adequate sleep, proper nutrition and hygiene, and activity
  Prepare desirable foods and foods client can self-feed; sit with client while eating.
  Monitor bowel elimination patterns; intervene with fluids and fibre or prompts.
  Remind client to urinate; provide incontinence pads as needed, checking and changing them frequently to avoid infection, skin irritation, unpleasant odours.
  Encourage mild physical activity such as walking.
- Structuring environment and routine
  Encourage client to follow regular routine and habits of bathing and dressing rather than imposing new ones.

Monitor amount of environmental stimulation and adjust when needed.
- Providing emotional support
  Be kind, respectful, calm, and reassuring; pay attention to client.
  Use supportive touch when appropriate.
  Encourage the safe expression of feeling.
- Promoting interaction and involvement
  Plan activities geared to client's interests and abilities.
  Reminisce with client about the past.
  If client is non-verbal, remain alert to non-verbal behaviour.
  Employ techniques of distraction, time away, going along or reframing to calm people who are agitated, suspicious or confused.

'Let's go and look in your room and see what's there.'

and help the client to locate the misplaced or hidden items (suggesting collaboration). If the client is in a room with other people and says, 'They're here to take me away!' the nurse might say,

'Those people are here visiting with someone else. Let's go for a walk and let them have their visit' (presenting reality/distraction).

The nurse then can take the client to a quieter and less stimulating place, which moves the client away from the environmental trigger (Cody *et al.*, 2002).

PROMOTING ADEQUATE SLEEP AND PROPER NUTRITION, HYGIENE AND ACTIVITY

People with dementia may require assistance to meet basic physiological needs. The nurse may need to monitor food and fluid intake to ensure adequacy. People may eat poorly because of limited appetite or distraction at mealtimes. In a residential or hospital environment, the nurse should address this problem by providing foods people like, sitting with them at meals to provide cues to continue eating, having nutritious snacks available whenever people are hungry and minimizing noise and undue distraction at mealtimes.

People who have difficulty manipulating utensils may be unable to cut meat or other foods into bite-sized pieces. The food should be cut up when it is prepared, not in front of people, to deflect attention from their inability to do so. Food that can be eaten without utensils, or finger foods such as sandwiches and fresh fruit, may be best. In contrast, people may eat too much, even ingesting inedible items. Providing low-calorie snacks such as carrot and celery sticks can satisfy the desire to chew and eat without unnecessary weight gain. Enteral nutrition often becomes necessary when dementia is most severe, although not all families choose to use tube feedings.

Adequate intake of fluids and food is also necessary for proper elimination. People may fail to respond to cues indicating constipation, so the nurse or carer monitors the client's bowel elimination patterns and intervenes with increased fluids and fibre or prompts as needed. Urinary elimination can become a problem if people do not respond to the urge to void or are incontinent. Reminders to urinate may be helpful when people are still continent but not initiating use of the bathroom. Incontinence pads can address dribbling or stress incontinence; pads, rather than indwelling catheters, are indicated for incontinence. The nurse checks disposable pads and diapers frequently and changes soiled items promptly to avoid infection, skin irritation and unpleasant odours. It is also important to provide good hygiene to minimize these risks.

Balance between rest and activity is an essential component of the daily routine. Mild physical activity such as walking promotes physical health but is not a cognitive challenge. Daily physical activity also helps people to sleep at night. The nurse provides rest periods so people can conserve and regain energy, but extensive daytime napping may interfere with night-time sleep. The nurse encourages people to engage in physical activity because they may not initiate such activities independently; many people tend to become sedentary as cognitive abilities diminish. People are often quite willing to participate in physical activities but unable to initiate, plan or carry out those activities without assistance.

STRUCTURING THE ENVIRONMENT AND ROUTINE

A structured environment and established routines can reassure people with dementia. Familiar surroundings and routines help to eliminate some confusion and frustration from memory loss. Providing routines and structure, however, does not mean forcing people to conform to the structure of the setting or routines that other people determine. Rather than impose new structure, the nurse encourages people to follow their usual routines and habits of bathing and dressing (Yuhas et al., 2006). For example, it is important to know whether a client prefers a bath or shower and washes at night or in the morning, and to include those preferences in the client's care. Research has shown that attempting to change the dressing behaviour of people may result in physical aggression as people make ineffective attempts to resist unwanted changes. Monitoring response to daily routines and making needed adjustments are important aspects of care.

The nurse needs to monitor and manage the client's tolerance of stimulation. Generally, people can tolerate less stimulation when they are fatigued, hungry or stressed. Also, with the progression of dementia, tolerance for environmental stimuli generally decreases. As this tolerance diminishes, people need a quieter environment with fewer people and less noise or distraction.

PROVIDING EMOTIONAL SUPPORT

The therapeutic relationship between client and nurse (in the context of person-centred care) involves 'empathic caring' (Hendry & Douglas, 2003), which includes being genuine, kind, respectful, calm and reassuring and paying full attention to the client. Nurses employ these same qualities with many different people in various settings. In most situations, people give positive feedback to the nurse or carer, but people with dementia may often seem to ignore the nurse's efforts and may even respond negatively with anger or suspicion. This may make it more difficult for the nurse or carer to sustain caring behaviour. Nevertheless, nurses and other carers *must* maintain all the qualities of the therapeutic relationship even when people do not seem to respond.

Because of their disorientation and memory loss, people with dementia often become anxious and require much patience and reassurance. The nurse can convey reassurance by approaching the client in a calm, supportive manner,

as if nurse and client are a team – a 'we can do it together' approach. The nurse reassures the client that he or she knows what is happening and can take care of things when the client is confused and cannot do so. For example, if the client is confused about getting dressed, the nurse might say,

'I'll be glad to help you with that shirt. I'll hold it for you while you put your arms in the sleeves' (offering self/suggesting collaboration).

Supportive touch is effective with many people. Touch can provide reassurance and convey caring when words may not be understood. Holding the hand of the client who is tearful and sad, and tucking the client into bed at night are examples of ways to use supportive touch. As with any use of touch, the nurse must evaluate each client's response. People who respond positively will smile or move closer toward the nurse. Those who are threatened by physical touch will look frightened or pull away from the nurse, especially if the touch is sudden or unexpected or if the client misperceives the nurse's intent.

PROMOTING INTERACTION AND INVOLVEMENT

In a psychosocial model of dementia care, the nurse or carer plans activities that reinforce the client's identity and keep him or her engaged and involved in the business of living (Yuhas et al., 2006). The nurse or carer tailors these activities – perhaps alongside occupational therapists or other staff – to the client's interests and abilities: they should *not* be routine group activities that 'everyone is supposed to do'. For example, a client with an interest in history may enjoy documentary programmes on television; a client who likes music may enjoy singing. People often need the involvement of another person to sustain attention in the activity and to enjoy it more fully. Those who have long periods without anything to engage their interest are more likely to become restless and agitated. People engaged in activities are more likely to stay calm.

Reminiscence therapy (thinking about or relating personally significant past experiences) can be an effective intervention for people with dementia if carried out in a co-operative, respectful and non-challenging way (Woods et al., 2005). Rather than lamenting that the client is 'living in the past', this therapy encourages family and carers also to reminisce with the client. Reminiscing uses the client's remote memory, which is not affected as severely or quickly as recent or immediate memory. Photo albums may be useful in stimulating remote memory, and they provide a focus on the client's past. Sometimes people like to reminisce about local or national events and talk about their roles or what they were doing at the time. In addition to keeping people involved in the business of living, reminiscence also can build self-esteem as people discuss accomplishments. Engaging in active listening, asking questions and providing cues to continue promote successful use of this technique.

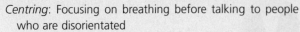

Box 21.4 **VALIDATION TECHNIQUES THAT CAN BE USED BY NURSES TALKING TO PEOPLE WITH DEMENTIA**

Centring: Focusing on breathing before talking to people who are disorientated

Using non-threatening, factual words to build trust: Using factual questions such as who, what, where, when and how

Rephrasing: Repeating the gist of what someone with dementia has said by using the same key words and tone of voice

Using polarity: Asking the person with dementia to think about the most extreme example of his or her complaint

Imagining the opposite: Asking the person with dementia to imagine the opposite to allow them to recollect a familiar solution to a problem

Reminiscing: Exploring the past can re-establish familiar coping methods that the disoriented person once used and can help people with dementia survive present-day losses

Maintaining genuine, close eye contact: Looking directly into the eyes of someone with dementia

Using ambiguity: Time-confused people often use words that have no meaning to others. By using ambiguity, nurses can communicate with people who are time-confused even when they do not understand what is being said

Using a clear, low, loving tone of voice: This can be very reassuring to people who are confused

Observing and matching the person's motion and emotions (Mirroring): Mimicking the physical movements of people with dementia as a means of promoting their understanding

Linking the behaviour with the unmet human needs: Most people need to be loved and nurtured, to be active and engaged and to express their deep emotions to someone who listens with empathy

Identifying and using the preferred sense: Communicating using a person's preferred sense- seeing, hearing, touching, smelling and tasting

Using music: When words have gone, familiar, early-learned melodies return

From Adams, T. (2008). Activities and interventions with people who have dementia and their families. In T. Adams (Ed.), *Dementia Care Nursing: promoting well-being in people with dementia and their families* (pp. 166–167). Basingstoke: Palgrave.

Validation therapy, developed by Naomi Feil, is, as Adams (2008, p. 166) says, focused on accomplishment and the validation of people's feelings, rather than (as in reminiscence therapy and reality orientation (frequently much used in the past)) risking a continued, reinforcing, therapeutic emphasis on cognitive deficits. Painful emotions can be expressed within a trusting environment and creative approaches taken to one-to-one sessions and group work.

People have increasing problems interacting with others as dementia progresses. Initially, people retain verbal language skills, but others may find them difficult to understand as words are lost or content becomes vague. The nurse must listen carefully to the client and try to determine the meaning behind what is being said. The nurse might say,

'Are you trying to say you want to use the bathroom?' or 'Did I get that right, you're hungry?' (seeking clarification).

It is also important not to interrupt people or to finish their thoughts. If a client becomes frustrated when the nurse cannot understand his or her meaning, the nurse might say,

'Can you show me what you mean or where you want to go?' (assisting to take action).

When verbal language becomes less coherent, the nurse should remain alert to the client's non-verbal behaviour. When nurses or carers consistently work with a particular client, they develop the ability to determine the client's meaning through non-verbal behaviour. For example, if the client becomes restless, it may indicate that he or she is hungry if it is close to mealtime, or tired if it is late in the evening. Sometimes it is impossible to determine exactly what the client is trying to convey, but the nurse can still be responsive. For example, a client is pacing and looks upset but cannot indicate what is bothering her. The nurse says,

'You look worried. I don't know what's wrong, but let's go for a walk' (making an observation/ offering self).

Interacting with people with dementia often means dealing with thoughts and feelings that are not based in reality but arise from the person's suspicion or chronic confusion. Rather than attempting to explain reality or allay suspicion or anger, it is often helpful to use the techniques of distraction, time away or going along to reassure the client.

Distraction involves shifting the client's attention and energy to a more neutral topic. For example, the client may display a catastrophic reaction to the current situation, such as jumping up from dinner and saying, 'My food tastes like poison!' The nurse might intervene with distraction by saying,

'Can you come to the kitchen with me and find something you'd like to eat?' or 'You can leave that food. Can you come and help me find a good pro- gramme on television?' (redirection/distraction).

People usually calm down when the nurse directs their attention away from the triggering situation.

'**Time away**' involves leaving people for a short period and then returning to them to re-engage in interaction. For example, the person may get angry and yell at the nurse for no discernible reason. The nurse can leave the client for about 5 or 10 minutes and then return without referring to the previous outburst. The client may have little or no memory of the inci- dent and may be pleased to see the nurse on his or her return.

'**Going along**' means providing emotional reassurance to people without correcting their misperception or delusion. The nurse does not engage in delusional ideas or reinforce them, but he or she does not deny or confront their exis- tence. For example, a client is fretful, repeatedly saying, 'I'm so worried about the children. I hope they're okay,' and speaking as though his adult children were small and needed protection. The nurse could reassure the client by saying,

'There's no need to worry; the children are just fine' (going along),

which is likely to calm the client. The nurse has responded effectively to the client's worry without addressing the reality of the client's concern. Going along is a specific intervention for people with dementia and should be used with great care with those experiencing delusions whose conditions are expected to improve: individual nurses and teams need to consider care- fully their feelings about the morality and ethics of doing this.

The nurse can use **reframing** techniques to offer people different points of view or explanations for situations or events. Because of their perceptual difficulties and confu- sion, people frequently interpret environmental stimuli as threatening. Loud noises often frighten and agitate them. For example, one client may interpret another's yelling as a direct personal threat. The nurse can provide an alternative explanation, such as

'That lady has lots of problems at the moment, and she yells sometimes because she's frustrated' (reframing).

Alternative explanations often reassure people with demen- tia and help them become less frightened and agitated.

Evaluation

Care and treatment outcomes change constantly as the dis- ease progresses. For example, in the early stage of dementia, maintaining independence may mean that the client dresses

with minimal assistance. Later, the same client may keep some independence by selecting what foods to eat. In the late stage, the client may maintain independence by wearing his or her own clothing rather than an institutional night- gown or pyjamas.

The nurse must assess people for changes as they occur and revise outcomes and interventions as needed. When a client is cared for at home, this includes provid- ing ongoing education to family members and carers while supporting them as the client's condition worsens. See the sections that follow on the role of the carer and community-based care.

RESIDENTIAL, INPATIENT AND COMMUNITY-BASED CARE

At least half of all nursing home residents have Alzheimer's disease or another illness that causes dementia. In addi- tion, for every person with dementia in a nursing home, two or three with similar impairments are receiving care in the community by some combination of family members, friends and paid carers.

Programmes and services for people with dementia and their families have increased – slowly and sporadically – with the growing awareness of Alzheimer's disease, the increas- ing numbers of older adults in the UK, and the fundraising efforts for education by noted figures (e.g. Terry Pratchett). Specialist psychiatric care is provided by multidisciplinary community mental health teams for the elderly (CMHTEs) who work closely with primary care teams (especially health visitors, GPs and district nurses). Home care is available through Social Services and voluntary agencies. These ser- vices offer assistance with bathing, food preparation and transportation as well as with other support. Periodic nurs- ing assessment may ensure that the level of care provided is appropriate to the client's current needs.

Older people's day care centres provide supervision, meals, support and recreational activities in group settings. People may attend the centre a few hours a week or full-time on weekdays if needed. Respite care offers in-home supervi- sion for people so that family members or carers can run errands or have social time of their own.

Residential facilities are available for people who do not have 'in-house' carers or whose needs have progressed beyond the care that could be provided at home. These people usu- ally require assistance with ADLs such as eating and taking medications. People in residential facilities are often referred for skilled nursing home placement as dementia progresses.

MENTAL HEALTH PROMOTION

Research continues to identify risk factors for dementia. People with elevated levels of plasma homocysteine are at increased risk for dementia. As levels of plasma homocysteine increase, so does the risk for dementia (Herrmann, 2006).

Because folate, vitamin B$_{12}$, and betaine are known to reduce plasma homocysteine levels, potential therapeutic strategies using these substances may modify or diminish the risk for dementia. Clinical trials are currently in progress to see if lowering homocysteine levels actually decreases the risk for dementia and whether taking high supplemental doses of B vitamins slows the progression of Alzheimer's disease.

People who regularly participate in brain-stimulating activities such as reading books and newspapers or doing crossword puzzles seem to be less likely to develop Alzheimer's disease than those who do not. Engaging in leisure-time physical activity during mid-life (Rovio *et al.*, 2005) and having a large social network (Bennett *et al.*, 2006) both seem to be associated with a decreased risk for Alzheimer's disease in later life.

ROLE OF THE CARER

According to the Alzheimer's Society (2008b), 'the value of services provided by all carers in 2001–2002 has been estimated at £57.4 billion. This is around the same level as the total amount spent in the UK on health. Nearly half (49 per cent) of all carers of people with dementia surveyed in Right From The Start, a survey of over 2,000 carers, were over 70-years-old, and 5 per cent were over 90-years-old. Unpaid carers deliver most of the care to people with dementia in the UK. Most carers are partners/spouses and many are elderly and frail themselves'.

Most family carers in dementia are women who are either adult daughters or wives of people with cognitive disorders. Sons and husbands still account for a smaller percentage of all carers. The trend toward caring for family members with dementia at home is largely the result of the high costs of institutional care, dissatisfaction with institutional care and difficulty locating suitable placements for people with behaviours that are sometimes disruptive and difficult to manage. Family members identify many other reasons for becoming primary carers, including the desire to reciprocate for past assistance, to provide love and affection, to uphold family values or loyalty, to meet duty or obligation and to avoid feelings of guilt.

Carers need to know about dementia and the required client care as well as how client care will change as the disease progresses. Carers may also be dealing with other family members who may or may not be supportive, or who may have differing expectations. Many carers have other demands on their time, such as their own families, careers and personal lives. Carers must deal with their feelings of loss and grief as the health of their loved ones continually declines (Mittelman *et al.*, 2004).

Caring for people with dementia can be emotionally and physically exhausting and stressful. Carers may need to drastically change their own lives, such as quitting a job, to provide care. Carers may have young children as well. They often feel exhausted and as if they are 'on duty' 24 hours a day. Carers caring for parents may have difficulty 'being in charge' of their mothers or fathers (role reversal). They may feel uncomfortable or depressed about having to bathe, feed or change diapers for parents.

'Role strain' is identified when the demands of providing care threaten to overwhelm a carer. Indications of role strain include constant fatigue that is unrelieved by rest, increased use of alcohol or other drugs, social isolation, inattention to personal needs and inability or unwillingness to accept help from others. Carers may feel unappreciated by other family members, as indicated by statements such as 'No one ever asks how I am!' (Mittelman *et al.*, 2004). In some situations, role strain can contribute to the neglect or abuse of people with dementia (see Chapter 11).

Supporting the carer is an important component of providing care at home to people with dementia. Carers must have an ongoing relationship with a knowledgeable health professional; the client's physician can make referrals to other health-care providers. Depending on the situation, that person may be a nurse, care manager or social worker. He or she can provide information, support and assistance during the time that home care is provided. Carers need education about dementia and the type of care that people need. Carers should use the interventions previously discussed to promote the client's well-being, deal with deficits and limitations and maximize the quality of the client's life. Because the care that people need changes as the dementia progresses, this education by the nurse, care manager or social worker is ongoing.

Carers need outlets for dealing with their own feelings. Support groups can help them to express frustration, sadness, anger, guilt or ambivalence; all these feelings are common. Attending a support group regularly also means that carers have time with people who understand the many demands of caring for a family member with dementia. The nurse can provide information about support groups and information and advocacy resources, including the Alzheimer's Society, Alzheimer Scotland and Carers UK.

Carers should be supported to seek and accept assistance from other people or agencies. Often, carers believe that others may not be able to provide care as well as they do, or they say they will seek help when they 'really need it'. Carers must maintain their own well-being and not wait until they are exhausted before seeking relief. Sometimes family members disagree about care for the client. The primary carer may believe other family members should volunteer to help without being asked, but other family members may believe that the primary carer chose to take on the responsibility and do not feel obligated to help out regularly. Whatever the feelings are among family members, it is important for them all to express their feelings and ideas and to participate in caring according to their own expectations. Many families need assistance from professionals, including CMHNs, to reach this type of compromise.

Finally, carers need support to maintain personal lives. They need to continue to socialize with friends and to engage in leisure activities or hobbies rather than focus solely on the client's care. Carers who are rested, happy and have met their own needs are better prepared to manage the rigorous demands of the carer role. Most carers need to be reminded to take care of themselves; this act is not selfish but really is in the client's best long-term interests.

RELATED DISORDERS

Amnestic disorders are characterized by a disturbance in memory that results directly from the physiological effects of a general medical condition or the persisting effects of a substance such as alcohol or other drugs (American Psychiatric Association, 2000). The memory disturbance is sufficiently severe to cause marked impairment in social or occupational functioning and represents a significant decline from previous functioning. Confusion, disorientation and attentional deficits are common. People with amnestic disorders are similar to those with dementia in terms of memory deficits, confusion and problems with attention. They do not, however, have the multiple cognitive deficits seen in dementia such as aphasia, apraxia, agnosia and impaired executive functions.

Several medical conditions can cause brain damage and result in an amnestic disorder – for example, stroke or other cerebrovascular events, head injuries and neurotoxic exposures such as carbon monoxide poisoning, chronic alcohol ingestion, and vitamin B_{12} or thiamine deficiency. Alcohol-induced amnestic disorder results from a chronic thiamine or vitamin B deficiency and is called **Korsakoff's syndrome**.

The main difference between dementia and amnestic disorders is that once the underlying medical cause is treated or removed, the client's condition no longer deteriorates. Treatment of amnestic disorders focuses on eliminating the underlying cause and rehabilitating the client, and includes preventing further medical problems. Some amnestic disorders improve over time when the underlying cause is stabilized. Other people have persistent impairment of memory and attention, with minimal improvement; this can occur in cases of chronic alcohol ingestion or malnutrition (Grossman, 2005). Nursing diagnoses and interventions are similar to those used when dealing with the memory loss, confusion and impaired attention abilities of people with dementia or delirium (see Nursing Interventions for Dementia).

Nursing Care Plan *Dementia*

Nursing Formulation

Impaired Memory: *Inability to remember or recall bits of information or behavioural skills.*

ASSESSMENT DATA

- Inability to recall factual information or events
- Inability to learn new material or recall previously learned material
- Inability to determine whether a behaviour was performed
- Agitation or anxiety regarding memory loss

EXPECTED OUTCOMES

Immediate
The client will
- Respond positively to memory cues
- Demonstrate decreased agitation or anxiety

Medium term
The client will
- Attain an optimal level of functioning with routine tasks
- Use long-term memory effectively as long as it remains intact
- Verbalize or demonstrate decreased frustration with memory loss

Longer term
The client will
- Maintain an optimal level of functioning
- Be, and feel, respected and supported

continued ···⟶

Nursing Care Plan: Dementia, cont.

IMPLEMENTATION

Nursing Interventions *denotes collaborative interventions	**Rationale**
Provide opportunities for reminiscence or recall of past events, on a one-to-one basis or in a small group.	Long-term memory may persist after loss of recent memory. Non-threatening and non-judgemental reminiscence is usually an enjoyable activity for the client.
Encourage the client to use written cues such as a calendar, lists or a notebook.	Written cues decrease the client's need to recall appointments, activities and so on from memory.
Minimize environmental changes. Determine practical locations for the client's possessions, and return items to this location after use. Establish a usual routine and alter the routine only when necessary.	There is less demand on memory function when structure is incorporated in the client's environment and daily routine.
Provide single step instructions for the client when instructions are needed.	People with memory impairment may not be able to remember 'multistep' instructions.
Provide verbal connections about using implements. For example, 'Here's a flannel to wash your face,' 'Here's a spoon you can use to eat your dessert,'	The client may not remember what an implement is for; stating its related function is an approach that compensates for memory loss.
Integrate reminders of previous events into current interactions such as 'Earlier you put some clothes in the washing machine; it's time to put them in the dryer.'	Providing links with previous behaviours helps the client to make connections that he or she may not be able to make independently.
Assist with tasks as needed, but do not 'rush' to do things for the client that he or she can still do independently.	It is important to maximize independent function, yet assist the client when memory has deteriorated further.
Use a matter-of-fact approach when assuming tasks the client can no longer perform. Do not allow the client to work unsuccessfully at a task for an extended time.	It is important to preserve the client's dignity and minimize his or her frustration with progressive memory loss.

Adapted from Schultz, J. M. & Videbeck, S. L. (2005). *Lippincott's manual of psychiatric nursing care plans* (7th edn). Philadelphia: Lippincott Williams & Wilkins.

SELF-AWARENESS ISSUES

Working with and caring for people with dementia can be exhausting and frustrating for both nurse and carer. Education is a fundamental role for nurses, but helping people who have dementia to learn can be especially challenging and frustrating. People often don't retain explanations or instructions, so the nurse must repeat the same things continually. The nurse must be careful not to lose patience and not to give up. He or she may begin to feel that repeating instructions or explanations does no good because people do not understand or remember them. Discussing these frustrations with others – in clinical supervision and informally – can help the nurse to avoid conveying negative feelings to people and families, or experiencing professional and personal burnout.

The nurse may get little or no positive response or feedback from people with dementia. It can be difficult to deal with feelings about caring for people who will never 'get better and go home'. As dementia progresses, people may seem not to hear or respond to anything the nurse does. It is sad and frustrating for the nurse to see people decline and eventually lose their abilities to manage basic self-care activities and to interact with others. Remaining positive and supportive to people and family can be difficult when the outcome is so bleak. In addition, the progressive decline may last months or years, which adds to the frustration and sadness. The nurse may need to deal with personal feelings of depression and grief as the dementia progresses; he or she can do so by discussing the situation with colleagues or even a counsellor.

Points to Consider When Working With People With Dementia

- Remember VIPS:
  V = a value base that asserts the absolute value of all human lives regardless of age or cognitive ability
  I = an individualized approach, recognizing uniqueness
  P = understanding the world from the perspective of the service user
  S = providing a social environment that supports psychological needs
- Remember how important it is to provide dignity for the client and family as the client's life ends.

- Remember that death is the last stage of life. The nurse can provide emotional support for the client and family during this period.
- People may not notice the caring, patience and support the nurse offers, but these qualities will mean a great deal to the family for a long time.

DELIRIUM

As stated earlier, it is vital to distinguish between delirium and dementia. **Delirium** is a syndrome that involves a disturbance of consciousness accompanied by a change in cognition. Delirium usually develops over a short period, sometimes a matter of hours, and fluctuates, or changes, throughout the course of the day. People with delirium have difficulty paying attention, are easily distracted and disoriented and may have sensory disturbances such as illusions, misinterpretations or hallucinations. An electrical cord on the floor may appear to them to be a snake (illusion). They may mistake the banging of a trolley in the hallway for a gunshot (misinterpretation). They may see 'angels' hovering above when nothing is there (hallucination). At times, they also experience disturbances in the sleep–wake cycle, changes in psychomotor activity and emotional problems such as anxiety, fear, irritability, euphoria or apathy (American Psychiatric Association, 2000).

An estimated 10% to 15% of people in the hospital for general medical conditions are delirious at any given time. Delirium is common in older, acutely ill people. An estimated 30% to 50% of acutely ill older adult people

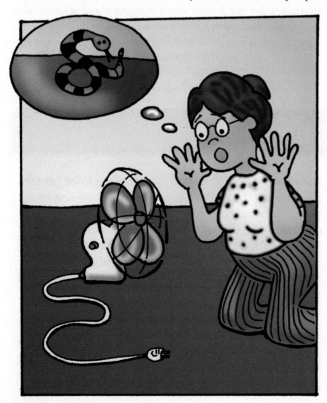

Illusion

become delirious at some time during their hospital stay. Risk factors for delirium include increased severity of physical illness, older age and baseline cognitive impairment such as that seen in dementia (Samuels & Neugroschl, 2005). Children may be more susceptible to delirium, especially that related to a febrile illness or certain medications, such as anticholinergics (American Psychiatric Association, 2000).

Aetiology

Delirium almost always results from an identifiable physiological, metabolic or cerebral disturbance or disease, or from drug intoxication or withdrawal. The most common causes are listed in Box 21.5. Often, delirium results from multiple causes and requires a careful and thorough physical examination and laboratory tests for identification.

Cultural Considerations

People from different cultural backgrounds may not be familiar with the information requested to assess memory, such as the name of former Prime Ministers. Other cultures may consider orientation to placement and location differently. Also, some cultures and religions, such as Jehovah's Witnesses, do not celebrate birthdays, so people may have difficulty stating their date of birth: the nurse should not mistake failure to know such information for disorientation (American Psychiatric Association, 2000).

Treatment and Prognosis

The primary treatment for delirium is to identify and treat any causal or contributing medical conditions. Delirium is almost always a transient condition that clears with successful treatment of the underlying cause. Nevertheless, some causes, such as head injury or encephalitis, may leave people with cognitive, behavioural or emotional impairments even after the underlying cause resolves.

PSYCHOPHARMACOLOGY

People with quiet, hypoactive delirium need no specific pharmacological treatment, aside from that indicated for the causative condition. Many people with delirium, however, show persistent or intermittent psychomotor agitation that can interfere with effective treatment or pose a risk to safety. Sedation to prevent inadvertent self-injury may be indicated. An antipsychotic medication such as haloperidol (Haldol) may be used in doses of 0.5 to 1 mg to decrease agitation. Sedatives and benzodiazepines are avoided because they may worsen delirium (Samuels & Neugroschl, 2005). People with impaired liver or kidney function could have

Box 21.5   MOST COMMON CAUSES OF DELIRIUM

Physiological or metabolic	Hypoxaemia, electrolyte disturbances, renal or hepatic failure, hypoglycaemia or hyperglycaemia, dehydration, sleep deprivation, thyroid or glucocorticoid disturbances, thiamine or vitamin B_{12} deficiency, vitamin C, niacin, or protein deficiency, cardiovascular shock, brain tumour, head injury, and exposure to gasoline, paint solvents, insecticides and related substances
Infection	Systemic: sepsis, urinary tract infection, pneumonia
	Cerebral: meningitis, encephalitis, HIV, syphilis
Drug-related	Intoxication: anticholinergics, lithium, alcohol, sedatives and hypnotics
	Withdrawal: alcohol, sedatives and hypnotics
	Reactions to anaesthesia, prescription medication or illicit (street) drugs

Compiled from Samuels, S. C. & Neugroschl, J. A. (2005). Delirium. In B. J. Sadock & V. A. Sadock (Eds.), *Comprehensive textbook of psychiatry, Vol. 1* (8th edn, pp. 1054–1068). Philadelphia: Lippincott Williams & Wilkins; and Ribby, K. J. & Cox, K. R. (1996). Development, implementation, and evaluation of a confusion protocol. *Clinical Nurse Specialist, 10*(5), 241–247.

difficulty metabolizing or excreting sedatives. The exception is delirium induced by alcohol withdrawal, which usually is treated with benzodiazepines (see Chapter 17).

OTHER MEDICAL TREATMENT

While the underlying causes of delirium are being treated, people may also need other supportive physical measures. Adequate nutritious food and fluid intake speed recovery.

Intravenous fluids or even total parenteral nutrition may be necessary if a client's physical condition has deteriorated and he or she cannot eat and drink.

If a client becomes agitated and threatens to dislodge intravenous tubing or catheters, physical restraints may be necessary so that needed medical treatments can continue. Restraints are used only when necessary and stay in place no longer than warranted because they may increase the client's agitation.

CLINICAL VIGNETTE: DELIRIUM

On a hot and humid August afternoon, the emergency services received a call requesting an ambulance for an elderly woman who had collapsed on the pavement in a residential area. According to neighbours gathered at the scene, the woman had been wandering around the area since early morning. No one recognized her and several people had tried to approach her to offer help or give directions. She would not or could not give her name or address; much of her speech was garbled and hard to understand. She was not carrying a purse or identification. She finally collapsed and appeared unconscious, so they dialled 999.

The woman was taken to A&E. She was perspiring profusely, was found to have a fever of 39.5°C, and was grossly dehydrated. Intravenous therapy was started to replenish fluids and electrolytes. A cooling blanket was applied to lower her temperature, and she was monitored closely over the next several hours. As the woman began to regain consciousness, she was confused and could not provide any useful information about herself. Her speech remained garbled and confused. Several times she attempted to climb out of the bed and remove her intravenous tube, so restraints were used to prevent injury and to allow treatment to continue.

By the end of the second day in the hospital, she could accurately give her name, address and some of the circumstances surrounding the incident. She remembered she had been gardening in her back yard in the sun and felt very hot. She remembered thinking she should go back in the house to get a cold drink and rest. That was the last thing she remembered.

APPLICATION OF THE NURSING PROCESS: DELIRIUM

Nursing care for people with delirium focuses on meeting their physiological and psychological needs and maintaining their safety. Behaviour, mood and level of consciousness of these people can fluctuate rapidly throughout the day. Therefore, the nurse must assess them continuously to recognize changes and to plan nursing care accordingly.

Assessment

HISTORY

Because the causes of delirium are often related to medical illness, alcohol or other drugs, the nurse needs to obtain a thorough history of these areas. He or she may need to obtain information from family members if a client's ability to provide accurate data is impaired.

Information about drugs should include prescribed medications, alcohol, illicit drugs and over-the-counter medications. Although many people perceive prescribed and over-the-counter medications as relatively safe, combinations or standard doses of medications can produce delirium, especially in older adults. Box 21.6 lists types of drugs that can cause delirium. Combinations of these drugs significantly increase risk.

GENERAL APPEARANCE AND MOTOR BEHAVIOUR

People with delirium often have a disturbance of psychomotor behaviour. They may be restless and hyperactive, frequently picking at bedclothes or making sudden, uncoordinated attempts to get out of bed. Conversely, people may have slowed motor behaviour, appearing sluggish and lethargic with little movement.

Speech also may be affected, becoming less coherent and more difficult to understand as delirium worsens. People may perseverate on a single topic or detail, may be rambling and difficult to follow or may have pressured speech that is rapid, forced and usually louder than normal. At times, people may call out or scream, especially at night.

MOOD AND AFFECT

People with delirium often have rapid and unpredictable mood shifts. A wide range of emotional responses is possible, such as anxiety, fear, irritability, anger, euphoria and apathy. These mood shifts and emotions usually have nothing to do with the client's environment. When people are particularly fearful and feel threatened, they may become combative to defend themselves from perceived harm.

THOUGHT PROCESS AND CONTENT

Although people with delirium have changes in cognition, it is difficult for the nurse to assess these changes accurately and thoroughly. Marked inability to sustain attention makes it difficult to assess thought process and content. Thought content in delirium often is unrelated to the situation, or speech is illogical and difficult to understand. The nurse may ask how people are feeling, and they will mumble about the weather. Thought processes often are disorganized and make no sense. Thoughts also may be fragmented (disjointed and incomplete). People may exhibit delusions, believing that their altered sensory perceptions are real.

SENSORY AND INTELLECTUAL PROCESSES

The primary and often initial sign of delirium is an altered level of consciousness that is seldom stable and

Box 21.6 DRUGS CAUSING DELIRIUM

Anaesthesia	Benzodiazepines
Anticholinergics	Cardiac glycosides
Anticonvulsants	Cimetidine
Antidepressants	Hypoglycaemic agents
Antihistamines	Insulin
Antihypertensives	Narcotics
Antineoplastics	Propranolol (Inderal)
Antipsychotics	Reserpine
Aspirin	Steroids
Barbiturates	Thiazide diuretics

Adapted from Samuels, S. C. & Neugroschl, J. A. (2005). Delirium. In B. J. Sadock and V. A. Sadock (Eds.), *Comprehensive Textbook of Psychiatry*, Vol. 1 (8th edn, pp. 1068–1093). Philadelphia: Lippincott Williams and Wilkins.

usually fluctuates throughout the day. People usually are oriented to person but frequently disoriented to time and place. They demonstrate decreased awareness of the environment or situation and instead may focus on irrelevant stimuli such as the colour of the bedspread or the room. Noises, people or sensory misperceptions easily distract them.

People cannot focus, sustain or shift attention effectively, and there is impaired recent and immediate memory (American Psychiatric Association, 2000). This means the nurse may have to ask questions or provide directions repeatedly. Even then, people may be unable to do what is requested.

People frequently experience misinterpretations, illusions and hallucinations. Both misperceptions and illusions are based on some actual stimuli in the environment: people may hear a door slam and interpret it as a gunshot, or see the nurse reach for an intravenous bag and believe the nurse is about to strike them. Examples of common illusions include people believing that intravenous tubing or an electrical cord is a snake and mistaking the nurse for a family member. Hallucinations are most often visual: people 'see' things for which there is no stimulus in reality. Some people, when more lucid, are aware that they are experiencing sensory misperceptions. Others, however, actually believe their misinterpretations are correct and cannot be convinced otherwise.

JUDGEMENT AND INSIGHT

Judgement is impaired. People often cannot perceive potentially harmful situations or act in their own best interests. For example, they may try repeatedly to pull out intravenous tubing or urinary catheters; this causes pain and interferes with necessary treatment.

Insight depends on the severity of the delirium. People with mild delirium may recognize that they are confused, are receiving treatment and will likely improve. Those with severe delirium may have no insight into the situation.

ROLES AND RELATIONSHIPS

People are unlikely to fulfil their roles during the course of delirium. Most regain their previous level of functioning, however, and have no longstanding problems with roles or relationships.

SELF-CONCEPT

Although delirium has no direct effect on self-concept, people are often frightened or feel threatened. Those with some awareness of the situation may feel helpless or powerless to do anything to change it. If delirium has resulted from alcohol, illicit drug use or overuse of prescribed medications, people may feel guilt, shame and humiliation, or think, 'I'm a bad person; I did this to myself.' This would indicate possible long-term problems with self-concept.

PHYSIOLOGICAL AND SELF-CARE CONSIDERATIONS

People with delirium most often experience disturbed sleep–wake cycles that may include difficulty falling asleep, daytime sleepiness, night-time agitation or even a complete reversal of the usual daytime waking/night-time sleeping pattern (American Psychiatric Association, 2000). At times, people also ignore or fail to perceive internal body cues such as hunger, thirst or the urge to urinate or defaecate.

Data Analysis

The primary nursing formulations for people with delirium are as follows:

- Risk of injury
- Acute confusion.

Additional diagnoses that are commonly selected, based on client assessment, include the following:

- Disturbed sensory perception
- Disturbed thought processes
- Disturbed sleep pattern
- Risk of deficient fluid volume
- Risk of imbalanced nutrition: less than body requirements.

Outcome Identification

Treatment outcomes for the client with delirium may include the following:

- The client will remain safe and be free of injury.
- The client will demonstrate increased orientation and reality contact.
- The client will maintain an adequate balance of activity and rest.
- The client will maintain adequate nutrition and fluid balance.
- The client will return to his or her optimal level of functioning.

Intervention

PROMOTING THE CLIENT'S SAFETY

Maintaining the client's safety is the primary focus of nursing interventions. Medications should be used judiciously because sedatives may worsen confusion and increase the risk for falls or other injuries (Samuels & Neugroschl, 2005).

The nurse teaches people to request assistance for activities such as getting out of bed or going to the bathroom. If people cannot request assistance, they require close supervision to prevent them from attempting activities they cannot perform safely alone. The nurse responds promptly to calls from people for assistance and checks people at frequent intervals.

If a client is agitated or pulling at intravenous lines or catheters, physical restraints may be necessary. Use of restraints, however, may increase the client's fears or feelings of being threatened, so restraints are a last resort. The nurse first tries other strategies such as having a family member stay with the client to reassure him or her.

MANAGING THE CLIENT'S CONFUSION

The nurse must approach these clients calmly and speak in a clear, low voice. It is important to give realistic reassurance to people, such as

'I know things are upsetting and confusing right now, but things should get clearer and easier as you get better' (validating/giving information).

Facing people while speaking helps to capture their attention. The nurse provides explanations that people can comprehend, avoiding lengthy or too detailed discussions. The nurse should phrase questions or provide directions to people in short, simple sentences, allowing adequate time for people to grasp the content or to respond to a question. He or she permits people to make decisions as they are able and takes care not to overwhelm or frustrate them.

The nurse provides orienting cues when talking with people, such as calling them by name and referring to the time of day or expected activity. For example, the nurse might say,

'Good morning, Mrs Jones. I see you're awake and look ready for breakfast' (giving information).

Reminding the client of the nurse's name and role repeatedly may be necessary, such as

'My name is Sheila, and I'm your nurse today. I'm here now to see if you want to go for a walk' (reality orientation).

Orienting objects such as a calendar and clock in the client's room are useful.

Often, the use of touch reassures people and provides contact with reality. It is important to evaluate each client's response to touch rather than to assume all people welcome it. A client who smiles or draws closer to the nurse when touched is responding positively. The fearful client may perceive touch as threatening rather than comforting and startle or draw away.

People with delirium can experience sensory overload, which means more stimulation is coming into the brain than they can handle. Reducing environmental stimulation is helpful because these people are distracted and over-stimulated easily. Minimizing environmental noises, including television or radio, should calm them. It is also important

to monitor response to visitors. Too many visitors or more than one person talking at once may increase the client's confusion. The nurse can explain to visitors that the client will best tolerate quiet talking with one person at a time.

The client's room should be well lit to minimize environmental misperceptions. When people experience illusions or misperceptions, the nurse corrects them matter-of-factly. It is important to validate the client's feelings of anxiety or fear generated by the misperception but not to reinforce that misperception. For example, a client hears a loud noise in the hall and asks the nurse, 'Was that an explosion?' The nurse might respond,

'No, that was a trolley banging in the hall. It was really loud, wasn't it? It startled me a bit when I heard it' (presenting reality/validating feelings).

PROMOTING SLEEP AND PROPER NUTRITION

The nurse monitors the client's sleep and elimination patterns and food and fluid intake. People may require prompting or assistance to eat and drink adequate food and fluids. It may be helpful to sit with people at meals or to frequently offer fluids. Family members also may be able to help people to improve their intake. Assisting people to the bathroom periodically may be necessary to promote elimination if people do not make these requests independently.

Promoting a balance of rest and sleep is important if people are experiencing a disturbed sleep pattern. Discouraging or limiting daytime napping may improve ability to sleep at night. It is also important for people to have some exercise during the day to promote night-time sleep. Activities could include sitting in a chair, walking in the hall or engaging in diversional activities (as possible).

CLIENT/FAMILY EDUCATION FOR DELIRIUM

- Monitor chronic health conditions carefully.
- Visit GP regularly.
- Tell all professionals what medications are taken, including over-the-counter medications, dietary supplements and herbal preparations.
- Check with GP before taking any non-prescription medication.
- Avoid alcohol and recreational drugs.
- Maintain a nutritious diet.
- Get adequate sleep.
- Use safety precautions when working with paint solvents, insecticides and similar products.

NURSING INTERVENTIONS FOR DELIRIUM

- **Promoting client's safety**
  Teach client to request assistance for activities (getting out of bed, going to bathroom).
  Provide close supervision to ensure safety during these activities.
  Promptly respond to client's call for assistance.
- **Managing client's confusion**
  Speak to client in a calm manner in a clear, low voice; use simple sentences.
  Allow adequate time for client to comprehend and respond.
  Allow client to make decisions as much as possible.
  Provide orienting verbal cues when talking with client.
  Use supportive touch if appropriate.
- **Controlling environment to reduce sensory overload**
  Keep environmental noise to a minimum (television, radio).

Monitor client's response to visitors; explain to family and friends that client may need to be visited quietly one-on-one.
Validate client's anxiety and fears, but do not reinforce misperceptions.
- **Promoting sleep and proper nutrition**
  Monitor sleep and elimination patterns.
  Monitor food and fluid intake; provide prompts or assistance to eat and drink adequate amounts of food and fluids.
  Provide periodic assistance to bathroom if client does not make requests.
  Discourage daytime napping to help sleep at night.
  Encourage some exercise during day, like sitting in a chair, walking in hall or other activities client can manage.

Evaluation

Usually, successful treatment of the underlying causes of delirium returns people to their previous levels of functioning. People and carers or family must understand what health-care practices are necessary to avoid a recurrence. This may involve monitoring a chronic health condition, using medications carefully or abstaining from alcohol or other drugs.

ONGOING CARE

Even when the cause of delirium is identified and treated, people may not regain all cognitive functions, or problems with confusion may persist. Because delirium and dementia frequently occur together, many people may have dementia. A thorough medical evaluation can confirm dementia, and appropriate treatment and care can be initiated (see the earlier section of this chapter).

When delirium has cleared and any other diagnoses have been eliminated, it may be necessary for the nurse or other health-care professionals to initiate referrals to health visitors, CMHNs or a rehabilitation programme if people continue to experience cognitive problems. Various community programes provide such care, including adult day care or residential care. People who have ongoing cognitive deficits after an episode of delirium may have difficulties similar to those of people with head injuries or mild dementia. People and family members or carers might benefit from support groups to help them deal with the changes in personality and remaining cognitive or motor deficits.

Critical Thinking Questions

1. The nurse is working in an elderly-care setting with people with dementia. One of the ancillary staff makes a joke about a client in the client's presence. The nurse tells the staff person that this is unacceptable behaviour. The staff person replies, 'Oh, he can't understand what I'm saying, and besides, he was laughing too. What's the big deal?' How should the nurse respond?

2. A client is newly diagnosed with dementia in the early stages. Can the client make decisions about future care and treatment? Why-or why not? At what point in the progression of dementia can the client no longer make decisions about their own life?

 KEY POINTS

- Cognitive disorders involve disruption or impairment in the higher functions of the brain. They include delirium, dementia and amnestic disorders.
- Compassionate, person-centred approaches to care are essential.
- Delirium is a syndrome that involves disturbed consciousness and changes in cognition. It is usually caused by an underlying, treatable medical condition such as physiological or metabolic imbalances, infections, nutritional deficits, medication reactions or interactions, drug intoxication or alcohol withdrawal.

Nursing Care Plan

Delirium

Nursing Diagnosis

Acute Confusion: *Abrupt onset of a cluster of global, transient changes and disturbances in attention, cognition, psychomotor activity, level of consciousness and/or sleep–wake cycle.*

ASSESSMENT DATA

- Poor judgement
- Cognitive impairment
- Impaired memory
- Lack of, or limited, insight
- Loss of personal control
- Inability to perceive harm
- Illusions
- Hallucinations
- Mood swings

EXPECTED OUTCOMES

Immediate
The client will
- Engage in a trusting relationship with staff and carers
- Be safe and remain free from injury
- Increase reality contact
- Co-operate with treatment

Medium-term
The client will
- Establish or follow a routine for activities of daily living
- Demonstrate decreased confusion, illusions or hallucinations
- Experience minimal distress related to confusion
- Validate perceptions with staff or caregiver before taking action

Longer-term
The client will
- Return to optimal level of functioning
- Manage health conditions, if any, effectively
- Seek medical treatment as needed

IMPLEMENTATION

Nursing Interventions *denotes collaborative interventions	**Rationale**
Do not allow the client to assume responsibility for decisions or actions if he or she is patently unsafe to do so.	The client's safety is a priority. He or she may be unable to determine harmful actions or situations.
If limits on the client's actions are necessary, explain limits and reasons respectfully and clearly, within the client's ability to understand.	The client has the right to be informed of any restrictions and the reasons limits are needed.
Involve the client in making plans or decisions as much as he or she is able to participate.	Compliance with treatment is enhanced if the client is emotionally invested in it.
In a matter-of-fact manner, give the client factual feedback on misperceptions, delusions or hallucinations (e.g. 'That is a chair') and convey that others do not share his or her interpretations (e.g. 'I don't see anyone else in the room').	When given feedback in a non-judgemental way, the client can feel validated for his or her feelings, while recognizing that his or her perceptions are not shared by others.
Assess the client daily, or more often if needed, for his or her level of functioning.	People with organically based problems tend to fluctuate frequently in terms of their capabilities.
Allow the client to make decisions as much as he or she is able.	Decision making increases the client's participation, independence and self-esteem.

continued ⋯⋗

Nursing Care Plan: Delirium, cont.

IMPLEMENTATION

Nursing Interventions *denotes collaborative interventions	**Rationale**
Assist the client to establish a daily routine, including hygiene, activities and so forth.	Routine or habitual activities do not require decisions about whether or not to perform a particular task.
Teach the client about underlying cause(s) of confusion and delirium.	Knowledge about the cause(s) of confusion can help the client seek assistance when indicated.

Adapted from Schultz, J. M. & Videbeck, S. L. (2005). *Lippincott's manual of psychiatric nursing care plans* (7th edn) Philadelphia: Lippincott Williams & Wilkins.

- The primary goals of nursing care for people with delirium are protection from injury, management of confusion and meeting their physiological and psychological needs.
- Dementia is a disease-process involving memory loss and multiple cognitive deficits such as language deterioration (aphasia), motor impairment (apraxia) or inability to name or recognize objects (agnosia).
- Dementia is usually progressive, beginning with prominent memory loss (mild stage) and confusion and loss of independent functioning (moderate), followed by total disorientation and loss of functioning (severe).
- Medications used to treat dementia, including donepezil (Aricept), can slow disease progression. Other medications such as antipsychotics, antidepressants and benzodiazepines help manage symptoms but do not affect the course of dementia.
- A psychosocial model for providing care for people with dementia addresses genuine involvement and choice, needs for safety, structure, support, interpersonal involvement and social interaction.

- Many people with dementia receive care at home rather than in institutional settings (e.g. nursing homes). The carer role (often assumed by a spouse or adult child) can be physically and emotionally exhausting and stressful; this contributes to strain on carers.
- To deal with the exhausting demands of this role, family carers need ongoing education and support from a health-care professional such as a nurse, social worker or case manager.
- Carers must learn how to meet the client's physiological and emotional needs and to protect him or her from injury. Areas for teaching include monitoring the client's health, avoiding alcohol and recreational drugs, ensuring adequate nutrition, scheduling regular check-ups, getting adequate rest, promoting activity and socialization and helping the client to maintain independence as much as possible.
- The therapeutic relationship with people with dementia is collaborative, supportive and protective and recognizes the client's individuality and dignity.

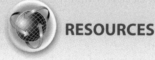

INTERNET RESOURCES

RESOURCES	**INTERNET ADDRESS**
Age Concern	http://www.ageconcern.org.uk/
Alzheimer Scotland	www.alzscot.org
Alzheimer's Society	http://www.alzheimers.org.uk/site/index.php
CARERS UK	http://www.carersuk.org/Home
Department of Health Older People's Policy Documents	http://www.dh.gov.uk/en/SocialCare/ Deliveringadultsocialcare/Olderpeople/index.htm
Help The Aged	http://www.helptheaged.org.uk/en-gb
Parkinson's Disease Society	http://www.parkinsons.org.uk/

REFERENCES

Adams, T. (2008). *Dementia care nursing*. Basingstoke: Palgrave Press

Alzheimer's Society. (2007). *Dementia UK*. Available: http://www.alzheimers.org.uk/downloads/Dementia_UK_Summary.pdf

Alzheimer's Society. (2008a). *Statistics*. Available: http://www.alzheimers.org.uk/site/scripts/documents_info.php?categoryID=200120&documentID=341

Alzheimer's Society. (2008b). *Carer support*. Available: http://www.alzheimers.org.uk/site/scripts/documents_info.php?categoryID=200167&documentID=546

Alzheimer's Society. (2008c). *Overprescription of antipsychotic drugs (2008)*. Available: http://www.alzheimers.org.uk/site/scripts/documents_info.php?categoryID=200149&documentID=389

American Psychiatric Association. (2000). *Diagnostic and statistical manual of mental disorders* (4th edn, text revision). Washington, DC: American Psychiatric Association.

Bennett, D. A., Schneider, J. A., Tang, Y., *et al.* (2006). The effect of social networks on the relation between Alzheimer's disease pathology and level of cognitive function in old people: A longitudinal cohort study. *Lancet Neurology, 5*(5), 406–412.

Brooker, W., Edwards, P., & Benson, S. (2004). *Dementia care mapping: Experience and insights into practice*. London: Hawker Publications.

Brooker, D. (2007). Person-centred dementia care: making services better. London: Jessica Kingsley Publications.

Brooker, D. (2008). Person-centred care. In R. Jacoby, C. Oppenheimer, T. Dening & A. Thomas (Eds.), *Oxford textbook of old age psychiatry*. Oxford: Oxford University Press.

Brooker, D., Woolley, R., & Lee, D. (2007). Enriching opportunities for people living with dementia in nursing homes: An evaluation of a multi-level activity-based model of care. *Aging & Mental Health, 11*(4), 361–370.

Cody, M., Beck, C., & Svarstad, B. L. (2002). Challenges to the use of non-pharmacologic interventions in nursing homes. *Psychiatric Services, 53*(11), 1402–1406.

CSIP Older Peoples Mental Health programme, (2007). *Strengthening the involvement of people with dementia*. Available: http://www.olderpeoplesmentalhealth.csip.org.uk/service-user-and-carer-engagement-tool.html

Davis, K. L. (2005). Cognitive disorders: Introduction and overview. In B. J. Sadock & V. A. Sadock (Eds.), *Comprehensive textbook of psychiatry, Vol. 1* (8th edn, pp. 1053–1054). Philadelphia: Lippincott Williams & Wilkins.

Geerlings, M., den Heijer, T., Koudstaal, P., Hofman, A. & Breteler, M. (2008). History of depression, depressive symptoms, and medial temporal lobe atrophy and the risk of Alzheimer disease. *Neurology, 70*, 1258–1264.

Goldsmith, M. (1996). Hearing the voice of people with dementia. London: Jessica Kingsley Publications.

Grossman, H. (2005). Amnestic disorders. In B. J. Sadock & V. A. Sadock (Eds.), *Comprehensive textbook of psychiatry, Vol. 1* (8th edn, pp. 1093–1106). Philadelphia: Lippincott Williams & Wilkins.

Hendry, K. C. & Douglas, D. H. (2003). Promoting quality of life for people diagnosed with dementia. *Journal of the American Psychiatric Nurses Association, 9*(3), 96–102.

Herrmann, W. (2006). Significance of hyperhomocysteinemia. *Clinical Laboratory, 52*(7–8), 367–374.

Kitwood, T. (1997). Dementia rediscovered. Buckingham: Open University Press.

Kitwood, T. and Bredin, K. (1992). Towards a theory of dementia care: personhood and well-being. *Ageing and Society, 12*, 269–287.

Mittelman, M. S., Roth, D. L., Coon, D. W., *et al.* (2004). Sustained benefit of supportive intervention for depressive symptoms in caregivers of patients with Alzheimer's disease. *American Journal of Psychiatry, 161*(5), 850–856.

Neugroschl, J. A., Kolevzon, A., Samuels, S. C., *et al.* (2005). Dementia. In B. J. Sadock & V. A. Sadock (Eds.), *Comprehensive textbook of psychiatry, Vol. 1* (8th edn, pp. 1068–1093). Philadelphia: Lippincott Williams & Wilkins.

Rovio, S., Kareholt, I., Helkala, E. L., *et al.* (2005). Leisure-time physical activity at midlife and the risk of dementia and Alzheimer's disease. *Lancet Neurology, 4*(11), 705–711.

Samuels, S. C. & Neugroschl, J. A. (2005). Delirium. In B. J. Sadock & V. A. Sadock (Eds.), *Comprehensive textbook of psychiatry, Vol.1* (8th edn, pp. 1054–1068). Philadelphia: Lippincott Williams & Wilkins.

Woods, B., Spector, A., Jones, C., *et al.* (2005). Reminiscence therapy for dementia. *Cochrane database of systematic reviews (online), 2* (CD001120).

Yuhas, N., McGowan, B., Fintaine, T., *et al.* (2006). Psychosocial interventions for disruptive symptoms of dementia. *Journal of Psychosocial Nursing, 44*(11), 34–42.

ADDITIONAL READING

Brooker, D. & Woolley, R. (2006). *Enriching opportunities; unlocking potential, searching for keys: Summary of development and evaluation*. University of Bradford. Available: www.brad.ac.uk/acad/health/dementia.

Brooker, D. J. & Woolley, R. J. (2007). Enriching opportunities for people living with dementia: The development of a blueprint for a sustainable activity-based model. *Aging & Mental Health, 11*(4), 371–383.

Brooker, D. & Woolley, R. (2008). Development and evaluation of a multi-level activity-based model of care. *Journal of Quality Research in Dementia, 5*, May 2008.

Chen, P., Ganguli, M., Mulsant, B., & DeKosky, S. (1999). The temporal relationship between depressive symptoms and dementia: a community-based prospective study. *Archives of General Psychiatry, 56*, 261–266.

CSIP. (2008). *Everybody's business (2005)*. Available: http://www.olderpeoplesmentalhealth.csip.org.uk/everybodys-business.html

Lipinska, D. (2009). Person-centred counselling for people with dementia: making sense of self. London: Jessica Kingsley Publications.

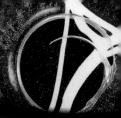

Chapter Study Guide

MULTIPLE-CHOICE QUESTIONS

Select the best answer for each of the following questions.

1. The nurse is talking with a woman who is worried that her mother has Alzheimer's disease. The nurse knows that the first sign of dementia is usually:
   a. Disorientation to person, place or time
   b. Memory loss that is more than ordinary forgetfulness
   c. Inability to perform self-care tasks without assistance
   d. Variable with different people

2. The nurse has been teaching a carer about Aricept. The nurse knows that teaching has been effective by which of the following statements?
   a. 'Let's hope this medication will stop the Alzheimer's disease from progressing any further.'
   b. 'It is important to take this medication on an empty stomach.'
   c. 'I'll be eager to see if this medication makes any improvement in concentration.'
   d. 'This medication will slow the progress of Alzheimer's disease temporarily.'

3. Which of the following statements by the carer of a client newly diagnosed with dementia might require further intervention – and possible challenge – by the nurse?
   a. 'I will remind Mother of things she has forgotten.'
   b. 'I will keep Mother busy with favourite activities as long as she can participate.'
   c. 'I will try to find new and different things to do every day.'
   d. 'I will encourage Mother to talk about her friends and family.'

4. A client with delirium is attempting to remove the intra-venous tubing from his arm, saying to the nurse, 'Get off me! Go away!' The client may be experiencing which of the following?
   a. Delusions
   b. Hallucinations
   c. Illusions
   d. Disorientation

5. Which of the following statements indicates the carer's accurate knowledge about the needs of a parent at the onset of the moderate stage of dementia?
   a. 'I need to give my parent a bath at the same time every day.'
   b. 'I need to postpone any holidays for 5 years.'
   c. 'I need to spend time with my parent doing things we both enjoy.'
   d. 'I need to stay with my parent 24 hours a day for supervision.'

6. Which of the following interventions is most appropriate in helping a client with early-stage dementia complete activities of daily living (ADLs)?
   a. Allow enough time for the client to complete ADLs as independently as possible.
   b. Provide the client with a written list of all the steps needed to complete ADLs.
   c. Plan to provide step-by-step prompting to complete the ADLs.
   d. Tell the client to finish ADLs before breakfast or the nursing assistant will do them.

7. A client with late moderate stage dementia has been admitted to a long-term care facility. Which of the following nursing interventions might help the client to maintain optimal cognitive function?
   a. Discuss pictures of children and grandchildren with the client.
   b. Do word games or crossword puzzles with the client.
   c. Provide the client with a written list of daily activities.
   d. Watch and discuss the evening news with the client.

FILL-IN-THE-BLANK QUESTIONS

Identify each of the following behaviours as occurring primarily in delirium or dementia.

_____ Change in level of consciousness

_____ Sudden acute confusion

_____ Loss of long-term memory

_____ Tactile hallucinations

_____ Slurred speech

_____ Loss of language abilities

_____ Change in personality traits

_____ Chronic confusion

GROUP DISCUSSION TOPICS

1. How important is memory to someone's sense of self-esteem?

2. How might depression and Alzheimer's be related?

CLINICAL EXAMPLE

Martha Smith, a 79-year-old widow with Alzheimer's disease, was admitted to a nursing home. The disease has progressed during the past 4 years to the point that she can no longer live alone in her own house. Martha has poor judgement and no short-term memory. She had stopped paying bills, preparing meals and cleaning her home. She had become increasingly suspicious of her health visitor and home help, finally refusing to allow them in the house.

   After her arrival at the home, Martha has been sleeping poorly and frequently wanders from her room in the middle of the night. She seems agitated and afraid in the dining room at meal-times, is eating very little and has lost weight. If left alone, Martha would wear the same clothing day and night and would not attend to her personal hygiene.

1. What additional assessments would the nurse want to make to plan care for this client?

2. What nursing formulation would the nurse identify for this client?

3. Write an expected outcome and at least two interventions for each nursing formulation.

Answers to
Chapter Study Guides

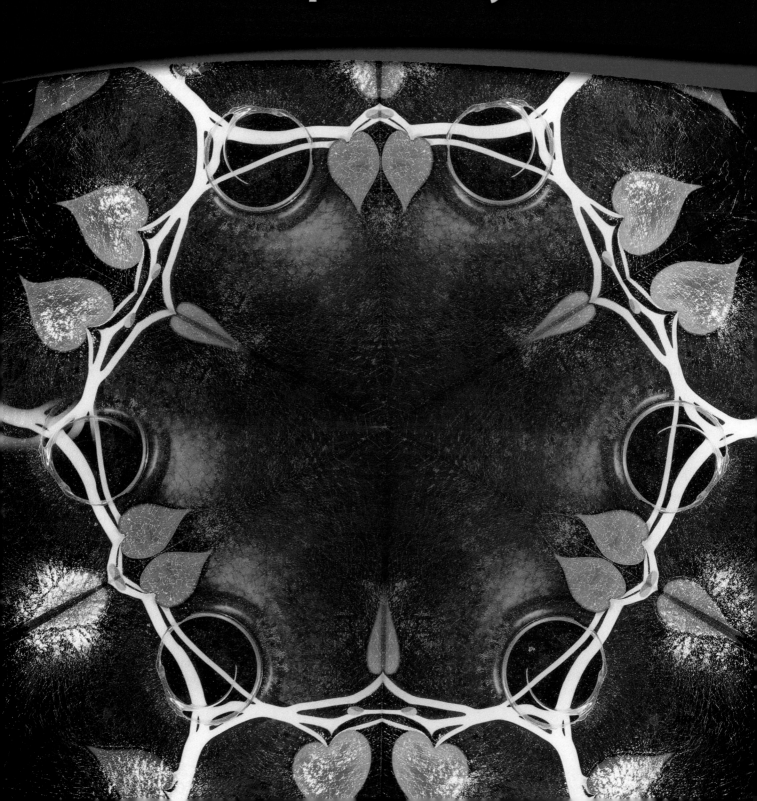

ANSWER KEY

CHAPTER 1

Multiple-Choice Questions

1. c
2. a
3. d
4. b

Fill-in-the-Blank Questions

Axis I: All major psychiatric disorders except 'mental retardation' (learning disabilities) and personality disorders

Axis II: 'Mental retardation' (learning disabilities), personality disorders, prominent maladaptive personality features, defence mechanisms

Axis III: Current medical conditions, contributing medical conditions

Axis IV: Psychosocial and environmental problems

Axis V: Global Assessment of Functioning (GAF) score

CHAPTER 2

Multiple-Choice Questions

1. c
2. d
3. c
4. b
5. a
6. a
7. a
8. a

Fill-in-the-Blank Questions

1. Carl Rogers
2. Erik Erikson
3. Ivan Pavlov
4. Albert Ellis
5. B. F. Skinner
6. Carl Rogers
7. Frederick Perls
8. Abraham Maslow
9. Viktor Frankl
10. Albert Ellis

CHAPTER 3

Multiple-Choice Questions

1. d
2. a
3. b
4. c
5. b

Fill-in-the-Blank Questions

1. Atypical antipsychotic
2. SSRI antidepressant
3. Tricyclic antidepressant
4. Anticholinergic
5. Stimulant
6. Anticonvulsant used as mood stabilizer
7. Benzodiazepine
8. Atypical antipsychotic

CHAPTER 4

Multiple-Choice Questions

1. d
2. d
3. c
4. d

Fill-in-the-Blank Questions

Psychiatrist
Occupational therapist
Community Mental Health Nurse
Clinical Psychologist

CHAPTER 5

Multiple-Choice Questions

1. a
2. a
3. c
4. b

Fill-in-the-Blank Questions

Empirical
Aesthetic
Personal
Ethical

Clinical Example

Mr V: 'I like to choose my student nurses; otherwise, I don't get chosen.'

Nurse: 'I'm honoured you chose me, Mr V. My name's Jodie Moore, and I'll be a student nurse here for the next 6 weeks. You seem to have had some experience with other students so I guess you know their role?' (Nurse clearly states information about herself and her role and acknowledges client's previous experience.)

Mr V: 'Oh, yeah, I've seen 'em come and go, but I never get picked to be their patient. I guess I'm too mad for them!' (laughs nervously)

Nurse: 'Well, I'm delighted you chose me. It makes me feel honoured.' (Nurse makes it clear she is glad to be with client.)

Mr V: 'Are you sure?'

Nurse: 'Yes. I'll be here on Tuesdays from 10 AM to 3 PM for the next 6 weeks. I hope we can have some helpful conversations about things that are important to you and I can work with you and other members of the team to make your stay here better.' (provides clear parameters for the relationship)

CHAPTER 6

Multiple-Choice Questions

1. c
2. a
3. b
4. b
5. b
6. c
7. a

Cues and Responses

1. Cue: I feel good.
   'Tell me one way you feel good?'
   'When did you start feeling good?'
   'What was going on around you just before you realized you felt good?'
2. Cue: I can't take it anymore.
   'What is it you can't take?'
   'How long have you had to take it?'
   ' What's going on that you feel you have to take?'
3. Cues: two children, my wife, my girlfriend
   Nurse: 'What are your children's names and ages?'
   Client: 'Taylor is 4, and Anita is 1.'
   Nurse: 'Tell me about the relationship between you and Taylor.' After discussion concludes, try, 'Tell me about your relationship with Anita.'
4. Cues: we, standing, corner
   'Who do you mean by 'we'?'
   'On what corner were you standing?'
   'What were you doing at the corner?'
5. Cues: my son, never going to understand, way his wife is ruining them
   Nurse: 'What's your son's name?'
   Client: 'Paul.'
   Nurse: 'What's his wife's name?'
   Client: 'Susan.'
   Nurse: 'How do you think Susan is ruining herself and Paul?'
   'How did you arrive at the conclusion that Paul will never understand something Susan is doing?'

CHAPTER 7

Multiple-Choice Questions

1. a
2. b
3. a
4. b
5. c
6. b

Fill-in-the-Blank Questions

Trust vs. Mistrust
Industry vs. Inferiority
Identity vs. Role diffusion
Intimacy vs. Isolation
Ego integrity vs. Despair

CHAPTER 8

Multiple-Choice Questions

1. b
2. d
3. c
4. b
5. b
6. c
7. a
8. c

Fill-in-the-Blank Questions

1. Automatism
2. Thought broadcasting
3. Psychomotor retardation
4. Word salad

Clinical Example

1. Give positive feedback for coming to the CMHT to get help.
   Tell her it is all right to cry.
   Tell the client that the nurse will sit with her until she's ready to talk.
   Validate the client's feelings (i.e. 'I can see you're very upset').
2. What's the problem as you see it? (to gain the client's perception of the situation)
   Have you ever felt this way before? (to determine if this is a new occurrence, or recurrent)
   Do you have thoughts of harming yourself or anyone else? (to determine safety)
   Have you been drinking alcohol, using drugs, or taking medication? (to assess client's ability to think clearly or if there is impairment)

What kind of help do you feel you need? (to see what kind of help the client wants, e.g. someone to listen, help to solve a specific problem, a referral)
3. The client may be in crisis.
   The client is seeking help/treatment.
   The client is feeling distressed
4. Tell the client that the nurse needs to know if the client is safe (from suicidal ideas or self-harm urges). If the client feels – or appears – unsafe but insists on leaving, the nurse should tell her she will contact her GP (or other involved professional) or – if really concerned – the police.

CHAPTER 9

Multiple-Choice Questions

1. a
2. b
3. d

Fill-in-the-Blank Questions

Veracity
Non-maleficence
Fidelity
Beneficence
Justice
Autonomy

CHAPTER 10

Multiple-Choice Questions

1. b
2. b
3. b
4. c
5. b

CHAPTER 11

Multiple-Choice Questions

1. b
2. c
3. c
4. c
5. d
6. b
7. a

Fill-in-the-Blank Questions

Child neglect
Self-neglect
Financial abuse
Psychological or emotional abuse

CHAPTER 12

Multiple-Choice Questions

1. c
2. b
3. c
4. d
5. a

Fill-in-the-Blank Questions

Emotional dimension
Behavioural dimension
Cognitive dimension
Spiritual dimension
Physiological dimension

Short Answer Questions

'This is unbearable. I can't believe she's gone.'
Nurse: 'This is a real shock for you. Sounds like it's incredibly difficult to believe it's happened?' (validates, reflects, encourages further verbalization)
'No one will want to hire me at this age.'
Nurse: 'Tell me more about that' (encourages exploration, helps understanding, hopefully moves conversation towards client's solutions)
'There's nowhere for me to turn.'
Nurse: 'Sounds like you're feeling alone in this?' (reflects, validates, encourages further exploration)
'Get out of here! Leave me alone! I don't need your help.'
Nurse: 'Could we get someone to be with you who might be helpful?' (Acknowledges anger without taking it personally; encourages collaboration and, if wanted by the client, more discussion of feelings)

CHAPTER 13

Multiple-Choice Questions

1. c
2. d
3. d
4. b
5. d
6. c
7. c
8. d

Fill-in-the-Blank

1. Severe
2. Mild
3. Panic
4. Moderate

Clinical Example

1. The nurse should validate Mrs Noe's feelings and thoughts and find ways to encourage her to come up with suggestions. She is more likely to take responsibility for, and act on, her own solutions to problems than on the suggestions of others.
2. Mrs Noe may be gaining in the short term from the attention and focus Mr Noe gives her and it may be reinforcing the problem. The nurse could recommend that both Mr and Mrs Noe attend an agoraphobic self-help group or other support group for clients and carers. Mr Noe might benefit from being given direct information about the cause and distress resulting from phobias, by having his experiences sincerely validated and by being gently and respectfully challenged about what the nurse's belief is about the influence of his behaviour on his wife.
3. CBT or other pyschotherapeutic approaches, individual or group relaxation training, mindfulness, yoga or meditation, or other measures designed to help her manage the anxiety response are available. Additionally, medication can sometimes reduce agoraphobic behaviours or the distress resulting from them, so referral to a psychiatrist or discussion with the GP may be appropriate.

CHAPTER 14

Multiple-Choice Questions

1. c
2. d
3. b
4. c
5. a
6. b
7. c

Fill-in-the-Blank Questions

1. Neologism
2. Verbigeration
3. Word salad
4. Clang association

Clinical Example

1. Additional assessment data (examples): discover content of any command hallucinations; ask about preferences for hygiene (for example, shower or bath); determine whether there is a thing or place that makes him feel safe and secure.
2. Disturbed thought processes: John will have 5-minute interactions that are reality-based; he will be gently encouraged to express feelings and emotions.
   Ineffective medication management (refusal): John will take medication as prescribed; he will verbalize difficulties in following medication regime.

Self-care deficit: John will shower or bathe, wash his hair, and clean his clothes every other day; he will wear appropriate clothing for the weather or activity.
3. Disturbed thought processes: engage John in present, here-and-now topics not related to delusional ideas; focus on his emotions and feelings.
   Ineffective medication management: offer scheduled medications in matter-of-fact manner; assess for side-effects and give medications or provide nursing interventions to relieve side-effects; provide factual information to John: 'This medication should help to decrease the voices you're hearing.'
   Self-care deficit: provide supplies and privacy for hygiene activities; give respectful feedback about body odour, dirty clothes and so forth; help John store extra clothing where he has access to it and believes it is safe.
4. John might benefit from referral to AOT or to the Crisis Team followed by CMHT support. CBT may be helpful. A care co-ordinator must be involved. Other social supports may be helpful, such as a day hospital or a voluntary day centre run by MIND or another local organization.

CHAPTER 15

Multiple-Choice Questions

1. d
2. a
3. a
4. c
5. a
6. d
7. b
8. d
9. a

Clinical Example

(*These are examples of correct answers; others are possible.*)

1. It is essential that the nurse directly ask if June is having suicidal thoughts. If so, the nurse would assess June's risk by finding out if she has a plan, if she has access to the means to carry out the plan, and details of her plan.
2. Ineffective coping; Ineffective Role Performance; and Impaired Social Interaction.
   Note: Risk of suicide would be a priority if the nurse determined June was having suicidal thoughts.
3. June will identify past successful coping strategies; she will carry out activities of daily living; she will verbalize her thoughts and feelings.
4. Spending 1:1 interaction time with June to discuss thoughts, feelings, past coping strategies and possible solutions; providing encouragement and support to get up, shower, get dressed, eat and so forth; educating June about depression and its treatment; assisting June to identify life stressors and possible sources of support.

CHAPTER 16

Multiple-Choice Questions

1. a
2. a
3. d
4. b
5. d
6. c
7. a
8. a

Fill-in-the-Blank Questions

Borderline personality disorder
Antisocial personality disorder
Schizoid personality disorder
Avoidant personality disorder

Clinical Example

(*These are examples of correct answers; others are possible.*)

1. Risk of Self-Mutilation, Ineffective Coping
2. Risk of Self-Mutilation: Susan will be safe and free from significant injury.
   Ineffective Coping: She will demonstrate increased control of impulsive behaviour.
3. Risk of Self-Mutilation: Discuss presence and intensity of self-harm urges with Susan; negotiate a no self-harm contract with her; help her to identify triggers for self-harm behaviour.
   Ineffective Coping: Help her to identify feelings by keeping a journal; discuss ways she can use distraction when gratification must be delayed; discuss alternative ways she can express feelings without an exaggerated response.
4. Psychotherapy: individual or group DBT; community support services – care co-ordinator/CMHT, vocational/career counselling, self-help group.

CHAPTER 17

Multiple-Choice Questions

1. b
2. b
3. b
4. a
5. c
6. a
7. c

Fill-in-the-Blank Questions

(*These are examples of correct answers; others are possible.*)

Stimulants: cocaine, amphetamines
Opioids: morphine, heroin

Hallucinogens: peyote, LSD
Inhalants: paint thinner, glue, petrol fumes

Clinical Example

1. Ineffective Denial: Ineffective Coping
2. Ineffective Denial: Sharon will abstain from alcohol or drug use.
   Ineffective Coping: Sharon will identify two non-chemical ways of coping with life stressors.
3. Ineffective Denial: Teach Sharon about alcoholism; work to dispel myths about alcoholism; ask her about recent life events (break-up, arrest) and the role of her drinking in those events.
   Ineffective Coping: Encourage Sharon to express feelings directly and openly; teach her relaxation techniques; role-play a situation (of her choice) that has been difficult for her to handle.

CHAPTER 18

Multiple-Choice Questions

1. b
2. c
3. a
4. b
5. a
6. b
7. d
8. a

Fill-in-the-Blank Questions

Bulimia
Both
Both
Anorexia
Bulimia

Clinical Example

(*These are examples of correct answers; others are possible.*)

1. Imbalanced Nutrition: Less Than Body Requirements and Ineffective Coping
2. (Nutrition) Judy will eat all of her meals and snacks with no purging. (Coping) She will identify two non–food-related mechanisms.
3. (Nutrition) Sit with Judy while eating; monitor her 1 to 2 hours after meals and snacks; supervise her use of the bathroom and toilet. (Coping) Ask her how she is feeling, and continue to focus on feelings (and thoughts) if she gives a somatic response; have Judy keep a journal including thoughts, feelings and food eaten; teach her the use of relaxation, mindfulness and distractions such as music and other activities.

CHAPTER 19

Multiple-Choice Questions

1. b
2. c
3. d
4. b
5. a
6. a
7. a
8. c

Fill-in-the-Blank Questions

Body dysmorphic disorder
Somatization disorder
Conversion disorder
Pain disorder
Hypochondriasis

Clinical Example

(*These are examples of correct answers; others are possible.*)

1. Ineffective Coping, Pain, Anxiety
2. Mary will identify the relationship between stress and increased pain; she will be able to perform activities of daily living satisfactorily.
3. Encourage Mary to keep a journal about her feelings and the quality or intensity of pain; teach her relaxation exercises; help her make a daily schedule of activities, beginning with simple tasks; encourage her to listen to music or engage in other distracting activities she may enjoy; talk with her about her feelings of frustration and anxiety in a sensitive and supportive manner.
4. Occupational therapists, pain management specialists, psychologists, practice nurses.
5. Support group for persons with chronic pain/pain disorder, exercise group, social or volunteer opportunities.

CHAPTER 20

Multiple-Choice Questions

1. a
2. c
3. a
4. a
5. b
6. d

Fill-in-the-Blank Questions

Pica
Rumination disorder
Reactive attachment disorder
Selective mutism

Clinical Example

(*These are examples of correct answers; others are possible.*)

1. Ritalin is a stimulant medication that may be at least partially effective for up to 70% to 80% of children with ADHD by decreasing hyperactivity and impulsivity and improving the child's attention. Ritalin can cause appetite suppression and should be given after meals to encourage proper nutrition. Substantial, nutritious snacks between meals are helpful. Giving the medication in the daytime helps avoid the side-effect of insomnia. Parents should notice improvements in a day or two. Notify clinicians at follow-up if no improvements in behaviour are noted.
2. The exact cause of ADHD is not known, but it is not due to faulty parenting or anything the parents have done. Taking medications may be helpful with behavioural symptoms, but other strategies are needed as well. The medication will help control symptoms so Lucy can participate in school, make friends and so forth.
3. Provide supervision when Lucy is with her brother, and help her learn to play gently with him. Do not forbid her to touch him, but teach her the proper ways to do so. Give Lucy directions in a clear, step-by-step manner, and assist her to follow through and complete tasks. Provide a quiet place with minimal distraction for activities that require concentration, such as homework. Try to establish a routine for getting up and dressing, eating meals, going to school, doing homework and playing; don't change the routine unnecessarily. Structured expectations will be easier for Lucy to follow. Remember to recognize Lucy's strengths and provide positive feedback frequently to boost her self-esteem and foster continued progress.
4. Family interventions and cognitive-behavioural input may be helpful. Clinicians and the parents should contact her GP, Lucy's teacher, headmaster/headmistress and school nurse to inform them of this diagnosis so that special education classes or tutoring can be made available. It would also be helpful to meet with the school nurse who may be giving Lucy her medication at noon on school days. The nurse can refer the parents to a local support group for parents of children with ADHD and provide pamphlets, books or other written materials, as well as Internet addresses.

CHAPTER 21

Multiple-Choice Questions

1. b
2. d
3. c
4. b
5. c
6. a
7. a

Fill-in-the-Blank Questions

Delirium
Delirium
Dementia
Delirium
Delirium
Dementia
Dementia
Dementia

Clinical Example

(*These are examples of correct answers; others are possible.*)

1. What does she like to eat? What were her usual personal hygiene practices? What are her favourite activities? What personal items does she value?
2. Chronic Confusion, Impaired Socialization, Disturbed Sleep Pattern, Self-Care Deficits, and Risk of Imbalanced Nutrition: Less Than Body Requirements
3. Martha will experience as little frustration as possible. *Interventions:* Gently and respectfully point out objects, people and the time of day to prompt her and decrease confusion. Do not ask her to make decisions when she is unable to; offer choices only when she can make them. Martha will interact with the nurse. She will participate in going for a walk with the group. *Interventions:* Involve the client in solitary activities with the nurse initially. Structure group activities that focus on intact physical abilities rather than those requiring cognition.
Martha will eat 50% of meals and snacks. *Interventions:* Provide foods Martha likes, and provide those foods in an environment where she will be likely to eat, such as her room or a table alone.
Martha will sleep 6 hours per night. *Interventions:* Provide a soothing night-time routine every night (for example, offering a drink, reading aloud, dimming lights). Decrease stimulation after dinner, and discourage daytime naps.
Martha will participate in hygiene routines with assistance. *Interventions:* Try to imitate her home hygiene routine (bath or shower, morning or evening), and develop a structured routine for hygiene.

Appendix

A

People With Learning Disabilities

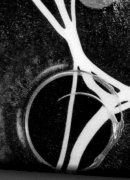

According to MENCAP (2008):

- 1.5 million people in the UK have a learning disability.
- 8 out of 10 people with a learning disability get bullied.
- Half of all families with children with a learning disability live in poverty.
- People with a learning disability are 58 times more likely to die aged under 50 than other people.
- 8 out of 10 families caring for children and adults with profound and multiple learning disabilities have reached 'breaking point' because of the lack of support they get in their caring roles.
- There are more than 29,000 people with a severe or profound learning disability who live at home with carers aged over 70.

The essential *diagnostic* feature (though not the essential *life* feature) of people with learning disabilities is below-average intellectual functioning (an intelligence quotient (IQ) less than 70) accompanied by significant limitations in areas of adaptive functioning such as communication skills, self-care, home living, social or interpersonal skills, use of community resources, self-direction, academic skills, work, leisure and health and safety (King *et al.*, 2005).

Causes of learning disability include hereditary conditions such as Tay–Sachs disease or fragile X chromosome syndrome; early alterations in embryonic development such as trisomy 21 or maternal alcohol intake, which causes fetal alcohol syndrome; pregnancy or perinatal problems such as foetal malnutrition, hypoxia, infections and trauma; medical conditions in infancy such as infection or lead poisoning; and environmental influences such as deprivation of nurturing or stimulation.

In the UK, people use a variety of terms including 'people with special needs' and 'people with learning needs' but the most widely accepted phrase currently is to talk about 'people with learning disabilities'. Fundamentally, as nurses we need to think in terms of individuals with strengths, qualities and 'different abilities' rather than

merely as patients or clients with deficits or disabilities. There has been a fundamental shift away from thinking in psychiatric or psychological terms about categorizing in the field of 'learning disabilities' (Department of Health, 2001), though many professionals (and some carers) still use this way of thinking about disabilities.

Children with 'mild-to-moderate' mental learning disabilities usually receive treatment in their homes and communities, and have periodic contact with primary care teams and learning disability teams. Those with a 'moderate' or 'severe' learning disability may require more intensive input from learning disability teams and, perhaps, residential placement or day-care services.

LEARNING DISABILITIES AND MENTAL HEALTH

Many people – children and adults – with learning disabilities also have mental health problems. According to the Royal College of Nursing (RCN) (2007), around a quarter of adults with learning disabilities have mental health problems, compared with 16% in the general population. Deb *et al.* (2001), cited by the RCN, suggest that 'the prevalence of schizophrenia in people with learning disabilities is three times that of the wider population' (p. 25) and prevalence rates for a whole range of child and adult mental disorders (from ADHD to depression, anxiety or bipolar disorder) is higher in those with a learning disability. This appears to be the case for a number of reasons – biological, psychological and social.

Traditionally, primary care services and child *and* adult mental health services and learning disability services (including nurses) have been poor at recognizing and helping those with the dual diagnoses of learning disability and mental disorder, and poor at working collaboratively (in a similar way to the difficulties between substance misuse and general mental health services). Frequently, those

INTERNET RESOURCES

RESOURCES	INTERNET ADDRESS
• British Institute of Learning Disabilities	http://www.bild.org.uk/
• Foundation for people with Learning Disabilities	http://www.learningdisabilities.org.uk
• Learning Disability Coalition	http://www.learningdisabilitycoalition.org.uk/
• MENCAP	http://www.mencap.org.uk/
• Valuing People	http://valuingpeople.gov.uk/index.jsp

with a mild learning disorder have found that this hasn't been recognized by the mental health services; those with a moderate or severe learning disability have often found their bipolar affective disorder, OCD, depression, PTSD, anxiety or psychosis haven't been recognized by learning disability services,

In terms of assessment, planning, implementation and evaluation of care, MHNs need to be aware of the impact a learning disability may have on someone's appearance, behaviour, speech, thought content, perception, mood, cognition and insight, and on the person's ability to communicate these, and to tailor their engagement appropriately (RCN, 2007). *Principles* of care and the essential skills of assessment, planning, intervention and evaluation nevertheless remain the same: there is a need for full client collaboration, the validation and acknowledgement of distress and suffering, respect, curiosity and an assumption of strength and resource.

The RCN guidance (2007) provides an excellent starting point for all MHNs working with people who may have a learning disability. Websites listed in the Internet resources offer insightful perspectives from the person's own point of view and from that of carers. The excellent books by Goward *et al.* (2005) and Cambridge and Carnaby

(2005) offer a good foundation for mental health students and nurses to start developing their empathy, skills and understanding.

REFERENCES

Cambridge, P. & Carnaby, S. (Eds.) (2005). *Person centered planning and care management with people with learning disabilities*. London: Jessica Kingsley.

Deb, S., Matthews, T., Holtn G., & Bouras, N. (2001). *Practice guidelines for the assessment and diagnosis of mental health problems in adults with intellectual disability*. Brighton: Pavilion Publishing.

Department of Health. (2001). *Valuing people: a new strategy for learning disability for the 21st century*. London: the Stationery Office.

Goward, P., Grant, G., Ramcharan, P., & Richardson, M. (2005). *Learning disability: a life cycle approach to valuing people*. Oxford: Oxford University Press.

King, B. H., Hodapp, R. M., & Dykens, E. M. (2005). Mental retardation. In B. J. Sadock & V. A. Sadock (Eds.), *Comprehensive textbook of psychiatry* (8th edn, pp. 3227–3236). Philadelphia: Lippincott, Williams and Wilkins.

MENCAP. (2008). *Facts about learning disability*. Available: http://www.mencap.org.uk/page.asp?id=1703)

Royal College of Nursing. (2007). *Mental health nursing of adults with learning disabilities*. Available: http://www.rcn.org.uk/__data/assets/pdf_file/0006/78765/003184.pdf

Mental Health (Care and Treatment) (Scotland) Act 2003

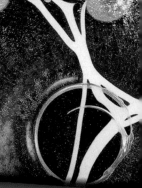

- **Compulsory detention**: In Scotland (as in England and Wales), you may hear the terms 'informal' when the client is admitted voluntarily, and 'formal' when the client is detained under the Mental Health (Care and Treatment) (Scotland) Act (2003).
- **'Nurse's holding power'**: Similar to Section 5:4 in England and Wales, this can be exercised by nurses 'of a prescribed class' (first-level registered nurses qualified in the fields of mental health or learning disability) by way of section 299 of the Act. If there is cause for concern, the nurse can use this holding power to detain a patient for up to 2 hours while awaiting a medical examination. If necessary, the detention may be extended by 1 hour while the medical examination is carried out.
- **Emergency detention** in Scotland is dealt with by way of a 72-hour provision under Section 36 of the Act (similar to Section 4 in England and Wales). Detention runs from the time of admission or granting of a certificate (if already an inpatient). No right of appeal is included but can be cancelled by a registered medical officer.
- **Short-term detention** is a 28-day provision under Section 44 of the Act (similar to Section 2 in England and Wales). A 72-hour window is included for removal to hospital and detention time is effective from admission. Appeal from the patient or their named person to the Mental Health Tribunal is allowed.

- **The Mental Welfare Commission** for Scotland (a body with similarities to the Mental Health Act Commission in England and Wales (which will become the Care Quality Commission in 2009)) is an independent organization that works to safeguard the rights and welfare of any person with a mental illness, learning disability or other mental disorder. The main purpose of the Mental Welfare Commission is to check that individual care and treatment is in line with the law and to monitor the use of mental health and incapacity law in Scotland.
- **Mental Health Tribunals**, broadly similar in function and range to those in England and Wales, were established under the 2003 Act and hear review, appeal and extension requests. Tribunals consist of three members – one each from medical, legal and lay panellists – and are held as close to the patient's location as possible (often hospital boardrooms or health centre facilities). They remove the burden and stress of Sheriff Court appearances for both service staff and patients from the previous statute.
- **Community Treatment Orders:** Section 64 Mental Health (Care and Treatment) (Scotland) Act 2003 (which have parallels with CTOs in England and Wales) offer the opportunity for inpatient or community treatment and care. Appeal from the patient or their named person to the Mental Health Tribunal is allowed.

Glossary of Psychiatric, Psychological and Nursing Terms

abstract thinking: ability to make associations or interpretations about a situation or comment

abuse: the harmful use and mistreatment of another person, animal or substance

acceptance: positive embracing of – and the avoidance of judgements of – oneself or another person, regardless of behaviour

acculturation: altering cultural values or behaviours as a way to adapt to another culture

acting out: in psychodynamic thought, an immature defence mechanism by which the person deals with emotional conflicts or stressors through actions rather than through reflection or feelings

active listening: concentrating exclusively on what the client says, whilst attempting to refrain from (or to notice and re-focus back from) other internal mental activities

active observation: watching the speaker's non-verbal actions as he or she communicates

acute inpatient units: specialist units committed to caring for the most acute clients, i.e. those most at risk to themselves and others. Alongside crisis teams, form part of acute care services

acute stress disorder: post-trauma response characterized by symptoms appearing within the first month after the trauma and persisting no longer than 4 weeks

adrenaline: derivative of noradrenaline, the most prevalent neurotransmitter in the nervous system, located primarily in the brain stem, and which plays a role in changes in attention, learning and memory, sleep and wakefulness and mood regulation

advocacy: the process of acting on the client's behalf when he or she cannot do so

affect: the outward expression of the client's emotional state or mood

agnosia: inability to recognize or name objects despite intact sensory abilities

akathisia: intense need to move about; characterized by restless movement, pacing, inability to remain still and the client's report of inner restlessness; a side-effect of some neuroleptic medications

alexithymia: difficulty identifying and expressing feelings

alogia: an apparent lack of any real meaning or substance in what the client says

alternative therapies: used *instead of* conventional practice

Alzheimer's disease: a progressive brain disorder that has a gradual onset but causes an increasing decline in functioning, including loss of speech, loss of motor function, and profound personality and behavioural changes such as those involving paranoia, delusions, hallucinations, inattention to hygiene and belligerence

amnestic disorder: characterized by a disturbance in memory that results directly from the physiological effects of a general medical condition or from the persisting effects of a substance such as alcohol or other drugs

anergia: lack of energy

anger: a normal human emotion involving a strong, uncomfortable, emotional response to a real or perceived provocation

anhedonia: having no pleasure or joy in life; losing any sense of pleasure from activities previously enjoyed

anorexia nervosa: an eating disorder characterized by the client's refusal or inability to maintain a minimally normal body weight, intense fear of gaining weight or becoming fat, significantly disturbed perception of the shape or size of the body and steadfast inability or refusal to acknowledge the existence or seriousness of a problem

anticholinergic effects: dry mouth, constipation, urinary hesitancy or retention, dry nasal passages and blurred near vision; commonly seen as side-effects of medication

anticipatory grieving: when people facing an imminent loss begin to grapple with the very real possibility of the loss or death in the near future

antidepressant drugs: primarily used in the treatment of major depressive disorders anxiety disorders, the depressed phase of bipolar disorder and psychotic depression

antipsychotic drugs: also known as *neuroleptics;* used to treat the symptoms of psychosis such as the delusions and hallucinations seen in schizophrenia, schizoaffective disorder and the manic phase of bipolar disorder

antisocial personality disorder: characterized by a pervasive pattern of disregard for, and violation of, the rights of others and with the central characteristics of deceit and manipulation

anxiety: a feeling of dread or apprehension; it is a response to external or internal stimuli that can have behavioural, emotional, cognitive and physical symptoms

anxiety disorders: a group of conditions that share a key feature of excessive anxiety, with ensuing behavioural, emotional, cognitive and physiological responses

anxiolytic drugs: used to treat anxiety and anxiety disorders, insomnia, OCD, depression, posttraumatic stress disorder and alcohol withdrawal

aphasia: deterioration of language function – in either understanding or communicating

apraxia: impaired ability to execute motor functions despite intact motor abilities

assault: involves any action that causes a person to fear being touched, without consent or authority, in a way that is offensive, insulting or physically injurious

assertive outreach: an approach to 'hard-to-engage' people which involves intensive, focused therapeutic work in the community

assertiveness training: a structured programme of cognitive-behavioural techniques using statements to identify feelings and communicate needs and concerns to others; helps the person negotiate interpersonal situations, fosters self-assurance and ultimately assists the person to take more control over life situations

asylum: a safe refuge or haven offering protection; became a term used to describe institutions for the 'mad' or 'mentally ill'

attachment behaviours: the expression of emotional bonds with significant people in one's life

attention deficit hyperactivity disorder (ADHD): characterized by inattentiveness, overactivity and impulsiveness. Also known as Attention Deficit Disorder (ADD) and hyperkinetic disorder

attention-seeking: a widely used but often destructive term frequently used to dismiss the inner experience of 'difficult' clients

attentive presence: being with the client and focusing intently on communicating with and understanding him or her

attitudes: general feelings or a frame of reference around which a person organizes knowledge about the world

autistic disorder: a pervasive developmental disorder characterized by impairment of growth and development milestones, such as impaired communication with others, lack of social relationships even with parents, and stereotyped motor behaviours

automatism: repeated, seemingly purposeless behaviours often indicative of anxiety, such as drumming fingers, twisting locks of hair or tapping the foot; unconscious mannerism

autonomy: the person's right to self-determination and independence

avoidance behaviour: behaviour designed to avoid unpleasant emotional or practical consequences or potentially threatening situations

avoidant personality disorder: characterized by a pervasive pattern of social discomfort and reticence, low self-esteem, and hypersensitivity to negative evaluation

behaviour modification: a method of attempting to strengthen a desired behaviour or response by reinforcement, either positive or negative

behaviourism: a school of psychology that focuses on observable behaviours and what one can do externally to bring about behaviour changes. It does not attempt to explain how the mind works

beliefs: ideas – about the self, others, the world or the supernatural – that one holds to be true

beneficence: refers to one's duty to benefit or to promote good for others

bereavement: the process by which a person experiences grief

binge eating: consuming a large amount of food (far greater than most people eat at one time) in a discrete period of usually 2 hours or less

bipolar (affective) disorder: a disorder – increasingly diagnosed and formerly called manic-depression – characterized by cyclical and dramatic changes in mood and behaviour – from depression to mania or hypomania

blackout: an episode during which the person continues to function but has no conscious awareness of his or her behaviour at the time nor any later memory of the behaviour; usually associated with alcohol consumption

blunted affect: showing little or a slow-to-respond facial expression; few observable facial expressions

body dysmorphic disorder: preoccupation with an imagined or exaggerated defect in physical appearance

body image: how a person perceives his or her body, i.e. a mental self-image

body image disturbance: occurs when there is extreme dissatisfaction with one's body image and an extreme discrepancy between one's body image and the perceptions of others

body language: a non-verbal form of communication: gestures, postures, movements and body positions

borderline personality disorder: pervasive and enduring pattern of unstable interpersonal relationships, self-image, affect; marked impulsivity; sometimes involves frequent self-harming behaviour

breach of duty of care: the nurse (or doctor) failed to conform to standards of care, thereby breaching or failing the existing duty. The nurse did not act as a reasonable, prudent professional would have acted in similar circumstances

broad affect: displaying a full range of emotional expressions

bulimia nervosa: an eating disorder characterized by recurrent episodes (defined by *DSM-IV* as at least twice a week for 3 months) of binge eating followed by inappropriate compensatory behaviours to avoid weight gain such as purging (self-induced vomiting or use of laxatives, diuretics, enemas or emetics), fasting, or excessively exercising

care co-ordination: the process of ensuring a named professional is responsible and accountable for the assessment, care-planning, intervention and evaluation aspects of a client's care

catatonia: psychomotor disturbance, the person either being completely motionless or exhibiting excessive motor activity; usually related to psychosis

catharsis: the release of strong feelings such as anger, rage, grief

character: consists of concepts about the self and the external world

child abuse: the intentional injury of a child

circumstantial thinking: term used when a client eventually answers a question but only after giving excessive, unnecessary detail

circumstantiality: the use of extraneous words and long, tedious descriptions- talking 'round the houses'

client-centered therapy: focused on the role of the client, rather than the therapist, as the key to the healing process

clinical supervision: a formal, structured process – either one-to-one or in a group – in which clinicians focus on their therapeutic work with clients and their professional development

closed body positions: non-verbal behaviour such as crossed legs and arms folded over chest that indicate the listener may be failing to listen, defensive or not accepting

closed group: structured to keep the same members in the group for a specified number of sessions

clubhouse model: community-based rehabilitation; an 'intentional community' based on the belief that men and women with serious and persistent psychiatric disability can and will achieve normal life goals when given the opportunity, time, support and fellowship

CMHT: community mental health team. A multidisciplinary team committed to working with longer-term and primary care clients

co-dependence: a maladaptive coping pattern on the part of family members or others that results from a prolonged relationship with the person who uses substances

cognitive-behavioural therapies (CBT): increasingly widespread, evidence-based therapeutic approaches to helping people with a range of psychological and psychiatric problems; involve a structured, collaborative and focused approach to shifting patterns of thinking, feeling and acting

command hallucinations: disturbed auditory sensory perceptions demanding that the client take action, often to harm self or others, and are considered dangerous; often referred to as 'voices'

communication: the processes that people use to exchange information

CMHN/CPN: community mental health nurse/community psychiatric nurse. A specialist nurse working in the community and focusing on primary and secondary care clients with acute and longer-term mental health problems

compassion: a sense of shared humanity that is manifested in attempts to relieve the suffering of another person

compensatory behaviours: for clients with eating disorders, actions designed to counteract food intake, such as purging (vomiting), excessively exercising, using/abusing laxatives and diuretics

complementary therapies: used *with* conventional practice

complicated grieving: a response outside the norm and occurring when a person may seem or feel devoid of emotion, grieves for prolonged periods or has expressions of grief that seem disproportionate to the event

compulsions: ritualistic or repetitive behaviours or mental acts that a person carries out continuously in an attempt to neutralize anxiety

computed (axial) tomography (CT/CAT): a diagnostic procedure in which a precise X-ray beam takes cross-sectional images (slices) layer by layer

concrete message: words that are as clear as possible when speaking to the client so that the client can understand the message; concrete messages are important for accurate information exchange

concrete thinking: in schizophrenia, for example, when a person gives a literal interpretation of a proverb or metaphor; abstraction is diminished or absent. More generally, a rigid, narrow view of people or things that lacks imagination or creativity

conduct disorder: characterized by persistent antisocial behaviour in children and adolescents that significantly impairs their ability to function in social, academic or occupational areas

confabulation: process in which people may make up answers/create narratives to fill in memory gaps; usually associated with organic brain problems

confidentiality: respecting the client's right to keep private any information about his or her mental and physical health and related care

confrontation: technique designed to highlight the incongruence between a person's verbalizations and actual behaviour; sometimes used to manage perceived manipulative or deceptive behaviour or to expose dissonance in someone's thinking

congruence: occurs when words and actions match

congruent message: when communication content and processes agree

context: the environment in which an event occurs; includes the time and the physical, social, emotional and cultural environments: vital for nurses to analyse in order to develop empathy and be effective

contract: a verbal or written agreement outlining the care the nurse will give, the times the nurse will be with the client and acceptance of these conditions by the client.

controlled substance: drug classified under the Controlled Substances Act; includes opioids, stimulants, benzodiazepines, anabolic steroids, cannabis derivatives, psychedelics and sedatives

conversion disorder: sometimes called conversion reaction; involves unexplained, usually sudden deficits in sensory or motor function related to an emotional conflict the client experiences but does not handle directly

counselling: a structured, focused, usually short-term process of therapeutic problem-solving (see *psychotherapy*)

countertransference: occurs when the therapist displaces onto the client attitudes or feelings from his or her past; process that can occur when the nurse responds to the client based on personal, unconscious needs and conflicts

CPA: care programme approach; a statutory process intended to ensure a rigorous, well-documented, person-centred and accountable programme of care for people with mental health problems

Creutzfeldt-Jakob disease: a central nervous system disorder that typically develops in adults 40 to 60 years of age and involves altered vision, loss of co-ordination or abnormal movements and dementia

crisis: a turning point in an individual's life that produces an overwhelming emotional response; individual is confronting life circumstance or stressor that cannot be managed through customary coping strategies

crisis intervention: includes a variety of techniques, based on the assessment of the individual in crisis, to assist in resolution or management of the stressor or circumstance

crisis resolution/home treatment teams: multidisciplinary teams committed to intensive support, care and treatment of people in acute mental health crises. Work as an alternative to – and gatekeepers for – acute inpatient admission

cues (overt and covert): verbal or non-verbal messages that signal key words or issues for the client

culturally competent: being sensitive to issues related to culture, race, gender, sexual orientation, social class, economic situation and other factors

culture: all the socially learned behaviours, values, beliefs and customs, transmitted down to each generation, as well as a population's ways of thinking, that guide its members' views of themselves and the world. Can be specific to families and sub-cultures as well as to wider groups and is influenced by age, class, ethnicity, gender and sexuality

curiosity: an essential element of nursing that requires the maintenance of an uncertain, interested and respectful approach to people's lives

cycle of violence: a typical pattern in domestic abuse: violence; honeymoon or remorseful period; tension-building; and, finally, violence; this pattern continually repeats itself throughout the relationship

date rape (acquaintance rape): sexual assault that may occur on a first date, on a ride home from a party or when the two people have known each other for some time

decatastrophizing: a technique that involves learning to assess situations realistically rather than always assuming a catastrophe will happen

defence mechanisms: in psychodynamic approaches, cognitive distortions that a person uses unconsciously to maintain a sense of being in control of a situation, to lessen discomfort and to deal with stress; also called ego defence mechanisms

deinstitutionalization: the deliberate shift in care of people with mental health problems that took place in the 1970s,1980s and 1990s from institutional care in hospitals to community-based facilities and through community-based services

delirium: a syndrome that involves a disturbance of consciousness accompanied by a change in cognition

delusion: a fixed, false belief not based on reality

dementia: a mental disorder that involves multiple cognitive deficits, initially involving memory impairment with progressive deterioration that includes all cognitive functioning

denial: defence mechanism; people may deny directly having any problems or may minimize the extent of problems or, for example, substance use

deontology: a theory that says ethical decisions should be based on whether or not an action is morally right with no regard for the result or consequences

dependent personality disorder: characterized by a pervasive and excessive need to be taken care of, which leads to submissive and clinging behaviour and fears of separation

depersonalization: feelings of being disconnected from himself or herself; the client feels detached from his or her behaviour

depot injection: a slow-release, injectable form of antipsychotic medication for maintenance therapy

depression: a debilitating mental disorder characterized by low mood, negativity, poor concentration, physiological changes such as disturbed sleep and appetite and lack of energy; concurrent anxiety symptoms are also extremely common

depressive personality disorder: characterized by a pervasive pattern of depressive cognitions and behaviours in various contexts

derealization: client senses that events and subjective experiences are not real, when, in fact, they are

detoxification: the process of safely withdrawing from a substance

Diagnostic and Statistical Manual of Mental Disorders (DSM-IV-TR): taxonomy published by the American Psychiatric Association. The *DSM-IV-TR* describes all mental disorders and outlines specific diagnostic criteria for each based on clinical experience and research. It is sometimes used in the UK and other countries alongside or instead of the *ICD-10*

diagnostic axes: the five axes that comprise diagnosis under *DSM-IV-TR* criteria; include major mental disorders, 'mental retardation' (learning disabilities) or personality disorders, medical illnesses, psychosocial stressors and global assessment of functioning (GAF)

dialectical-behaviour therapy (DBT): a therapeutic approach to helping people with difficulties with self-harm, addictions and mood disorders that combines elements of CBT, mindfulness and psychodynamic therapy with the concept of dialectics

directive role: asking direct, yes/no questions and using problem solving to help the client develop new coping mechanisms to deal with present, here-and-now issues

disease conviction: preoccupation with the fear that one has a serious disease

disease phobia: preoccupation with the fear that one will get a serious disease

disenfranchised grief: grief over a loss that is not or cannot be mourned publicly or supported socially

disorganization and despair: the point in the grieving process when the bereaved person is distressed as they begin to understand the loss's permanence

dissociation: a subconscious defence mechanism that helps a person protect his or her emotional self from recognizing the full effects of some horrific or traumatic event by allowing the mind to forget or remove itself from the painful situation or memory

dissociative disorders: have the essential feature of a disruption in the usually integrated functions of consciousness, memory, identity or environmental perception; include amnesia, fugue and dissociative identity disorder

distance zones: amount of physical space between people during communication; in the UK and Ireland, United States, Canada, Australia and New Zealand and many Eastern European nations, four distance zones are generally observed: intimate zone, personal zone, social zone and public zone

distraction: involves shifting the client's attention and energy to a different topic

dopamine: a neurotransmitter located primarily in the brain stem; has been found to be involved in the control of complex movements, motivation, cognition and regulation of emotional responses

dream analysis: a primary method used in psychoanalysis; involves discussing a client's dreams to discover their true meaning and significance

dual diagnosis: a term referring to clients with both substance misuse problems and a mental disorder such as schizophrenia, bipolar affective disorder or a personality disorder

duty: existence of a legally recognized relationship, i.e. doctor to client, nurse to client

duty to warn: the exception to the client's right to confidentiality; when health-care providers are legally obligated to warn another person who is the target of the threats or plan by the client, even if the threats were discussed during therapy sessions otherwise protected by confidentiality

dysfunctional grieving: extended, unsuccessful attempts to working through the grieving process

dysphoric: mood that involves unhappiness, restlessness and malaise

dystonia: extrapyramidal side-effect to antipsychotic medication; includes acute muscular rigidity and cramping, a stiff or thick tongue with difficulty swallowing, and, in severe cases, laryngospasm and respiratory difficulties; also called dystonic reactions

early intervention teams: teams dedicated to working proactively with those young people who are at risk of developing a long-term psychotic disorder

echolalia: repetition or imitation of what someone else says; echoing what is heard

echopraxia: imitation of the movements and gestures of someone an individual is with

education/psychoeducational group: a therapeutic group; provides information to members on a specific issue: for instance, stress management, medication management or assertiveness training

effectiveness: the achievement of identified client goals

efficacy: refers to the maximal therapeutic effect a drug can achieve

ego: in psychoanalytic theory, the balancing or mediating force between the id and the superego; represents mature and adaptive behaviour that allows a person to function successfully in the world

elder abuse: the maltreatment of older adults by family members or caretakers

electroconvulsive therapy (ECT): used to treat depression (and, sometimes, other disorders) in select groups such as clients who are severely depressed and not responsive to antidepressants or those who experience intolerable medication side-effects at therapeutic doses

empathy: the cognitive ability to perceive the meanings and feelings of another person and to communicate that understanding to that person: developed as a result of a conscious effort

enabling: behaviours that seem helpful on the surface but actually perpetuate the substance use of another, e.g. a wife who calls to report her husband has the flu and will miss work when he is actually drunk or hungover

encopresis: the repeated passage of faeces into inappropriate places, such as clothing or the floor, by a child who is at least 4 years of age either chronologically or developmentally

enmeshment: lack of clear role boundaries between people

enuresis: the repeated voiding of urine during the day or at night into clothing or bed by a child at least 5 years of age either chronologically or developmentally

environmental control: a client's ability to control the surroundings or direct factors in the environment

ethical dilemma: a situation in which ethical principles conflict or when there is no one clear course of action in a given situation

ethics: a branch of philosophy that deals with values of human conduct related to the rightness or wrongness of actions and to the goodness and badness of the motives and ends of such actions

ethnicity: concept of people identifying with one another (or being identified) based on a shared heritage

euthymic: normal or level mood

evidence-based: an intervention, programme or service approach that is supported by research

executive functioning: the ability to think abstractly and to plan, initiate, sequence, monitor and stop complex behaviour

exploitation: phase of nurse–client relationship, identified by Peplau, when the nurse guides the client to examine feelings and responses and to develop better coping skills and a more positive self-image; this encourages behaviour change and develops independence; part of the working phase

exposure: behavioural technique that involves having the client deliberately confront the situations and stimuli that he or she is trying to avoid

extrapyramidal side-effects: reversible movement disorders induced by antipsychotic or neuroleptic medication

eye contact: looking into the other person's eyes during communication

factitious disorders: characterized by physical symptoms that are feigned or inflicted for the sole purpose of drawing attention to oneself and gaining the emotional benefits of assuming the sick role

false imprisonment: the unjustifiable detention of a client, such as the inappropriate use of restraint or seclusion

family therapy: a form of group therapy in which the client and his or her family members participate to deal with mutual issues

family violence: encompasses domestic or partner abuse; neglect and physical, emotional or sexual abuse of children; elder abuse; and marital rape

fear: feeling afraid or threatened by a clearly identifiable, external stimulus that represents danger to the person

flat affect: showing no facial expression

flight of ideas: excessive amount and rate of speech composed of fragmented or unrelated ideas; racing, often unconnected, thoughts

flooding: a form of rapid desensitization in which a therapist confronts the client with the phobic object (either a picture or the actual object) until it no longer produces anxiety

flushing: a reddening of the face and neck as a result of increased blood flow

free association: a method in psychoanalysis used to gain access to subconscious thoughts and feelings in which the therapist tries to uncover the client's true thoughts and feelings by saying a word and asking the client to respond quickly with the first thing that comes to mind

genuine interest: truly paying attention to the client, caring about what he or she is saying; only possible when the nurse is comfortable with himself or herself and aware of his or her strengths and limitations

going along: technique used with clients with dementia; providing emotional reassurance to clients without correcting their misperceptions or delusions

grief: subjective emotions and affect that are a normal response to the experience of loss

grieving: the process by which a person experiences grief

grounding techniques: helpful to use with the client who is dissociating or experiencing a flashback; grounding techniques remind the client that he or she is in the present, as an adult and is safe

group therapy: therapy during which clients participate in sessions with others. The members share a common purpose and are expected to contribute to the group to benefit others and to receive benefit from others in return

half-life: the time it takes for half of the drug to be eliminated from the bloodstream

hallucinations: false sensory perceptions or perceptual experiences that do not really exist

hallucinogen: substances that distort the user's perception of reality and produce symptoms similar to psychosis, including hallucinations (usually visual) and depersonalization

hardiness: the ability to resist illness when under stress

hierarchy of needs: a pyramid used to arrange and illustrate the basic dr   ds that motivate people; devel   low

histrio   r: characterized by a pe   e emotionality and 'att

**home   um or balance

hostility: an emotion expressed through verbal abuse, lack of co-operation, violation of rules or norms or threatening behaviour; also called verbal aggression

humanism: often used interchangeably with 'client-centred' or 'person-centred', humanistic approaches to care and treatment focus on a person's positive qualities, his or her capacity to change (human potential) and the promotion of self-esteem; more broadly, a non-theistic philosophical and practical approach to life that is based on reason, compassion and evidence

Huntington's disease ('Huntington's chorea'): an inherited, dominant gene disease that primarily involves cerebral atrophy, demyelination and enlargement of the brain ventricles

hypertensive crisis: a life-threatening condition that can result when a client taking MAOIs ingests tyramine-containing foods and fluids or other medications

hypochondriasis: preoccupation with the fear that one has a serious disease or will get a serious disease

hypomania: a period of abnormally and persistently elevated, expansive or irritable mood lasting 4 days; does not significantly impair the ability to function and does not usually involve psychotic features

hysteria: refers to multiple, recurrent physical complaints with no organic basis

ICD-10: the World Health Organisation's International Classification of Diseases; often used as an alternative to *DSM-IV*

id: in psychoanalytic theory, the part of one's nature that reflects basic or innate desires such as pleasure-seeking behaviour, aggression and sexual impulses. The id seeks instant gratification; causes impulsive, unthinking behaviour; and has no regard for rules or social convention

ideas of reference: client's inaccurate interpretation that general events are personally directed to him or her, such as hearing a speech on the news and believing the message has personal meaning

impulse control: the ability to delay gratification and to think about one's behaviour before acting

inappropriate affect: displaying a facial expression that is incongruent with mood or situation; often silly or giddy regardless of circumstances

incongruent message: when the communication content and process disagree

individual psychotherapy: a method of bringing about change in a person by exploring his or her feelings, attitudes, thinking and behaviour. It involves a one-to-one relationship between the therapist and the client

inhalant: a diverse group of drugs including anaesthetics, nitrates and organic solvents that are inhaled for their effects

insight: the ability to understand the true nature of one's situation and accept some personal responsibility for that situation

interdisciplinary (multidisciplinary) team: treatment group comprised of individuals from a variety of fields or disciplines; the most useful approach in dealing with the multifaceted problems of clients with mental illness

intergenerational transmission process: explains that patterns of violence are perpetuated from one generation to the next through role modelling and social learning

internalization: keeping stress, anxiety or frustration inside rather than expressing them outwardly

intimate relationship: a relationship involving two people who are emotionally committed to each other. Both parties are concerned about having their individual needs met and helping each other to meet needs as well. The relationship may include sexual or emotional intimacy as well as sharing of mutual goals

intimate zone: space of 0 to 18 inches between people; the amount of space comfortable for parents with young children, people who mutually desire personal contact or people whispering. Invasion of this intimate zone by anyone else can be threatening and produce anxiety

intoxication: use of a substance that results in maladaptive behaviour

judgment: refers to the ability to interpret one's environment and situation correctly and to adapt one's behaviour and decisions accordingly

justice: refers to the concept of treating all people fairly and equally without regard for social or economic status, race, sex, marital status, religion, ethnicity or cultural beliefs

kindling process: the snowball-like effect seen when minor seizure activity seems to build up into more frequent and severe seizures

Korsakoff's syndrome: type of dementia caused by long-term, excessive alcohol intake that results in a chronic thiamine or vitamin B deficiency

la belle indifférence: a seeming lack of concern or distress; a key feature of conversion disorder

labile: rapidly changing or fluctuating, such as someone's mood or emotions

latency of response: refers to hesitation before the client responds to questions

learning disability: a restriction on a person's intellectual and social functioning, present from before the age of 18 and resulting from an hereditary condition, alterations in embryonic development, pregnancy or perinatal problems, medical conditions in infancy or an extreme lack of nurturing or stimulation

least restrictive environment: treatment appropriate to meet the client's needs with only necessary or required restrictions

limbic system: an area of the brain located above the brain stem that includes the thalamus, hypothalamus, hippocampus and amygdala (although some sources differ regarding the structures that this system includes)

limit-setting: an effective technique that involves three steps: stating the behavioural limit (describing the unacceptable behaviour); identifying the consequences if the limit is exceeded; and identifying the expected or desired behaviour

loose associations: disorganized thinking that jumps from one idea to another with little or no evident relation between the thoughts

magnetic resonance imaging (MRI): diagnostic test used to visualize soft tissue structures; energy field is created with a magnet and radio waves, then converted into a visual image

malingering: the intentional production of false or grossly exaggerated physical or psychological symptoms

malpractice: a type of negligence that refers specifically to professionals such as nurses and doctors

mania: a distinct period during which mood is abnormally and persistently elevated, expansive or irritable

mental disorder: defined by *DSM-IV-TR* as a clinically significant behavioural or psychological syndrome or pattern that occurs in an individual and that is associated with present distress (e.g. a painful symptom) or disability (i.e. impairment in one or more important areas of functioning) or with a significantly increased risk of suffering death, pain, disability or an important loss of freedom

mental health: a state of emotional, psychological and social wellness evidenced by satisfying relationships, effective behaviour and coping, positive self-concept and emotional flexibility and stability

mild anxiety: an uncomfortable sensation that something is different, potentially threatening and warrants special attention

milieu therapy: the concept involves clients' interactions with one another; i.e. practicing interpersonal relationship skills, giving one another feedback about behaviour and working co-operatively as a group to solve day-to-day problems

mindfulness: both an approach to living and a series of skills that help people stay in the 'here-and-now', stay fully awake to their internal and external world and relate to themselves and others non-judgementally and effectively

moderate anxiety: the disturbing feeling that something is definitely wrong; the person becomes nervous or agitated

mood: refers to a person's relatively pervasive and enduring emotional state

mood disorders: pervasive alterations in emotions that are manifested by depression, mania or both

mood-stabilizing drugs: used to treat bipolar disorder by stabilizing the client's mood, preventing or minimizing the highs and lows that characterize bipolar illness and treating acute episodes of mania

mourning: the outward expression of grief

Munchausen's by proxy: a controversial diagnosis sometimes made when a person inflicts illness or injury on someone else to gain the attention of emergency medical personnel or to be a hero for 'saving' the victim

Munchausen's syndrome: a factitious disorder where the person intentionally causes injury or physical symptoms to self to gain attention and sympathy from health care providers, family and others

narcissistic personality disorder: characterized by a pervasive pattern of grandiosity (in fantasy or behaviour), need for admiration and lack of empathy

negative reinforcement: involves removing a stimulus immediately after a behaviour occurs so that the behaviour is more likely to occur again

neglect: malicious or ignorant withholding of physical, emotional, or educational necessities for a child or vulnerable adult's well-being

negligence: an unintentional tort that involves causing harm by failing to do what a reasonable and prudent person would do in similar circumstances

neologisms: invented words that have meaning only for the person themselves

neuroleptic malignant syndrome (NMS): a potentially fatal, idiosyncratic reaction to an antipsychotic (or neuroleptic) drug

neuroleptics: antipsychotic medications

neurotransmitter: the chemical substances manufactured in the neuron that aid in the transmission of information throughout the body

non-directive role: using broad openings and open-ended questions to collect information and help the client to identify and discuss the topic of concern

non-maleficence: the requirement to do no harm to others either intentionally or unintentionally

non-verbal communication: the behaviour that accompanies verbal content, such as body language, eye contact, facial expression, tone of voice, speed and hesitations in speech, grunts and groans, and distance from the listener

noradrenaline: the most prevalent neurotransmitter in the nervous system

numbing: beginning of the grieving process; the common first response to the news of a loss is to be stunned, as though not able to take in reality

obsessions: recurrent, persistent, intrusive and unwanted thoughts, images or impulses that cause marked anxiety and interfere with interpersonal, social or occupational function

obsessive-compulsive disorder (OCD): an anxiety-based disorder in which the person's functioning is severely hampered by recurrent and distressing obsessions and a consequent behavioural response to those internal experiences

obsessive-compulsive personality disorder: characterized by a pervasive pattern of preoccupation with perfectionism, mental and interpersonal control and orderliness at the expense of flexibility, openness and efficiency

open group: an ongoing group that runs indefinitely; members join or leave the group as they need to

operant conditioning: the theory which says people learn their behaviour from their history or past experiences, particularly those experiences that were repeatedly reinforced

opioid: controlled drugs; often abused because they desensitize the user to both physiological and psychological pain and induce a sense of euphoria and well-being; some are prescribed for analgesic effects but others are illegal

orientation phase: the beginning of the nurse–client relationship; begins when the nurse and client meet and ends when the client begins to identify problems to examine

pain disorder: has the primary physical symptom of pain, which generally is unrelieved by analgesics and greatly affected by psychological factors in terms of onset, severity, exacerbation and maintenance

palilalia: repeating words or sounds over and over

panic attack: short-term (usually 5-10 minutes) experience of extreme anxiety symptoms (including hyperventilation, dizziness, sweating and feeling of terror and/or depersonalization), caused by prolonged high levels of adrenaline

panic disorder: composed of discrete episodes of panic attacks, that is, 15 to 30 minutes of rapid, intense, escalating anxiety in which the person experiences great emotional fear as well as physiological discomfort

paranoid personality disorder: characterized by pervasive mistrust and suspiciousness of others

parataxic mode: begins in early childhood as the child begins to connect experiences in sequence; the child may not make logical sense of the experiences and may see them as coincidence or chance events; the child seeks to relieve anxiety by repeating familiar experiences, although he or she may not understand what he or she is doing

Parkinson's disease: a slowly progressive neurological condition characterized by tremor, rigidity, bradykinesia and postural instability

participant observer: the therapist both participates in and observes the progress of the relationship

passive-aggressive personality disorder: characterized by a negative attitude and a pervasive pattern of passive resistance to demands for adequate social and occupational performance

patterns of knowing: the four patterns of knowing in nursing are empirical knowing (derived from the science of nursing), personal knowing (derived from life experiences), ethical knowing (derived from moral knowledge of nursing) and aesthetic knowing (derived from the art of nursing); provide the nurse with a clear method of observing and understanding every client interaction

personal zone: space of 18 to 36 inches, a comfortable distance between family and friends who are talking

personality: an ingrained, enduring pattern of behaving and relating to self, others and the environment; includes perceptions, attitudes and emotions

personality disorders: diagnosed when personality traits become inflexible and maladaptive and significantly interfere with how a person functions in society or cause the person emotional distress

pervasive developmental disorders: characterized by pervasive and usually severe impairment of reciprocal social interaction skills, communication difficulties and restricted, stereotypical behavioural patterns

phenomena of concern: describe the 12 areas of concern that mental health nurses focus on when caring for clients

phobia: an illogical, intense, persistent fear of a specific object or social situation that causes extreme distress and interferes with normal functioning

physical abuse: ranges from shoving and pushing to severe battering and choking and may involve broken limbs and ribs, internal bleeding, brain damage, even homicide

physical aggression: behaviour in which a person attacks or injures another person or that involves destruction of property

pica: persistent ingestion of non-nutritive substances such as paint, hair, cloth, leaves, sand, clay or soil

Pick's disease: a degenerative brain disease that particularly affects the frontal and temporal lobes and results in a clinical picture similar to that of Alzheimer's disease

polydipsia: excessive water intake

polysubstance abuse: abuse of more than one substance

positive reframing: a cognitive behavioural technique involving turning negative messages into positive messages

positive regard: unconditional, non-judgemental attitude that implies respect for the person

positive reinforcement: a reward immediately following a behaviour to increase the likelihood that the behaviour will be repeated

positive self-talk: a cognitive behavioural technique in which the client changes thinking about the self from negative to positive

positron emission tomography (PET): a diagnostic test used to examine the function of the brain by monitoring the flow of radioactive substances that are injected into the bloodstream

posttraumatic stress disorder (PTSD): a disturbing pattern of behaviour demonstrated by someone who has experienced a traumatic event: for example, a natural disaster, combat or an assault

potency: describes the amount of a drug needed to achieve maximum effect

preconception: the way one person expects another to behave or speak; often a roadblock to the formation of an authentic relationship

pressure of speech: unrelenting, rapid, often loud talking without pauses (common in bipolar disorder and schizophrenia)

primary gain: the relief of anxiety achieved by performing the specific anxiety-driven behaviour; the direct external benefits that being sick provides, such as relief of anxiety, conflict or distress

problem identification: part of the working phase of the nurse–client situation, when the client identifies the issues or concerns causing problems

process: in communication, denotes all non-verbal messages that the speaker uses to give meaning and context to the message

prototaxic mode: characteristic of infancy and childhood that involves brief, unconnected experiences that have no relationship to one another. Adults with schizophrenia exhibit persistent prototaxic experiences

proxemics: the study of distance zones between people during communication

pseudoparkinsonism: a type of extrapyramidal side-effect of antipsychotic medication; drug-induced parkinsonism; includes shuffling gait, mask-like face, muscle stiffness (continuous) or cogwheeling rigidity (ratchet-like movements of joints), drooling and akinesia (slowness and difficulty initiating movement)

psychoanalysis: focuses on discovering the causes of the client's unconscious and repressed thoughts, feelings and conflicts believed to cause anxiety and helping the client to gain insight into and resolve these conflicts and anxieties; pioneered by Sigmund Freud, not commonly seen today, at least in its original form

psychodynamic: approaches – developed from psychoanalytic principles – to understanding the internal and external worlds of people and groups that assume the existence of both conscious and unconscious psychological energy and forces

psychoimmunology: examines the effect of psychosocial stressors on the body's immune system

psychological abuse (emotional abuse): includes name-calling, belittling, screaming, yelling, destroying property and making threats, as well as subtler forms such as refusing to speak to or ignoring the victim

psychomotor agitation: increased body movements and thoughts

psychomotor retardation: overall slowed movements; a general slowing of all movements; slow cognitive processing and slow verbal interaction

psychopharmacology: the use of medications to treat mental disorders

psychosis: cluster of experiences that may include delusions, hallucinations and disordered thinking and behaviour and that set someone aside from the reality perceived by those around them; the many precipitating factors include substance misuse, neurological disorders, infections, severe acute stress reactions, schizophrenia, bipolar disorder and depression

psychosocial interventions: activities that enhance the client's social and psychological functioning and improve social skills, interpersonal relationships and communication; a term particularly used when referring to interventions in schizophrenia

psychosomatic: used to convey the connection between the mind (*psyche*) and the body (*soma*) in states of health and illness

psychotherapy: a structured programme of therapeutic interaction between a qualified, supervised clinician and individual or group, designed to benefit people experiencing emotional distress, impairment or mental disorder; the therapist's approach is based on a theory or combination of theories and tends to look at longer-term, broader, more 'in-depth' and underlying issues than counselling, although the distinction between the two is blurred and controversial

psychotropic drugs: drugs that affect mood, behaviour and thinking that are used to treat mental disorder

public zone: space of 12 to 25 feet; the acceptable distance between a speaker and an audience, between small groups and among others at informal functions

purging: compensatory behaviours designed to eliminate food by means of self-induced vomiting

race: a (controversial and contested) division of mankind possessing traits that are transmitted by descent and sufficient to identify it as a distinct human type

rape: a crime of violence, domination and humiliation of the victim expressed through sexual means

rebound: temporary return of symptoms; may be more intense than original symptoms

recovery: a set of principles for effective, compassionate mental health care that are underpinned by optimism, collaboration and respect; an approach that seeks to empower and help people achieve their full potential

reflection: the process of – informally or in a structured way – reviewing one's interaction with a client

reframing: cognitive behavioural technique in which alternative points of view are examined to explain events

rehabilitation: services designed to promote the recovery process for clients with mental health problems; should not be limited to medication management and symptom control, includes personal growth, reintegration into the community, increased independence and improved quality of life

religion: an organized system of beliefs about one or more powerful, supernatural forces that govern the universe and offer guidelines for living in harmony with the universe and with others

reminiscence therapy: thinking about, or relating, personally significant past experiences in a purposeful manner to benefit the client (sometimes used with people with dementia)

reorganization: at the end of the grieving process, when the bereaved person begins to re-establish a sense of personal identity, direction and purpose for living

repressed memories: memories that are buried deeply in the subconscious mind or repressed because they are too painful for the person to acknowledge; often relate to childhood abuse

resilience: having healthy responses to stressful circumstances or risky situations

resourcefulness: involves using problem-solving abilities and believing that one can cope with adverse or novel situations

respect: an attitude of sensitivity towards another human being in which that person is treated as an equal and worthy of consideration and care

response prevention: behavioural technique that focuses on delaying or avoiding performance of rituals in response to anxiety-provoking thoughts

restraining order: legal order of protection obtained to prohibit contact between a victim and perpetrator of abuse

restraint: the direct application of physical force to a person, without his or her permission, to restrict his or her freedom of movement

restricted affect: displaying one type of emotional expression, usually serious or sombre

ruminate: to repeatedly go over the same thoughts

satiety: satisfaction of appetite

schizoid personality disorder: characterized by a pervasive pattern of detachment from social relationships and a restricted range of emotional expression in interpersonal settings

schizophrenias: a cluster of mental disorders that encompass 'positive' characteristics such as delusions and hallucinations and/or 'negative' characteristics such as anergia, lack of motivation and social withdrawal

schizotypal personality disorder: characterized by a pervasive pattern of social and interpersonal deficits marked by acute discomfort with, and reduced capacity for, close relationships, as well as by cognitive or perceptual distortions and behavioural eccentricities

seasonal affective disorder (SAD): mood disorder in which people experience depressive symptoms beginning in late autumn or (more rarely) from late spring or early summer

seclusion: the involuntary confinement of a person in a specially constructed, locked room, often equipped with a security window or camera for direct visual monitoring; legal, organizational and professional restrictions restrict its use

secondary gain: the internal or personal benefits received from others because one is sick, such as attention from family members, comfort measures, being excused from usual responsibilities or tasks

self-actualization: in Maslow's hierarchy, the development of one's fullest potential in life

self-awareness: an ongoing process by which a person gains recognition of his or her own feelings, beliefs, and attitudes; the process of developing an understanding of one's own values, beliefs, thoughts, feelings, attitudes, motivations, prejudices, strengths and limitations, and how these qualities affect others

self-concept: the way one views oneself in terms of personal worth and dignity

self-disclosure: revealing personal information such as biographical information and personal experiences, ideas, thoughts and feelings about oneself

self-efficacy: a belief that personal abilities and efforts affect the events in our lives

self-help group: members share a common experience, but the group is not a formal or structured therapy group

self-monitoring: a cognitive-behavioural technique designed to help clients manage their own behaviour

sense of belonging: the feeling of connectedness with, or involvement in, a social system or environment of which a person feels an integral part: its absence may be seen as a sign of mental ill-health

serotonin: a neurotransmitter found only in the brain

serotonin (serotonergic) syndrome: uncommon but potentially life-threatening disorder characterized by agitation, sweating, fever, tachycardia, hypotension, rigidity, hyperreflexia, confusion and, in extreme cases, coma and death; most commonly results from a combination of two or more medications with serotonin-enhancing properties, such as taking MAOI and SSRI antidepressants at the same time or too close together

severe anxiety: an increased level of anxiety when more primitive survival skills take over, defensive responses ensue and cognitive skills decrease significantly; person with severe anxiety has trouble thinking and reasoning

sexual abuse: involves sexual acts performed by one person in a position of power over another (often by an adult on a child)

social network: groups of people whom one knows and with whom one feels connected

social organization: refers to family structure and organization, religious values and beliefs, ethnicity and culture, all of which affect a person's role and, therefore, his or her health and illness behaviour

social relationship: primarily initiated for the purpose of friendship, socialization, companionship or accomplishment of a task

social support: emotional sustenance that comes from friends, family members and even health-care providers who help a person when a problem arises

social zone: a space of 4 to 12 feet, which is the distance acceptable for communication in social, work and business settings

socioeconomic status: refers to one's income, education and occupation

sodomy: anal intercourse

solution-focused therapy: a therapeutic approach that emphasizes preferred futures, strengths, resources, exceptions and solutions rather than a focus on the past, problems, causes, pathology and deficits

somatization : the transference of mental experiences and states into bodily symptoms (i.e. the development of psychosomatic disorders)

somatization disorder: characterized by multiple, recurrent physical symptoms in a variety of bodily systems that have no organic or medical basis

somatoform disorders: characterized as the presence of physical symptoms that suggest a medical condition without a demonstrable organic basis to account fully for them

spirituality: a client's beliefs about life, health, illness, death, self and one's relationship to the universe; involves the essence of a person's being and his or her beliefs about the meaning of life and the purpose for living

spontaneous remission: natural recovery that occurs without treatment of any kind

spouse or partner abuse: the mistreatment or misuse of one person by another in the context of an intimate relationship

stalking: repeated and persistent attempts to impose unwanted communication or contact on another person

standards of care: authoritative statements by professional organizations such as the NMC that describe the responsibilities for which nurses are accountable; the care that nurses provide to clients meets set expectations and is what any nurse in a similar situation would do

stereotypical movements: repetitive, seemingly purposeless movements; may include waving, rocking, twirling objects, biting fingernails, banging the head, biting or hitting oneself or picking at the skin or body orifices

stimulants: drugs that stimulate or excite the central nervous system

stress: strictly, the wear and tear that life causes on the body; more popularly, used as a catch-all term for any psychological or social event or series of events that impose pressure on the person's capacity to function effectively

substance abuse/misuse: can be defined as using a drug in a way that is inconsistent with medical or social norms and despite negative consequences

substance dependence: includes problems associated with addiction, such as tolerance, withdrawal and unsuccessful attempts to stop using the substance

suicidal ideation: thinking about killing oneself

suicide: the intentional act of killing oneself

superego: in psychoanalytic theory, the part of a person's nature that reflects moral and ethical concepts, values and parental and social expectations; it is, therefore, often in direct opposition to the id

support group: organized to help members who share a common problem to cope with it

supportive touch: the use of physical touch to convey support, interest, caring; may not be welcome or effective with all clients

survivor: view of the client as a survivor of trauma or abuse rather than as a 'victim'; helps to refocus client's view of him- or herself as being strong enough to survive the ordeal and 'move on', a more empowering self-image than that of victim

sympathy: an emotional response of sadness, pity or connection to another person; emerges spontaneously

syntaxic mode: begins to appear in school-aged children and becomes more predominant in pre-adolescence; the person begins to perceive him- or herself and the world within the context of the environment and can analyse experiences in a variety of settings

systematic desensitization: behavioural technique used to help overcome irrational fears and anxiety associated with a phobia

tangential thinking: wandering off the topic and never providing the information requested

tapering: administering decreasing doses of a medication leading to discontinuation of the drug

tardive dyskinesia: a late-onset, irreversible neurological side-effect of antipsychotic medications; characterized by abnormal, involuntary movements such as lip smacking, tongue protrusion, chewing, blinking, grimacing and choreiform movements of the limbs and feet

temperament: refers to the biological processes of sensation, association and motivation that underlie the integration of skills and habits based on emotion

termination or resolution phase: the final stage in the nurse–client relationship. It begins when the client's goals are achieved, and it concludes when the relationship ends

therapeutic communication: an interpersonal interaction between the nurse and client during which the nurse focuses on the client's specific needs to promote an effective exchange of information

therapeutic community or milieu: a consciously beneficial environment; interaction among clients is seen as beneficial, and treatment emphasizes the role of this client-to-client interaction

therapeutic nurse–client relationship (or 'therapeutic alliance'): professional, planned relationship between client and nurse that focuses on client needs, feelings, problems and ideas; interaction designed to promote client growth, discuss issues and resolve problems; includes the three phases of orientation, working (identification and exploitation) and termination (resolution)

therapeutic play: techniques used to understand a child's thoughts and feelings and to promote communication

therapeutic relationship: see *therapeutic nurse–client relationship*

therapeutic use of self: nurses use themselves – their experiences, personal qualities, skills and knowledge – as a therapeutic tool to establish a relationship with clients and to help clients grow, change and heal

thought blocking: stopping abruptly in the middle of a sentence or train of thought; sometimes client is unable to continue the idea

thought broadcasting: a delusional belief that others can hear or know what the client is thinking

thought content: what a person seems to be thinking, elicited from what they actually say

thought insertion: a delusional belief that others are putting ideas or thoughts into the client's head: that is, the ideas are not those of the client

thought stopping: a cognitive-behavioural technique to alter the process of negative or self-critical thought patterns

thought withdrawal: a delusional belief that others are taking the client's thoughts away and the client is powerless to stop it

tic: a sudden, rapid, recurrent, non-rhythmic, stereotyped motor movement or vocalization

time away: involves leaving clients for a short period then returning to them to re-engage in interaction; used in dementia care

time orientation: whether or not one views time as precise or approximate; differs among cultures

time-out: retreat to a neutral place to give the opportunity to regain self-control

tolerance: the need for increased amount of a substance to produce the same effect

tort: a wrongful act that results in injury, loss or damage

Tourette's disorder: characterized by multiple motor tics and one or more vocal tics, which occur many times a day for more than 1 year

transference: in psychodynamic theories, occurs when the client displaces on to the therapist attitudes and feelings that the client originally experienced in other relationships; it is common for the client unconsciously to transfer to the nurse feelings he or she has for significant others

twelve–step programme: based on the philosophy that total abstinence is essential and that people addicted to alcohol or other substances need the help and support of others to maintain sobriety

unknowing: uncertainty; when the nurse admits he or she does not know the client or the client's subjective world, this opens the way for a truly authentic encounter. The nurse in a state of unknowing is open to seeing and hearing the client's views without imposing any of his or her values or viewpoints

utilitarianism: a theory that bases ethical decisions on the 'greatest good for the greatest number'; primary consideration is on the outcome of the decision rather than its inherent morality

values: abstract standards that give a person a sense of right and wrong and establish a code of conduct for living

vascular dementia: has symptoms similar to those of Alzheimer's disease, but onset is typically abrupt and followed by rapid changes in functioning, a plateau or levelling-off period, more abrupt changes, another levelling-off period and so on

veracity: the duty to be honest or truthful

verbal communication: the words a person uses to speak to one or more listeners

waxy flexibility: maintenance of posture or position over time even when it is awkward or uncomfortable

withdrawal: new symptoms resulting from discontinuation of drug or substance

withdrawal syndrome: refers to the negative psychological and physical reactions that occur when use of a substance ceases or dramatically decreases

word salad: flow of unconnected words that convey no meaning to the listener; sometimes referred to as schizophasia

working phase: in the therapeutic relationship, the phase where issues are addressed, problems identified, solutions explored; nurse and client work to accomplish goals; contains Peplau's phases of problem identification and exploitation

yearning and searching: the point in the grieving process when the person begins to recognize the reality of the loss

Index

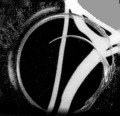

Page numbers followed by b indicates box; those followed by f indicates figure; those followed by t indicates table.